Contraception and mechanisms of endometrial bleeding

Books in this series contain the edited proceedings of symposia arranged by the WHO Special Programme of Research, Development and Research Training in Human Reproduction. The purpose of the series is to explore current knowledge in areas of biomedical science which have potential in the development of improved methods of fertility regulation. The series contains invited and uniformly edited contributions from scientists in molecular and cell biology, and from leading clinicians, and will find a wide audience among all those involved with reproductive biology and fertility control.

Already published
Safety Requirements for Contraceptive Steroids
Edited by F. Michal

Cellular and Molecular Events in Spermiogenesis
Edited by D.W. Hamilton and G.M.H. Waites

Contraception and Mechanisms of Endometrial Bleeding
Edited by C. d'Arcangues, I.S. Fraser, J.R. Newton and V. Odlind

Forthcoming
Growth Factors in Fertility Regulation
Edited by F.P. Haseltine and J.K. Findlay

Vaccines for Fertility Regulation: Safety and Efficacy
Edited by G. Ada and D. Griffin

Contraception and mechanisms of endometrial bleeding

Proceedings of a symposium organized by the Special Programme of Research, Development and Research Training in Human Reproduction of the World Health Organization in Geneva on 28 November–2 December 1988

EDITED BY

C. D'ARCANGUES
WHO Special Programme of Research, Development and Research Training in Human Reproduction, Geneva, Switzerland

I.S. FRASER
Department of Obstetrics and Gynaecology, University of Sydney, Sydney, Australia

J.R. NEWTON
Department of Obstetrics and Gynaecology, Queen Elizabeth Medical Centre, Birmingham, England

V. ODLIND
Department of Obstetrics and Gynaecology, University Hospital, Uppsala, Sweden

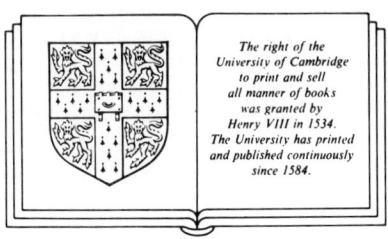

The right of the
University of Cambridge
to print and sell
all manner of books
was granted by
Henry VIII in 1534.
The University has printed
and published continuously
since 1584.

Published on behalf of the World Health Organization
CAMBRIDGE UNIVERSITY PRESS
CAMBRIDGE
NEW YORK   PORT CHESTER
MELBOURNE   SYDNEY

Published by the Press Syndicate of the University of Cambridge
The Pitt Building, Trumpington Street, Cambridge CB2 1RP
40 West 20th Street, New York, NY10011, USA
10 Stamford Road, Oakleigh, Melbourne 3166, Australia

First published 1990

Printed in Great Britain by Redwood Press Limited, Melksham, Wiltshire

British Library cataloguing in publication data

Scientific basis of fertility regulation: contraception and
mechanisms of endometrial bleeding.
1. Women. Uterus, endometrium. Effects of contraceptives.
I. Arcangues, Catherine d'
616.62

Library of Congress cataloguing in publication data

Scientific basis of fertility regulation: contraception and
mechanisms of endometrial bleeding: proceedings of a symposium /
organized by the Special Programme of Research, Development, and
Research Training in Human Reproduction of the World Health
Organization in Geneva on 28 November–2 December 1988 ; edited by
Catherine d'Arcangues . . . [et al.].
    p.   cm.
'Published on behalf of the World Health Organization.'
ISBN 0 521 39025 7
1. Contraceptive drugs–side effects–Congresses.   2. Endometrium
–Effect of drugs on–Congresses.   3. Endometrium–Physiology
–Congresses.   4. Menstruation–Congresses.   I. D'Arcangues,
Catherine   II. Special Programme of Research, Development, and
Research Training in Human Reproduction (World Health Organization).
III. World Health Organization.
[DNLM: 1. Contraceptive Agents–adverse effects–congresses.
2. Endometrium–drug effects–congresses.   3. Endometrium
–physiology–congresses.   4. Menstruation–drug effects–congresses.
WP 550 S416   1988]
RG137.4.S43   1990
615′.766–dc20   90-1333   CIP

ISBN 0 521 39025 7 hardback

Contents

Participants

Dr Biran Affandi
Klinik Raden Saleh
University of Indonesia
Jakarta Pusat, Indonesia

Dr Mats Åkerlund
Department of Obstetrics &
   Gynaecology
University of Lund
Lund, Sweden

Dr David Archer
Department of Obstetrics &
   Gynecology
Contraceptive Research and
   Development Programme
Eastern Virginia Medical School
   Norfolk, USA

Dr David T. Baird
Department of Obstetrics &
   Gynaecology
University of Edinburgh
Centre for Reproductive Biology
Edinburgh, UK

Dr Stephen C. Bell
Department of Obstetrics &
   Gynaecology
University of Leicester School of
   Medicine
Leicester Royal Infirmary
Leicester, UK

Dr Paul Bischof
Service de Gynécologie et d'Obstétrique
Université de Genève
Genève, Switzerland

Dr Peter Böhlen
Lederle Laboratories

N. Middletown Road
Pearl River, USA

Dr Philippe Bouchard
Service d'Endocrinologie et des
   Maladies de la Reproduction
Hôpital de Bicêtre
Bicêtre, France

Dr Ivo Brosens
St Elizabeth Clinic
Bruxelles, Belgium

Dr M. Linette Casey
The University of Texas Southwestern
   Medical School
Dallas, USA

Dr David A. Clark
Department of Medicine
McMaster University
Hamilton, Canada

Dr Ian D. Cooke
Department of Obstetrics &
   Gynaecology
University of Sheffield
Jessop Hospital for Women
Sheffield, UK

Dr Frederick J. Cornillie
Department of Obstetrics &
   Gynaecology
Universitaire Ziekenhuizen
Leuven, Belgium

Dr Pierre Courtoy
International Centre of Pathology
Sint Lambrechts Woluwe, Belgium

Dr Marie-Carmen Cravioto
Department of Reproductive Biology

Instituto Nacional de la Nutricion
Mexico DF, Mexico

Dr Soledad Diaz
Consultorio de Planificación Familiar
Instituto Chileno de Medicina
    Reproductiva
Santiago, Chile

Dr Yves Eeckhout
International Centre of Pathology
Sint Lambrechts Woluwe, Belgium

Dr Murdo G. Elder
Institute of Obstetrics and Gynaecology
University of London
Hammersmith Hospital
London, UK

Dr Jock K. Findlay
Medical Research Centre
Prince Henry's Hospital
Melbourne, Australia

Dr Ian S. Fraser
Department of Obstetrics &
    Gynaecology
University of Sydney
Sydney, Australia

Dr Elisabeth Granström
Department of Physiological Chemistry
Karolinska Sjukhuset
Stockholm, Sweden

Dr Erlio Gurpide
Department of Obstetrics &
    Gynecology
Mount Sinai Medical Center
New York, USA

Dr Michael Harper
Department of Obstetrics &
    Gynecology
The University of Texas Health Science
    Center
San Antonio, USA

Dr David L. Healy
Medical Research Centre
Prince Henry's Hospital
Melbourne, Australia

Dr Fusao Hirata
The Johns Hopkins University School
    of Hygiene and Public Health
Baltimore, USA

Dr Helena Hourihan
Department of Obstetrics &
    Gynaecology
Universitaire Ziekenhuizen
Leuven, Belgium

Dr Elisabeth Johannisson
Clinic of Sterility and Gynecologic
    Endocrinology
Department of Obstetrics & Gynecology
University Hospital
Genève, Switzerland

Dr Dennis O. Johnsen
International Health Attaché
United States Mission to the United
    Nations Office and other
    International Organizations at
    Geneva
Chambésy, Switzerland

Dr Roger J. B. King
Hormone Biochemistry Department
Imperial Cancer Research Fund
London, UK

Dr Hans Ludwig
Department of Obstetrics &
    Gynaecology
University Women Clinic
Basel, Switzerland

Dr Tapani Luukkainen
Department of Medical Chemistry
University of Helsinki
Steroid Research Laboratory
Helsinki, Finland

Dr Frederick Naftolin
Department of Obstetrics &
    Gynecology
Yale University School of Medicine
New Haven, USA

Dr John R. Newton
Department of Obstetrics &

Gynaecology
Queen Elizabeth Medical Centre
Birmingham, UK

Dr Viveca Odlind
Department of Obstetrics &
  Gynaecology
University Hospital
Uppsala, Sweden

Dr Qiu Shu-hua
Science Research Office
State Family Planning Commission
Beijing, People's Republic of China

Dr Margaret C. P. Rees
Department of Obstetrics &
  Gynaecology
John Radcliffe Hospital
Oxford, UK

Dr Catherine Rice-Evans
Department of Biochemistry &
  Chemistry
Royal Free Hospital School of
  Medicine
London, UK

Dr Markku Seppälä
Department of Obstetrics &
  Gynaecology
University Central Hospital
Helsinki, Finland

Dr Brian L. Sheppard
Central Pathology Building
St James' Hospital
Dublin, Ireland

Dr Régine Sitruk-Ware
Central Medical Affairs
CIBA-GEIGY
Basel, Switzerland

Dr Steven K. Smith
Department of Obstetrics &

Gynaecology
University of Cambridge
School of Clinical Medicine
The Rosie Maternity Hospital
Cambridge, UK

Dr Mokhtar Toppozada
Department of Obstetrics &
  Gynaecology
University of Alexandria
Shatby Maternity Hospital
Alexandria, Egypt

Dr Reijo Vihko
Department of Clinical Chemistry
University of Oulu
Oulu, Finland

Dr Pramuan Virutamasen
Department of Obstetrics &
  Gynaecology
Chulalongkorn Hospital Medical
  School
Bangkok, Thailand

Dr Jonathan Weintraub
Centre de Cytologie
Université de Genève
Genève, Switzerland

Dr John White
Institute of Obstetrics & Gynaecology
University of London
Hammersmith Hospital
London, UK

Secretariat

C. d'Arcangues
J. Barzelatto
E. Diczfalusy
P. Hall
E. Wilson

Authors alone are responsible for the views expressed in the Proceedings. The mention of specific companies or of certain manufacturers' products does not imply that they are endorsed or recommended by the World Health Organization in preference to others of a similar nature that are not mentioned.

Acknowledgement

A special note of thanks is due to Ms Katherine Macham for her outstanding work in preparing this volume for publication.

Welcoming address

J. BARZELATTO

Director, Special Programme of Research, Development and Research Training in Human Reproduction.

It is a great pleasure for me to welcome you all on behalf of the Director-General of the World Health Organization to this important symposium. I would also like to thank you for accepting the invitation to assist us with the in-depth assessment of a problem which is of major concern to the entire field of contraception.

The suggestion to organize this symposium came from the Steering Committee of the Task Force on Long-Acting Systemic Agents for Fertility Regulation. This task force is engaged, among other things, in the development of progestogen-only contraceptives, which offer several advantages, but have a major drawback: bleeding irregularities. However, the importance of bleeding irregularities goes far beyond injectable contraceptives, since it has relevance to several other areas of fertility regulation, be it oral contraceptives, intrauterine devices, or post-ovulatory methods. Hence, the problem is a major concern to the Special Programme since we do not know how to cope with bleeding irregularities due to contraceptive use.

The importance of the problem has been recognized by the Programme since its inception. Ten years ago, the Programme focused the attention of the international scientific community on our incomplete knowledge in this area by organizing a symposium on this subject. The book *Endometrial Bleeding and Steroidal Contraception*, published in 1980, remains one of the authoritative reviews of the state of art in this field. During the past decade, considerable advances have been made in our understanding of a number of fundamental mechanisms. However, it is not yet clear how these advances can be used in the solution of the 'bleeding problems' due to contraceptives in general and to steroidal contraceptives in particular.

It is of interest to note that many of the questions asked at the symposium a decade ago are still relevant today. What is the sequence of events leading to normal menstrual bleeding? Is there any difference in this respect among populations with different nutritional status? What are the mechanisms inducing different bleeding irregularities, e.g. spotting, prolonged bleeding, amenorrhea? What kind of basic information is needed to provide us with a more rational approach to the management of bleeding irregularities and how can such information guide us in the development of improved contraceptive methods?

After a decade of research efforts, the questions posed above are still unresolved, so much so that we might start wondering whether it is possible at all to develop steroidal contraceptives which do not cause any bleeding irregularities. Steroids affect the hypothalamic–pituitary–ovarian axis and they also affect the endometrium, and it is questionable whether these effects can ever completely be dissociated from each other. It is therefore possible that after the development of three generations of more and more potent contraceptive steroids, we are approaching the end of the road of steroidal contraception, and I must confess that I am not optimistic as to whether satisfactory answers can be provided today to the questions posed a decade ago. My suspicion is that the future of contraception is beyond the 'classical' hormonal interference with the function of the hypothalamic–pituitary–gonadal axis; I feel rather that the future lies in specific interference with biochemical mechanisms involved in gamete maturation, fertilization and implantation.

Nevertheless, I also feel that we have an obligation to look again into the questions raised a decade ago and see if it is possible today to propose at least improved therapeutic measures for dealing with bleeding irregularities.

I would also like to make another comment in this introduction, in which I am just talking very informally about the things that, during the years, have been a matter of concern to all of us. Looking back to the 1950s and 1960s, our major concern at that time was demographic – population explosion, human numbers – and our goal was to find the magic bullet, the 'perfect' contraceptive to solve the problem of unbalanced population growth. Since then, we have realized that the problems of population are far more complex and are intimately interrelated with resources, development and environment. Similarly, we have realized that reproductive health is also much more complex than just contraception and fertility regulation. A number of components – family planning, safe motherhood, infant and child survival and, if we wish to use more slogans, 'safe sex' – are all parts of a complex interaction, which is greatly influenced by socio-economic conditions. Unless we are willing to take a holistic approach, we cannot solve the problem of population and provide an optimal approach to fertility regulation.

This change in focus to assess real life situations rather than to look only for technological breakthroughs has also made a significant impact on our priorities in contraceptive research and development and has influenced our views on irregular bleeding.

When we assessed a contraceptive in the past, we used to say 'the bleeding is acceptable'. What did we mean by saying this? We meant that no anemia appeared and that there was no need for blood transfusion, or iron replacement therapy. However, the new focus, the emphasis on the quality of life, helped us to realize that with this former approach we were simply banking on the well-known tolerance of women. Women who have decided not to have more children will go through anything in order not to have another child, and this 'going through anything' is a reality. In developing countries they will resort to illegal abortions, although they do realize that they are risking their lives. By the same token, women accept the use of a number of contraceptives despite the fact that the existence of major bleeding irregularities cannot be considered as a small nuisance, an 'acceptable disturbance' in the daily life of a normal person. Hence, the importance of this side-effect of hormonal contraceptives, which was previously regarded as 'minor', has grown considerably within the new conceptual framework of modern contraceptive research.

I hope, Ladies and Gentlemen, that from this brief introduction you realize that to me the present symposium is of particular importance. Can we solve the problem of bleeding irregularities caused by steroidal contraceptives? Or are we pursuing a wrong track and therefore must look for a completely new approach? I also hope that you do not consider my remarks as an exercise in philosophy, but appreciate that the problem we are addressing is not only the concern of the scientific community at present. It is also the concern of all our governing bodies.

Contraception and menstrual bleeding disturbances: a clinical overview

VIVECA ODLIND* AND IAN S. FRASER**

*Department of Obstetrics and Gynaecology, University of Uppsala, Uppsala, Sweden.
**Department of Obstetrics and Gynaecology, University of Sydney, Sydney, Australia.

Abstract

Acceptability of modern methods for fertility regulation depends to a large extent on the degree of menstrual bleeding disturbances that these methods induce. With the injectable methods, depot-medroxyprogesterone acetate (DMPA) and norethisterone enanthate (NET-EN), as well as with Norplant[R] subdermal implants, the 1-year discontinuation rates for bleeding problems constitute around one-half or more of all terminations. Among women using progestogen-only oral pills or low-dose levonorgestrel vaginal rings, around 30–40% of all terminations are for bleeding-related reasons. The proportion of terminations for bleeding disturbances in relation to all terminations is usually somewhat lower among women using combined oral contraceptive pills (OCs) or monthly injectable preparations, both estrogen-containing methods. The degree of menstrual disruption with various progestogen-only methods of contraception seems to correspond to the effects that the methods exert upon ovarian function, although many studies indicate that direct effects on the endometrium also constitute an important explanation for the abnormal bleeding patterns. Further studies are needed to clarify those mechanisms. There is little indication in the literature that different progestogens exert different effects on the bleeding pattern when equipotent doses have been administered. Counselling has been reported to be the most important tool to improve acceptability with methods that commonly cause major menstrual disturbances. Women have to be reassured that amenorrhea or irregular or prolonged bleeding episodes are expected side-effects of a particular method rather than signs of disease or pregnancy. Treatment regimens have been suggested, particularly with estrogens, for the management of bleeding disturbances. None of these has yet been properly tested in a controlled trial. Further studies need to be performed to evaluate the effects of various treatment regimens on bleeding patterns and method acceptability.

Introduction

One of the most important factors that determine acceptability of modern methods for fertility regulation is the disturbance of menstrual bleeding pattern that these methods induce. An extensive WHO study has demonstrated that, irrespective of socio-cultural background, most women wish to have a regular and unchanged pattern of vaginal bleeding while using a contraceptive (Snowden & Christian, 1983). This study has also demonstrated that women's perceptions of their menstrual bleeding patterns vary considerably with socio-cultural background.

Different contraceptive methods are associated with different types as well as degrees of menstrual disturbances and these patterns also seem to vary between populations. Contraceptive methods may either produce bleeding pattern changes that remain the same for the entire period of method use or there may be considerable changes over the time during which the method is used.

Detailed analyses of bleeding patterns in large-scale studies may serve several useful purposes:

1. when comparing different methods of contraception, i.e. when changes in composition or dose of established methods have been made, when new methods are being developed, or when different modes of administration are being studied.
2. to generate knowledge in order to provide good counselling for women about the bleeding pattern changes that can be expected to result from use of a particular method.
3. to generate background knowledge to form a basis for research in order to increase understanding of the etiology of some of the bleeding disturbances associated with use of contraceptive methods.

The purposes of this chapter are to review and summarize what is reported in the literature concerning some of the characteristic bleeding pattern disturbances associated with various hormonal and intrauterine methods for fertility regulation and to discuss the influence that such disturbances may have on acceptability of the methods.

Collection of menstrual data

The first prerequisite for an appropriate evaluation of vaginal bleeding patterns is the accurate collection of menstrual data. Retrospectively collected menstrual data, based on the ability of the woman to recall past events, have been shown to be unreliable (Rodriguez *et al.*, 1976; Snowden, 1977). Menstrual data are therefore best recorded prospectively on a day-to-day basis by the woman on a specially designed menstrual diary card. Such cards usually ask for some distinction between a scanty bleed, often referred to as 'spotting', and a more normal bleed. Sometimes more information is sought, i.e. days of contraceptive use and non-use, concomitant symptoms and/or medication. The woman is asked to bring the card to the clinic at follow-up visits. Special types of menstrual diary cards for use by illiterate women, using symbols instead of text, have been developed. In their collection of menstrual data from women in eight different countries, Snowden and Christian (1983) recognized the difficulties with diary cards, and had to apply different procedures, using local interviewers in some populations and letting the women themselves complete their cards in others. They reported that the differing data collection techniques did not seem to introduce a serious bias into the analysis.

The perception of volume of menstrual bleeding

Quantitation of menstrual flow has always been a difficult problem in spite of its unquestionable importance in gynaecological symptomatology. Many women using intrauterine devices will complain of excessively heavy bleeding. Quantitation of flow is generally of lesser importance in relation to bleeding disturbances with hormonal contraception where unpredictable, irregular, frequent, prolonged or absent bleeding are the usual complaints. When assessed by objective measurements, the difference in perception of volume of flow between individuals is enormous (Fraser *et al.*, 1984).

Methods of analysis

Different methods that have been proposed for the analysis of menstrual data were recently reviewed by Belsey and Farley (1988). In papers evaluating OCs, the method of analysis was usually based on the 28-day menstrual cycle, and any bleeding that was not classified as menstrual was described as intermenstrual. When contraceptive methods that cause major disturbances of the cycle, particularly long-acting progestogen-only methods, were introduced, it was no longer possible to use the menstrual cycle as the unit of analysis. The method of analysis that has proven most useful in assessing long-acting methods of contraception and when comparing methods, is that involving a reference period, first suggested by Rodriguez *et al.* (1976). The reference period method uses the woman as the unit of analysis and describes the bleeding events as they happen. The reference period is the number of days on which the analysis is to be based. In order to allow description of the different characteristics of menstrual bleeding and its disturbances, data from sufficiently long periods of time have to be collected. Since the menstrual bleed occurs cyclically at approximately monthly intervals a reference period is usually a multiple of months or 30-day periods. The number of 30-day periods to be included in one reference period may be decided according to the contraceptive method studied and the duration of the study. Rodriguez *et al.* suggested that the minimum length of a reference period should be 90 days.

Based on several consultations with clinicians and statisticians by WHO, Belsey *et al.* (1986) recommended the reference period method of analysis and suggested modifications in terminology and improvement of the statistical methods. The definitions used in the reference period method of analysis are found in Table 1. The bleeding pattern indices listed in Table 2 are those that were suggested as the most appropriate for between-method comparison. In a

Table 1. *Reference period analysis: definitions (Belsey* et al., *1986)*

Bleeding
Any bloody vaginal discharge that requires the use of such protection as pads or tampons.

Spotting
Any bloody vaginal discharge that is not large enough to require sanitary protection.

Bleeding/spotting episode
One or more consecutive days on which bleeding or spotting has been entered on the diary card.

Bleeding/spotting-free interval
One or more consecutive days on which no bleeding or spotting has been entered on the diary card.

Bleeding/spotting segment
One bleeding/spotting episode and the immediately following bleeding/spotting-free interval.

Reference period
The number of consecutive days upon which the analysis is based.

Table 2. *Reference period analysis: bleeding pattern indices as suggested by WHO (Belsey* et al., *1986)*

Number of bleeding/spotting (b/s) days
Number of b/s episodes
Mean, range and maximum value of lengths of b/s episodes
Mean, range and minimum value of lengths of b/s-free intervals
Number of spotting days
Number of spotting-only episodes

subsequent analysis following the recommendations of WHO, the number of indices was found to be too large and it was suggested that the separate calculation of spotting days and episodes be omitted, since those were indices that added little information to the overall analysis (Belsey *et al.*, 1988a).

The reference period analysis may appear artificial to clinicians and difficult to translate into terms that are easily comprehensible to the patients. WHO therefore recommended the identification of different clinically important patterns to be calculated and described during each reference period, as shown in Table 3 (Belsey *et al.*, 1986). Assessment of these clinically important patterns in women who continue or discontinue for various reasons, and assessment of changes throughout successive reference periods, may prove useful for counselling purposes.

Bleeding problems as a reason for termination

Changes in the bleeding pattern constitute one of the most common reasons for discontinuation, both with hormonal methods and with intrauterine

Table 3. *Clinically important bleeding patterns: definitions using 90-day reference periods (Belsey* et al., *1986)*

No bleeding
No days of bleeding/spotting entered throughout the reference period

Prolonged bleeding
Bleeding/spotting episodes lasting more than 14 days during one reference period.

Frequent bleeding
More than 5 bleeding/spotting episodes in a reference period.

Infrequent bleeding
1-2 bleeding/spotting episodes in a reference period.

Irregular bleeding
3-5 bleeding/spotting episodes and fewer than 3 bleeding/spotting-free intervals of 14 days or more in a reference period.

devices (IUDs). The proportion of women discontinuing method use for menstrual reasons as a percentage of all reasons for discontinuation is shown in Tables 4 and 5.

With the injectable methods DMPA and NET-EN as well as Norplant[R] subdermal implants, the 1-year discontinuation rates for bleeding problems constitute around one-half or more of all terminations with these methods (Table 4). The percentage of women who terminate use of the monthly injectable preparations, which contain both estrogen and progestogen, and cyclically used vaginal rings, releasing progestogen/estrogen combinations, for bleeding-related problems is lower and closer to what is reported for combined OCs (Table 4). The proportion of bleeding problems as a reason for IUD termination seems to be very variable between studies. The character of the disturbances that may lead to discontinuation is, however, quite different with non-medicated or copper IUDs than it is with progestogen-releasing IUDs and other hormonal methods.

There may be a whole range of reasons, apart from those related to bleeding, that could lead to termination of use of a contraceptive method, i.e. side-effects, fear of side-effects, opposition from husband, wish to become pregnant, no more need for contraception etc. The reason given by the woman to the investigators may not always be the true one, although several studies have shown that the menstrual reasons for discontinuation of a method given by a woman usually reflect her menstrual bleeding pattern as recorded on her diary card (Belsey *et al.*, 1988b).

In studies of contraceptive methods, the overall termination rates as well as those for bleeding and amenorrhea vary considerably between centres in multicentre studies and the variability of termination rates between studies is even greater. This suggests that several factors determine whether or not a woman will continue with a contraceptive method, some of which are

Table 4. *Termination rates per 100 women at 1 year for all reasons and bleeding-related reasons, and bleeding-related reasons as a proportion of all reasons for termination with different hormonal methods of contraception. (Figures within brackets indicate references.)*

Method	(Ref.)	All reasons	Menstrual reasons		Menstrual/ all (%)
			Amenorrhea	Bleeding	
Injectable (3-monthly)					
DMPA 150	(WHO, 1986)	41.2	12.5	15.5	68
DMPA 100	(WHO, 1986)	40.2	7.2	13.8	52
DMPA 150	(WHO, 1983)	51.4	11.9	15.0	52
DMPA 150	(WHO, 1977)	28.8	11.5	9.3	72
NET-EN 200	(WHO, 1977)	24.4	1.8	10.3	50
Injectable (2-monthly)					
NET-EN	(WHO, 1983)	49.7	6.8	13.6	41
Injectable (monthly)					
HRP 112	(WHO, 1988)	35.5	2.1	6.3	24
HRP 102	(WHO, 1988)	36.8	1.6	7.5	25
Implants					
Norplant[R]	(Sivin, 1983)	22.9		9.5	41
Norplant[R]	(Olsson et al., 1988)	40.6		26.1	64
Vaginal rings					
LNG 20	(WHO, 1989b)	50.4		17.2	34
LNG/E₂	(Sivin et al., 1981a)	49.6		8.9	18
Oral pills (combined)					
LNG/EE₂	(Sivin et al., 1981a)	61.8		5.8	9
LNG/EE₂	(WHO, 1982a)	52.6		9.7	18
NE/Mestranol	(WHO, 1982a)	61.0		23.2	38
Oral pills (progestogen only)					
LNG 30	(WHO, 1982a)	60.9		26.0	43
NE 350	(WHO, 1982a)	57.7		24.2	42

Notes:
DMPA   Depot-medroxyprogesterone acetate.
E₂   Estradiol.
EE₂   Ethinyl estradiol.
LNG   Levonorgestrel.
NE   Norethisterone.
NET-EN Norethisterone enantate.

probably not directly related to the method. Population differences as well as protocol differences could explain some of the large variation between studies. Counselling is an important determinant for method continuation and counselling procedures may vary from one country to another, from one centre to another and from one individual to another. For example, it appears that counselling on the management of amenorrhea is particularly variable and the sometimes high discontinuation rates for amenorrhea may reflect the

Table 5. *Termination rates per 100 women at 1 year for all reasons and bleeding-related reasons, and bleeding-related reasons as a proportion of all reasons for termination reported from studies of different intrauterine devices*

Device	(Ref)	All reasons	Menstrual reasons	Menstrual/ all (%)
TCu-380	(Sivin *et al.*, 1987)	20.2	7.0	35
LNG-20	(Sivin *et al.*, 1987)	26.5	10.9	41
Nova-T	(Luukkainen *et al.*, 1987b)	17.8	7.5	42
LNG-20	(Luukkainen *et al.*, 1987b)	20.3	8.7	43
Nova-T	(Luukkainen *et al.*, 1983)	23.9	11.9	50
TCu-200Ag	(Luukkainen *et al.*, 1983)	23.3	12.2	52
TCu-220C	(WHO, 1982b)	23.7	2.2	9
Lippes	(WHO, 1982b)	31.2	4.5	14
Cu-7	(WHO, 1982b)	29.4	3.6	12

counsellor's acceptability of amenorrhea rather than that of the woman. Therefore, the continuation rates with contraceptive methods, as usually presented in the literature, should be considered a crude and insensitive instrument for determination of method acceptability.

Factors that may influence bleeding patterns

It is apparent from many studies that the bleeding pattern with hormonal contraceptive methods depends on both the exogenous and endogenous steroid influences and on their effects on the ovarian function and on the endometrium. Since the initiation of normal menstruation depends on withdrawal of estrogen and progesterone, any fluctuation of the endogenous or exogenous steroid concentrations is likely to contribute to irregular bleeding. Markee (1948) reported that a fall in progesterone always resulted in bleeding, whereas a fall in estrogen did not always result in a bleed if progesterone remained high. In general, methods that contain estrogens produce fewer bleeding disturbances than do progestogen-only methods.

It seems likely that a variety of mechanisms exist in the endometrium, which may be triggered under certain circumstances and contribute to bleeding disturbances. Amenorrhea appears fairly easy to explain in women exposed to high-dose progestogens where the endometrium is thin, highly suppressed and histologically 'stable'. Episodes of erratic, unpredictable and frequent bleeding are among the most troublesome disturbances with progestogen-only methods. It seems that in these women there must be one or more mechanisms within the endometrium which can be easily triggered – or self-triggered – to release substances which cause vascular or tissue destruction. These mechanisms could involve the arachidonic acid cascade, activated macrophages releasing any one of a number of potentially destructive substances (free

Table 6. *Classification of ovarian response to low-dose progestogens according to Landgren and Diczfalusy (1980)*

Reaction type	Ovarian response
A	No cyclic follicular activity No luteal activity
B	Cyclic follicular activity No luteal activity
C	Cyclic follicular activity Inadequate luteal activity
D	Ovulatory-like ovarian function

oxygen radicals, tumour necrosis factor-α, various enzymes etc.), other migratory white cells, endometrial lysosomes and other tissue enzymes. Once tissue breakdown has begun, a number of processes may be activated which amplify the local destruction. A variety of factors may limit the extent of tissue destruction and bleeding. Prolonged bleeding, sometimes for several weeks, is another troublesome symptom among progestogen-only users. This symptom obviously also requires some mechanism to initiate bleeding. Following this, disturbances of the hemostatic and/or fibrinolytic mechanisms, and of tissue remodelling and regeneration, may contribute to the prolongation of bleeding. A greater understanding of the complex interaction of all these processes seems essential in order to develop better means of preventing or treating these clinical disturbances.

There is a great range of individual difference in ovarian sensitivity to a given dose of a progestogen. Landgren and Diczfalusy (1980) investigated women before and during treatment with a norethisterone 0.3 mg minipill and could distinguish between four ovarian reaction patterns (Table 6). They found no significant correlation between bleeding patterns and ovarian reaction in the four groups, which they explained by the small number of subjects in each subgroup. In subsequent studies Landgren *et al.* (1982) monitored women with vaginal rings releasing 0.02 mg levonorgestrel (LNG), or 0.2 mg or 0.5 mg norethisterone at a zero-order rate and reported that those who were anovulatory (reactions A and B) had significantly more days of bleeding than those with some luteal activity (reactions C and D), irrespective of type or dose of progestogen. They also found that even those who had ovulatory-like cycles (D) during treatment reported significantly more bleeding days than before treatment, irrespective of dose or type of progestogen, suggesting direct effects on the endometrium. Thus, there is little evidence that one progestogen is different from another in its effects on the bleeding pattern, if equipotent doses are compared. In general, those progestogen-only methods that invariably induce pronounced effects on ovulatory function more often result in menstrual disturbances than do those with which the ovary is less suppressed.

Combined oral contraceptive pills

Use of combined oral contraceptive pills inhibits ovulation in the majority of women by effects on hypothalamic–pituitary function. Bleeding episodes with OCs occur as a result of the withdrawal of the exogenous hormones. If occasional pills are forgotten or taken at irregular intervals, erratic bleeding is common. The bleeding pattern with OCs is usually extremely predictable, but unexpected bleeding episodes do occur and are usually referred to as episodes of intermenstrual spotting or bleeding. Gray (1980), reviewing bleeding patterns with different methods of steroidal contraception, reported that intermenstrual bleeding was more common with pills containing less than 0.05 mg ethinyl estradiol (EE) compared with higher doses and that intermenstrual bleeding/spotting with OCs seems to occur most frequently during the first few cycles and then the frequency declines. Breakthrough bleeding and/or spotting is usually reported to occur in around 2–20% and amenorrhea in around 1–8% of the treatment cycles. In a study comparing a triphasic pill (LNG 0.05 mg, 0.075 mg, 0.125 mg + EE 0.03 mg, 0.04 mg, 0.03 mg) with a monophasic (LNG 0.15 mg + EE 0.03 mg), women on the triphasic formulation had significantly fewer episodes of spotting or breakthrough bleeding than did women on the monophasic formulation during the first two treatment cycles. This difference between formulations, however, almost disappeared in treatment cycles 3 to 6 (Zador, 1979). In another study, the same triphasic formulation was compared to a monophasic formulation (containing 0.03 mg EE and 0.15 mg desogestrel) and no difference between bleeding patterns was found, nor did the bleeding patterns differ considerably from what had been reported by Zador for the monophasic levonorgestrel formulation (Cullberg *et al.*, 1982).

Bleeding disturbances are usually not a major problem or reason for discontinuation with OCs. In a recent analysis of bleeding patterns using WHO recommendations with one natural and eight hormonal methods of contraception, three different pill formulations were included (LNG 0.15 mg + EE 0.03 mg, LNG 0.25 mg + EE 0.05 mg, norethisterone acetate (NA) 1.0 mg + EE 0.05 mg; Belsey *et al.*, 1988a). All three formulations produced bleeding episodes that were shorter than in untreated women and there were only minor differences between formulations. Episodes of spotting and patterns classified as irregular bleeding were found more often in women on NA + EE and the low dose LNG + EE formulations. Around 90% of pill users had no disturbance in their bleeding patterns. Infrequent bleeding was reported by 2–7% of the pill users and probably reflected occasional failure of a withdrawal bleed (Belsey *et al.*, 1988a).

Progestogen-only oral contraceptives

These formulations were originally developed to act on the cervical mucus to form a hormonal barrier method and were not designed to inhibit ovulation.

The majority of investigators of progestogen-only pills, however, report cycle changes, such as shortening of the cycles, intermenstrual bleeding and/or spotting and absence of bleeding, suggesting effects other than just on the cervical mucus (Gray, 1980). Subsequent studies have shown that ovarian function is affected in many women using a minipill. Only 40% of women on a daily norethisterone 0.3 mg minipill had unchanged ovulatory patterns (reaction D) during treatment in the study by Landgren and Diczfalusy (1980); complete ovulatory suppression (reaction A) was found in 16%, cyclic follicular activity but no luteal activity (reaction B) was found in 23% and normal follicular but insufficient luteal activity (reaction C) in 21%.

Gray (1980), reviewing bleeding patterns with hormonal contraceptive methods, found that in the early clinical studies of various progestogen-only pills, the frequency of cycles with 'normal' (25–35 days) cycle lengths was reported to be between 50% and 70%. Amenorrhea, here defined as no bleeding for 45 days or more, was reported in 5–10% of cycles. 'Short' cycles, usually defined as bleeding-free intervals less than 25 days, were reported to occur in approximately 25% of cycles, with large variation between studies. In a recent report by Belsey *et al.* (1988a), menstrual data obtained from WHO studies of one natural and eight hormonal methods of contraception were analyzed according to the WHO recommendations. Two progestogen-only pills were included in the analysis, LNG 0.03 mg and NA 0.35 mg. Around 70% of women on each preparation had no bleeding pattern disturbance at all. Since both preparations resulted in shorter bleeding-free intervals and since shorter mean episode lengths were found in women on LNG, but not on NA, the segment lengths were shorter, which seems to be in accordance with the previously described 'shortening of the cycles' associated with progestogen-only pill use. In the recent analysis, the bleeding pattern met the definition of 'frequent bleeding' in around 10% of NA users and around 13% of LNG users during the first reference period. Older studies often reported an improvement of bleeding patterns with increasing duration of use. There is little evidence that the ovarian or endometrial response would change considerably over time if a woman continued with the same progestogen-only pill, and the recent WHO analysis did not show a change in bleeding pattern when the four consecutive reference periods of 90 days were analyzed (Belsey *al.*, 1988a). The previously reported 'improvement' could possibly reflect that those women who had the most chaotic bleeding patterns would discontinue first, leaving those with more acceptable patterns in the study.

Injectable progestogen-only methods for contraception

When given in the usual dose (150 mg every 90 days) DMPA completely suppresses ovulation in the vast majority of women for the whole treatment period. After a single injection of DMPA, a peak of plasma MPA is usually found after 7–10 days and then there is a slow decline of MPA levels that is very variable from one individual to another. MPA is almost invariably measurable in plasma after 90 days and occasionally after 200 days (Fotherby *et al.*, 1980).

Pharmacodynamic studies have not reported progesterone rises until well beyond the 90-day post-injection period and not until plasma levels of MPA have become undetectable. Rises in estradiol are sometimes seen towards the end of the 90-day post-injection period in response to decreasing levels of MPA (Fotherby *et al.*, 1980; Bassol *et al.*, 1984). Thus, women on DMPA exhibit ovarian reaction type A most of the time, and sometimes, shortly before the next injection is due, reaction B may be seen.

In comparative studies of 150 mg and 100 mg DMPA, there were no significant differences in serum peak levels of MPA or the serum levels measured 90 days after the injection, between the two doses, nor was there a difference in the ability of either dose to inhibit ovulation for a minimum of 90 days. Women treated with the lower dose exhibited signs of follicular activity (as judged by rises in estradiol) slightly earlier than those treated with 150 mg (Fotherby *et al.*, 1980; Bassol *et al.*, 1984). Although this difference was not statistically significant, presumably due to the small number of subjects studied, a difference in time before resumption of follicular activity may explain the significantly lower incidence of amenorrhea found among women treated with the lower dose (100 mg) as compared with those receiving 150 mg in a recent multicentre phase III clinical study of the two DMPA doses, given every 90 days (WHO, 1986, 1987a).

The bleeding pattern with DMPA shows the greatest aberration from the 'normal' of all contraceptive methods. Only around 10% of patterns were classified as 'no disturbance' in the first reference period in a recent comparative analysis of bleeding patterns with nine methods of contraception (Belsey *et al.*, 1988a). Almost 10% had amenorrhea in the first and around 40% in the fourth reference period. The analysis highlighted the total unpredictability of bleeding patterns with DMPA, showing great inter-individual as well as intra-individual variations. There is no tendency for the bleeding pattern in users of DMPA to 'normalize' with time. The effect is rather for women on DMPA to have fewer bleeding/spotting days and a tendency to develop amenorrhea with increasing duration of use (Belsey *et al.*, 1988a). Most studies report that around 30–50% of DMPA users have amenorrhea after 1 year. In extreme long-term users of DMPA the rate of amenorrhea has anecdotally been reported to be close to 90%.

Clinical trials of NET-EN in doses of 200 mg, given every 90 days, demonstrated a significantly higher pregnancy rate than did 150 mg DMPA, whereas, when given every 60 days, the pregnancy rate with NET-EN was low and similar to that of DMPA (WHO, 1977, 1983). This clinical difference probably reflects the difference in pharmacokinetics between the two injectable contraceptive methods. After a single injection of NET-EN there is an early plasma peak of NET within a week and a rapid decline of plasma NET levels over a period that may vary between 8 and 12 weeks before NET is undetectable in plasma (Sang *et al.*, 1981). Pharmacodynamic studies have demonstrated ovulatory suppression throughout a 60-day post-injection interval, and rises in progesterone are usually not seen until 90 days or later, but follicular activity, as reflected by rises in estradiol, has been demonstrated 30–50 days after an injection (Fotherby *et al.*, 1980). Using the classification suggested by Landgren and Diczfalusy, reaction A is mostly found during the first post-injection month, followed by reaction B until the next injection is due after 60 days. If the next injection is further delayed, occasional women might exhibit some luteal or ovulatory-like activity (reaction C or D).

The bleeding patterns in women treated with NET-EN every 60 days are not unlike those of women treated with DMPA. However, comparative clinical studies have shown that significantly fewer women on NET-EN than on DMPA report amenorrhea or discontinue method use for that reason (WHO 1978, 1983). In a 24-month study, comparing DMPA 150 mg, given every 90 days, with NET-EN 200 mg, given either every 60 days (NET-EN 60), or NET-EN 200 mg, given every 60 days for 6 months and then every 84 days (NET-EN 84), the frequency of amenorrhea at 12 months with the two NET-EN regimens was around 30% and significantly lower than that with DMPA, which was around 50%. At 24 months, the frequency of amenorrhea in the NET-EN 84 group remained the same, whereas it had increased to 40% in the NET-EN 60 group and to 60% in the DMPA group. Women on either dose regimen of NET-EN reported fewer days of spotting than did women on DMPA (WHO, 1983). The bleeding patterns probably reflect differences in pharmacodynamic effects of the three regimens, with more ovulatory-like cycles in women on NET-EN 84, a regimen that was associated with a higher pregnancy rate (WHO, 1983).

Monthly injectable preparations

Injectable preparations containing a progestogen plus an estrogen to be given once a month have long been available on trial in Latin America and in the People's Republic of China (Hall, 1984). It has been reported that the inconvenience of the frequent injections often is outweighed by a more 'normal' bleeding pattern and a more rapid return to fertility in comparison with longer-acting injectable formulations (Hall, 1984). Two injectable preparations for monthly administration, HRP 112 (DMPA, 25 mg, and estradiol cypionate, 5 mg) and HRP 102 (NET-EN, 50 mg, and estradiol valerate, 5 mg) have recently been tested in clinical trials and found to offer highly effective and acceptable methods for contraception (WHO, 1988).

Aedo *et al.* (1985) reported that after a single injection of HRP 112 there was a peak of MPA within a few days and then plasma levels of MPA declined over the next 30–50 days. All women studied had detectable low levels of MPA at the time of the next injection. After an injection of HRP 102, NET levels were detectable in all subjects as long as 90 days after the last injection. With both preparations, there was a peak of estradiol 2–4 days after the injection, followed by a decrease to a minimum after approximately 15 days, or slightly earlier with HRP 102, followed by a more pronounced, second estradiol peak 40–60 days after the injection. The first peak is apparently due to the exogenous estradiol, whereas the second peak reflects the return of follicular activity with endogenous production of estradiol. This second estradiol peak was followed by a slight rise in progesterone in some of the volunteers but progesterone levels suggestive of ovulation were not recorded until 60–90 days after the last injection. Regardless of preparation, the first bleed occurred around 15 days after the injection, apparently in response to the first estradiol peak. Thus, during an injection interval of 30 days, both HRP 112 and HRP 102 produce inhibition of ovulation (ovarian reaction A-B).

In a recent clinical multicentre study, both formulations were reported to be highly effective contraceptives (WHO, 1988). There were no statistically significant differences between the two formulations. Both the total 1-year termination rates and terminations for menstrual reasons were lower than usually reported for long-acting injectable preparations (see Table 4). An analysis of the bleeding pattern showed no difference between the drugs (WHO, 1989a). There were significantly more bleeding/spotting days and more episodes in the first reference period, presumably reflecting the pharmacokinetics of the drugs, the first bleed occurring approximately 15 days after the first injection as an estradiol withdrawal bleed. In the consecutive reference periods around 70% of the women had 'normal' patterns. Among the 30% who were classified as having unacceptable bleeding patterns, the most common abnormalities were infrequent bleeding and irregular bleeding. Both prolonged bleeding and amenorrhea were very uncommon and found only in around 1% of the women. Except for an improvement in bleeding pattern from the first to the second reference period, the analysis could not detect any particular trend throughout the year. The analysis also showed a good correlation between the reasons for discontinuation given by the women and the bleeding pattern as recorded in their diary cards, with the exception that most of the women discontinuing for amenorrhea rather fell under the category of infrequent bleeding.

Methods providing constant steroid release

One disadvantage of long-acting injectable methods is the type of pharmaco-kinetics they provide, whereby the woman has to be given a high dose initially to allow the steroid load to last for a particular time. By use of constant release systems, such as Silastic[R] subdermal implants or vaginal rings, the total steroid load can be kept lower, presumably with fewer side-effects and metabolic effects than with higher steroid doses.

Subdermal implants

Several clinical studies have been performed on biodegradable or non-biodegradable implants, releasing various progestogens. The implant system that is by far the most widely used and best studied is that consisting of six Silastic[R] capsules releasing levonorgestrel, Norplant[R]. A similar system, Norplant[R]-2, consisting of two solid Silastic[R] rods, has been tested in clinical studies, but is not yet widely used. Norplant[R] is a highly effective method for contraception for at least 5 years and Norplant[R]-2 is highly effective for at least 3 years. With Norplant[R], levonorgestrel diffuses through the Silastic[R] membrane at a slow and steady rate. The daily release of levonorgestrel is between 0.05 mg and 0.08 mg during the first year of use, after which it declines to around 0.03 mg per day for the next 5 years (Robertson *et al.*, 1983). During the first year of use, ovulations are suppressed in the majority of women, after which approximately half of the women have ovulatory-like cycles (Weiner & Johansson, 1976; Croxatto *et al.*, 1982; Brache *et al.*, 1985; Alvarez *et al.*, 1986). In a study of five volunteers with Norplant[R] during a year, Weiner and Johansson (1976) found signs of follicular activity (reaction B) in all, and occasional luteal activity (reaction C) in three. Brache *et al.* (1985) reported ovulatory-like cycles in 40% of users during the second to the fifth year of Norplant[R] use. It appears that the ovarian function in women with Norplant[R] is more suppressed during the first year of use, reflecting a slightly higher release of levonorgestrel in the beginning. From the second through the fifth year of use the release is fairly constant and around half of the women exhibit some luteal activity (reaction C and D).

Unlike the situation with most other progestogen-only contraceptive methods the bleeding pattern with Norplant[R] improves with increasing duration of use, the most aberrant patterns and most of the terminations for menstrual reasons being reported in the first year (Sivin *et al.*, 1983). This progressive improvement of bleeding patterns probably reflects the return of ovulatory-like cycles, which, in turn, probably reflects the decrease in release rate. In one study, 26% of the women terminated method use for menstrual problems during the first year and an additional 6% during the second year, whereas there were no terminations for menstrual problems during the third year of use (Olsson *et al.*, 1988). The bleeding pattern in many users of Norplant[R] is characterized by frequent, irregular and/or prolonged bleeding, particularly during the first 12 months of use (Faundes *et al.*, 1978). An analysis of diary cards from 43 Norplant[R] users in Sweden showed that around 40% of women had 'normal' bleeding patterns and around 10% had bleeding-free intervals of more than 90 days (amenorrhea) during the first year

Table 7. *Clinically important bleeding patterns in 43 users of Norplant^R (%) analyzed according to WHO recommendations. Note that the last four parameters are not mutually exclusive, and the percentages may sum to more than 100*

| | Reference period (90 days each) | | | |
	I	II	III	IV
No disturbance	31.6	41.7	42.4	42.8
Amenorrhea	5.3	16.7	9.1	7.1
Infrequent	23.7	13.9	9.1	10.7
Frequent	15.8	5.6	15.2	3.6
Irregular	5.3	8.3	15.1	32.2
Prolonged	26.3	22.3	12.1	10.8

(Table 7). Sivin (1984) was able to analyze bleeding pattern indices in 105 women who kept diaries for 4 full years of continuing Norplant^R use and reported a decrease in the number of bleeding episodes and number of bleeding days and shortening of bleeding episode lengths when the first year was compared to the fourth. Bardin *et al.* (1987) reported that the mean number of bleeding/spotting days in a group of women, continuing Norplant^R use through 5 years, was 92.3 during the first year and then gradually decreased to 70.2 during the fifth year. Sivin (1984) reported from multicentre studies that 34% of Norplant^R users had 97 or more bleeding days and 15% had at least one episode longer than 15 days in the first year. The corresponding figures for the third year were 19% and 7%, respectively. Amenorrhea, defined as no bleeding for 90 days, was reported by 26% in year 1 and 15% in year 3.

There have been no large studies correlating the bleeding pattern with the endocrine response. In one study, 15 women who had been using Norplant^R-2 for more than 3 years were monitored for 6 weeks with ultrasonography and endocrine parameters for assessment of ovarian function. Six (40%) had ovulatory-like patterns (D), 6 (40%) had signs of follicular activity (B) and 3 (20%) had signs of inadequate luteal activity (C) (Table 8). All women, irrespective of endocrine pattern, had had regular menses with a mean segment length of 28 days. The range of segment lengths was slightly larger in women with reaction type B (Olsson & Odlind, unpublished data).

Vaginal rings

Silastic vaginal rings releasing either a progestogen alone or estrogen/progestogen combinations have been widely investigated and reported to be a highly acceptable constant-release system for contraception. Contraceptive

Table 8. *Type of ovarian reaction (classi-*
fied according to Landgren & Diczfalusy)
and segment lengths in 15 women who had
used Norplant^R-2 rods for more than 3
years

Ovarian reaction	N	Range of segment lengths (mean)
(B)	6/15	22–32 (28)
(C)	3/15	25–28 (27)
(D)	6/15	25–33 (28)

steroids are efficiently absorbed through the vaginal mucosa. Different steroids, doses, combinations and ring types have been tested, some in large phase III studies, some in small-scale studies. There are two types of rings that have been more widely tested than others, the low-dose progestogen-only ring for continuous use and the progestogen/estrogen combination ring for cyclical use.

Low-dose progestogen-only vaginal ring

WHO has developed a vaginal ring that has an estimated daily release of levonorgestrel of 0.02 mg. The ring is used continuously and each ring can be used for 90 days. With this particular ring a 1-year pregnancy rate of 3.7 per 100 was reported from a recent multicentre clinical study (WHO, 1990a). The effects of the ring on ovarian function have been described in detail by Landgren *et al.* (1982). They reported from a study of 20 women using the ring for 90 days that around 40% of the '30-day treatment segments' were anovulatory (reactions A-B), 10% were classified as inadequate luteal function (reaction C), and around 50% were classified as ovulatory-like patterns (reaction D). In 40% of the women, the same ovarian pattern was found in the three consecutive '30-day treatment segments' studied, whereas in the others the ovarian reaction pattern varied from one segment to the next, usually between A and B, between B and C or between C and D.

The 1-year discontinuation rate for menstrual problems was reported to be 15.2% in the recent multicentre study (WHO, 1990a). Approximately half of the women had bleeding patterns that were classified as 'normal' and the most commonly observed abnormal pattern was irregular bleeding, which was recorded among one-quarter of the women (WHO, 1990b). Amenorrhea was very uncommon and only found in 1% of the users (WHO, 1990b). In the comparative analysis between nine methods of contraception, women using the vaginal ring had slightly more bleeding/spotting days per 90-day period than women in any of the other groups (Belsey *et al.*, 1988a).

Vaginal rings containing estradiol

Combination vaginal rings releasing a progestogen and an estrogen, estradiol or ethinyl estradiol, have been developed and tested in clinical trials. The International Committee for Contraception Research of the Population Council performed a clinical multicentre study of rings releasing 0.25–0.29 mg levonorgestrel and 0.15–0.18 mg estradiol-17-beta administered cyclically, used for 21 days with 7 ring-free days. Women on a combined OC containing levonorgestrel 0.15 mg and ethinyl estradiol 0.03 mg were recruited as a comparison group. Both regimens inhibited ovulation (Sivin *et al.*, 1981a). As a result of the cyclical administration the bleeding patterns were basically regular and 'cyclical'. Intermenstrual spotting or bleeding was reported by 20–25% of ring users and by around 12% of pill users. Analysis of diaries, however, showed no significant difference in the number of bleeding/spotting days between regimens and it was concluded that both regimens produced similar bleeding patterns (Sivin *et al.*, 1981b).

Intrauterine devices

One of the most common complaints with IUDs is increased menstrual bleeding, sometimes associated with pain. Recent studies of modern copper-releasing IUDs show that bleeding and/or pain account for around 40% of all terminations (see Table 5). The removal rates for bleeding and pain with copper IUDs vary between 4% and 15% in most studies. The type of problems reported are both increased number of bleeding days and increased volume of blood loss (Andrade & Orchard, 1987). Most reports suggest at least a doubling of the menstrual blood loss with large non-medicated devices such as Lippes loop and other plastic IUDs. With copper IUDs the increase is usually reported to be around 40% (Andrade & Orchard, 1987).

Exposure to an IUD causes a localized trauma in the endometrium with a foreign body response and impaired hemostasis (Sheppard, 1987). The changes are particularly pronounced in the areas in direct contact with or adjacent to the IUD. Studies of the endometrium of IUD users have demonstrated superficial erosion leading to microvascular bleeding into the cavity and increased vascular permeability leading to interstitial hemorrhage (Sheppard, 1987). The precipitating mechanism for this reaction is poorly understood, but changes in a number of factors have been reported in IUD users, such as high levels of plasminogen activator, increased fibrinolytic activity, increases in macrophages, mast cells and various prostaglandins.

Progestogen-releasing IUDs have been shown substantially to reduce menstrual blood loss (Andrade & Orchard, 1987). The Progestasert, releasing progesterone at a daily rate of around 0.65 mg, has been associated with a 40% reduction in menstrual blood loss. IUDs releasing different doses of LNG have been developed and tested in clinical trials, the most widely tested being the one releasing approximately 0.02 mg per 24 hours. This IUD has been shown to be highly effective and acceptable in most clinical studies (Luukkainen *et al.*, 1987a). One of the most common reasons for termination in the trials was amenorrhea, which was the reason for termination given by 1.6–4.9% of users in the first 12 months in different studies (Luukkainen *et al.*, 1984; Luukkainen *et al.*, 1987b). It has been pointed out that a large proportion of the removals for amenorrhea took place early in the studies and that later, when the counselling was modified, amenorrhea became a desirable 'side-effect' that was quite acceptable to many women. Apart from a high number of bleeding/spotting days during the first 3 months of use, all women using the LNG-IUD reported a reduction both in number of bleeding days and in amount of bleeding. Nilsson *et al.* (1984) studied the ovarian function in women with or without amenorrhea, using the LNG-IUD, and found that 75% had signs of luteal activity (reaction C or D), irrespective of menstrual status. They concluded that the ovarian function is affected only in occasional women and that the important mechanism behind the amenorrhea is a local effect of LNG on the endometrium. The endometrium of LNG-IUD users is characterized by total loss of cyclical changes. The endometrium becomes strongly suppressed and appears atrophic with few glands and a thin, decidualized stroma (Luukkainen *et al.*, 1984).

Comparison between methods

From data available, it seems that among progestogen-only methods of contraception, the oral 'minipill' causes the least disruptive bleeding pattern, followed by the vaginal ring and Norplant[R]. The 2- and 3-monthly injectable methods cause disruption with 'chaotic' patterns in the majority of users. This progression of disruption seems to be in parallel with the effects that the different methods have on ovarian function. There are some indications that bleeding patterns with low-dose progestogen-only methods are influenced by body weight. Among women using the LNG 0.02 mg vaginal ring, a higher ponderal index was associated with shorter and less variable episodes and longer bleeding-free intervals than was found among lighter women (Belsey *et al.*, 1988c). This suggests that ovarian function is less affected in heavy women than in light, which is further supported by the fact that there was a statistically significant positive correlation between body weight and pregnancy rate in a recent study of the vaginal ring (WHO, 1990c). A similar correlation between body weight and risk of pregnancy has been reported for Norplant[R] (Sivin, 1988). There has been no study in women using Norplant[R] correlating body weight and bleeding patterns. Diaz *et al.* (1986), however, reported that all women who had become pregnant during Norplant[R] use and who had kept a bleeding record, had regular menses for the 180-day interval preceding pregnancy. These findings support the concept that the endocrine effects induced by progestogen-only methods of contraception to some extent are reflected in the bleeding pattern and this knowledge can be used for counselling purposes. Different endocrine responses do not, however, explain why some women using a particular method develop amenorrhea whereas others, using the same method and exhibiting the same endocrine pattern, report prolonged bleeding periods. There are presumably other mechanisms operating directly on the endometrium that are responsible for part of the effects that are expressed as severe disturbances of the normal menstrual bleeding pattern.

Among other factors that may affect bleeding patterns, cigarette smoking has been proposed. In a recent study, Brown *et al.* (1988) reported a positive association between self-perceived menstrual abnormalities and cigarette smoking that was independent of contraceptive method.

Management of bleeding disturbances

It is important to point out that, although most of the bleeding disturbances associated with hormonal contraception are due to the treatment, other possible causes for abnormal bleeding should always be ruled out. Such possible causes include neoplasia and infection, and management should therefore always include both a thorough history with as detailed bleeding data as possible and a pelvic examination.

Heavy bleeding in women using non-medicated or copper IUDs has been reported to respond favourably to treatment with antifibrinolytic agents and to non-steroidal anti-inflammatory drugs (NSAIDs) (Toppozada, 1987). Treatment with NSAIDs is usually reported also to improve dysmenorrhea, associated with IUD use.

Heavy bleeding in association with progestogen-only contraception is rare. Hormonal contraception is usually associated with reduced blood loss and/or increased hemoglobin levels, although few studies have objectively measured blood loss (Nilsson & Holma, 1981). Curettage is seldom justified and need usually be performed only to rule out neoplasia.

The influence of infection was demonstrated in an study of 700 sexually active young users of combined OCs, where 27% of those who reported intermenstrual bleeding during the last month were Chlamydia culture positive in the cervix in comparison to 11% of those who did not report any bleeding abnormalities (Rahm & Odlind, unpublished observations).

Many different approaches are known among clinicians for the management of abnormal uterine bleeding in association with use of hormonal contraception, few of which have been subject to controlled clinical trials (Koetsawang, 1980). Johannisson *et al.* (1982) studied the effects of a 7-day course of oral EE, 0.05 mg, on bleeding patterns and endometrial histology in women who bled during use of a norethisterone 0.3 mg minipill, and reported no significant difference in number of bleeding days in comparison with those who received placebo.

From a questionnaire to experienced clinicians on the management of menstrual disturbances with injectable contraceptive methods, mainly DMPA and NET-EN, Fraser (1983) reported different approaches. Counselling appeared to be the most important and, in many centres, the only activity for the management both of prolonged and/or frequent bleeding and of amenorrhea. Active therapy for prolonged and/or frequent bleeding consisted of either early repeat injection of the progestogen or various forms of estrogens.

Early repeat injection of DMPA could be expected to have the effect on ovarian function that any follicular activity, resulting from decreasing plasma MPA levels, would be inhibited. As there is some evidence from dose-finding studies that the incidence of amenorrhea is greater in those who have little or no follicular activity (reaction A), early repeat injections would theoretically promote the development of amenorrhea. In practice, a transient improvement is seen, but this is not always maintained (Gray, 1980).

Estrogen regimens, oral or injectable, have sometimes been reported to appear effective if the duration of treatment was as long as 14–21 days (Fraser, 1983). It should be pointed out, however, that even if a course of estrogen could stop a single episode of bleeding, the original bleeding pattern may return after the end of the estrogen treatment. Well-designed clinical studies of the effects of various estrogen regimens on prolonged bleeding with long-acting progestogen-only methods need to be performed.

Until there is good evidence that a specific treatment regimen is effective in the management of bleeding disturbances in women on progestogen-only contraception, counselling will remain the most important tool. Most of the bleeding disturbances described in this paper are of a nature that is previously unknown to the woman and may remind her of either pregnancy or ill-health. Therefore, counselling should be provided both before and during use of the method and be given in a reproductive health perspective, i.e. the significance of any potential bleeding abnormality should be explained, efficacy and possible effects of other contraceptive methods as well as the risk of an unwanted pregnancy should be discussed. The development of amenorrhea may be equated with the physiological amenorrhea which usually accompanies lactation. The quality of counselling depends among other things on such factors as level of education, personal experience of and attitudes towards contraceptive methods and some of their expected side-effects among method providers, attitudes within the local society, media activities etc. Good counselling requires the method provider to have experience, confidence and good theoretical understanding of all available methods of contraception and to be familiar with their potential side-effects and effects on the bleeding pattern. Bleeding disturbances may remain the price to be paid for safe and effective contraception, and it is important that those who want to encourage women to pay this price are sensitive to the queries and needs of their clients, the women.

References

Aedo, A.-R., Landgren, B.-M., Johannisson, E. & Diczfalusy, E. (1985). Pharmacokinetic and pharmacodynamic investigations with monthly injectable contraceptive preparations. *Contraception*, 31:453–469.

Alvarez, F., Brache, V., Tejada, A.S. & Faundes, A. (1986). Abnormal endocrine profile among women with confirmed or presumed ovulation during long-term Norplant[R] use. *Contraception*, 33:111–119.

Andrade, A.T.L. & Pizarro-Orchard, E. (1987). Quantitative studies on menstrual blood loss in IUD users. *Contraception*, 36:129–144.

Bardin, C.W., Sivin, I., Nash, H., Robertson, D., Croxatto, H.B., Diaz, S., Alvarez, F., Faundes, A., Holma, P., Luukkainen, T., Olson, S.E., Odlind, V., Johansson, E. & Mishell, D.R. Jr. (1987). Norplant[R] contraceptive implants. (In) *Fertility Regulation Today and Tomorrow* (Diczfalusy, E. & Bygdeman, M., eds.), Vol. 36, pp.143–152. New York, Raven Press.

Bassol, S., Garza-Flores, J., Cravioto, M.-C., Diaz-Sanchez, V., Fotherby, K., Lichtenberg, R. & Perez-Palacios, G. (1984). Ovarian function following a single administration of depot-medroxyprogesterone acetate (DMPA) at different doses. *Fertility and Sterility*, 42:216–222.

Belsey, E.M., d'Arcangues, C., Carlson, N. and Task Force on Long-acting Systemic Agents for Fertility Regulation (1988c). Determinants of menstrual bleeding patterns among women using natural and hormonal methods of contraception. II. The influence of individual characteristics. *Contraception*, 38:243–257.

Belsey, E.M. & Farley, T.M.M. (1988). The analysis of menstrual bleeding patterns: A review. *Contraception*, 38:129–156.

Belsey, E.M., Machin, D. & d'Arcangues, C. (1986). The analysis of vaginal bleeding patterns induced by fertility regulating methods. *Contraception*, 34:253–260.

Belsey, E.M. and Task Force on Long-acting Systemic Agents for Fertility Regulation (1988a). Vaginal bleeding patterns among women using one natural and eight hormonal methods of contraception. *Contraception*, 38:181–206.

Belsey, E.M. and Task Force on Long-acting Systemic Agents for Fertility Regulation (1988b). The association between vaginal bleeding patterns and reasons for discontinuation of contraceptive use. *Contraception*, 38:207–225.

Brache, V., Faundes, A., Johansson, E. & Alvarez, F. (1985). Anovulation, inadequate luteal phase and poor sperm penetration in cervical mucus during prolonged use of Norplant[R] implants. *Contraception*, 31:261–273.

Brown, S., Vessey, M. & Stratton, I. (1988). The influence of method of contraception and cigarette smoking on menstrual patterns. *British Journal of Obstetrics and Gynaecology*, 95:905–910.

Croxatto, H.B., Diaz, S., Pavez, M., Miranda, P. & Brandeis, A. (1982). Plasma progesterone levels during long-term treatment with levonorgestrel Silastic implants. *Acta Endocrinologica*, 101:307–311.

Cullberg, G., Samsioe, G., Finstad Andersen, R., Bredesgaard, P., Boe Andersen, N., Ernerot, H., Fanöe, E., Fylling, P., Haack-Sörensen, P.E., Klottrup, P., Pedersen, J.H. & Sandager, T. (1982). Two oral contraceptives, efficacy, serum proteins, and lipid metabolism. A comparative multicentre study on a triphasic and a fixed dose combination.*Contraception*, 26:229–243.

Diaz, S., Pavez, M., Herreros, C., Johansson, E.D.B. & Croxatto, H.B. (1986).

Bleeding pattern, outcome of accidental pregnancies and levonorgestrel plasma levels associated with method failure in Norplant[R] implant users. *Contraception*, **33**:347–356.

Faundes, A., Sivin, I. & Stern, J. (1978). Long acting implants. An analysis of menstrual bleeding patterns. *Contraception*, **18**:355–365.

Fotherby, K., Koetsawang, S. & Mathrubutham, M. (1980). Pharmacokinetic study of different doses of Depo Provera. *Contraception*, **22**:527–536.

Fraser, I.S. (1983). A survey of approaches to management of menstrual disturbances in women using injectable contraceptives. *Contraception*, **28**:385–397.

Fraser, I.S., McCarron, G. & Markham, R. (1984). A preliminary study of factors influencing perception of menstrual blood loss volume. *American Journal of Obstetrics and Gynecology*, **149**:788–793.

Gray, R.H. (1980). Patterns of bleeding associated with the use of steroidal contraceptives. (In) *Endometrial Bleeding and Steroidal Contraception* (Diczfalusy, E., Fraser, I.S. & Webb, F.T.G., eds.), pp.14–49. Bath, England, Pitman Press.

Hall, P.E. (1984). Clinical trial of the monthly injectable contraceptives Cycloprovera and HRP 102. (In) *Long-acting contraceptive delivery systems* (Zatuchni, G.I., Goldsmith, A., Shelton, J.D. & Sciarra, J.J., eds.), pp.515–522. Philadelphia, Harper & Row.

Johannisson, E., Landgren, B.-M. & Diczfalusy, E. (1982). Endometrial morphology and peripheral steroid levels in women with and without intermenstrual bleeding during contraception with the 300 μg norethisterone (NET) minipill. *Contraception*, **25**:13–30.

Koetsawang, S. (1980). Present management of abnormal bleeding associated with steroidal contraceptives. (In) *Endometrial Bleeding and Steroidal Contraception* (Diczfalusy, E., Fraser, I.S. & Webb, F.T.G., eds.), pp.50–64. Bath, England, Pitman Press.

Landgren, B.-M. & Diczfalusy, E. (1980). Hormonal effects of the 300 μg norethisterone (NET) minipill. *Contraception*, **21**:87–113.

Landgren, B.-M., Johannisson, E., Masironi, B. & Diczfalusy, E. (1982). Pharmacokinetic and pharmacodynamic investigations with vaginal devices releasing levonorgestrel at a constant, near zero order rate. *Contraception*, **26**:567–585.

Luukkainen, T., Allonen, H., Haukkamaa, M., Holma, P., Pyörälä, T., Terho, J., Toivonen, J., Batar, I., Lampe, L., Andersson, K., Atterfeldt, P., Johansson, E.D.B., Nilsson, S., Nygren, K.G., Odlind, V., Olsson, S.E., Rybo, G., Sikström, B., Nielsen, N.C., Buch, A., Osler, M., Steier, A. & Ulstein, M. (1987b). Effective contraception with the levonorgestrel-releasing intrauterine device: 12-month report of a European multicenter study. *Contraception*, **36**:169–179.

Luukkainen, T., Allonen, H., Nielsen, N.-C., Nygren, K.G. & Pyörälä, T. (1983). Five years' experience of intrauterine contraception with the Nova-T and the Copper-T-200. *American Journal of Obstetrics and Gynecology*, **147**:885–892.

Luukkainen, T., Nilsson, C.G., Allonen, H., Haukkamaa, M. & Toivonen, J. (1984). Intrauterine release of levonorgestrel. (In) *Long-acting Contraceptive Delivery Systems* (Zatuchni, G.I., Goldsmith, A., Shelton, J.D. & Sciarra, J.J., eds.), pp. 601–612. Philadelphia, Harper and Row.

Luukkainen, T., Toivonen, J. & Lähteenmäki, P. (1987a). Medicated intrauterine devices. (In) *Fertility Regulation Today and Tomorrow* (Diczfalusy, E. & Bygdeman, M., eds.), Vol.36, pp.153–163. New York, Raven Press.

Markee, J.E. (1948). Morphological basis for menstrual bleeding. Relation of regression to the initiation of bleeding. *Bulletin of the New York Academy of Medicine*, **24**:253–268.

Nilsson, C.G. & Holma, P. (1981). Menstrual blood loss with contraceptive subdermal levonorgestrel implants. *Fertility and Sterility*, **35**:304–306.

Nilsson, C.G., Lähteenmäki, P.L.A. & Luukkainen, T. (1984). Ovarian function in amenorrheic and menstruating users of a levonorgestrel-releasing intrauterine device. *Fertility and Sterility*, **41**:52–55.

Olsson, S.E., Odlind, V., Johansson, E.D.B. & Sivin, I. (1988). Contraception with Norplant^R implants and Norplant^R-2 implants (two covered rods). Results from a comparative clinical study in Sweden. *Contraception*, **37**:61–73.

Robertson, D.N., Sivin, I., Nash, H.A., Braun, J. & Dinh, J. (1983). Release rates of levonorgestrel from Silastic^R capsules, homogeneous rods and covered rods in humans. *Contraception*, **27**:483–495.

Rodriguez, G., Faundes-Latham, A. & Atkinson, L.E. (1976). An approach to the analysis of menstrual patterns in the critical evaluation of contraceptives. *Studies in Family Planning*, **7**:42–51.

Sang, G.W., Fotherby, K., Howard, G., Elder, M. & Bye, P.G. (1981). Pharmacokinetics of norethisterone oenanthate in humans. *Contraception*, **24**:15–27.

Sheppard, B.L. (1987). Endometrial morphological changes in IUD users: a review. *Contraception*, **36**:1–10.

Sivin, I. (1983). Clinical effects of Norplant^R subdermal implants for contraception. (In) *Long-Acting Steroid Contraception* (Mishell, D.R., ed.), pp.89–116. New York, Raven Press.

Sivin, I. (1984). Findings in phase III studies of Norplant implants. (In) *Long-Acting Contraceptive Delivery Systems* (Zatuchni, G.I., Goldsmith, A., Shelton, J.D. & Sciarra, J.J., eds.), pp.488–500. Philadelphia, Harper and Row.

Sivin, I. (1988). International experience with Norplant^R and Norplant^R-2 contraceptives. *Studies in Family Planning*, **19**:81–94.

Sivin, I., Alvarez-Sanchez, F., Diaz, S., Holma, P., Coutinho, E., McDonald, O., Robertson, D.N. & Stern, J. (1983a). Three-year experience with Norplant subdermal contraception. *Fertility and Sterility*, **39**:799–808.

Sivin, I., Alvarez-Sanchez, F., Diaz, S., Holma, P., Coutinho, E., McDonald, O., Robertson, D.N. & Stern, J. (1983). Three-year experience with Norplant subdermal contraception. *Fertility and Sterility*, **39**:799–808.

Sivin, I., Mishell, D.R., Victor, A., Diaz, S., Alvarez-Sanchez, F., Nielsen, N.C., Akinla, O., Pyörälä, T., Coutinho, E., Faundes, A., Roy, S., Brenner, P.F., Åhren, T., Pavez, M., Brache, V., Giwa-Osagie, O.F., Fasan, M.O., Zausner-Guelman, B., Darze, E., Da Silva, J.C.G., Diaz, J., Jackanicz, T.M., Stern, J. & Nash, H.A. (1981a). A multicenter study of levonorgestrel-estradiol contraceptive vaginal rings. I. Use–effectiveness. An international comparative trial. *Contraception*, **24**:341–358.

Darze, E., Da Silva, J.C.G., Diaz, J., Jackanicz, T.M., Stern, J. & Nash, H.A. (1981b). A multicenter study of levonorgestrel–estradiol contraceptive vaginal rings: III – Menstrual patterns. An international comparative trial. *Contraception*, **24**:377–392.

Sivin, I., Stern, J., Diaz, J., Diaz, M.M., Faundes, A., El Mahgoub, S., Diaz, S., Pavez, M., Coutinho, E., Mattos, C.E., McCarthy, T., Mishell, D.R., Shoupe, D., Alvarez, F., Brache, V. & Jimenez, E. (1987). Two years of intrauterine contraception with levonorgestrel and with copper: a randomized comparison of the TCu 380Ag and levonorgestrel 20 mcg/day devices. *Contraception*, **35**:245–255.

Snowden, R. (1977). The statistical analysis of menstrual bleeding patterns. *Journal of Biosocial Science*, **9**:107–120.

Snowden, R. & Christian, B. (1983). *Patterns and Perceptions of Menstruation.* London, Croom Helm.

Toppozada, M. (1987). Treatment of increased menstrual blood loss in IUD users. *Contraception*, **36**:145–157.

Weiner, E. & Johansson, E.D.B. (1976). Plasma levels of d-norgestrel, estradiol and progesterone during treatment with Silastic implants containing d-norgestrel. *Contraception*, **14**:81–92.

WHO Expanded Programme of Research, Development and Research Training in Human Reproduction. Task Force on Long-acting Systemic Agents for the Regulation of Fertility (1977). Multinational comparative clinical evaluation of two long-acting injectable contraceptive steroids: norethisterone oenanthate and medroxyprogesterone acetate. I. Use–effectiveness. *Contraception*, **15**:513–533.

WHO Special Programme of Research, Development and Research Training in Human Reproduction. Task Force on Long-acting Systemic Agents for Fertility Regulation (1978). Multinational comparative clinical evaluation of two long-acting injectable contraceptive steroids: norethisterone oenanthate and medroxyprogesterone acetate. 2. Bleeding patterns and side-effects. *Contraception*, **17**:395–406.

WHO Special Programme of Research, Development and Research Training in Human Reproduction. Task Force on Intrauterine Devices for Fertility Regulation (1982b). Interval IUD insertion in parous women: a randomized multicentre comparative trial of the Lippes Loop D, TCu220C and the Copper-7. *Contraception*, **26**:1–22.

WHO Special Programme of Research, Development and Research Training in Human Reproduction. Task Force on Long-acting Systemic Agents for Fertility Regulation (1983). Multinational comparative clinical trial of long-acting injectable contraceptives: norethisterone enanthate given in two dosage regimens and depot-medroxyprogesterone acetate. Final Report. *Contraception*, **28**:1–20.

WHO Task Force on Oral Contraceptives. Special Programme of Research, Development and Research Training in Human Reproduction. WHO Task Force on Oral Contraceptives. (1982a). A randomized, double-blind study of two combined and two progestogen-only oral contraceptives. *Contraception*, **25**:243–252.

WHO Task Force on Long-acting Systemic Agents for Fertility Regulation. Special Programme of Research, Development and Research Training in Human Reproduction. (1986). A multicentred phase III comparative clinical trial of depot-medroxyprogesterone acetate given three-monthly at doses of 100 mg or 150 mg: I. Contraceptive efficacy and side effects. *Contraception*, **34**:223–235.

WHO Task Force on Long-acting Systemic Agents for Fertility Regulation. Special Programme of Research, Development and Research Training in Human Reproduction. (1987a). A multicentred phase III comparative clinical trial of depot-medroxyprogesterone acetate given three-monthly at doses of 100 mg or 150 mg: II. The comparison of bleeding patterns. *Contraception*, **35**:591–610.

WHO Task Force on Long-acting Systemic Agents for Fertility Regulation. Special Programme of Research, Development and Research Training in Human Reproduction. (1988). A multicentred phase III comparative study of two hormonal contraceptive preparations given once-a-month by intramuscular injection: I. Contraceptive efficacy and side effects. *Contraception*, **37**:1–20.

WHO Task Force on Long-acting Systemic Agents for Fertility Regulation (1989a). A multicentred phase III comparative study of two hormonal contraceptive preparations given once-a-month by intramuscular injection: II. The comparison of bleeding patterns. *Contraception*, **40**:531–551.

WHO Task Force on Long-acting Systemic Agents for Fertility Regulation (1990a). Microdose intravaginal levonorgestrel contraception: A multicentre clinical trial. I. Contraceptive efficacy and side-effects. *Contraception*, **41**: 105–124.

WHO Task Force on Long-acting Systemic Agents for Fertility Regulation (1990b). Microdose intravaginal levonorgestrel contraception: A multicentred clinical trial. IV. Bleeding patterns. *Contraception*, **41**:151–167.

WHO Task Force on Long-acting Systemic Agents for Fertility Regulation (1990c). Microdose intravaginal levonorgestrel contraception: A multicentred clinical trial. III. The relation between pregnancy rate and body weight. *Contraception*, **41**: 143–150.

Zador, G. (1979). Fertility regulation using 'triphasic' administration of ethinyl estradiol and levonorgestrel in comparison with the 30 plus 150 μg fixed dose regime. *Acta Obstetricia et Gynecologica Scandinavica*, Supplement, **88**:43–48.

Discussion

Cooke. The point stressed in this review was that the monthly injectables and the levonorgestrel-containing IUDs seem to be superior methods with respect to minimum number of bleeding episodes. Is that such an important consideration as one would infer from Dr Barzelatto's introduction? Should reduction of bleeding be one of the guiding principles behind the strategy? How is the Task Force reacting to the sort of data that you presented this morning?

Odlind. Well, maybe it came across too strongly, because I think I made the point that amenorrhea may also be a problem, and one of the important solutions to any bleeding problem is good counselling and good preparation of the patient. I think the acceptability is quite good if you provide good counselling. There are so many aspects to acceptability that it is difficult to pick one or two methods and say that they are superior. There are certainly advantages, particularly, I think, with the levonorgestrel IUD.

Sheppard. Studies that have been carried out in our department would suggest that the triphasic oral contraceptives, particularly those containing levonorgestrel, are better at balancing the increased peripheral coagulation and fibrinolysis (Bonnar, 1987). Are there any large studies which show the bleeding disturbances which are associated with the triphasic pills?

Odlind. There was a study (Zador, 1979) in which the monophasic levonorgestrel pill was compared to the triphasic levonorgestrel pill, and the bleeding patterns were better with the triphasic pill during the 2 or 3 initial months of use. But this difference disappeared within 6 months.

Naftolin. I was interested in your emphasis on ovulatory disturbance as the basis for the bleeding and wondered whether that is always the case. For example, if one uses Norplant[R] and then adds to it a progesterone-containing IUD, what happens to the bleeding?

Odlind. If you treat the endometrium directly with levonorgestrel, you will have the highest dose directly on the end-organ and this will result in amenorrhea. Dr Nilsson and his co-workers (1984) have shown that, irrespective of the bleeding pattern, 75% of levonorgestrel-releasing IUD users have ovulatory cycles whether or not there is amenorrhea. So with the levonorgestrel-releasing IUD you can have ovulatory amenorrhea, which you cannot have with any other method.

Naftolin. Is that not the point, that in fact if the attempt is to avoid bleeding, we may be defeating ourselves. My point is that we should let the women decide what method is best for them, and we should then offer methods to stop bleeding when this occurs and the women complain. In some cases it will be sufficient to block ovulation, in some cases it will be sufficient to block directly the menstrual process at the local level, and in some cases it may be necessary to combine the two.

Hall. Continuing the discussion on what is the Task Force's strategy in relation to development of new methods and how that relates to bleeding, the first part of this strategy is to develop safe, effective methods which broaden women's choice of contraceptive methods. However, that is qualified by saying that we have been looking at delivery systems to reduce the actual amount of steroid delivered, and secondly, actively pursuing preparations which might reduce the problem associated with menstrual bleeding. We have had a lot of pressure over the past, in fact over the whole life-time of the Programme to try to get away from bleeding irregularities, as has been implied in this discussion and in Dr Barzelatto's introduction. Women do put up with an immense amount, but they do not always put up with bleeding disturbances and we need to offer choices that are better.

They will often discontinue for reasons that appear not to be related to bleeding irregularities, but when you have the possibility of actively looking at objective data that have been collected on menstrual diary patterns, then you will find that women often have difficult bleeding patterns. But women sometimes give another reason to the physician that they feel is acceptable in that clinic. A once-a-month injectable creates the necessity of going back for 12 injections in a year as opposed to 4 with DMPA, yet in introductory trials, the overall continuation rates are greater with the once-a-month injectable than have been seen with DMPA. Secondly, you often hear from the physician in the central clinic: 'We do not have many drop-outs for menstrual bleeding with DMPA, we counsel the women very well, they do not come back and they do not complain'. If you talk to the midwives and the field-auxiliaries, they tell you that the women come back all the time, they want treatment and they are complaining.

Fraser. We have heard so far discussion on amenorrhea and irregular bleeding. A particularly important problem for women is in fact prolonged episodes of bleeding, not usually heavy but prolonged sometimes for many, many weeks on end. This will sometimes continue, particularly with the long-acting injectables, over many injection intervals. This has been one of the areas that we have been particularly concerned about because many of these women do drop out from treatment and if we did have some simple way of stopping or preventing those episodes, then it would directly enhance the acceptability of the method. We have heard from Dr Odlind that estrogen can be used but in fact there are very few objective data in the literature showing the value of estrogen in this situation and the Long-Acting Task Force has set up a placebo controlled double-blind study to actually look at how effective estrogen is in stopping a particular episode and also hopefully at improving the long-term pattern of bleeding. But in addition to that WHO study, I am aware of data from Chile from Dr Diaz who has actually carried out a study looking at estrogen as well as two other treatment modalities for this type of prolonged bleeding problems with Norplant[R].

Diaz. We did a double blind study trying to treat prolonged bleeding that occurs in the first year of Norplant[R] use. We used four different treatments: oral levonorgestrel, ethinyl estradiol, ibuprofen and a placebo as a control group. Treatments were to be initiated every time a bleeding episode exceeded 7 days. The groups were of 45 to 47 women. Not all the women completed the study year, for different reasons, such as they were not able to comply with the study protocol, they did not return to the clinic and so on. So only about 35 women completed the first year of the study in each group.

In those women who were treated, the number of bleeding and spotting days in the first 330 days of use was significantly lower in the ethinyl estradiol group than in the placebo group. And it was also lower for levonorgestrel users and ibuprofen users. Women who were never treated had a significantly higher number of bleeding plus spotting days throughout the first year.

I wonder if the interpretation Dr Odlind gave about the change in the bleeding pattern in Norplant[R] users is correct. You said that probably the large number of bleeding irregularities during the first year may be due to a higher degree of ovarian suppression and the more regular pattern that is observed after the first year is due to the fact that ovulatory cycles are more frequent. We have observed that bleeding irregularities do not occur in the first year of implants which release a higher dose of levonorgestrel, where ovarian suppression is stronger than in Norplant[R] users. We used the rods that delivered twice the dose and there were no bleeding irregularities and the pattern was more like that of the LNG-IUD users. So if the ovary is fully suppressed, you do not get bleeding irregularities, but amenorrhea. The appearance of the endometrium in long-term users is that of a suppressed endometrium, and it does not follow the ovarian pattern.

Odlind. I do not think we are in disagreement, Dr Diaz. I am just saying that the lower the dose the higher the frequency of ovulatory cycles and the more regular bleedings you can get. But if you increase the dose, you get a higher frequency of amenorrhea as a result of complete ovarian suppression.

Diaz. The real question is the one raised by the subject: 'What do I do doctor? I am bleeding too long or too much.' And that is the question I would like to have an answer to, and I hope that we can find some answers.

References

Bonnar, J. (1987). Coagulation effects of oral contraception. *American Journal of Obstetrics and Gynecology*, **157**:1042–1048.

Nilsson, C.G., Lähteenmäki, P.L.A. & Luukkainen, T. (1984). Ovarian function in amenorrheic and menstruating users of a levonorgestrel-releasing intrauterine device. *Fertility and Sterility*, **41**:52–55.

Zador, G. (1979). Fertility regulation using 'triphasic' administration of ethinyl estradiol and levonorgestrel in comparison with the 30 plus 150 μg fixed dose regime. *Acta Obstetricia et Gynecologica Scandinavica*, Supplement, **88**:43–48.

The physiology of menstruation

S.K. SMITH

Department of Obstetrics and Gynaecology, University of Cambridge School of Clinical Medicine, The Rosie Maternity Hospital, Cambridge, UK.

Abstract

Menstruation is the mechanism which has evolved in primates whereby the endometrium undergoes remodelling to be prepared for the implantation of the blastocyst which will arrive in the uterine cavity during the ensuing cycle. Menstruation usually arises after orderly changes occur in both the histological and biochemical development of the endometrium, under the regulation of the ovarian steroids. Specific changes in the endometrial vasculature have been described which precede menstruation, and alterations in the normal hemostatic process arise in the uterus. The widespread need for fertility regulation has encouraged the use of steroidal contraceptives. These drugs have variable effects on the ovarian cycle which further complicates the ovarian regulation of endometrial function. Menstrual disorders of endogenous cycles are an important cause of ill-health in women and irregular bleeding is an important factor in reducing the acceptability of steroidal contraception. Disturbances of prostaglandin synthesis have been demonstrated in endometrium of women with menstrual disorders, and exogenous steroids alter prostaglandin release. This has been suggested to affect the endometrial blood vessels. Regulation of endometrial growth by growth factors is just becoming to be appreciated as another mechanism which may influence endometrial bleeding, particularly with respect to regeneration. A greater understanding of endometrial physiology is likely to lead to more effective regulation of endometrial bleeding.

Introduction

In a strictly evolutionary sense, menstruation is the mechanism whereby the primate endometrium undergoes a process of remodelling which prepares it for the implantation of the blastocyst which arises from the ensuing ovarian cycle. In the past the presence of the menstrual bleed was heralded as a good sign that it was an indication of fertility. It is only in the latter half of the 20th century that menstruation has become a considerable problem for a variety of reasons.

Widespread use of fertility regulation has reduced the numbers of children carried by women during their reproductive life. This has resulted in an increase in the average number of periods experienced by each woman from 40 to 400 during her reproductive life. Most strategies of fertility regulation in women have almost inevitably had consequences for the menstrual loss. The combined oral contraceptive pill reduces menstrual blood loss (MBL) (Andrade *et al.*, 1979), whereas the intrauterine contraceptive device (IUD) increases MBL (Guillebaud *et al.*, 1978). With large-scale sterilization many women experience endogenous ovarian and menstrual cycles in place of periods regulated by oral contraceptives. This experience may lead to perceptual changes which exaggerate this return to endogenous cycles. Certainly in the Western world, the changing role of women within society has further aggravated this problem. The greater involvement of women in activities outside of the home has furthered views of social embarrassment and uncleanliness long associated with menses (Snow & Johnson, 1977).

In addition to the problems of abnormal cyclical menstrual bleeding, has now been added the disorder of breakthrough bleeding, usually associated with the use of combined oral contraceptives, oral or intramuscular progestogen administration or the use of the IUD (Tietze & Lewit, 1970; Guillebaud *et al.*, 1978; Landgren & Diczfalusy, 1980; Fraser, 1983; Van der Vange, 1988). Little is known about the mechanism of menstruation and even less is known about breakthrough bleeding. However, problems with menstruation cost the National Health Service in the United Kingdom about £500 million per annum and irregular bleeding is one of the commonest reasons for women to change their method of contraception. This area of reproduction has received little attention over recent years and is long overdue for the kind of investigation and resources necessary for the eradication of this problem.

The ovarian cycle and menstrual bleeding

The relationship between the ovarian steroids and menstrual bleeding has been known for over 50 years. Withdrawal of progesterone from an estrogen-primed endometrium will induce menstrual bleeding which can be prevented by the continued administration of progesterone. Withdrawal of estrogen will usually induce menstrual bleeding but not if the withdrawal is gradual. Removal of progesterone from a non-estrogen primed endometrium will not result in menstrual bleeding.

Menstruation arising from withdrawal of the combined oral contraceptive is reduced in volume. However, the main problem of steroid contraception is breakthrough bleeding which can occur with either combined pills or progestogens, administered orally or by intramuscular injection. The mechanism underlying this type of bleeding is poorly understood. It is not known whether the bleeding that occurs during the course of taking the pills is the same as that which occurs when the pills are stopped or even compared to a normal period when steroids have not been taken.

The situation is further complicated by endogenous release of steroids during the course of other medication. Smith *et al.* (1986) found plasma levels of estradiol in excess of 500 pmol/l in 5 out of 14 women during the first 2 weeks of administration of a triphasic levonorgestrel/ethinyl estradiol oral combined contraceptive (Trinordiol). In one woman plasma estradiol levels were in excess of 2000 pmol/l. In two of these cases, plasma estradiol levels dropped from 500 to less than 100 pmol/l and from 1000 to less than 500 pmol/l. Women taking Microgynon (levonorgestrel 150 μg and ethinyl estradiol 30 μg) did not demonstrate follicular activity, defined as a level of estradiol greater than 500 pmol/l in blood. Women taking the progesterone-only pill show even greater variability of hypothalamo–pituitary–ovarian suppression. Landgren and Diczfalusy (1980) studied the hormonal profiles of 43 women taking norethisterone, 300 μg/day. They demonstrated four types of response. Seventeen (40%) of the women continued to have regular cycles which demonstrated luteinization and levels of progesterone consistent with pretreatment levels. Nine (21%) women had progesterone rises consistent with inadequate or short luteal phases. Ten (23%) of the women showed active follicular development but failed to luteinize. Seven (16%) women appeared to show effective suppression of follicular activity. Bleeding during the course of medication was associated with estrogen and progesterone withdrawal in most of the well-luteinized group but also occurred in response to the withdrawal of estradiol alone. However, breakthrough bleeding may arise in the absence of clearly defined changes in systemic levels of hormone and these are not characterized by significant changes in endometrial morphology (Johannisson *et al.*, 1982). A further complication is that of compliance, as bleeding may occur because of irregular ingestion of the contraceptive.

Histological changes throughout the menstrual cycle and in response to exogenous steroids

Endometrium

The histological changes that arise in endometrium during the menstrual cycle have been extensively described and reviewed (Noyes *et al.*, 1950; Wynn, 1977). When menstruation is preceded by ovulatory menstrual cycles, the endometrium undergoes proliferative and secretory changes. To characterize endometrial changes as simply proliferative or secretory is inadequate. Proliferation is characterized by the presence of mitotic figures in both glands and stroma. The early proliferative endometrium is 1–2 mm thick. The superficial endometrium is composed of cuboidal cells and the glands are short, straight and narrow. The stroma is compact and the stromal cells stellate or spindle shaped. Shortly after ovulation, subnuclear vacuoles appear in the columnar cells of the glandular epithelium which disappear in the mid-secretory phase of the cycle. At this stage of the cycle, the most prominent feature of the endometrium is the edema of the stroma. In the last week of the menstrual cycle, the three distinct layers of the endometrium can be identified. The zona compacta is the most superficial layer and is so called because of the densely packed stromal cells situated beneath the epithelium. Below this layer is the zona spongiosa which comprises the convoluted and dilated glands.

These two layers constitute the functional layer. The deepest layer of the endometrium is the basal layer which is next to the myometrium. This zone contains the basal arteries, the bases of the glands and dense stroma.

Ultrastructural changes have been described in endometrium (Wynn, 1977). In the proliferative phase of the cycle, the cells are characterized by ciliogenesis and mitosis, whereas in the secretory phase they have large mitochondria, polyribosomes, rough endoplasmic reticulum, well-developed Golgi apparatus and large intracellular accumulations of glycoproteins.

Differentiation of the endometrium is characterized by changes in the immunohistochemical staining for various enzymes which are present in the glandular or stromal fractions. Glandular cells stain for alkaline phosphatase, γ-glutamyltransferase, peptidase, peroxidase and β-glucuronidase. Stromal cells stain for leucine aminopeptidase and also secrete the glycoproteins, fibronectin and laminin (Siegfried *et al.*, 1984). Some enzymes, such as acid phosphatase, lactate dehydrogenase, succinate dehydrogenase and nonspecific esterase, are found in both glandular and stromal cells. Most importantly, species with hemochorial placentation have endometrium which undergoes decidual change under the influence of the ovarian steroids, unlike rodents in which a further stimulus is required for decidualization to occur (Finn, 1977; Bell, 1985). The earliest signs of decidualization occur around the 21st day of the cycle, when large glycogen-containing predecidual cells accumulate around the spiral arterioles supplying the endometrium. These decidual cells begin to synthesize prolactin (Markoff *et al.*, 1983). Recently, the infiltration of the endometrium by leukocytes has been characterized. Macrophages are present in endometrium throughout the cycle and have been reported to rise before the onset of menses (Kamat & Isaacson, 1987). This rise was not found by Bulmer and Ritson (1988). The other type of leukocytes present in the endometrium are lymphocytes which are probably the previously described endometrial stromal granulocytes and are now thought to be large granular lymphocytes (LGLs). These cells infiltrate the stroma in the secretory phase of the cycle and are particularly abundant in the premenstrual phase of the cycle (Bulmer *et al.*, 1986). Their function remains unclear, but they could be transforming natural killer cells which could be required during menstruation to facilitate the removal of cellular debris. Nothing is known of the role of these cells during menses.

Uterine vasculature

On entering the myometrium, arteries coalesce to form the arcuate sheath. Radial arteries pass perpendicular to the arcuate sheath to enter the deeper layers of the myometrium and the endometrium. Shortly after entering the endomyometrial junction, the radial artery gives off a short straight artery, the basal artery, which supplies the basal layer of the endometrium. The superficial two-thirds of the endometrium, the functional layer, is supplied by the continuation of the radial artery which is now termed the spiral artery. As will be described, the spiral arteries undergo various degrees of coiling during the cycle but are effectively end-arterioles. A continuous network of superficial capillaries is supplied by the spiral arteries, each vessel being responsible for about 4–7 mm² of endometrium (Markee, 1940). These capillaries are lost at menstruation. The basal capillaries do not branch in the same way as the superficial vessels. A network of veins drains the superficial capillaries and these pass towards the myoendometrial junction. Contraction of venular endothelial cells occurs in endometrium of women taking norethisterone (Johannisson *et al.*, 1982).

Menstruation

Vascular changes

Knowledge of the changes that arise in endometrium during menstruation is largely based on studies undertaken over 40 years ago. These studies included the work of Markee (1940), who examined endometrium of rhesus monkeys explanted to the anterior chamber of the eye of rabbits, and the histological work of Bartelmez (1937).

Markee described a period of regression of the endometrium which occurred 2–6 days before the onset of bleeding and which was associated with the decline of ovarian steroid levels. The explant was reduced by between 25% to 75% of its original size. Different explants in the same eye regressed at different rates. Most of the regression arose from the resolution of the stromal edema. During this time, the spiral arterioles became more coiled and stasis of blood was observed until erythrocyte flow was nearly or on occasions completely stopped. Red cells may not move for 60–90 seconds. After regression, the arterioles were seen to constrict for between 4 and 24 hours before bleeding began. This was observed before every episode of bleeding. The arterioles were tightly constricted and red cells were unable to pass the area of constriction.

Menstrual bleeding arose when the vessels dilated after a period of intense vasoconstriction. Several different types of bleeding were noted. Firstly, blood could pass out of a damaged arteriole and form a hematoma which would then rupture into the uterine cavity. Secondly, blood would pass directly from a ruptured arteriole into the uterine cavity. Thirdly, red cells could pass through the walls of capillaries by a process of diapedesis. Finally, blood could pass out of veins, either directly through damaged walls or by reflex drainage following extravasation from arterioles. Markee estimated that 75% of the bleeding arose from the arterioles, and the remainder from the venules. Cessation of bleeding was caused by the return of constriction of the vessel.

It is not known whether bleeding following exogenous steroid withdrawal in women follows this pattern, nor if breakthrough bleeding occurs by similar mechanisms. To date, no satisfactory model has been developed to study the mechanism of breakthrough bleeding.

Tissue loss

The amount of tissue lost at menstruation remains a point of contention. Most authors suggest that the superficial two-thirds of the endometrium is lost at menstruation (Ferenczy, 1976a, 1976b). Others suggest that some areas of the zona spongiosa are retained and assist with the regeneration that occurs at the beginning of the new cycle (McLennan & Rydell, 1965). Flowers and Wilborn (1978) have proposed the controversial view that little tissue is lost at menstruation. The most likely explanation for these divergent views is that endometrial loss varies throughout the uterus, with most tissue being shed from the corpus and fundus and with little loss in other areas of the uterine cavity (Bartelmez, 1937).

Regeneration

Transmission and scanning electron microscopic studies have examined the process of regeneration in the endometrium (Ferenczy, 1976a, 1976b; Ludwig & Metzger, 1976). Regeneration appears to arise from the denuded stumps of the glands in the zona basalis and from in-growing of surface epithelium which has not been shed. This process appears to begin around the second day of bleeding and is well established by the fourth day, indeed to such a degree that most of the surface will be re-epithelialized by that time. Regeneration involves both replication and migration of cells. Recent advances in the field of cellular biology of cellular remodelling have not been applied to the mechanisms of endometrial regeneration.

Regeneration of the vascular system begins with relaxation of the constricted spiral arterioles. Blood re-enters the vessels and new capillary formation arises from these vessels in the middle third of the functional zone. Increased looping of the capillaries and a greater thickening of the bases result in the re-establishment of the capillary network.

Hemostasis

Menstrual blood does not clot (Sixma & Wester, 1977). It appears to coagulate and be rapidly anticoagulated as it passes through the uterus. Reduced amounts of coagulation factors are present in menstrual blood compared to peripheral blood, there being no or very little activatable prothrombin and factor X, low levels of free thrombin and thrombin-generating activity and low antithrombin levels (Rees *et al.*, 1985). Conversely, menstrual blood contains fibrin, fibrin degradation products (Sheppard *et al.*, 1983), inactive α_2-antiplasmin and elevated levels of plasminogen activator and enzymatically active plasmin (Rees *et al.*, 1985).

Lysosomes

The lysosomal theory of menstruation as espoused by Henzl *et al.* (1972) suggests that lysosomal membranes become more 'leaky' during the cycle on withdrawal of progesterone. This results in the release of a large number of enzymes which initiate intracellular digestion (e.g. acid phosphatases), hydrolyse ground substance (β-glucuronidase) and degrade collagen fibres (acid cathepsin D).

Prostaglandins and menstruation

Introduction

The relationship between the ovarian and menstrual cycles has been outlined above, but this does not provide an explanation for the mechanism whereby withdrawal of steroids results in menstrual bleeding.

The identification in the early 1960s of large amounts of prostaglandins (PGs) in menstrual fluid and endometrium raised the prospect of a local agent which could be involved in the mechanism of menstruation. Subsequent investigations linking the capacity of tissue to synthesize PGs to the influence of ovarian steroids further enhanced the possible role of PGs in menstruation.

Menstruation

The effect of steroids on endometrial PG synthesis will be discussed in another chapter, but the evidence that PGs are involved in menstruation will be considered here. Instillation of PGs into the cavity of the uterus of the rhesus monkey reduces endometrial blood flow (Einer-Jensen, 1973). Instillation of PGs into the uterine cavity of women induces a light menstrual bleed (Wiqvist *et al.*, 1971; Toppozada *et al.*, 1980). Administration of analogues of PGs induces bleeding and abortion when given to women in early pregnancy (Karim, 1983). Enhanced synthesis of PGs by endometrium is associated with increased uterine work and dysmenorrhea which is reduced by the administration of cyclo-oxygenase inhibitors. Alteration of the capacity of endometrium to synthesize PGs reduces the volume of menstrual blood loss. The PG levels in menstrual fluid of women on the pill are reduced, as is the blood loss (Chan *et al.*, 1979). Menstrual blood loss (MBL) in women using the IUD is reduced by non-steroidal anti-inflammatory drugs (NSAIDs) (Guillebaud *et al.*, 1978) and women with menorrhagia have a reduction of MBL of about 30% when given NSAIDs (Anderson *et al.*, 1976; Fraser *et al.*, 1981). Further evidence for a role of altered synthesis of PGs in promoting changes in MBL is the observation that endometrium taken from women with heavy periods has an altered capacity to synthesize relatively more vasodilatory PGs than normal endometrium (Smith *et al.*, 1981; Makarainen & Ylikorkala, 1986).

This evidence is only circumstantial, although PG administration to endometrial explants maintained in the immunoprotected site of the hamster cheek pouch did alter capillary tonicity (Abel, 1985). The capacity of tissue to release PGs resides predominantly in the glandular cells and is greatest in the proliferative phase of the cycle (Smith & Kelly, 1988). Progesterone reduces the synthesis and release of PGs by the endometrium (Kelly & Smith, 1987). Withdrawal of progesterone removes this 'block', but progesterone also increases the potential of endometrium to synthesize PGs (Smith *et al.*, 1982). The hypothesis is that the capacity of the tissue to release PGs increases during the cycle, but that it is only with the removal of progesterone that this capacity becomes expressed in the endometrial cells. This would explain the premenstrual pain that many women experience and would provide the link between the steroid withdrawal and the onset of bleeding. Prostaglandin $F_{2\alpha}$ induces vasoconstriction and could be the local factor which initiates vasospasm in response to progesterone withdrawal. Once the tissue destruction has begun, large amounts of PGs might be expected to be released in response to the trauma of menstruation.

Endogenous steroids do alter the capacity of endometrium to synthesize PGs, both when the agents are being given and when menstrual bleeding arises from the withdrawal of the drug (Chan *et al.*, 1979). This hypothesis is consistent with the observations of the effects of progesterone on PG synthesis but would not explain menstrual bleeding in response to estrogen withdrawal. Thus far, the speculative role for PGs in menstruation has concentrated on potential vascular and anticoagulatory properties of PGs, but this is almost certainly too naive a view.

Growth factors and endometrial function

Inhibition of PG synthesis in the rabbit is associated with abolition of proliferation of endometrial growth (Orlicky *et al.*, 1987). The poor response of endometrial tissue to grow *in vitro* in the presence of estradiol raised the prospect of other growth factors which might be important in the proliferation and differentiation of endometrial growth. Human glandular and stromal cells have receptors for epidermal growth factor (EGF) (Lin *et al.*, 1988), estradiol mediates the expression of the message for the receptor (Lingham *et al.*, 1988) and glandular cells synthesize the pre-pro message for EGF (DiAugustine *et al.*, 1988). Recently, EGF has been shown to stimulate growth of the glandular endometrial cells of human proliferative and secretory endometrium, but only in the presence of estradiol (Haining *et al.*, 1988). Surprisingly, EGF does not promote the growth of stromal cells despite these cells expressing the receptor for this growth factor. The role of growth factors in regulating re-epithelialization and mediating the effects of exogenous and endogenous steroids on endometrial growth are not known. Human endometrium does express the message for transforming growth factor β (TGFβ) and can secrete tumour necrosis factor α (TNFα) into culture media (Smith, unpublished observation). The observation that EGF stimulates prostaglandin E_2 (PGE$_2$) synthesis in human amnion (Casey *et al.*, 1988) raises the prospect of important interactions in the endometrium between growth factors, PGs, steroids and endometrial function which could have important consequences for the mechanism of menstruation.

Conclusion

The mechanism of menstruation remains one of the great conundrums of reproductive physiology, yet disorders of menstruation are an important cause of ill-health in women and are a significant factor in reducing the acceptability of steroid contraception. Recent advances in molecular biology may lead to a greater understanding of endometrial function which lies at the base of this problem. It is likely that a concerted and combined approach from several specialties will eventually yield the knowledge to deal with this problem effectively.

References

Abel, M.H. (1985). Prostanoids and menstruation. (In) *Mechanism of Menstrual Bleeding* (Baird, D.T. & Michie, E.A., eds.), pp. 139–156. New York, Raven Press.

Anderson, A.B.M., Haynes, P.J., Guillebaud, J. & Turnbull, A.C. (1976). Reduction of menstrual blood-loss by prostaglandin-synthetase inhibitors. *Lancet*, i:774–776.

Andrade, A.T.L., Souza, J.P., Rowe, P.J. & Shaw, S.T. (1979). Effect of prior pregnancy and combined oral contraceptives on baseline menstrual blood loss and bleeding response to intrauterine devices. *Contraception*, **20**:19–27.

Bartelmez, G.W. (1937). Menstruation. *Physiological Review*, **17**:28–72.

Bell, S.C. (1985). Comparative aspects of decidualization in rodents and human cell types, secreted products and associated function. (In) *Implantation of the Human Embryo* (Edwards, R.G., Purdy, J.M. & Steptoe, P.C., eds.), pp.71–121. London, Academic Press.

Bulmer, J.N., Hagin, S.V., Browne, C.M. & Billington, W.D. (1986). Localization of immunoglobulin-containing cells in human endometrium in the first trimester of pregnancy and throughout the menstrual cycle. *European Journal of Obstetrics, Gynecology and Reproductive Biology*, **23**:31–44.

Bulmer, J.N. & Ritson, A. (1988). The decidua in early pregnancy. (In) *Early Pregnancy Loss Mechanisms and Treatment* (Beard, R.W. & Sharp, F., eds.) pp. 171–180. London, Royal College of Obstetricians and Gynaecologists.

Casey, M.L., Korte, K. & MacDonald, P.C. (1988). Epidermal growth factor stimulation of prostaglandin E_2 biosynthesis in amnion cells. Induction of prostaglandin H_2 synthase. *Journal of Biological Chemistry*, **263**:7846–7854.

Chan, W.Y., Dawood, M.Y. & Fuchs, F. (1979). Relief of dysmenorrhoea with the prostaglandin synthetase inhibitor ibuprofen: effect on prostaglandin levels in menstrual fluid. *American Journal of Obstetrics and Gynecology*, **135**:102–108.

DiAugustine, R.P., Petrusz, P., Bell, G.I., Brown, C.F., Korach, K.S., McLachlan, J.A. & Teng, C.T. (1988). Influence of estrogens on mouse uterine epidermal growth factor precursor protein and messenger ribonucleic acid. *Endocrinology*, **122**:2355–2363.

Einer-Jensen, N. (1973). Decreased endometrial blood flow and plasma progesterone level after instillation of 10 μg prostaglandin $F_{2\alpha}$ into the lumen of the uteri of rhesus monkeys. *Prostaglandins*, **4**:517–522.

Ferenczy, A. (1976a). Studies on the cytodynamics of human endometrial regeneration. I. Scanning electron microscopy. *American Journal of Obstetrics and Gynecology*, **124**:64–74.

Ferenczy, A. (1976b). Studies on the cytodynamics of human endometrial regeneration. II. Transmission electron microscopy and histochemistry. *American Journal of Obstetrics and Gynecology*, **124**:582–595.

Finn, C.A. (1977). The implantation reaction. (In) *Biology of the Uterus* (Wynn, R.M., ed.), pp.245–308. New York, Plenum Press.

Flowers, C.E. & Wilborn, W.H. (1978). New observations on the physiology of menstruation. *Obstetrics and Gynaecology*, **51**:16–24.

Fraser, I.S. (1983). A survey of different approaches to management of menstrual disturbances in women using injectable contraceptives. *Contraception*, **28**:385–397.

Fraser, I.S., Pearse, C., Shearman, R.P., Elliott, P.M., McIlveen, J. & Markham, R. (1981). Efficacy of mefenamic acid in patients with a complaint of menorrhagia. *Obstetrics and Gynaecology*, **58**:543–551.

Guillebaud, J., Anderson, A.B.M. & Turnbull, A.C. (1978). Reduction by mefenamic acid of increased menstrual blood loss associated with intra-uterine contraception. *British Journal of Obstetrics and Gynaecology*, **85**:53–62.

Haining, R.W., Frazer, H.M. & Smith, S.K. (1988). Effect of epidermal growth factor (EGF) on proliferation of separated cells of human endometrium. *Journal of Reproduction and Fertility*, Abstract No. 56.

Henzl, M.R., Smith, R.E., Boost, G. & Tyler, E.T. (1972). Lysosomal concept of menstrual bleeding in humans. *Journal of Clinical Endocrinology and Metabolism*, **34**:860–875.

Johannisson, E., Landgren, B.M. & Diczfalusy, E. (1982). Endometrial morphology and peripheral steroid levels in women with and without intermenstrual bleeding during contraception with the 300 μg norethisterone (NET) minipill. *Contraception*, **25**:13–30.

Kamat, B.R. & Isaacson, P.G. (1987). The immunocytochemical distribution of leukocytic sub-populations in human endometrium. *American Journal of Pathology*, **127**:66–73.

Karim, S.M.M. (1983). Clinical applications of prostaglandins in obstetrics and gynaecology. (In) *Cervagem: A New Prostaglandin in Obstetrics and Gynaecology* (Karim, S.M.M., ed.), pp.15–34. Lancaster, England, MTP Press.

Kelly, R.W. & Smith, S.K. (1987). Progesterone and anti-progestins, a comparison of their effect on prostaglandin production by human secretory phase endometrium and decidua. *Prostaglandins, Leukotrienes and Medicine*, **29**:181–186.

Landgren, B.M. & Diczfalusy, E. (1980). Hormonal effects of the 300 μg norethisterone (NET) minipill. I. Daily steroid levels in 43 subjects during a pretreatment cycle and during the second month of NET administration. *Contraception*, 21:87–113.

Lin, T.H., Mukku, V.R., Verner, G., Kirkland, J.L. & Stancel, G.M. (1988). Autoradiographic localization of epidermal growth factor receptors to all major uterine cell types. *Biology of Reproduction*, 38:403–411.

Lingham, R.B., Stancel, G.M., Loose-Mitchell, D.S. (1988). Estrogen regulation of epidermal growth factor receptor messenger ribonucleic acid. *Molecular Endocrinology*, 2:230–235.

Ludwig, H. & Metzger, H. (1976). The re-epithelialization of endometrium after menstrual desquamation. *Archiv für Gynaekologie*, 221:51–60.

Makarainen, L. & Ylikorkala, 0. (1986). Primary and myoma-associated menorrhagia: role of prostaglandins and effects of ibuprofen. *British Journal of Obstetrics and Gynaecology*, 93:974–978.

Markee, J.E. (1940). Menstruation in intraocular endometrial transplants in the rhesus monkey. *Contributions to Embryology*. Carnegie Institution of Washington Publication No. 518, 28(No. 177):219–308.

Markoff, E., Zeitler, P., Peleg, S. & Handwerger, S. (1983). Characterization of the synthesis and release of prolactin by an enriched fraction of human decidual cells. *Journal of Clinical Endocrinology and Metabolism*, 56:962–968.

McLennan, C.E. & Rydell, A.H. (1965). Extent of endometrial shedding during normal menstruation. *Obstetrics and Gynaecology*, 26:605–621.

Noyes, R.W., Hertig, A.T. & Rock, J. (1950). Dating the endometrial biopsy. *Fertility and Sterility*, 1:3–25.

Orlicky, D.J., Lieberman, R., Williams, C. & Gerschenson, L.E. (1987). Requirement for prostaglandin $F_{2\alpha}$ in 17β-estradiol stimulation of DNA synthesis in rabbit endometrial cultures. *Journal of Cell Physiology*, 130:292–300.

Rees, M.C.P., Cederholm-Williams, S.A. & Turnbull, A.C. (1985). Coagulation factors and fibrinolytic proteins in menstrual fluid collected from normal and menorrhagic women. *British Journal of Obstetrics and Gynaecology*, 92:1164–1168.

Sheppard,B.L., Docheray, C.J. & Bonnar, J. (1983). An ultrastructural study of menstrual blood in normal menstruation and dysfunctional uterine bleeding. *British Journal of Obstetrics and Gynaecology*, 90:259–265.

Siegfried, J.M., Nelson, K.G., Martin, J.L. & Kaufman, D.G. (1984). Histochemical identification of cultured cells from human endometrium. *In Vitro*, 20:25–32.

Sixma, J.J. & Wester, J. (1977). The hemostatic plug. *Seminars in Hematology*, 14:265–299.

Smith, S.K., Abel, M.H., Kelly, R.W. & Baird, D.T. (1981). Prostaglandin synthesis in the endometrium of women with ovular dysfunctional uterine bleeding. *British Journal of Obstetrics and Gynaecology*, 88:434–442.

Smith, S.K., Abel, M.H., Kelly, R.W.. & Baird, D.T. (1982). The synthesis of prostaglandins from persistent proliferative endometrium. *Journal of Clinical Endocrinology and Metabolism*, 55:284–289.

Smith, S.K. & Kelly, R.W. (1988). The release of $PGF_{2\alpha}$ and PGE_2 from separated cells of human endometrium and decidua. *Prostaglandins, Leukotrienes and Essential Fatty Acids*, 33:91–96.

Smith, S.K., Kirkman, R.J.E., Arce, B.B., McNeilly, A.S., Loudon, N.B. & Baird,

D.T. (1986). The effect of deliberate omission of Trinordiol or Microgynon on the hypothalamo–pituitary–ovarian axis. *Contraception*, **34**:513–522.

Snow, L.F. & Johnson, S.M. (1977). Modern day menstrual folklore. Some clinical implications. *Journal of the American Medical Association*, **237**:2736–2739.

Tietze, C. & Lewit, S. (1970). Evaluation of intrauterine devices; 9th progress report of the cooperative statistical program. *Studies in Family Planning*, **55**:1–40.

Toppozada, M., El-Attar, A., El-Ayyat, M.A. & Khamis, Y. (1980). Management of uterine bleeding by PGs or their synthesis inhibitors. *Advances in Prostaglandin and Thromboxane Research*, **8**:1459–1463.

Van der Vange, N. (1988). Ovarian activity during low dose oral contraceptives. (In) *Contemporary Obstetrics and Gynaecology* (Chamberlain, G., ed.), pp.315–326. London, Butterworths.

Wiqvist, N., Bygdeman, M., & Kirton, K. (1971). Non-steroidal antifertility agents in the female. (In) *Nobel Symposium 15: Control of Human Fertility* (Diczfalusy, E. & Borell, B. eds.). **1**:137–149.

Wynn, R.M. (1977). Histology and ultrastructure of the human endometrium. (In) *Biology of the Uterus* (Wynn, R.M., ed.), pp.341–376. New York, Plenum Press.

Discussion

Sheppard. I agree with you on the patient's perception of menstruation. In a study that we are carrying out at the moment in three Dublin gynecology clinics we find that approximately 60% of patients referred for excessive menstrual bleeding in fact have a menstrual loss of less than 80 ml per cycle. With your experience in the prostaglandin area would you consider that leukotrienes have a role to play in the physiological process of menstruation?

Smith. If you look at mammary epithelial cells, the proliferation of those tissues is dependent upon an interplay between prostaglandins and leukotrienes, so there is a link between both pathways of eicosanoid synthesis and proliferation, which I think is probably quite relevant. So, yes, I think leukotrienes are important.

Rees. The highest levels of leukotrienes are found during menstruation itself, and that might correlate with the influx of leukocytes at that stage. They are elevated mainly in dysmenorrhea, and there does not seem to be any clear elevation in menorrhagia. So leukotrienes are more involved with pain rather than with bleeding. Another point: we have been looking at EGF receptors and I know that in the rat they are found in all cells. In fact, there were some studies in a limited number of human specimens, where they also were found in all uterine cells using autoradiography. We have been using immunohistochemistry with G15, which is one of the antibodies made by Dr A.R. Rees in Oxford, and we can find receptors mainly in the glands rather than in the stroma. So that would fit in with your findings.

Fraser. We know that menstruation is an event which only occurs in primates, in the human and some subhuman primates, but there has been some work done over the years on animal models. I have been interested in some of the work of Colin Finn and his group in Liverpool (Finn & Pope, 1984), where they have managed to produce a model which has some resemblance to menstruation by manipulating the endocrinology. They have treated mice with estradiol and progesterone, in order to produce decidualization of the endometrium, which does not normally occur in animals that do not menstruate before the end of the cycle. They have also seen a very large influx of migratory white cells. They seem to feel that decidualization and the influx of various white cell types may well be important in this event of menstruation which does seem to be entirely related to primates. I would also like to make the comment that many other animal species do achieve a considerable amount of remodelling of the endometrium at the end of the ovarian cycle without menstruation and I still find it very difficult to understand why the Good Lord should have produced this process of endometrial breakdown and bleeding in primates, when the same sort of thing can be achieved in subprimates without the inconvenience of bleeding.

Smith. To come back to the white cell infiltration, I think this is again another area where the interplay of cytokines and reproductive function is something which we have alluded to and is now an important area because of the availability of recombinant cytokines and also methods of assessing their production. Perhaps we are only just beginning on that era of studies of the role of cytokines in reproductive function, which in the mouse, in both the pregnant and non-pregnant cycles, seems to be an important feature of endometrial function. So, I would strongly agree that the lymphokines are important.

Johannisson. I would just like to make a comment on your finding *in vitro* that there was a difference in growth activity between glands and stroma. When you are looking at mitoses, you will find almost the same thing: there is a difference in the frequency of mitoses in the glands and in the stroma.

Bischof. I would like to suggest a new candidate for the study of the initiation of menstruation. As you know, cells are embedded in an extracellular matrix, which influences the functioning and the shape of these cells. As it has been reported recently that the endometrium is capable of producing heparin sulphate, I wonder if heparin sulphate could be a candidate, because as you probably know, these glycosaminoglycans are polysulphated molecules. They have a great capacity for absorbing water, which means that in the matrix one of the first things which will happen is edema. Now, Markee (1940) has shown that one of the first signs in the initiation of menstruation is a decrease in edema in the 4 or 5 days before menstruation. And I wonder if, in fact, regulation is not achieved by glycosaminoglycans.

Smith. Yes, the observations of Markee on the regression are fairly well substantiated and certainly any change in the extracellular matrix might make a difference. As you know, there are studies already looking at factors like laminin, showing that there is a difference between the stroma and the glands which might be important in terms of the eventual decidualization of the tissue. On the other hand, my own feeling is that we should always view menstruation in terms of a post event, i.e. that the physiology of the endometrium is essentially to allow for implantation. One of the difficulties with laminin is that there is a relationship with progesterone, but it is not consistent with the continued secretion of progesterone in early pregnancy. So I would agree that in general terms the extracellular matrix almost certainly is an important part of the eventual breakdown of the endometrium that occurs. But I think it is unlikely to be an initiating event in menstruation. It might be part of the control and subsequent remodelling that occurs once the bleeding has started.

Rees. I think that menstruation does seem to be limited to a certain number of species that have coiled spiral arterioles in their endometrium. I tried to mimic a hormonal menstruum in sheep, which have a different anatomy in their endometrium, and I did this by castrating the sheep and then using a series of implants. And I never ever managed to induce them to bleed when the progesterone was withdrawn.

Cornillie. I would like to add another candidate: hyaluronic acid, which is also in the matrix. But I have two questions for Dr Smith. In your culture system, are these crude populations of cells or are you working with really 100% epithelial and 100% stromal cells? Did you separate the glands, and are there still some stromal cells sticking to the basement membrane region of the glands and are these cells proliferating? I have some experience in the culture of endometrium and what happens when I do cultures of epithelial cells starting with proliferative phase endometrium is that I usually end up with a secretory endometrium. So, my second question is: are the proliferative endometria which you are putting in cultures still in a proliferative phase, or do they differentiate into secretory cells?

Smith. In answer to your first question: no. These are enriched preparations, if you like. So, there is some contamination between the two and on average I would say that the contamination is something in the order of about 20%. It is very difficult to get specific cells to grow. However, coming back to your point about the interplay between mesenchyme and epithelium, we have also done studies in which we have used conditioned medium of stromal tissue, which is shown to have no effect on the proliferation of the epithelial cells. So, I cannot accept that the cells which are growing in our glandular preparation are stromal cells. Anyway, they would have grown in the stromal culture, so that when we use conditioned medium, there does not appear, unlike other systems, to be an increase in growth of the glandular cells over and above that of the contaminated stromal cells. So I think that these probably do reflect the glandular cells closely.

The second point was whether the proliferative cells become secretory. What system did you use to describe that? Do you mean histological changes in the monolayers? How do you know they have become secretory cells?

Cornillie. Well, I used a system of organ culture. But if I put proliferative endometrium in culture using 10% and 5% serum, even within 24 hours this proliferative endometrium differentiates histologically into tissue which looks like secretory endometrium.

King. Could I also inject two notes of caution over interpretation of these culture data. Firstly, the effects you are seeing are minute. You are seeing a fraction of one cell division difference, and at that level I think interpretation is very difficult. And, secondly, it is well known from the literature (Kirk & Irwin, 1980), that when using these preparations, the first thing you start seeing from this is a process of polyploidization. And this can be influenced by hormones. You can get a lot of changes occurring biochemically in these systems that have got nothing to do with the components you are adding, but are simply a reflection of the cells going diploid, tetraploid, polyploid.

Smith. Could I ask you on that, if there was any difference in the cell growth, would that not be a random event throughout all the different treatment preparations?

King. Yes, but if I interpret it correctly, I think you are getting about a quarter of a division difference. With that minute difference I think caution is the word.

Ludwig. I would like to comment on two items. Firstly, the topographical view. We always examine hysterectomy specimens which are dated according to the cycle. We were interested to find out whether there was any chronological order in shedding; for instance, is the most fundal endometrium shedded first and the isthmic endometrium second? What we saw is that there is no time sequence and the premenstrual changes are distributed over the whole endometrium. Secondly, you discussed the remodelling of the endometrium after menstrual desquamation. We confirmed that around 90% of remodelling of the lining surface epithelium is coming from the glandular stumps. But there are islands of lining epithelial cells which take part in the remodelling of the endometrium. These islands can be detected between the second and the sixth day of the cycle. They have fewer ciliated cells, they show cilioneogenesis in a more immature phase than the glandular epithelium. So now we are investigating the true relation between regeneration coming from the glands and that from the remaining islands of lining epithelial cells.

Healy. My comment concerns our endeavours in Melbourne to look at what we have called a receptive endometrium based on a series of clinical approaches to people on our in-vitro fertilization programme who had no ovaries. In that programme it would seem that a receptive endometrium, as defined by scanning electronmicroscopy (EM), is one in which the so-called ciliated cells of the endometrium have very short microvilli and have a bulging appearance to the apices of the cells. Initially we could reproduce that process by trying to reconstruct artificial cycles in these women. But it is now clear, both on the scanning EM work as well as in clinical results with oocyte donation, that repetition of the menstrual cycle is quite unnecessary. By giving a constant low dose of estradiol, for example for a period of about 3 weeks followed by 2 days of vaginal progesterone, it is quite possible to support an early pregnancy and also to reproduce the scanning EM changes. My question is whether in the 40 years since Markee, there have been any scanning EM studies of the non-human primate endometrium at the time of the implantation, and what are its appearances?

Naftolin. In the rat, Dr Szego has now mounted a series of incontrovertible studies on the rapid effects of estrogen on the endometrial cell, and shows changes in microvilli within 30 seconds of administration of systemically physiologic levels of estradiol (Szego *et al.*, 1988). These are accompanied by changes in microtubules that are the reverse, and as she has shown therefore, and I think in a way it is very cleverly linked, changes in the cytoskeleton that make endometrial cells in the rat make these microtubules.

Gurpide. In studying endometrial cancer cells, we found that carbachol or acetylcholine has an effect on phosphoinositol (PI) in the production of inositol phosphates (Weiss & Gurpide, 1988), and we are also finding that it has an effect on mucin production (unpublished observations). And I have read that there is some histological evidence that there could be cholinergic innervation. Could that have any relevance?

Smith. Yes, I read your paper and acknowledge it. Yes, Bonney and Franks (1987) had shown before that phospholipase C (PLC) activity in the endometrium appears to be very profound, and certainly in the sheep, Flint *et al.* have shown that oxytocin stimulates PI hydrolysis (Flint *et al.*, 1986), so we have spent many years looking at phospholipase A2 activity, and clearly PLC activity might be just as important. There is now evidence in the rat for adrenoreceptors in the endometrium, and that raises the prospect of a whole extra batch of potential local paracrine effectors of endometrial function, either in terms of proliferation or in terms of secretion, which again would be closely in touch with ideas on PI hydrolysis and its possible roles. I think the problem with that at the moment is trying to distinguish the differences in the second message as to how different stimuli can produce different second messages. The work in that area is relatively new and hopefully one will be able to distinguish or discriminate between different intercellular responses to agents like carbachol in endometrial function, although I think it is still at the stage where cell lines are required to make those observations. I am not so sure that we will at this stage be able to apply those directly to primary cultures of endometrium. Transformed cell lines are important in the initial understanding of the mechanisms, but might not be, in a similarly critical way, similar to primary cultures nor to the situation *in vivo*.

Brosens. You have discussed the work of Markee and discussed the vasoconstriction at the base of the spiral arteries at the level of the endometrial/myometrial junction. Is there any evidence that this mechanism is controlled by hormones? Because, after all, it is in the non-hormonal responsive layer of the endometrium, and you have shown that bleeding may occur even before the fall of the steroids.

Smith. As with most things in menstruation, it is not direct evidence. I hope to show that if you withdraw steroids there is an increased capacity of endometrium to synthesize prostaglandins. So at least potentially, a steroid withdrawal mechanism does exist. There is some work that David Baird looked at, in endometrial explants in the hamster cheek pouch (Abel *et al.*, 1982) showing an effect of prostaglandins on microvasculature and I think Mats Åkerlund has also done work looking at endometrial blood flow in which, certainly, changes in prostaglandin amounts and other agents can affect the blood supply of the endometrium (Åkerlund, 1980, 1990). So even that is not a direct steroid effect; I think that the second message is certainly present. However, there is also work, in the sheep, in which estrogen was shown to increase blood flow. So there is evidence that steroids do alter blood flow; whether they affect spiral arterial contractility, I do not think there is evidence on that.

Rice-Evans. I would like to come back to the damage at the capillary endothelial cell level and talk about what happens when prolonged vasoconstriction followed by vasodilatation occurs. Oxygen radicals are generated from a variety of sources including activated leukocytes, and superoxide radicals that can be generated from the capillary endothelial cells. Superoxide is dismutated to hydrogen peroxide, which can interact with diapedesed red cells. The consequences of this and other factors are the generation of highly toxic hydroxyl radicals, which then start to damage the endothelial cells. What we have not addressed are the effects of the activated leukocytes and macrophages.

Clark. Is it possible for hormonally dependent cells to die if we remove the hormone? Hormone-induced cellular hypertrophy will regress if the agonist is removed. If blood vessels must constrict in order to kill hormone-dependent endometrial cells, or some other factor released following ischemia is required, then clearly what you are proposing is appropriate. On the other hand, perhaps hormonally dependent cells might not survive if we remove their hormonal support. Could we address that issue?

King. Most cells do not require estrogens or progestogens for viability. Steroids are required for alteration or modulation of various functions. On the other hand, all cells certainly require oxygen and nutrients. If you remove blood supply, the cells will die. But if the question is whether removal of a direct effect of steroids on the cells is cytotoxic, the answer is no.

Rice-Evans. It depends where your cells are and the time period and extent of the vasoconstriction.

Casey. And, related to that is the generation of superoxide radicals, the generation of tumour necrosis factor-α, and other potentially cytotoxic factors.

References

Abel, M.H., Zhu, C. & Baird, D.T. (1982). An animal model to study menstrual bleeding. *Research and Clinical Forums*, **4**(4):25–34.

Åkerlund, M. (1980). Non-prostaglandin factors influencing the microcirculation of the endometrium. (In) *Endometrial Bleeding and Steroidal Contraception* (Diczfalusy, E., Fraser, I.S. & Webb, F.T.G., eds.), pp.246–265. Bath, England, Pitman Press.

Åkerlund, M. (1990). Function of endometrial blood vessels. (In) *Contraception and Mechanisms of Endometrial Bleeding* (d'Arcangues, C., Fraser, I.S., Newton, J. & Odlind, V., eds), pp.81–89. Cambridge, England, Cambridge University Press.

Bonney, R.C. & Franks, S. (1987). Phospholipase C activity in human endometrium: its significance in endometrial pathology. *Clinical Endocrinology*, **27**:307–320.

Finn, C.A. & Pope, M. (1984). Vascular and cellular changes in the decidualized endometrium of the ovariectomized mouse following cessation of hormone treatment: a possible model for menstruation. *Journal of Endocrinology*, **100**:295–300.

Flint, A.P., Leat, W.M., Sheldrick, E.L. & Stewart, H.J. (1986). Stimulation of phosphoinositide hydrolysis by oxytocin and the mechanism by which oxytocin controls prostaglandin synthesis in the ovine endometrium. *Biochemical Journal*, **237**:797–805.

Kirk, D. & Irwin, J.C. (1980). Normal human endometrium in cell culture. *Methods in Cell Biology*, **21B**:51–77.

Markee, J.E. (1940). Menstruation in intraocular endometrial transplants in the rhesus monkey. *Contribution to Embryology*. Carnegie Institution of Washington Publication No. 518, **28**(No. 177):219–308.

Szego, C.M., Sjöstrand, B.M., Seeler, B.J., Baumer, J.W., Sjöstrand, F.S. (1988). Microtubule plasmalemmal reorganization: acute response to estrogen. *American Journal of Physiology*, **254**:E775–E785.

Weiss, D.J. & Gurpide, E. (1988). Regulation of phosphoinositide hydrolysis in transformed human endometrial cells. *Endocrinology*, **123**:981–990.

Endometrial morphology during the normal cycle and under the influence of contraceptive steroids

ELISABETH JOHANNISSON

Clinic of Sterility and Gynecologic Endocrinology, Department of Obstetrics and Gynecology, University Hospital, Genève, Switzerland.

Abstract

The morphological changes of the human endometrium during the normal cycle and following the use of contraceptive steroids are reviewed, in particular with regard to the vascularization and to other structures which may predispose to intermenstrual bleeding.

With regard to the changes during the normal menstrual cycle, new evidence has shown that biopsies timed in relation to the LH surge give a more accurate basis for histologic dating than if timed in relation to the date of onset of the menstrual bleeding at the beginning and at the end of the cycle. The cellular events in the glandular epithelium during the first 6 days after ovulation seem to be precisely regulated with small interindividual variation, as shown by light-microscopic and electron-microscopic studies. The morphometric assessment of the changes occurring in the glands and stroma also offers possibilities to quantitate the histologic events and to assess the effect of various contraceptive steroids on the endometrium in quantitative terms using statistical methods. The administration of progestogens as contraceptives is followed by significant changes in the surface lining epithelium, the glands and the stroma, depending upon dosage and duration of exposure.

The spiral arteries and the subepithelial capillary plexus have been reported to undergo hormone-regulated changes during the normal menstrual cycle. Recent studies have revealed the presence of estrogen and progesterone receptors in the muscle cells of the uterine arteries. The synthesis of Factor VIII in the endometrial endothelial cells may also be hormone regulated. Like other components of the endometrium, the endometrial vessels are influenced by the administration of contraceptive steroids. A significant increase in the number of dilated venules as well as an increase in proliferative activity of the endothelial cells have been reported. Submicroscopic structures of the endometrial capillary endothelial cells such as plasmalemmal vesicles and cytoplasmic contraction have been described to be significantly increased following the use of norethisterone (300 μg daily by oral administration). It is likely that these endothelial cell patterns are connected to specific functions of the surrounding tissue (e.g. the local blood–interstitial fluid exchanges). Further studies of the structure and function of the endometrial vessels may contribute to a better understanding of the endometrial bleeding mechanism.

Introduction

Irregular bleeding and amenorrhea are phenomena frequently described in relation to the use of long-acting contraceptive steroids, in particular those containing a progestogen as the active contraceptive substance. Irregular bleeding occurs irrespective of the mode of administration; it has been described with the use of minipills (Fotherby, 1977), of injectable long-acting formulations (Gray, 1980), of implants (Segal, 1982) or when the progestogen has been released from an intrauterine (Aznar & Giner, 1984; Luukkainen *et al.*, 1984), intracervical (Lähteenmäki *et al.*, 1984) or a vaginal delivery system (Diczfalusy & Landgren, 1981). The balance of evidence indicates that the contraceptive steroids induce characteristic changes in the infrastructure of the human endometrium and that these changes may represent a potential predisposing factor for intermenstrual bleeding and spotting. To better evaluate these changes, it may be important to review the morphological findings during the normal menstrual cycle and compare these with the morphological changes following the use of steroidal contraceptives.

This is not an easy task. A plethora of data has been accumulated during the last 30 years and it is impossible to give credit to all studies published during this period on this topic in the present review. However, it may be useful to review some of the most recent data in the field, in particular with regard to the changes occurring in the endometrial vascularization, the glands, the stroma and the epithelium lining the uterine cavity before and during the use of contraceptive steroids.

There are several ways to describe the morphology of the human endometrium. One of the ways is to describe the histology of the basal layer and then compare the findings with those observed in the functional layer. This may be the classical way to deal with the subject. Another approach would be to deal with the individual components of the endometrium such as the lining epithelium, the glands, the stroma and the vessels and to describe the morphological changes observed in each component before and after the use of various contraceptive steroids. A number of recent studies have reported on specific properties of endometrial glands and stroma. Morphometric measurements of biopsy specimens also open new avenues to deal with the specific endometrial structures as separate components. Although the whole endometrium as such must be considered as a target organ for endogenous and exogenous steroids where the structural components are likely to interact closely with each other, it is felt that the present review of the endometrial morphology might yield some new information if each structural component could be dealt with under a separate heading. Four endometrial components will therefore be described: the lining surface epithelium, the endometrial glands, the stroma, and the vasculature.

Lining surface epithelium

The endometrial surface epithelium has been considered to have its own special role to play in most mammals. In general, it has been considered to be involved in the attachment of a blastocyst to the wall of the endometrium.

Light microscopic (Hamperl, 1950) and transmission electron microscopic studies (Borell *et al.*, 1959) of the human endometrium have revealed that cyclic changes occur in the lining epithelium during the normal menstrual cycle and that some epithelial cells are ciliated. More recent studies using a scanning electron microscope confirmed the previous findings of cyclic changes occurring in the ciliated as well as in the non-ciliated cells of the lining epithelium (Johannisson & Nilsson, 1972; Ludwig & Metzger, 1976). The cilia were reported to be well developed in the preovulatory phase, whereas clods were formed from the cilia and the microvilli of the cell surfaces during the postovulatory phase. The function of ciliated cells is not clearly understood. They are unevenly distributed in the surface epithelium. A scanty number of ciliated cells are found in the tubal corners whereas ciliated cells are scattered all over the epithelial surface of the fundus area with a concentration around the gland openings. The number of ciliated cells increases towards the endocervix.

The distribution of ciliated cells seems, however, to support the theory that cilia are involved in the transport of endometrial secretory products. Changes similar to those described in the lining epithelium of the human endometrium have been reported to occur in baboons (Wilborn *et al.*, 1984). In these non-human primates, comparative scanning and transmission electron microscopic studies revealed cyclic changes not only in the ciliated cells but also in the cellular cytoplasm, indicating formation of secretory granules during the preovulatory phase and release of secretory products in the postovulatory phase. Secretory activity has also been demonstrated in the human surface epithelial cells, e.g. acid mucus glycoproteins (Hester *et al.*, 1968). The type and amount of endometrial surface glycoproteins seem to be dependent on the circulating steroid levels. It is likely that acid mucus glycoproteins participate in the formation of the glycocalyx of the surface epithelial cells. Membrane glycoproteins are rich in the amino acids threonine and serine, the hydroxyl groups of which carry oligosaccharide side-chains similar to those of the mucus glycoproteins. Cyclic changes take place in the composition of the glycocalyx of the lining epithelium with an increase in the postovulatory phase (Thor *et al.*, 1987) or, more precisely, the increase suddenly appears on day LH + 3 of the normal menstrual cycle (Jansen *et al.*, 1985). Permeability factors of the surface lining epithelium, with a possible passage of substances between the endometrial vessels and the uterine lumen, are likely to exist (Luukkainen *et al.*, 1984), but such factors have not been sufficiently studied during the normal menstrual cycle.

The fact that changes in the surface lining epithelium are mediated by ovarian hormones suggests that exogenous steroids may interfere with the physiologic events during the normal menstrual cycle. In particular, the ciliated cells seem to be a sensitive indicator reflecting even minor changes in the hormonal environment. Defects in the ciliogenesis have been reported already after 2 months use of 0.35 mg norethisterone daily (Ludwig, 1982). A decreased number of ciliated cells was also found in the endometrium of women having been exposed to long-term administration of oral progestogens.

Furthermore, some short-term high-dose treatments (e.g. gestonorone caproate 200 mg weekly for 1 month) were reported to produce a significant degeneration and 'holes' in the lining epithelium (Ludwig, 1982). Similar changes were reported by Wilborn et al. (1984) in baboons. Long-term administration of norethisterone (NET) in a dose of 50 mg daily or medroxyprogesterone acetate (37.5 mg and 100 mg injections) resulted in degeneration of the surface epithelial cells of the endometrium, epithelial denudation with exposure to the stroma, detached epithelial cells and breakthrough bleeding. The changes observed in the lining epithelium by Wilborn et al. (1984) could be related to specific properties of the progestogen compound used. Norethisterone seemed to cause detachment of the lining epithelium whereas norgestimate given intramuscularly in dosages of 25 mg and 50 mg for 3–6 months did not seem to produce significant degenerative changes of the surface epithelium. The authors did not find any 'gross or microscopic evidence of bleeding with norgestimate'. The combined estrogen–progestogen contraceptives have been reported to modify the structure of the lining epithelium in a way similar to that of the progestogen-only preparations. A decrease in the number of ciliated cells has been found by some (Fedele et al., 1987), whereas studies by Rabe et al. (1986) in women using norgestimate combined with 0.35 mg ethinyl estradiol for 6 months showed a well-preserved lining epithelium corresponding to midcycle or early secretory phase of the normal menstrual cycle.

The endometrial glands

During the normal menstrual cycle characteristic changes occur in the endometrial glands. The changes of the basal layer of the endometrium differ from those of the functional layer but the present review will be limited to the description of the functional layer since this part of the endometrium is most frequently represented in the biopsies. The morphological changes occurring in the endometrial glands are easy to identify and can be assessed quantitatively by morphometric methods. The number of glands per mm^2 is approximately 20 and the number does not vary significantly during the cycle (Johannisson et al., 1987) (Fig. 1). The number of glandular mitoses varies greatly during the proliferative phase, showing a significant decrease between days LH-3/-2 and LH-1/0(p $\langle$0.05). During the period preceding LH-3/-2 the glandular epithelial cells are characterized by a rapid growth and from day LH-11 through LH + 6 the epithelial cell height increases from 20.9 μm to 24.2 μm (geometric mean 22.5 μm). The size of the glands does not keep pace with this growth and the tall columnar epithelial cells finally pile up against each other with their nuclei at different levels giving rise to pseudostratification. The glandular lumen remains fairly constant (below 50 μm) throughout the

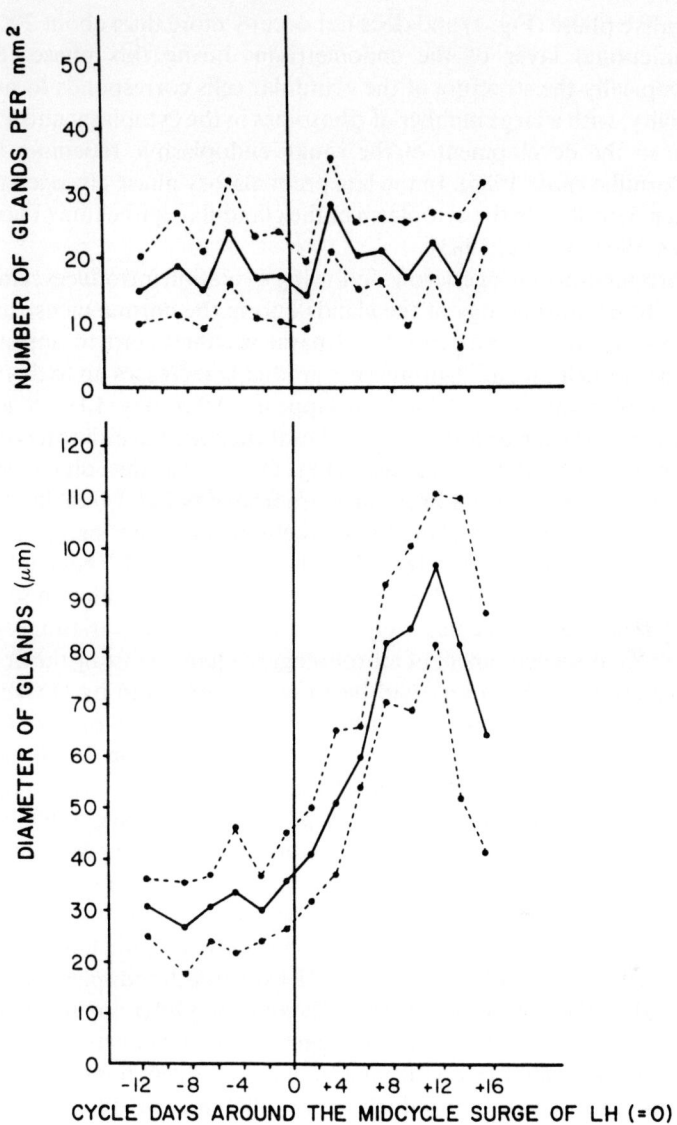

Fig. 1 Number of glands per mm² and diameter of glands expressed in μm in 90 women. Mean values of 48-hour periods ± SD grouped around the midcycle surge of LH.

proliferative phase (Fig. 1) and does not occupy more than about 20% of the total functional layer of the endometrium during this phase. Electron microscopically the structure of the glandular cells corresponds to proliferative activity, with a large number of ribosomes in the cytoplasm and a gradual increase in the development of the rough endoplasmic reticulum (Verma, 1983; Cornillie et al., 1985). In the late preovulatory phase glycogen particles have been described in the cytoplasm of the glandular epithelium (Themann & Schünke, 1963; Verma, 1983).

The production of progesterone following ovulation introduces remarkable changes in the morphology of the glands during the normal menstrual cycle. Between day LH-1/0 and LH + 1/ + 2 basal vacuoles start to appear in the glandular epithelium and their number gradually increases up to day LH + 4. The glandular mitoses gradually disappear. After day LH + 6 no more glandular mitoses can be found and the basal vacuoles have almost completely disappeared. The glandular diameter (Fig. 1) as well as the volume density of the glandular lumen show a linear increase from day LH-1/0 to day LH + 11/ + 12, and the height of the glandular epithelium diminishes significantly from day LH + 3/ + 4 to LH + 15/ + 16 (Johannisson et al., 1987). The cellular events in the glandular epithelium during the first 6 days after ovulation seem to be precisely regulated, with a relatively small interindividual variation. A similar regularity in the development of morphological changes during the first 6 days after ovulation has been reported by Li et al. (1988) and by Dockery et al. (1988b) using morphometric analysis of endometrial biopsies. Electron-microscopic studies of the glandular structure during the first 6 days after ovulation revealed the development of a nuclear channel system composed of 2–5 tubules (Clyman, 1963; Ancla et al., 1965; Terzakis, 1965; Wynn & Woolley, 1967; Dockery et al., 1988a). During this period glycogen particles were found throughout the cytoplasm and also in large accumulations close to the nucleus (Cornillie et al., 1985). On day LH + 4 giant mitochondria and subnuclear 'vacuoles' were observed in the glandular epithelium (Dockery et al., 1988a). In biopsies obtained at day LH + 6, smooth endoplasmic reticulum was found in the apical part of the cells and the Golgi apparatus was well developed with a vesicular structure suggesting secretory activity (Dockery et al., 1988a). After day LH + 6 the nuclear channel system has been reported to disappear and secretory products were observed in apical cytoplasmic protrusions bulging into the glandular lumen as well as in the glandular lumen itself (Verma, 1983; Cornillie et al., 1985). During the late secretory phase, giant lysosomes have been reported to be present in the cytoplasm of the glandular cells (Verma, 1983) and both basal and apical intercellular spaces became distended, with an increased complexity of interdigitations between the glandular cells (Cornillie et al., 1985). These changes have been postulated to play a role in menstruation (Davie et al., 1977).

The morphological changes of the human endometrial glands during the menstrual cycle coincide with the changing levels of estradiol and progesterone in plasma but there does not seem to be any simple relationship between the plasma hormone levels and the morphometric indices. The concentration and localization of estradiol and progesterone receptors have therefore been considered an important mediating factor between the circulating levels of steroids and the histologic changes of the endometrium. Immunocytochemical studies have shown that approximately 50% of the glandular cells stained positively for estrogen receptors in the early proliferative phase, whereas only a small portion stained positively for progesterone receptors (Garcia *et al.*, 1988). A marked staining for progesterone receptors was reported in the majority of glandular cells (75%) at the time of ovulation (Garcia *et al.*, 1988; Lessey *et al.*, 1988). During the postovulatory phase the estradiol and the progesterone receptor content declined or disappeared in the glandular cell (Garcia *et al.*, 1988; Lessey *et al.*, 1988). The varying concentration in the immunocytochemical localization of the estrogen receptors during the normal menstrual cycle suggests that they play an important role in the development of the glandular epithelium during the preovulatory phase. The estrogen receptors have also been reported to be associated with the initiation of transcription and protein synthesis as well as with the synthesis of progesterone receptors (Milgrom *et al.*, 1970).

The endometrial glands are a sensitive indicator for gauging the effect of contraceptive steroids. In women using progestogens as their contraceptive agent the glands respond by very definite histologic changes depending on the dosage and the duration of use.

Table 1 shows the effect of vaginal rings releasing norethisterone at two dose levels (50 μg and 200 μg/24 hours) and levonorgestrel at three dose levels (10 μg, 20 μg and 25 μg/24 hours). The control biopsies were all taken in the midsecretory phase. Endometrial biopsies were obtained after 6 and 10 months use of the device. While the release of 50 μg norethisterone/24 hours did not seem to have any significant effect on the number of glands per mm^2 nor on the size of glands, the release of 200 μg/24 hours significantly diminished the number of glands (p$\langle$0.05) after 10 weeks and their size (p$\langle$0.01) after only 6 weeks. With levonorgestrel, the release of 10 μg per 24 hours did not seem to have any significant effect on the number and size of glands when compared with the control specimens. However, at a release of 20 μg/24 hours the diameter of the glands was significantly smaller than in the control samples (p$=$0.02) after 6 weeks use. After 6 and 10 weeks use of a ring releasing levonorgestrel at a rate of 25 μg/24 hours, the size of the glands was significantly smaller than in the control specimens (p$\langle$0.001). A similar effect on the glandular component of the endometrium was found in women using norethisterone minipills at a dose of 300 μg daily (Johannisson *et al.*, 1982). Electron-microscopic studies of the endometrium following combined estrogen–progestogen administration give further support to the light-microscopic findings. The glandular nuclei contain small nucleoli, and no nuclear channel system was observed in the second half of the cycle (Clyman, 1963). The

Table 1. *Mean (± SD) morphological changes in the endometrium before and during the use of a vaginal device releasing norethisterone at a rate of 50 and 200 µg/24 hours and levonorgestrel at 10, 20 and 25 µg/24 hours. Biopsies obtained in a control cycle (C) and after 6 and 10 weeks' use*

Type of device	Number of glands/mm²			Diameter of glands (µm)			Glandular epithelial height (µm)		
	C	6	10	C	6	10	C	6	10
Norethisterone 50 µg/24 hours (n=7)	21.1 ±10.5	22.1 ±11.3	28.4 ±15.9	42.7 ±16.0	30.7 ±13.9	49.1 ±22.2	21.8 ±5.1	19.9 ±1.8	18.6 ±5.1
Norethisterone 200 µg/24 hours (n=7)	19.4 ±6.6	16.5 ±10.0	9.5[a] ±5.9	54.4 ±18.7	25.6[b] ±17.3	23.7[b] ±10.8	20.0 ±3.4	18.3 ±2.9	18.5 ±3.5
Levonorgestrel 10 µg/24 hours (n=5)	25.2 ±9.9	16.0 ±10.3	15.5 ±4.5	61.1 ±6.5	41.9 ±12.1	29.9 ±16.6	16.9 ±3.0	18.4 ±3.4	18.7 ±2.0
Levonorgestrel 20 µg/24 hours (n=5)	15.5 ±2.5	11.6 ±5.6	13.7 ±8.0	58.6 ±25.2	28.4[a] ±11.4	25.9[a] ±5.3	19.1 ±5.2	23.4 ±5.8	19.2 ±3.6
Levonorgestrel 25 µg/24 hours (n=15)	22.8 ±9.6	16.9 ±9.8	16.0 ±13.2	54.4 ±17.2	21.4[c] ±11.6	24.4[c] ±12.7	18.0 ±4.9	19.2 ±3.4	18.2 ±3.6

Notes:
[a] $p < 0.05$ when compared with the control sample.
[b] $p < 0.01$ when compared with the control sample.
[c] $p < 0.001$ when compared with the control sample.

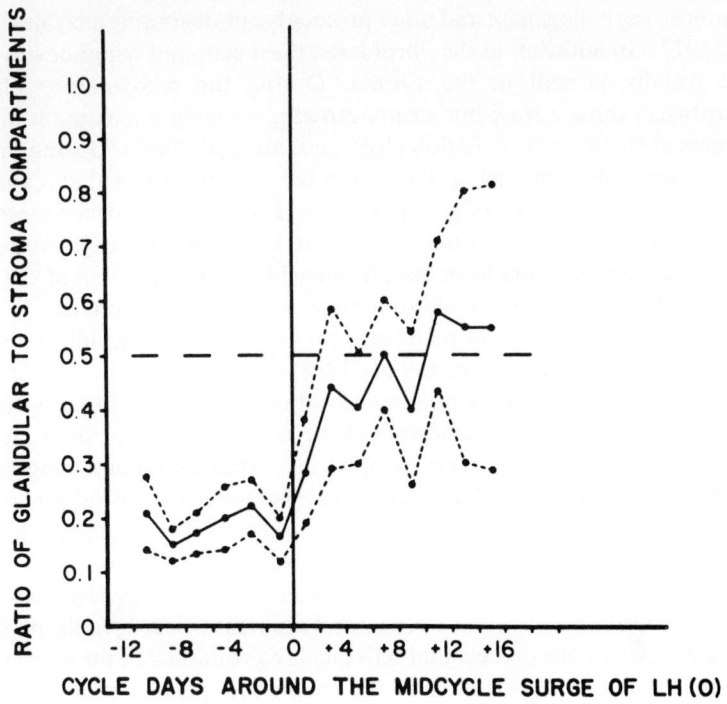

Fig. 2 Ratio of the glandular to stromal compartments based on volume density of the stroma and of the glands as a percentage of the total endometrial volume in 79 women. Mean values ±SD grouped around the midcycle surge of LH.

cytoplasmic structures remained poorly developed (Ancla *et al.*, 1965; Friedrich, 1967).

The endometrial stroma

Figure 2 shows the ratio between the stroma and the glandular component during the normal menstrual cycle. The stroma is predominant throughout the preovulatory phase whereas the glands gradually increase in volume during the postovulatory phase. The endometrial stroma is a complex structure which consists of mesenchymal cells with pluripotential properties. During the proliferative phase it is mainly composed of fibroblasts which produce macromolecular precursors of collagen and elastic fibres. Later, during the normal menstrual cycle, they also participate in the production of glycoproteins of the extracellular matrix as well as in the degradation of this matrix synthesizing collagenase and other proteoglycan-degrading enzymes (Werb *et al.*, 1977). In addition to the fibroblasts, mast cells and lymphocytes (T & B) are usually present in the stroma. During the preovulatory phase the· fibroblasts show a slow but steady growth, reaching a maximum of mitotic figures at the time of ovulation (Johannisson *et al.*, 1987). During this phase the cytoplasm contains a large number of ribosomes but cytoplasmic organelles such as the Golgi apparatus and the mitochondria remain poorly developed (Sengel & Stoebner, 1970). It is noteworthy that estradiol and progesterone receptors have been localized in a small portion of the stromal cells during the early preovulatory phase, whereas approximately 50% of the stromal cells are stained positively for progesterone and estradiol receptors at the time of ovulation (Garcia *et al.*, 1988).

Following ovulation, a number of submicroscopic changes occur in the stromal cells. The mitochondria and the endoplasmic reticulum increase in number and size and some cytoplasmic extensions containing glycogen granules have been described in the extracellular matrix (Cornillie *et al.*, 1985). However, the major changes in the morphology of the stroma take place 8–10 days after ovulation when the stroma becomes edematous and starts to develop predecidual changes. Light microscopically the predecidual cells are characterized by a vesicular nucleus and abundant clear cytoplasm. Electron microscopically the predecidual cells display a rounding of the nucleus as well as an increase and dilatation of the rough endoplasmic reticulum and the Golgi apparatus (Verma, 1983; Cornillie *et al.*, 1985). An accumulation of glycogen and various lysosomal enzymes has also been described (Schmidt-Matthiesen, 1963a). Laminin and type IV collagen have been detected around the stromal cells in the late secretory phase and it has been suggested that this accumulation is a progesterone/progestogen-dependent process (Bulletti *et al.*, 1988).

In this respect, it is noteworthy that a significant progesterone receptor content has been reported to be maintained in the nuclei of the stromal cells during the late secretory phase (Lessey *et al.*, 1988), whereas no positive staining has been observed in the glands.

The administration of contraceptive steroids, both in combined formulations and as progestogen-only compounds, clearly interferes with the morphologic events of the stroma during the normal menstrual cycle. The major alteration is a shift of the ratio of glands to stroma in favour of the stroma (Johannisson *et al.*, 1987).

Depending upon the dosage of progestogen, the stroma displays predecidual or decidual transformation. In women using high doses of a 19-nor steroid progestogen, a strong predecidual reaction was found in the stroma and ultrastructurally the rough and smooth endoplasmic reticulum was hyperplastic (Wienke *et al.*, 1969). In newer preparations where the 19-nor steroid is considerably reduced, the decidual reaction is not observed or is only observed in patches (Landgren *et al.*, 1979). Norgestrel, when released in small amounts from a vaginal ring, either produces an arrested proliferation or irregular secretory changes in the endometrium (Landgren *et al.*, 1985). Progestogens with an acetate radical have been reported to produce only patchy or poorly developed decidual reaction (Abell, 1975). Norgestimate (0.25 mg) in combination with ethinyl estradiol (0.035 mg) produces either no decidual response or an ill-developed decidua after 5–6 months use (Rabe *et al.*, 1986). It is noteworthy that no correlation has been found between the circulating endogenous or exogenous steroid levels and the endometrial morphologic changes of the stroma. For instance, in women using long-acting progestogens, bleeding irregularities have been observed even when the release of the steroid was kept at such a low level as 20 μg/24 hours and the hormonal profile indicated some luteal activity (Landgren *et al.*, 1982).

Endometrial vascularization

The anatomy of the endometrial vessels has been described in detail in the literature (see Schmidt-Matthiesen, 1963b). Figure 3 shows a diagram of the localization of the arteries and capillaries of the human endometrium. The vessels of the myometrium and the basal layer of the endometrium have been reported to be little influenced by hormonal changes. This segment of the spiral arteries passing through the basal layer of the endometrium is characterized by a thick muscular layer containing an elastic lamina. No major changes have been described in this lower part of the spiral arteries during the normal cycle.

On the other hand, the vessels of the functional layer are likely to be highly sensitive to hormones and have been reported to undergo significant changes during the menstrual cycle (Schmidt-Matthiesen, 1963b). This sensitivity includes the distal part of the spiral arteries, the arterioles, the capillaries, the venous lakes and the veins. In the early proliferative phase the arterial wall is thin with poorly developed elastic lamina. The spiral arteries continue to grow and extend further into the functional layer during the late proliferative phase. Using intraocular endometrial transplants in rhesus monkeys, Markee (1940) described a five-fold increase in the length of the spiral arteries during the proliferative phase when the increase in the endometrial thickness was only doubled. The increase of the endometrial stroma therefore seemed to determine the extent of coiling of the arteries. The most distal part of the spiral arteries becomes connected to the subepithelial capillary plexus via arterioles, but they also develop small branches at irregular intervals in the functional layer (Fanger & Barker, 1961; Ramsey, 1977). The endothelial cells of all endometrial arteries and arterioles show a strong positive staining for alkaline phosphatase, which is not the case with the venous vessels (Schmidt-Matthiesen, 1963b). At the time of ovulation the adventitia and the media of the spiral arteries increase, as do the amounts of collagen, elastin and acid mucopolysaccharides (Schmidt-Matthiesen, 1963b). During the second half

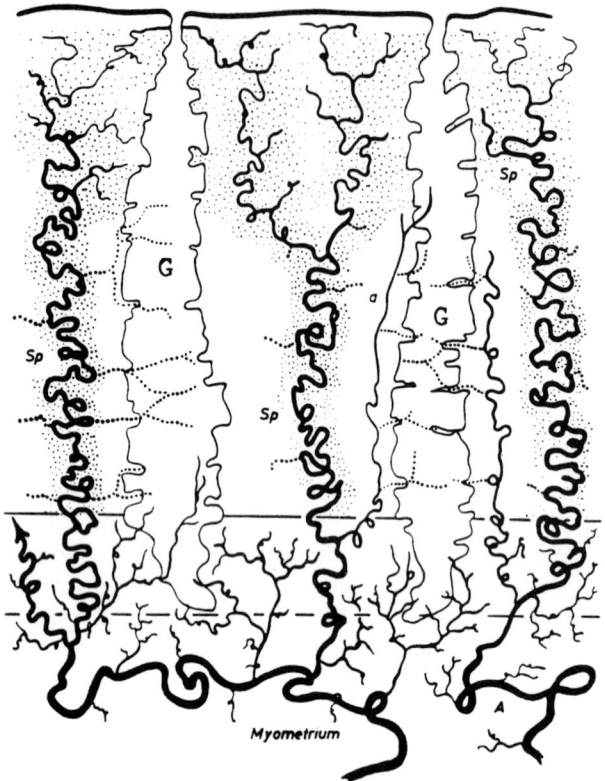

Fig. 3 Diagram of the vascularization of the endometrium showing arteries of the basal layer (A), spiral arteries (Sp) and ascending capillaries (a) supplying the glands (G). (Taken from Schmidt-Matthiesen (1963b), p.234.)

of the menstrual cycle the spiral arteries grow larger and longer and the tortuosity develops further.

The subepithelial capillary plexus also undergoes changes during the normal menstrual cycle. During the proliferative phase the capillaries are thin with a narrow lumen. However, the lumen progressively increases in diameter (Sheppard & Bonnar, 1980) and later in the secretory phase a complex meshwork of capillaries is present in the upper functional layer of the endometrium. There is a close connection between the thin capillaries and the arterioles as well as with the venules, which often are dilated and form venous lakes. These lakes are probably dilated venules, the function of which has been claimed to be the regulation of the blood volume and the rate of blood flow in the superficial part of the endometrium (Ramsey, 1977). Arteriovenous shunts have also been described as a factor responsible for the formation of the venous lakes (Schlegel, 1945; Dalgaard, 1945). However, this theory could not be confirmed by Bartelmez (1956).

In spite of the fact that a number of morphological studies have provided valuable information on the events in the endometrial vasculature, the relationship between the influence of ovarian steroids and the growth and differentiation of the endometrial vessels is still poorly understood and so is the mechanism triggering the onset of menstruation or causing intermenstrual bleeding. One of the models for the mechanism of the onset of menstrual bleeding in the normal cycle has been presented by Markee (1940). In intraocular endometrial transplants, Markee (1940) reported that during the late proliferative phase the blood flow rate increased and reached its maximum 10–16 days after the menstruation. The blood flow then gradually decreased during the secretory phase, probably due to a strong dilatation of the vessels observed prior to the onset of menstruation. The menstrual bleeding in these transplants started in relation to a sudden strong vasoconstriction in the distal segment of the spiral arteries. It was suggested that the bleeding took place through gaps in the cellular lining of the arterioles giving a calculated blood loss in endometrial transplants of 12.5 ml, through gaps in the capillaries giving a blood loss of 5 ml, by rupture of the venules with a blood loss of 6.25 ml and by diapedesis giving rise to a minor blood loss of 1.25 ml. Vessel lesions and disintegration of endometrial tissue have nevertheless been reported as a constant morphological finding during endometrial bleeding episodes (Sixma *et al.*, 1980).

It is generally assumed that endometrial bleeding and desquamation of the uterine mucosa during the normal menstrual cycle are a consequence of decreasing circulating levels of ovarian steroids. However, in normally menstruating women the onset of menstruation is not invariably associated with very low circulating estradiol and progesterone levels and the mechanism responsible for the onset of endometrial bleeding episodes may therefore be more complex than previously believed (Johannisson & Landgren, 1980). Recent immunocytochemical studies by Perrot-Applanat *et al.* (1988) revealed the presence of estrogen and progesterone receptors in the muscle cells (tunica media) of the uterine arteries. However, these authors could not detect any immunoreactivity in the endothelium of the uterine arteries nor in the uterine capillaries or veins. On the other hand, Press and Greene (1988) could not localize any progesterone receptors in vascular smooth muscle or endothelial cells. Disagreement therefore still exists regarding the direct effect of sex steroid hormones on the uterine blood vessels in the regulation of the uterine blood flow. The prostaglandins may also play a role in the endometrial bleeding.

The endothelium lining the endometrial vessels has only been sporadically studied during the normal menstrual cycle. Nevertheless, cyclic changes have been reported to occur also in these cells. Immunocytochemical studies of Factor VIII – an important component in the process of blood coagulation –

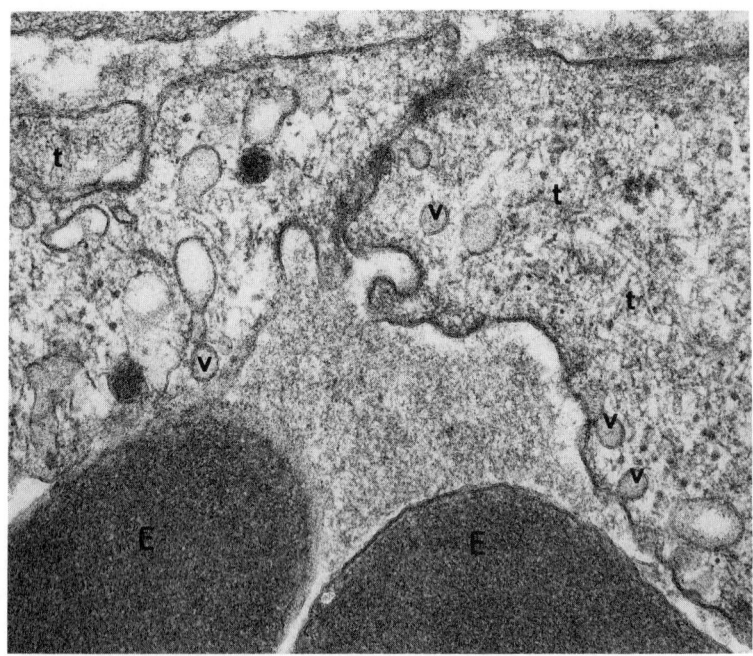

Fig. 4 Part of the cytoplasm of endometrial capillary endothelial cells showing plasmalemmal vesicles (v) scattered in the periphery and tonofilaments (t) exhibiting a criss-cross pattern. E = erythrocytes. (× 86000).

have revealed a gradual increase in the proliferative phase. No activity was observed in the late secretory phase nor in the menstrual phase (Zhu & Gu, 1988). In this respect it may be noteworthy that capillary fragility has been reported at the time of menstruation (Salvatore, 1952).

Bleeding irregularities have been reported in most clinical studies on steroidal contraceptives (see Odlind & Fraser, 1990). The endometrial vessels have also been reported to undergo a number of morphological changes in relation to the use of exogenous steroids. The spiral arteries of the functional layer of the endometrium fail to develop or develop prematurely or incompletely (Dallenbach-Hellweg, 1971). Intense dilatation of stromal vessels and thromboses have been reported by several authors (see Maqueo, 1980). In 1970, Maqueo *et al.* reported significant morphological changes of endometrial venules in the endometrium of women using various types of contraceptive steroids. When compared to a control group of normal cyclic women, the percentage of specimens showing venule dilatation was significantly larger in the women using contraceptive steroids. The frequency of dilated venules increased with the time of exposure but the incidence of venule dilatation decreased in samples with moderate or marked predecidual reaction. Maqueo (1980) also reported important proliferation of the endothelial cells and

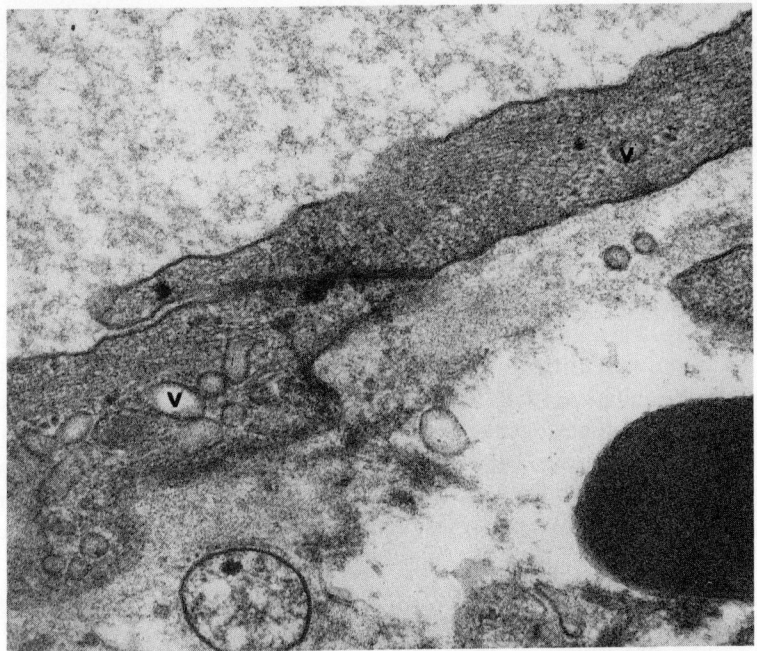

Fig. 5 Part of the cytoplasm of endometrial capillary endothelial cells showing contraction. The cytoplasmic matrix shows a high optical density and contains a few plasmalemmal vesicles (v) scattered at the periphery. ($\times 86000$).

thickening of the arterial media. Proliferation of the endothelial cells was also found by Ancla *et al.* (1965) and by Blaustein *et al.* (1968), who demonstrated vascular proliferation in 48% of endometria of women using the combined preparation. Changes in the ultrastructure of the endothelial cells following the use of 300 μg oral norethisterone daily have been reported (Johannisson *et al.*, 1982). Following treatment with norethisterone for 2 months, a significant increase was found in the plasmalemmal vesicles of endothelial cells ($p < 0.001$) (Fig. 4) and the number of contracted endothelial cells was significantly increased ($p < 0.05$) (Fig. 5). There is reason to believe that the endothelial cells of the endometrium undergo significant changes in relation to the use of steroidal contraceptives. The possibility cannot be excluded that these changes play an important role in the occurrence of irregular intermenstrual bleeding so frequently reported in users of long-acting progestational contraceptive steroids. Although not in the field of human reproduction, important research has been carried out on the structure and function of the endothelium, in various organs. In a comprehensive review of the endothelium, Majno and Joris (1978) state that 'it has become more and more obvious that endothelia differ in structure, function and metabolic properties not only in different organs, but in different parts of the same organ and even in different segments of a single microcirculatory loop'. Thus the endothelium is a markedly heterogeneous membrane. The data published have provided some information of the morphological events of the endothelium during the menstrual cycle and following the use of steroidal contraceptives. However, they have also pointed out serious gaps in our knowledge of the endometrial vascularization, in particular with regard to the dynamic function of the endothelial cells and their role in endometrial bleeding mechanism.

Conclusion

Bleeding irregularities represent one of the most important reasons for women to discontinue using long-acting progestogen contraception. The balance of evidence indicates that women using delivery systems that release small amounts of progestogens during prolonged periods of time bleed significantly less during periods characterized by some luteal function and more in anovulatory periods. And women using the combined formulations have fewer bleeding irregularities than those using the 'progestogen-only' formulation.

The human endometrium is a sensitive indicator of an altered hormonal environment. When compared to the normal menstrual cycle, significant changes are found in endometrial morphology in relation to the use of contraceptive steroids, in particular the long-acting progestogen-only formulations. Morphological changes are found at all levels: in the lining surface epithelium, in the glands, in the stroma and in the vessels. During the last 10 years new techniques have been developed to assess the effect of steroids at the cellular level, e.g. the assessment of the steroid receptors and the use of monoclonal antibodies to localize these receptors by immunocytochemical methods. A number of new sophisticated biochemical techniques are also available. All these techniques can certainly help us increase our knowledge with regard to the factor(s) which may be responsible for irregular endometrial bleeding in women using steroidal contraceptives. There is also a need for the development of an interdisciplinary research effort, where scientists representing research fields not directly related to human reproduction could contribute their expertise to a better understanding of the intriguing problem of endometrial bleeding and could give their advice for new areas of research in this field.

References

Abell, M.R. (1975). Endometrial biopsy: normal and abnormal diagnostic characteristics. (In) *Gynecologic Endocrinology* (Gold, J.J., ed.), pp.156–190. New York, Harper and Row.

Ancla, M., Simon, P., De Brux, J. & Robey, M. (1965). Modifications endométriales après administration prolongée de lynestrenol. Etude au microscope optique et électronique. *Gynécologie et Obstétrique*, **64**:231–249.

Aznar, R. & Giner, J. (1984). Development of the intrauterine progesterone-releasing system. (In) *Long-acting Contraceptive Delivery Systems* (Zatuchni, G.L., Goldsmith, A., Shelton, J.D. & Sciarra, J.J., eds.), pp.613–620. Philadelphia, Harper and Row.

Bartelmez, G.W. (1956). Premenstrual and menstrual ischemia and myth of endometrial arteriovenous anastomoses. *American Journal of Anatomy*, **98**:69–95.

Blaustein, A., Shenker, L. & Post, R.C. (1968). The effects of oral contraceptives on the endometrium. I. Blood vessels. *International Journal of Fertility*, **13**:466–475.

Borell, U., Nilsson, O. & Westman, A. (1959). The cyclical changes occurring in the epithelium lining the endometrial glands. An electron-microscopical study in the human being. *Acta Obstetricia et Gynecologica Scandinavica*, **38**:364–377.

Bulletti, C., Galassi, A., Jasonni, V.M., Martinelli, G., Tabanelli, S., Flamigni, C. (1988). Basement membrane components in normal, hyperplastic and neoplastic endometrium. *Cancer*, **62**:142–149.

Clyman, M.J. (1963). A new structure observed in the nucleolus of the human endometrial epithelial cell. *American Journal of Obstetrics and Gynecology*, **86**:430–432.

Cornillie, F.J., Lauweryns, J.M. & Brosens, I.A. (1985). Normal human endometrium. An ultrastructural survey. *Gynecologic and Obstetric Investigation*, **20**:113–129.

Dalgaard, J.B. (1945). The blood vessels of the human endometrium. *Acta Obstetricia et Gynecologica Scandinavica*, **26**:342–378.

Dallenbach-Hellweg, G. (1971). *Histopathology of the Endometrium*, pp.188–189. New York, Springer-Verlag.

Davie, R., Hopwood, D. & Levison, D.A. (1977). Intercellular spaces and cell junctions in endometrial glands: their possible role in menstruation. *British Journal of Obstetrics and Gynaecology*, **84**:467–476.

Diczfalusy, E. & Landgren, B.-M. (1981). New delivery systems: Vaginal devices. (In) *Recent Advances in Fertility Regulation* (Chang, C.F., Griffin, D. & Woolman, A., eds.), pp.43–69. Geneva, Atar SA.

Dockery, P., Li, T.C., Rogers, A.W., Cooke, I.D. & Lenton, E.A. (1988a). The ultrastructure of the glandular epithelium in the timed endometrial biopsy. *Human Reproduction*, **3**:826–834.

Dockery, P., Li, T.C., Rogers, A.W., Cooke, I.D., Lenton, E.A. & Warren, M.A. (1988b). An examination of the variation in timed endometrial biopsies. *Human Reproduction*, **3**:715–720.

Fanger, H. & Barker, B.E. (1961). Capillaries and arterioles in normal endometrium. *Obstetrics and Gynecology*, **17**:543–550.

Fedele, L., Marchini, M., Cavalli, G., Baglioni, A. & Taccagni, G.L. (1987). Marked deciliation and insufficient secretory modification of endometrial surface during treatment with a new progestogen–estrogen combination. *Contraception*, **35**:497–505.

Fotherby, K. (1977). Low doses of gestagens as fertility regulating agents. (In) *Regulation of Human Fertility* (Diczfalusy, E. ed.), pp.283–321. Copenhagen, Scriptor.

Friedrich, E.R. (1967). Effects of contraceptive hormone preparations on the fine structure of the endometrium. *Obstetrics and Gynecology*, **30**:201–219.

Garcia, E., Bouchard, P., De Brux, J., Berdah, J., Frydman, R., Schaison, G., Milgrom, E. & Perrot-Applanat, M. (1988). Use of immunocytochemistry of progesterone and estrogen receptors for endometrial dating. *Journal of Clinical Endocrinology and Metabolism*, **67**:80–87.

Gray, R.H. (1980). Patterns of bleeding associated with the use of steroidal contraceptives. (In) *Endometrial Bleeding and Steroidal Contraception* (Diczfalusy, E., Fraser, I.S. & Webb, F.T.G., eds.), pp.14–49. Bath, England, Pitman Press.

Hamperl, H. (1950). Über die 'hellen' Flimmerepithelzellen der menschlichen Uterusschleimhaut. *Virchows Archiv. A, Pathological Anatomy and Histopathology*, **319**:265–281.

Hester, L.L. Jr., Kellett, W.W. IIIrd, Spicer, S.S., Williamsson, H.O. & Pratt-Thomas, H.R. (1968). Effects of a sequential oral contraceptive on endometrial enzyme and carbohydrate histochemistry. *American Journal of Obstetrics and Gynecology*, **102**:771–783.

Jansen, R.P., Turner, M., Johannisson, E., Landgren, B.-M. & Diczfalusy, E. (1985). Cyclic changes in human endometrial surface glycoproteins: a quantitative histochemical study. *Fertility and Sterility*, **44**:85–91.

Johannisson, E. & Landgren, B.-M. (1980). Bleeding irregularities with steroidal contraceptives in relation to changes in circulating hormones. (In) *Endometrial Bleeding and Steroidal Contraception* (Diczfalusy, E., Fraser, I.S. & Webb, F.T.G., eds.), pp.291–317. Bath, England, Pitman Press.

Johannisson, E., Landgren, B.-M. & Diczfalusy, E. (1982). Endometrial morphology and peripheral steroid levels in women with and without intermenstrual bleeding during contraception with the 300 μg norethisterone (NET) minipill. *Contraception*, **25**:13–30.

Johannisson, E., Landgren, B.-M., Rohr, H.P. & Diczfalusy, E. (1987). Endometrial morphology and peripheral hormone levels in women with regular menstrual cycles. *Fertility and Sterility*, **48**:401–408.

Johannisson, E. & Nilsson, L. (1972). Scanning electron microscopic study of the human endometrium. *Fertility and Sterility*, **23**:613–625.

Lähteenmäki, P., Kurunmäki, H., Luukkainen, T., Lähteenmäki, P.L.A., Ratsula, K. & Toivonen, J. (1984). Development of intracervical steroid-releasing system. (In) *Long-acting contraceptive delivery systems* (Zatuchni, G.L., Goldsmith, A., Shelton, J.D. & Sciarra, J.J., eds), pp.595–600. Philadelphia, Harper & Row.

Landgren, B.-M., Johannisson, E., Masironi, B. & Diczfalusy, E. (1979). Pharmacokinetic and pharmacodynamic effects of small doses of norethisterone released from vaginal rings continuously during 90 days. *Contraception*, **19**:253–271.

Landgren, B.-M., Johannisson, E., Masironi, B. & Diczfalusy, E. (1982). Pharmacokinetic and pharmacodynamic investigations with vaginal devices releasing levonorgestrel at a constant, near zero order rate. *Contraception*, **26**:567–585.

Landgren, B.-M., Johannisson, E., Xing, S., Aedo, A.-R. & Diczfalusy, E. (1985). A clinical pharmacological study of a new type of vaginal delivery system for levonorgestrel. *Contraception*, **32**:581–601.

Lessey, B.A., Killam, A.P., Metzger, D.A., Haney, A.F., Greene, G.L. & McCarty, K.S. Jr. (1988). Immunohistochemical analysis of human uterine estrogen and progesterone receptors throughout the menstrual cycle. *Journal of Clinical Endocrinology and Metabolism*, **67**:334–340.

Li, T.C., Rogers, A.W., Dockery, P., Lenton, E.A. & Cooke, I.D. (1988). A new method of histologic dating of human endometrium in the luteal phase. *Fertility and Sterility*, **50**:52–60.

Ludwig, H. (1982). The morphologic response of the human endometrium to long-term treatment with progestational agents. *American Journal of Obstetrics and Gynecology*, **142**:796–808.

Ludwig, H. & Metzger, H. (1976). *The Human Female Reproductive Tract: A Scanning Electron Microscopic Atlas.* New York, Springer-Verlag.

Luukkainen, T., Nilsson, C.G., Allonen, H., Haukkamaa, M. & Toivonen, J. (1984). Intrauterine release of levonorgestrel. (In) *Long-acting Contraceptive Delivery Systems* (Zatuchni, G.L., Goldsmith, A., Shelton, J.D. & Sciarra, J.J., eds.), pp.601–612. Philadelphia, Harper & Row.

Majno, G. & Joris, I. (1978). Endothelium 1977: a review. *Advances in Experimental Medicine and Biology*, **104**:169–225.

Maqueo, M. (1980). Vascular and perivascular changes in the endometrium of women using steroidal contraceptives. (In) *Endometrial Bleeding and Steroidal Contraception* (Diczfalusy, E., Fraser, I.S. & Webb, F.T.G., eds.), pp.138–149. Bath, England, Pitman Press.

Maqueo, M., Rice-Wray, E., Gorodovsky, J. & Goldzieher, J.W. (1970). The effect of contraceptive steroids on endometrial sinusoids and the failure of these changes to correlate with breakthrough bleeding or systemic vascular effects. *Contraception*, **2**:283–288.

Markee, J.E. (1940). Menstruation in intraocular endometrial transplants in the Rhesus monkey. *Contributions to Embryology*. Carnegie Institution of Washington Publication No. 518, **28**(No. 177):219–308.

Milgrom, E., Atger, M. & Baulieu, E.E. (1970). Progesterone in uterus and plasma. IV. Progesterone receptor(s) in guinea pig uterus cytosol. *Steroids*, **16**:741–754.

Odlind, V. & Fraser, I.S. (1990). Contraception and menstrual bleeding disturbances: a clinical overview. (In) *Contraception and Mechanisms of Endometrial Bleeding* (d'Arcangues, C., Fraser, I.S., Newton, J.R. & Odlind, V., eds.) pp.5–29. Cambridge, England, Cambridge University Press.

Perrot-Applanat, M., Groyer-Picard, M.T., Garcia, E., Lorenzo, F. & Milgrom, E. (1988). Immunocytochemical demonstration of estrogen and progesterone receptors in muscle cells of uterine arteries in rabbits and humans. *Endocrinology*, **123**:1511–1519.

Press, M.F. & Greene, G.L. (1988). Localization of progesterone receptor with monoclonal antibodies to the human progestin receptor. *Endocrinology*, **122**:1165–1175.

Rabe, T., Leppien, G., Kiesel, L., Runnebaum, B., Heinrich, D., Johannisson, E. & Ludwig, H. (1986). Licht- und elektronen-mikroskopische Veränderungen des Endometriums unter Einnahme eines norgestimathaltigen oralen Kontrazeptivums (Cilest). *Geburtshilfe und Frauenheilkunde*, **46**:883–891.

Ramsey, E.M. (1977). Vascular anatomy. (In) *Biology of the Uterus* (Wynn, R.M., ed.), pp.59–76. New York, Plenum Press.

Salvatore, C.A. (1952). Capillary fragility and menstruation. *Surgery, Gynecology and Obstetrics*, **95**:13–16.

Schlegel, J.U. (1945). Arteriovenous anastomoses in endometrium in man. *Acta Anatomica*, **1**:284–325.

Schmidt-Matthiesen, H. (1963a). Histochemie. (In) *Das Normale Menschliche Endometrium* (Schmidt-Matthiesen, H., ed.), pp.149–224. Stuttgart, Thieme.

Schmidt-Matthiesen, H. (1963b). Vaskularisierung. (In) *Das Normale Menschliche Endometrium* (Schmidt-Matthiesen, H., ed.), pp.225–244. Stuttgart, Thieme.

Segal, S.J. (1982). Contraceptive subdermal implants. (In) *Advances in Fertility Research* (Mishell, D.R., ed.), pp.117–127. New York, Raven Press.

Sengel, A. & Stoebner, P. (1970). Ultrastructure de l'endomètre humain normal. I. Le chorion cytogène. *Zeitschrift für Zellforschung und Mikroskopische Anatomie*, **109**:245–259.

Sheppard, B.L. & Bonnar, J. (1980). The development of vessels of the endometrium during the menstrual cycle. (In) *Endometrial Bleeding and Steroidal Contraception* (Diczfalusy, E., Fraser, I.S. & Webb, F.T.G., eds.), pp.65–77. Bath, England, Pitman Press.

Sixma, J.J., Christiaens, G.C.M.L. & Haspels, A.A. (1980). The sequence of haemostatic events in the endometrium during normal menstruation. (In) *Endometrial Bleeding and Steroidal Contraception* (Diczfalusy, E., Fraser, I.S. & Webb, F.T.G., eds.), pp.86-96. Bath, England, Pitman Press.

Terzakis, J.A. (1965). The nucleolar channel system of human endometrium. *Journal of Cell Biology*, **27**:293–304.

Themann, H. & Schünke, W. (1963). Die Feinstruktur der Drüsenepithelien des menschlichen Endometriums. Elektronenoptische Morphologie. (In) *Das Normale Menschliche Endometrium* (Schmidt-Matthiesen, H., ed.), pp.111–148. Stuttgart, Thieme.

Thor, A., Viglione, M.J., Muraro, R., Ohuchi, N., Schlom, J. & Gorstein, F. (1987). Monoclonal antibody B72.3 reactivity with human endometrium: a study of normal and malignant tissues. *International Journal of Gynecological Pathology*, **6**:235–247.

Verma, V. (1983). Ultrastructural changes in human endometrium at different phases of the menstrual cycle and their functional significance. *Gynecologic and Obstetric Investigation*, **15**:193–212.

Werb, Z., Mainardi, C.L., Vater, C.A. & Harris, E.D. (1977). Endogenous activation of latent collagenase by rheumatoid synovial cells. Evidence for a role of plasminogen activator. *New England Journal of Medicine*, **296**:1017–1023.

Wienke, E.C. Jr., Cavazos, F., Hall, D.G. & Lucas, F.V. (1969). Ultrastructural effects of norethynodrel and mestranol on human endometrial stroma cell. *American Journal of Obstetrics and Gynecology*, **103**:102–111.

Wilborn, W.H., Hyde, B.M., Pope, V.Z., Beck, L.R., Hahn, D.W., McGuire, J. & Cohn, R. (1984). Comparative effects of norgestimate, norethisterone and medroxyprogesterone acetate on the microanatomy of baboon endometrium. (In) *Long-acting Contraceptive Delivery Systems* (Zatuchni, G.L., Goldsmith, E., Shelton, J.D. & Sciarra, J.J., eds.), pp.296–315. Philadelphia, Harper & Row.

Wynn, R.M. & Woolley, R.S. (1967). Ultrastructural cyclic changes in the human endometrium. II. Normal post-ovulatory phase. *Fertility and Sterility*, **18**:721–738.

Zhu, P.D. & Gu, Z. (1988). Observation of the activity of Factor VIII in the endometrium of women with regular menstrual cycles. *Human Reproduction*, **3**:273–275.

Discussion

Fraser. Dr Johannisson, you have used the term endometrial atrophy. To me this is a term which means complete absence of stimulation of the endometrium by estrogen and progestogen, as we find in a woman with ovarian failure. These women who have been exposed to relatively high doses or prolonged use of progestogen have in fact gone through a stage of initial decidualization, suppression of proliferation, and what we are seeing is the end-result of a very excessive suppression of proliferation. I suspect that some biochemical mechanisms within these endometria are probably different. I wonder if you can distinguish between these two different types of endometria, the true atrophy and the marked suppression morphologically.

Another question relates to migratory white cells within the endometrium. I wondered if you would comment about the timing of appearance of some of these white cells within the endometrium in relation to the late luteal phase and the onset of menstruation.

Johannisson. Well, to answer your first question, I would say that the methods we have do not allow us to differentiate between the atrophic endometrium and the atrophy which occurs following excessive exposure to progestogen. We only have a biopsy to look at, and it may be different in other parts of the endometrium but I doubt it. I do not have a good explanation for that, but I wonder if it is perhaps related to the lack of development of steroid receptors due to the exposure to progestogens.

When it comes to your second question, in the normal material, we found that the invasion of neutrophils occurs a maximum of 2 days before the onset of menstruation, while lymphocytes are always a part of the endometrium.

Cornillie. I would like to comment on the term 'atrophy'. If you mean by atrophy a decreased height in the endometrium, it is an anatomical description. On the other hand, in our study with the ring releasing 20 μg/day of levonorgestrel (Cornillie *et al.*, 1990), we noticed a significant decrease in cellular protein content, after 3 months of use. This indicates cytoplasmic atrophy. There was no difference in DNA content due to the levonorgestrel, which meant that the number of cells was unchanged but the volume of cytoplasm of each cell was smaller. Cellular atrophy was due to the decrease of the volume of the cytoplasm in each cell and this is something different.

Johannisson. I agree with you, but in many cases we see an atrophic appearance of the glands, but not of the stroma. When we have what I call atrophy, we have both. We also have what I think is at least a microscopic atrophy in the stroma as well as in the glands, and this really makes the difference. Of course, I agree that the decrease of protein synthesis, and perhaps the inhibition of DNA synthesis, is the beginning of an atrophy.

Brosens. You made the distinction between the functional and basal endometrium in relation to the cycle, but in the human, placentation is a deep interstitial implantation, and in pregnancy you will see a lot of changes in the inner third of the endometrium. So, after all, it is the inner third of the endometrium which is going to be very functional. So I wonder whether this basal layer of the endometrium has not been forgotten and been considered non-functional.

Johannisson. I couldn't agree more, but it is very difficult, at least in a normal biopsy, to get the basal layer. But I agree that it is very important for the regeneration of the endometrium.

Ludwig. Dr Johannisson, I hope you will agree with me that it is very difficult to draw conclusions from biopsies. We can use biopsies for some morphological aspects such as glandular structure, cytoplasm, nuclear relationships, stromal cells and so on. But for others such as the number and width of gland openings, the relation between the upper part of the endometrium and the vasculature, it is extremely difficult to draw conclusions and to put them in a morphometric scheme from biopsies. We need the whole specimen of a uterus to observe the number of glands, the width of glands, the relation between vasculature and stroma, etc.

Johannisson. Yes, a biopsy specimen has many limitations. But we orientate ourselves towards the surface epithelium, which we think is an important part of the endometrium, and then what is just below is the functional level.

Sheppard. I would like to go further, in fact, than Dr Brosens in saying that some of the factors that are affecting the endometrium may, in fact, be produced in the myometrium, even further back than the basal endometrium. But regarding morphometry, I would like to know if the method has reached the stage now that it could be used in any laboratory?

Johannisson. Well, I can't tell you. But I think it would be extremely interesting to get a comparative evaluation of the same slides by different centres, based on at least the simplest morphometric methods.

Cooke. I might just comment that we have ourselves been able to reproduce a good deal of Dr Johannisson's data. And there is a scheme in WHO at the moment for a quality control multi-observer approach to a standard set of slides for morphometric analysis.

Baird. We are always told classically that the basal layer of the endometrium is not hormonally sensitive and we are told that these 'stumpy' arteries that supply that area are not responsive to hormones. In light of new technology, such as the ability to demonstrate estradiol and progestogen receptors, either they are defective in these receptors or there is something quite peculiar about the stromal and glandular cells which are situated in this area. Now I would like to ask two questions. (1) Is this dogma actually true? Are there really no changes in the cells in response to quite marked changes in the endocrine environment? And (2) Do we have any information, if that is the case, as to how it is that these cells avoid a change in response to a change of hormone environment?

Sheppard. I think that the changes you are describing are probably not occurring at the basal level, at the endometrial/myometrial junction. The straight basal arteries do not respond morphologically to any change, while the spiral arterioles undergo dramatic changes.

Baird. Do we know whether they respond to vasoconstrictor substances?

Johannisson. I do not think that we have really been able to study the basal layer enough. We are mainly referring to very early work where modern techniques were not available. Also, I think, another factor which may be important is the desquamation which occurs during the menstruation and shedding which sometimes approaches the basal layer. It would be difficult to understand that there is no reaction to hormones in the basal layer which could explain this desquamation and the growth of endometrium following menstruation.

Ludwig. Before menstrual shedding, we observe perivascular erythrocyte aggregation and diapedesis. Have you seen signs of intravascular coagulation, or vessel wall platelet aggregation and diapedesis in your studies?

Sheppard. Dr Christiaens and Dr Sixma (Sixma *et al.*, 1980) have described platelet plug formation, and various vascular defects, but without specific identification of the type of vessel where the bleeding was occurring. Structurally, examining their vessels and our own material, it very much looks as if these are not arteries or arterioles; the majority of these vessels do not have a media of smooth muscle of any kind. The small hemorrhages and the hemostatic plug formation you are describing occur mainly in the dilated capillaries of the subepithelial capillary plexus.

Luukkainen. I would like to continue Dr Baird's question. Let us consider the woman who is fully lactating, is hypo-estrogenic and who has a very small uterus. She then stops lactation, starts follicular activity, and estrogen secretion increases. Do you see any action of these estrogens in the vessels? It is very difficult to find good histological work which is done during lactation.

Sheppard. I believe that the amount of information you can get from biopsies, particularly endometrial biopsies during lactation, is very limited, and that 90% of the observations that I feel happy about are hysterectomy samples where I have the whole uterus. It is only under these conditions that all the layers of the endometrium and the myometrium may be adequately studied.

Brosens. I should like to make two comments. The first: when we looked at the spiral vessels at the endometrium/myometrium junction, within the first trimester of pregnancy, we found changes in these vessels before they were really invaded by the endovascular trophoblast, which moves up the vessels from the intervillous space against the stream (Brosens, 1977). So, it seems to me that the modifications deep in the so-called basal layer and also within the inner part of the myometrium are there from the moment that there is trophoblast in the interstitial tissue invading stroma. So, the addition of interstitial trophoblast in what is going to be the placenta bed will modify these vessels and one of the changes which we saw was decidualization in the intimal cells of the spiral arteries and other arterioles.

The second point is that the whole inner part of the myometrium and the decidua underlying the placenta will be modified completely during pregnancy into vessels which no longer have any resemblance to an artery due to the association with intravascular trophoblast. And then, when pregnancy comes to an end, during the period of post-partum lactation, when there are no estrogens present, you will see a full regeneration of spiral arteries in their original condition, starting from vessels which have been completely modified. So there is quite an amazing process going on in that area – maybe in some way linked to the increase of steroids by paracrine secretion by trophoblast. I do not know. And then there is postpartum regeneration, even in the absence of estrogens and progesterone.

Sheppard. I am fully aware of your work in that area (Pignenborg *et al.*, 1980), and I think it is one of the few times when the basal endometrium undergoes such changes. But I think your group has also shown that this occurs in two stages and the myometrial sectors only really undergo these modifications later on in pregnancy. It is not the initial event, and it is the endometrium where primary decidualization occurs. So, I think that what happens in the myometrium is more a response to trophoblast invasion, rather than a response to the decidualized stromal cells.

King. What is known about the mechanism for producing this coiling, and is there any information, between ovulatory cycles and anovulatory cycles, that might give us clues to some of the components that are involved?

Johannisson. I can only mention what is described in the literature (Dallenbach-Hellweg, 1971), and the general idea is that there is a discrepancy between the growth of the stroma and gland components and the growth of the vessels. This means that the vessels are growing more rapidly than the stroma. Then, in the late secretory phase, the stroma component begins to collapse and, therefore, the spiral arteriole becomes even more coiled.

Rees. In answer to Professor Baird's question, the arteries in the basal layer probably do constrict during menstruation, and this is based on injection studies, where you cannot fill the endometrial blood vessels at all with contrast material down to myometrium. However, you can fill them completely in the luteal phase of the cycle.

Baird. I do not know what causes the blood vessels to coil. But I do know you do not have to have the vessels inside the uterus with a bit of myometrium round them, because in Markee's experiments the vessels in endometrial explants coiled (Markee, 1940).

Fraser. It is my understanding that there is fairly extensive morphological information on changes in spiral arterioles under different conditions of hormonal stimulation of the endometrium, including women who are anovulatory and women who are exposed to different exogenous steroids (Maqueo, 1980). It is also my understanding that, in fact, the spiral arterioles do not develop extensively if a woman is exposed to estrogen alone – there is some spiralling, but nothing like the extent that you get in the normal menstrual cycle. Additionally, with exposure to combined estrogen/progestogen pills, there is very suppressed development of the spiral arterioles. Perhaps one of our histologists or pathologists might like to comment on that.

Sheppard. In our studies of the endometrium of patients on low-dose oral progestogens (Hourihan *et al.*, 1986), we found a retardation in the development of the spiral arteries compared to the control group.

Cornillie. The basic question seems to be whether basal endometrium is different from superficial endometrium? We are focusing on the superficial endometrium because it is in our biopsies. But maybe Dr

Bouchard has had opportunities to look at some basal endometrial specimens with receptor localization techniques?

Bouchard. I do not have any personal data because I work in biopsies, but data are available in the literature from Dr Greene's group in Chicago who published several papers showing that steroid receptors are there (Press *et al.*, 1984; Press & Greene, 1988). But they seem to be present in smaller amounts than in the superficial layer. There are a number of publications on immunocytochemistry and fragments collected at hysterectomy.

Baird. If the steroid receptor is there, it would seem likely that the tissue is hormone sensitive.

Böhlen. It is not quite clear to me why, within this audience, there seems to be an emphasis on the spiral arteriole versus the capillary bed in a role in endometrial bleeding. Without being in the field of endometrial bleeding, I would like to ask the question: is there really a consensus that the arterioles are the structures to look at rather than the capillaries?

Ludwig. In terms of microcirculation, the capillary bed is much more important than the arterial layer. In histological terms, the premenstrual endometrium is like a 'shock-organ' 2 or 3 days before shedding. There are intravascular changes as in other organs in shock and we always see that in the capillary bed and not in the arteries.

Sheppard. I agree that if we are talking about breakthrough bleeding, we must move away from thinking purely about spiral arterioles because it is not going to be the arterioles that bleed but rather the capillaries and small venules.

Bischof. I would like to put forward a provocative hypothesis. Could we think that in fact coiling of these spiral arteries is an in-born phenomenon, and that continued growth and coiling of these arteries would lead to rupture and that coiling and rupture can be avoided, providing that either progesterone or estradiol is there?

Smith. I will make two points. The first is that I would strongly agree with Dr Sheppard. The spiral arteriolar constriction is probably a phenomenon of steroid withdrawal bleeding whereas breakthrough bleeding as you see with progestogens is probably a phenomenon of the capillaries. Secondly, in response to Dr Bischof's comment, it is important to remember that exaggerated coiling is only the first part of the mechanism of regression, that in fact it is not the coiling that produces the intense vasoconstriction or stops the blood getting through the vessel, it is the intense vasoconstriction which is a second phenomenon within the spiral arterioles. Withdrawal of steroids, particularly withdrawal of progesterone, does result in an increased capacity of endometrial glandular tissues to release prostaglandins, for example; and if we are keeping the simple model of steroid withdrawal inducing vasoconstriction, you can almost forget the concept of the increased coiling because you have a clear and simple mechanism, i.e. steroid withdrawal stimulates prostaglandin production which produces vasoconstriction which does not actually require coiling. I would be just as provocative and suggest that the coiling is not a phenomenon relevant to menstruation, but it is a phenomenon which is actually relevant to implantation and the subsequent invasion of those spiral arterioles by trophoblast, and the increase in size of the uterus that is required with placentation, and that is why the vessels are coiled.

Baird. Certainly, we are interested in what happens to the capillaries, but we are also interested in why the capillaries are damaged. The best working hypothesis is still that it is a response to intense vasoconstriction of the spiral arteries which has been observed to occur prior to the onset of menstruation.

Sheppard. To address the problem of breakthrough bleeding, we should decide which vessels we are going to be investigating. We know that the spiral arterioles are involved in the process of menstruation. But do we know that the spiral arterioles are behaving in any way abnormally in an episode of breakthrough bleeding, or is it just a simple fact of having underdeveloped spiral arterioles, coupled with an increase in the number of dilated vessels with a more fragile endothelial lining in the subepithelial capillary plexus of atrophic endometrium as a result of the progestogen treatment? I think one could probably investigate this by looking at hemorrhagic and non-hemorrhagic areas of the uterine wall in cases where patients are having a breakthrough bleeding episode at the time of hysterectomy.

King. I would agree with this completely. We must define what we are talking about. I am getting the feeling that what is happening at menstruation seems to be different to what is happening with breakthrough bleeding. So once we know which blood vessels we should be looking at for the one mechanism, and which blood vessels we should be looking at for the other, then I think we can make more constructive suggestions as to which biochemical parameters might be the most important.

Ludwig. I am fully in agreement with Dr Sheppard when he says that we have to look for hysterectomy specimens. If endometrium is sustained by steroids, we have to look at the uteri of very old women, where there is no functional sex steroid present. They still have an endometrium, they still have vessels, they still have coiled arterial vessels, but what they do not have are the shock signs of the terminal vascular bed just beneath the lining of the epithelium. In future research on this topic we should apply the most recent morphological methods to uteri from patients who are followed very closely so that we know their endocrine status at the time of hysterectomy. It is not necessary to have plenty of specimens, a few thorough examinations by all the methods available will solve many of the questions yet unanswered.

References

Brosens, I.A. (1977). Morphological changes in the utero-placental bed in pregnancy hypertension. *Clinics in Obstetrics and Gynaecology*, **4**:573–579.

Cornillie, F.J., Brosens, I.A., Marbaix, E., Vael, T., Baudhuin, P. & Courtoy, P.J. (1990). A biochemical study of lysosomal enzymes in control and levonorgestrel-treated human endometria: analysis of total activity and evidence for secretion. (In) *Contraception and Mechanisms of Endometrial Bleeding* (d'Arcangues, C., Fraser, I.S., Newton, J.R. & Odlind, V., eds.), pp.383–406. Cambridge, England, Cambridge University Press.

Dallenbach-Hellweg, G. (1971). *Histopathology of the Endometrium*. New York, Springer-Verlag.

Hourihan, H.M., Sheppard, B.L. & Bonnar, J. (1986). A morphometric study of the effect of oral norethisterone or levonorgestrel on endometrial blood vessels. *Contraception*, **34**:603–612.

Maqueo, M. (1980). Vascular and perivascular changes in the endometrium of women using steroidal contraceptives. (In) *Endometrial Bleeding and Steroidal Contraception* (Diczfalusy, E., Fraser, I.S. & Webb, F.T.G., eds.), pp.138–149. Bath, England, Pitman Press.

Markee, J.E. (1940). Menstruation in intraocular endometrial transplants in the rhesus monkey. *Contribution to Embryology*. Carnegie Institution of Washington Publication No. 518, **28**(No. 177):219–308.

Pignenborg, R., Dixon, J., Robertson, W.B. & Brosens, I.A. (1980). Trophoblastic invasion of human decidua from 8 to 10 weeks of pregnancy. *Placenta*, **1**:3–20.

Press, M.F. & Greene, G.L. (1988). Localization of progesterone receptor with monoclonal antibodies to the human progestin receptor. *Endocrinology*, **122**:1165–1175.

Press, M.F., Nousek-Goebl, N., King, W.J., Herbst, A.L. & Greene, G.L. (1984). Immunohistochemical assessment of estrogen receptor distribution in the human endometrium throughout the menstrual cycle. *Laboratory Investigation*, **51**:495–503.

Sixma, J.J., Christiaens, G.C.M.L. & Haspels, A.A. (1980). The sequence of haemostatic events in the endometrium during normal menstruation. (In) *Endometrial Bleeding and Steroidal Contraception* (Diczfalusy, E., Fraser, I.S. & Webb, F.T.G., eds.), pp.86–96. Bath, England, Pitman Press.

Function of endometrial blood vessels

MATS ÅKERLUND

Department of Obstetrics and Gynaecology, University Hospital, Lund, Sweden.

Abstract

During recent years, in-vivo data from humans on the function of endometrial vessels have been obtained mainly by ^{133}Xe clearance studies, giving numerical measures of flow, and by a thermistor technique based on continuous recording of thermoconduction locally, in the endometrium. With the former technique blood flows ranging from 10 ml/100 g to 70 ml/100 g tissue/minute were found in healthy women of fertile age. Cyclical variation was seen with peak values before ovulation and in late secretory phase. With the thermistor recordings, pulse-synchronous variations in blood flow were seen in the endometrium and substantial reduction of flow occurred at the well-demarcated uterine contractions of the menstrual period. Vasopressin reduced the endometrial circulation *in vivo* with effects both on the smooth muscle of arterial walls and via an increase in myometrial activity, effects which were counteracted by a uterine oxytocin and vasopressin receptor-blocking agent. Histochemical studies of branches of uterine arteries showed nerves of adrenergic and cholinergic nature, as well as fibres containing neuropeptide-Y (NPY) and vasoactive intestinal peptide (VIP). The most potent stimulator of the contractility of smooth muscle of the arterial wall was arginine vasopressin, followed in order by oxytocin, noradrenalin together with NPY, noradrenalin alone and dopamine. A change in response of human uterine arteries as they enter the myometrium and decrease in diameter was seen with prostaglandins (PG) $F_{2\alpha}$ and PGE_2. Both PGs, particularly $PGF_{2\alpha}$ in higher doses, stimulated contractions of extramyometrial arteries, whereas these two PGs caused relaxation of the smaller intramyometrial ones. A change in the magnitude of response was also seen with other vasoactive substances. The studies of the function of endometrial blood vessels indicate a complexity of the regulation of uterine blood flow involving effects of ovarian hormones, myometrial activity and, most probably, also different neuropeptides and circulating vasoactive substances. Further research in this area should focus on the mechanisms regulating the activity of the smallest intramyometrial vessels as well as that of the coiled arteries of the endometrium.

Introduction

Knowledge of the function of human endometrial blood vessels, of crucial importance for the understanding of menstrual disturbances, is still limited. The most important reason for this is the anatomical location of the endometrium within the body leading to technical difficulties in performing in-vivo studies. However, some new information has been obtained since this topic was reviewed during the previous WHO symposium on mechanisms of endometrial bleeding (Åkerlund, 1980).

Methodological considerations

During recent years, new data on the function of endometrial blood vessels in the human have been derived from studies with the ^{133}Xe clearance method (Fraser et al., 1987). By this technique, it is possible to obtain measures of absolute rates of flow in the human. Information has been obtained about blood flow during the menstrual cycle and in women with dysfunctional bleeding. The drawback of clearance methods is that they do not allow the continuous recording of blood flow over long periods. Furthermore, these methods are comparatively complicated. However, more precise information can now be obtained with modern computer analysis techniques (Fraser et al., 1987).

A newly developed instrument for continuous measurement of thermoconduction, reflecting blood flow locally in the endometrium, has also provided new in-vivo information (Hansson et al., 1987; Hauksson et al., 1988). This instrument is based on measuring the power needed to keep a constant temperature difference between two thermistor probes in the endometrium, one of body temperature and one at a constantly elevated temperature. In that way drift due to variation in body temperature, frequently a problem with the previous thermistor technique (Åkerlund et al., 1975), can be avoided. The measure of added power gives a relative measure of local flow.

Another method used for in-vivo studies of the function of endometrial blood vessels in the non-pregnant human is microhysteroscopy (Van Herendael et al., 1987), whereas ultrasonic technique has mainly been used during pregnancy (Turner & Carroll, 1979). New data on the function of uterine blood vessels in the human have also been obtained by in-vitro techniques for vasomotor studies and by immunohistochemical investigation of branches of uterine arteries (unpublished data).

Most previous studies of isolated vessels from the human uterus were performed on the uterine artery or its main branches. However, such large vessels are probably inappropriate for the elucidation of the mechanisms controlling peripheral vascular resistance. Only the smallest arteries appear to be actively involved in this regulation and functional differentiation with different dimensions of the vessels may exist (Tulenko, 1979). In-vitro studies on human material have therefore also included segments of intramyometrial arteries (Maigaard et al., 1985a, 1985b).

Some new data on endometrial blood flow have also been obtained from animal experiments (Einer-Jensen, 1980; Brown et al., 1985; Zhang et al., 1987). However, since the endometrium of the human differs markedly from that of other species, with respect both to function and structure, results of animal studies cannot easily be extrapolated to the human.

Ovarian steroids and endometrial circulation: long-time variations during the menstrual cycle

Endometrial blood flow studies by the ^{133}Xe technique showed blood flows ranging from 10 ml/100 g to 70 ml/100 g tissue/minute in healthy women of fertile age (Fraser *et al.*, 1987). When results obtained at different days of the menstrual cycle were compared, a significant correlation between plasma estradiol levels and endometrial blood flow in the follicular phase was seen, with a significant elevation in late follicular phase. This is in agreement with previous studies indicating a potent vasodilatory effect of estrogens on uterine arteries (for references, see Åkerlund, 1980). In the luteal phase there was no correlation between blood flow and estradiol levels (Fraser *et al.*, 1987), but a gradual increase until the onset of menstruation, when a fall was observed. Women with anovulatory, dysfunctional bleeding exhibited exceedingly variable flow rates.

Variations in endometrial blood flow during the menstrual cycle were also described in the classic reports by Markee (1950) and Prill and Götz (1961). However, the quantitative estimations by Fraser *et al.* (Fig. 1) do not fully correspond with these previous reports. This discrepancy may result from the different techniques employed. Fraser and co-workers investigated the endometrium of non-pregnant women *in vivo*, whereas Markee studied endometrial transplants in the eye chamber of monkeys and Prill and Götz, although studying humans, used a primitive thermodilution technique.

Microhysteroscopic studies (Van Herendael *et al.*, 1987) revealed changes in the vascularization pattern of the endometrium during the menstrual cycle, which allowed the definition of different phases of the cycle. These were early proliferative, late proliferative, early secretory, late secretory and premenstrual–menstrual phases.

Spontaneous blood flow of endometrial vessels: influence of the activity of myometrium and of the vascular wall muscle on the flow

With the thermoconduction–thermistor technique (Hansson *et al.*, 1987; Hauksson *et al.*, 1988), pulse-synchronous variations in flow of the endometrial arteries were recorded (Fig. 2). During spontaneous, well-demarcated uterine contractions, blood flow generally decreased, presumably as a result of a compressing effect of the increased intrauterine pressure on uterine vessels (Hauksson *et al.*, 1988).

The importance of the influence of uterine contractions on the endometrial blood flow in non-pregnant women, compared with the effects of the smooth muscle of the uterine vessels, is difficult to assess in the light of available data. However, it might be anticipated that the influence of myometrial activity is more important in the non-pregnant than in the pregnant condition because of

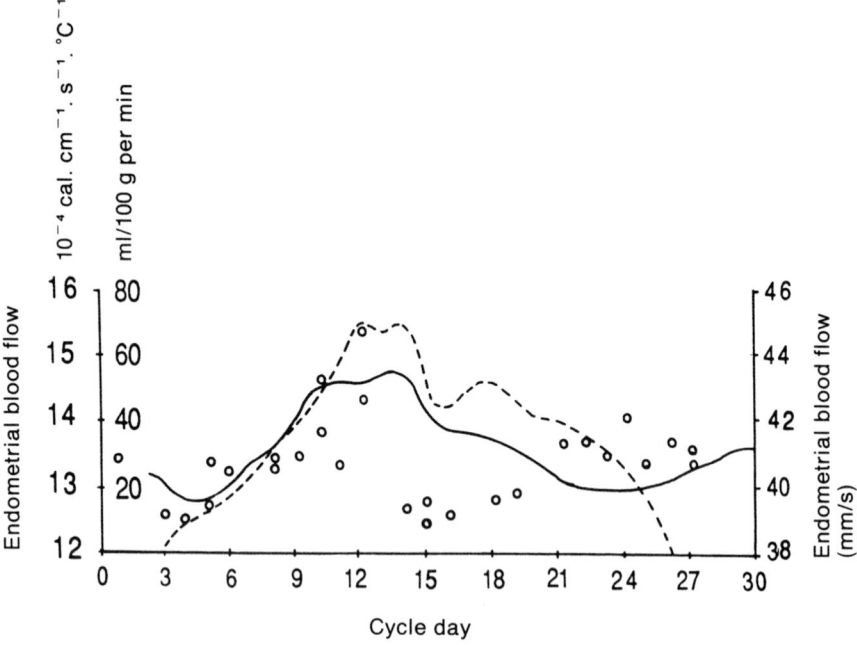

Fig. 1 Comparison of endometrial blood flow at different stages of the menstrual cycle measured by ^{133}Xe clearance (Fraser et al., 1987) in normal women (ml/100 g per min; circles), compared with the data of Markee (1950) in rhesus monkeys (mm/s; dashed line) and Prill and Götz (1961), using a heat clearance technique in women (10^{-4} cal × cm^{-1} s^{-1} × °C^{-1}; solid line).

the differences in diameter of the uterine cavity. Much higher intrauterine pressures can occur in non-pregnant women.

Effects of vasoactive substances on human uterine blood flow *in vivo*

Vasopressin has a potent effect on endometrial blood flow during early menstruation (Fig. 3), as shown by thermistor technique recordings during intrauterine pressure studies (Hansson et al., 1987; Hauksson et al., 1988). During the menstrual period, the effect on the flow is more or less constant. When the vasopressin effect was inhibited by a newly developed oxytocin and vasopressin receptor blocker, 1-deamino-2-D-Tyr(OEt)-4-Thr-8-Orn-oxytocin (dDETO-OXY), the blood flow rose markedly and the uterus relaxed.

In-vitro studies confirmed the inhibitory effect of this analogue also on the smooth muscle of the uterine arteries. For other vasoactive substances, new

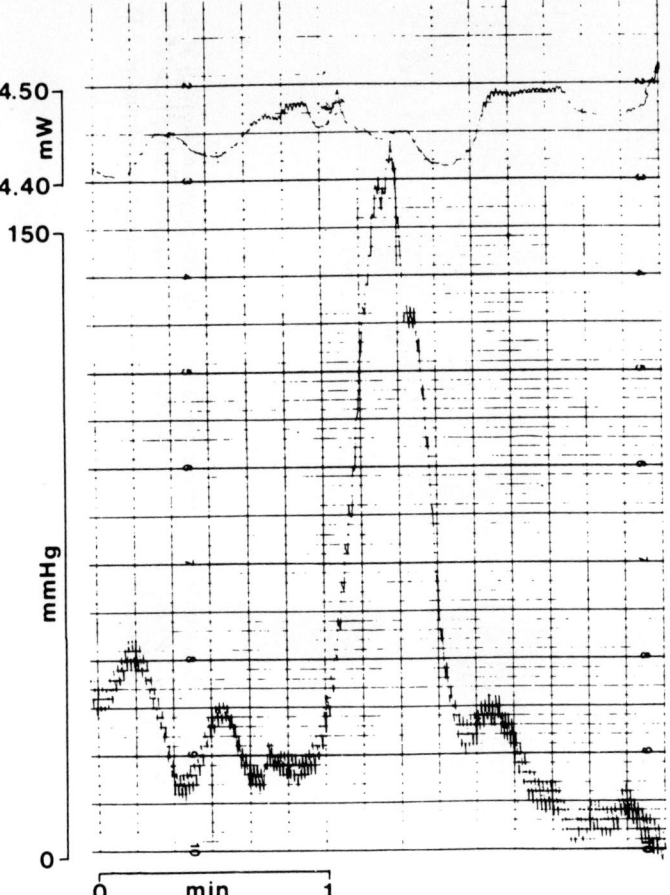

Fig. 2 Recording with high paper speed of pulse-mediated changes in added power reflecting uterine blood flow in a non-pregnant woman at the onset of menstruation. Pulse-synchronous changes in intrauterine pressure were also recorded.

data from in-vivo studies in the human are not available.

When considering agents which influence endometrial blood flow, the implication of myometrial effects must be taken into account when the endometrial circulatory effects are investigated. These substances can act both via effects on myometrial activity and by directly influencing the vessel walls. The relative importance of these two mechanisms remains to be settled for each factor.

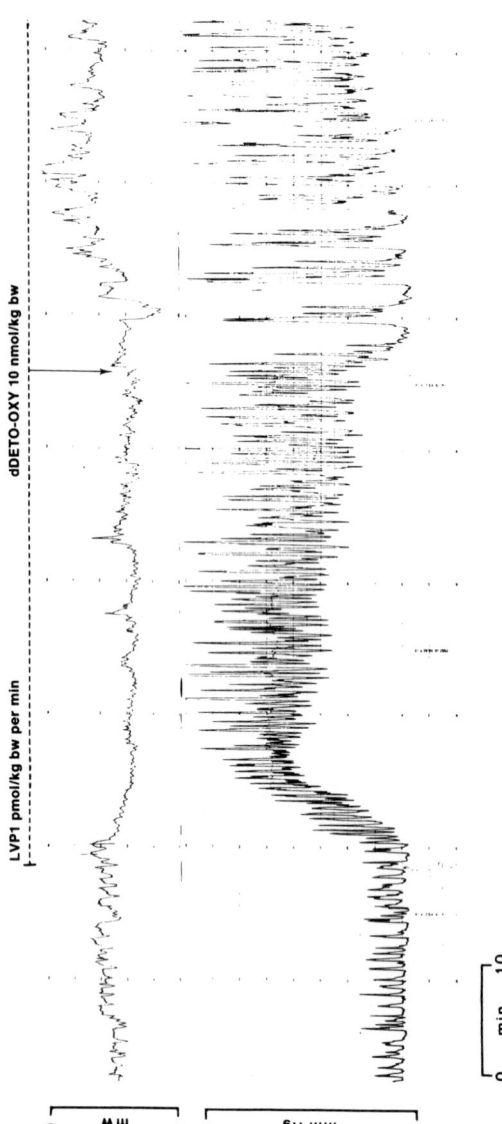

Fig. 3 Recording of intrauterine pressure and added power reflecting uterine blood flow in a non-pregnant woman at the onset of menstruation. Infusion of lysine vasopressin (LVP) induced uterine hyperactivity, reduction of blood flow and dysmenorrhea-like pain, which was counteracted by injection of the oxytocin and vasopressin antagonist 1-deamino-2-D-Tyr(OEt)-4-Thr-8-Orn-oxytocin (dDETO-OXY).

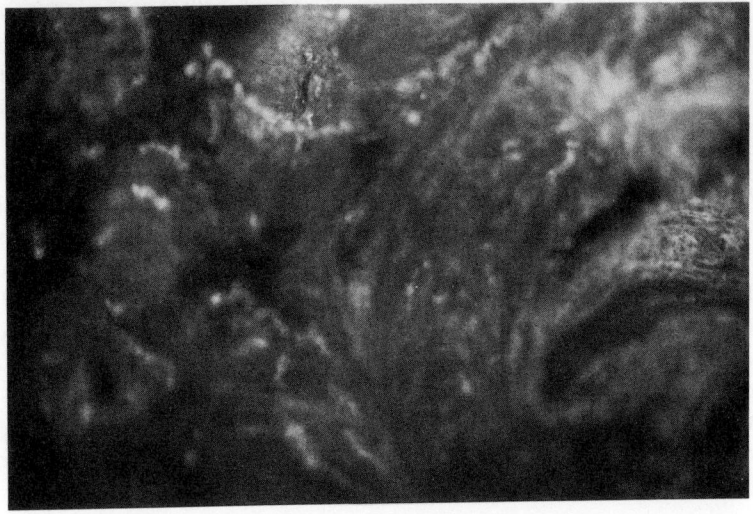

Fig. 4 Innervation of a branch of the human uterine artery as demonstrated by the protein gene product methodology, visualizing cytoplasmic protein in nerves.

Innervation of the human uterine artery and motor responses to neuropeptides and other vasoactive substances *in vitro*

The presence of adrenergic and cholinergic innervation of uterine arteries is well known (Fig. 4). Recent immunohistochemical studies of peptide-containing nerves in the smooth muscle of uterine arterial walls (unpublished data) also revealed the presence of fibres with only vasoactive intestinal peptide (VIP), peptide histidine methionine, neuropeptide-Y (NPY) and, to some extent, leu-enkephalin.

The order of potency of the peptides which were tested and of other important humoral factors or neuropeptides on the small branches of uterine arteries was:

1. Arginine vasopressin
2. Oxytocin
3. Noradrenalin together with neuropeptide-Y
4. Noradrenalin alone
5. Dopamine

No effect was seen with acetylcholine or tyrosine, and VIP caused relaxation of contractile activity induced by prostaglandin (PG) $F_{2\alpha}$.

However, the importance of these peptides for the function of endometrial blood vessels remains to be settled. The effects on the myometrium also need to be assessed, e.g. vasopressin is one of the most potent uterine stimulators that exist in the non-pregnant condition at the onset of menstruation (Åkerlund, 1980).

The important role of prostaglandins in the regulation of menstrual bleeding is discussed by other authors in this book. Several reviews of their role in endometrial bleeding were also published previously (Christiaens *et al.*, 1981; Granström *et al.*, 1983). With respect to the function of endometrial blood vessels, an interesting recent finding (Maigaard *et al.*, 1985a,b) was the difference in response to $PGF_{2\alpha}$ and PGE_2 of extra- and intramyometrial arteries. Both PGs, particularly $PGF_{2\alpha}$ in higher dose, stimulated contractions of extramyometrial uterine arteries. By contrast, both compounds caused relaxation of the intramyometrial arteries of smaller diameter. Changes in the magnitude of response were also seen with other vasoactive substances (Åkerlund, unpublished data).

Conclusion

Studies of the function of endometrial blood vessels reveal a complex regulation of uterine blood flow involving effects of ovarian hormones, myometrial activity and, most certainly, also of different neuropeptides and circulating vasoactive substances. Further research in this area should, in particular, focus on the mechanisms regulating the activity of the smallest myometrial vessels as well as of the coiled arteries of the endometrium. Additional in-vivo data from human studies are also needed.

References

Åkerlund, M. (1980). Non-prostaglandin factors influencing the microcirculation of the endometrium. (In) *Endometrial Bleeding and Steroidal Contraception* (Diczfalusy, E., Fraser, I.S. & Webb, F.T.G., eds.), pp.246–265. Bath, England, Pitman Press.

Åkerlund, M., Bengtsson, L.-P. & Carter, A.M. (1975). A technique for monitoring endometrial or decidual blood flow with an intra-uterine thermistor probe. *Acta Obstetricia et Gynecologica Scandinavica*, **54**:469–477.

Brown, B.W., Fraser, I.S. & Mattner, P.E. (1985). Capillary blood flow in the endometrium and myometrium of conscious sheep: effect of catheterization of uterine arteries. *Australian Journal of Biological Sciences*, **38**:209–214.

Christiaens, G.C.M.L., Sixma, J.J. & Haspels, A.A. (1981). Haemostasis in menstrual endometrium in the presence of an intrauterine device. *British Journal of Obstetrics and Gynaecology*, **88**:825–837.

Einer-Jensen, N. (1980). Lack of effect of a progesterone-containing silastic IUD on endometrial blood flow in rats. *Hormone Research*, 12:233–236.

Fraser, I.S., McCarron, G., Hutton, B. & Macey, D. (1987). Endometrial blood flow measured by [133]Xenon clearance in women with normal menstrual cycles and dysfunctional uterine bleeding. *American Journal of Obstetrics and Gynecology*, 156:158–166.

Granström, E., Swahn, M.-L. & Lundström, V. (1983). The possible roles of prostaglandins and related compounds in endometrial bleeding. A mini-review. *Acta Obstetricia et Gynecologica Scandinavica*, Supplement, 113:91–99.

Hansson, G.-Å., Hauksson, A., Strömberg, P. & Åkerlund, M. (1987). An instrument for measuring endometrial blood flow in the uterus, using two thermistor probes. *Journal of Medical Engineering and Technology*, 11:17–22.

Hauksson, A., Åkerlund, M. & Melin, P. (1988). Uterine blood flow and myometrial activity at menstruation, and the action of vasopressin and a synthetic antagonist. *British Journal of Obstetrics and Gynaecology*, 95:898–904.

Maigaard, S., Forman, A. & Andersson, K.-E. (1985a). Differences in contractile activation between human myometrium and intramyometrial arteries. *Acta Physiologica Scandinavica*, 124:371–379.

Maigaard, S., Forman, A. & Andersson, K.-E. (1985b). Different responses to prostaglandin $F_{2\alpha}$ and E_2 in human extra- and intramyometrial arteries. *Prostaglandins*, 30:599–607.

Markee, J.E. (1950). The relation of blood flow to endometrial growth and the inception of menstruation. (In) *Menstruation and its Disorders* (Engle, E.T., ed.), pp.165–185. Springfield, Illinois, Charles C Thomas.

Prill, H.J. & Götz, F. (1961). Blood flow in the myometrium and endometrium of the uterus. *American Journal of Obstetrics and Gynecology*, 82:102–108.

Turner, R.J. & Carroll, B.A. (1979). Ultrasound appearance of decidual reaction in the uterus during normal pregnancy. *American Journal of Roentgenology*, 133:493–496.

Tulenko, T.N. (1979). Regional sensitivity to vasoactive polypeptides in the human umbilicoplacental vasculature. *American Journal of Obstetrics and Gynecology*, 135:629–636.

Van Herendael, B.J., Stevens, M.J., Flakiewicz-Kula, A. & Hansch, C.H. (1987). Dating of the endometrium by microhysteroscopy. *Gynecological and Obstetrical Investigation*, 24:114–118.

Zhang, M., Wang, H.-F., Meng, Z. & Huang, H.-Y. (1987). The effect of copper IUD on microcirculation of blood flow in rabbit uterus.*Contraception*, 36:677–685.

Discussion

Naftolin. My questions have to do with whether you believe that these 'messages' are coming from the vessels or from the surroundings of the vessels to the vessels, or both; whether the prostaglandin data deal with a second messenger passed on by a triggered receptor in the vessels, or whether it is prostaglandin coming from outside of the vessels that is doing this; whether you have information about those receptors and the effect of sex steroids on those receptors; whether you have information about where these actions are – small, spiral or straight arteries, or are they veins; and where do typical vasoconstrictors, like angiotensin, and others fit in?

Åkerlund. If we start with the messengers, we know that several neurotransmitters are there. If they are there only by chance, because they are present in other arteries, or whether they have a particular role in the uterus, I do not know. Obviously they could play a role because they are active in low concentrations. There are substances other than neuronal factors which could be important as well: circulatory vasoactive substances such as vasopressin, angiotensin, bradykinins, serotonin, prostaglandins.

With respect to receptors for the messengers, there are several questions which have to be answered. What is the steroid hormonal effect on the receptors? Is there an interaction between estrogen and progesterone, which also have receptors in the uterus, and these vasoactive substances? To what extent do ovarian hormones influence receptor affinity, receptor concentration, release, plasma and tissue concentrations of vasoactive substances? All this has to be studied in the human, since there are marked species differences. Regarding prostaglandins, they certainly play a role as local tissue hormones or local messengers, but that role is difficult to define.

At which level of the arteries vasoactive substances have effects, I do not know. However, it is too simple to look at the main human uterine artery. You have to go down into the tissue to see the responses of the finer branches. I am sure the technique can be improved so that we can soon study very small intramyometrial arteries, and hopefully even the spiral arteries. Not until then will we know whether they really contract or not.

Casey. Let me take this opportunity to tell the group about another factor that we have not heard about yet. Endothelin, a newly described peptide, is a very potent vasoconstrictor that is produced in endothelial cells. It was cloned, the sequence was elucidated and the factor itself was purified by a group of Japanese investigators (Itoh *et al.*, 1988; Kimura *et al.*, 1988; Yanagisawa *et al.*, 1988a, 1988b). Recently, we found that this factor will stimulate contraction of strips of myometrial smooth muscle; it also causes an increase in intracellular calcium concentration in myometrial smooth muscle cells. Until last week, endothelin was known to be produced only by endothelial cells. But we found that mRNA for preproendothelin is expressed in human amnion cells, which are epithelial cells. Thus, with the potential for production in various cell types, this substance may be important in vasoconstriction of endometrial vessels.

King. I am not quite clear how these studies relate to the topic of the meeting, i.e. the components of the contraceptive pill.

Åkerlund. Ovarian steroids can have an important influence on the actions of a peptide. We have shown that the vasopressin concentration in plasma varies throughout the menstrual cycle with a peak level at ovulation in healthy women. We have also shown that estrogen stimulates the secretion of vasopressin, and that progestogens counteract that stimulatory effect. We have also shown by in-vivo recordings of intrauterine pressure that the effects of this peptide as well as of $PGF_{2\alpha}$ are modulated by ovarian steroids. In women with dysmenorrhea, oral contraceptives modulate both the spontaneous contractile activity and the effect of prostaglandin $F_{2\alpha}$ and vasopressin.

King. So does that mean we should interpret effects of estrogen and progestogen on these systems as being indirect effects by other agents or can one still think in terms of them as a direct effect on the vessels? For example, is estrogen influencing the production of vasopressin or analogous compounds?

Åkerlund. Obviously, the effect can be two sided. Ovarian hormones can influence both the secretion and the responsivity, that is mainly receptor concentration and affinity in technical terms.

Findlay. I refer to your comment about the differential response of uterine artery. I think this is an interesting and important point because if we are going to study the function of those cells, particularly *in vitro* in isolated systems, are we going always to have to use uterine vessels and, in particular, are we going to have to use vessels from specific segments in the endometrium? Is one piece of the spiral artery going to respond differently from another one?

Åkerlund. No, the difference seems to be between extra- and intrauterine arteries. When you dissect out arteries from within the myometrial tissue, they respond differently from the main branches of the uterine artery.

Baird. I also think that it is important to consider whether these responses to variations are really involved with the mechanisms of menstruation. I would like to put forward the view that really we would have to look very hard to find a better candidate than the prostaglandins. If we are going to think of substances which induce menstruation, they have to be able to produce the changes which occur in the blood vessels at the time of menstruation and their production has to be responsive to changes in steroid hormones that are known to produce menstruation. We have used an in-vitro model to study the effects of prostaglandins and other substances on the endometrial blood vessels, namely the explant of endometrium in the immunologically privileged site of the hamster cheek pouch. Dr Cheng Zhu from China and Dr Margaret Abel developed this model when they were in Edinburgh some years ago (Abel *et al.*, 1982), and as far as I know nobody has repeated it, largely because it requires a great deal of dedication to carry out this sort of work.

If I might just summarize the evidence that prostaglandins are involved in the changes in blood vessels that occur at menstruation, I think there is little doubt that the endometrium can produce prostaglandins F_{2a} and E_2 in response to changes in steroid hormones. In this model it is possible to induce menstruation by steroid treatment with estradiol and progesterone followed by withdrawal of progesterone. Menstruation will occur and the changes in endometrial blood flow which occur in response to this withdrawal of progesterone are, first, a vasoconstriction, as Markee described in the monkey model, followed by vasodilatation and bleeding. Now, that change in endometrial blood vessel can be produced by the local administration of prostaglandin F_{2a} onto those explants. I think until somebody comes up with a better candidate, a good working hypothesis is that the vasoconstriction which precedes the onset of bleeding is induced by PGF_{2a} released by the endometrium in response to withdrawal of progesterone.

Granström. If we are discussing the effects on vasodilatation or vasoconstriction of prostanoids, are we not forgetting the more potent compounds thromboxane and prostacyclin?

Åkerlund. Yes, but the effects of these compounds are more straightforward and well known. The topic of my talk was new information obtained since 1979.

Cornillie. In the WHO publication of 1980 you mentioned that histamine could be important (Åkerlund, 1980). It has been shown at least in venules of several tissues, that the endothelial cells have histamine receptors. After the histamine binds to the receptor, vasodilatation seems due to the opening of the junctions. Do you have any good reason for not mentioning or not using histamine in your techniques or does histamine have no effect on arteries and just acts on venules?

Åkerlund. We have not studied histamine, but I agree, it would be worthwhile doing so.

Naftolin. I understand what Dr Baird is saying, but I think that it becomes very important to separate experiments on vessels from experiments on menstruation. The evidence that we have indicates that any vessel given enough stimulus responds to estrogen the same way as any other vessel does. This evidence is in the cardiovascular system, e.g. cerebral blood flow, cardiac blood flow, muscle blood flow. The same things that affect vessels affect them throughout the body and respond to sex steroids. Studies on vessels need not be restricted to studies on uterine blood vessels to have implications for menstruation.

Baird. Dr Åkerlund, I just wonder how relevant those in-vitro studies are to the mechanism of menstruation. You have demonstrated that during a uterine contraction there is a marked diminution in blood flow *in vivo*. If you place prostaglandin $F_{2\alpha}$ into the uterus, you get a contraction and a decrease in uterine blood flow. So how do you explain the dilatation of uterine blood arteries when exposed to $PGF_{2\alpha}$ *in vitro*?

Åkerlund. There are two major mechanisms by which $PGF_{2\alpha}$ could influence uterine blood flow: by effects on the myometrial activity and by effects on the smooth muscle of the vessel walls. The first mechanism of uterine contractions could be important, since in the non-pregnant uterus much higher intrauterine pressures can occur than in the pregnant uterus. To this should be added that uterine arteries can respond differently to $PGF_{2\alpha}$.

Baird. But it is not only an effect on myometrial contractility because we can demonstrate a direct effect on endometrial blood vessels in the endometrial explants in hamster cheek pouches, where there is no myometrium present at all.

References

Abel, M.H., Zhu, C. & Baird, D.T. (1982). An animal model to study menstrual bleeding. *Research and Clinical Forums*, **4**(4):25–34.

Åkerlund, M. (1980). Non-prostaglandin factors influencing the microcirculation of the endometrium. (In) *Endometrial Bleeding and Steroidal Contraception* (Diczfalusy, E., Fraser, I.S., Webb, F.T.G., eds.), pp.246–265. Bath, England, Pitman Press.

Itoh, Y., Yanagisawa, M., Ohkubo, S., Kimura, C., Kosaka, T., Inoue, A., Ishida, N., Mitsui, Y., Onda, H., Fujino, M. *et al.* (1988). Cloning and sequence analysis of cDNA encoding the precursor of a human endothelium-derived vasoconstrictor peptide, endothelin: identity of human and porcine endothelin. *FEBS Letters*, **231**:440–444.

Kimura, S., Kasuya, Y., Sawamura, T., Shinmi, O., Sugita, Y., Yanagisawa, M., Goto, K. & Masaki, T. (1988). Structure-activity relationships of endothelin: importance of the C-terminal moiety. *Biochemical and Biophysical Research Communications*, **156**:1182–1186.

Yanagisawa, M., Inoue, A., Ishikawa, T., Kasuya, Y., Kimura, S., Kumagaye, S.-I.,

Nakajima, K., Watanabe, T.X., Sakakibara, S., Goto, K. & Masaki, T. (1988a). Primary structure, synthesis, and biological activity of rat endothelin, an endothelium-derived vasoconstrictor peptide. *Proceedings of the National Academy of Science USA*, **85**:6964–6967.

Yanagisawa, M., Kurihara, H., Kimura, S., Tomobe, Y., Kobayashi, M., Mitsui, Y., Yazaki, Y., Goto, K. & Masaki, T. (1988b). A novel potent vasoconstrictor peptide produced by vascular endothelial cells. *Nature*, **332**:411–415.

Endometrial hemostasis

H.M. HOURIHAN, B.L. SHEPPARD* AND I.A. BROSENS

Department of Obstetrics and Gynaecology, University Hospital, Leuven, Belgium.
**TCD Department of Obstetrics and Gynaecology, Sir Patrick Dun Research Centre,
St James's Hospital, Dublin, Ireland.*

Abstract

Changes which occur in endometrial hemostatic properties throughout the menstrual cycle are reviewed, as are the effects of steroid hormones and intrauterine devices on endometrial hemostasis. The results of a study investigating the effects of levonorgestrel (20 μg/day) administered via a vaginal ring are also discussed.

It has been shown that the level of fibrinolytic activity varies throughout the menstrual cycle: it rises during the proliferative phase, reaches a maximum at midcycle, declines during the secretory phase, and rises again premenstrually. Little is known about the endometrial levels of the various coagulation factors apart from Factor VIII which appears to respond to changes in the levels of the ovarian hormones, increased activity being present during the proliferative phase and decreased activity during the secretory phase.

In patients with IUDs, increased bleeding has been attributed to a higher level of fibrinolytic activity. Vascular defects showing little or no hemostatic response may be due to increased fibrinolytic activity.

Mast cells have been associated with increased endometrial bleeding; they contain histamine and heparin which may play a role in this bleeding. Significantly higher levels of histamine are found in menstrual fluid than in peripheral blood and higher levels of heparin-like activity have been found in the uterine fluid of women with menorrhagia.

A study of the effects of levonorgestrel administered via a vaginal ring showed that endometrial levels of tissue plasminogen activator (tPA) did not change significantly following treatment. Significantly higher levels of tPA were found in normal premenstrual endometrium when compared with mid/late secretory phase endometrium. Following treatment with levonorgestrel, the endometrium was found to have significantly fewer arterioles. Treatment patients who had longer bleeding episodes had significantly lower numbers of endometrial mast cells. Increased numbers of hemostatic plugs were found in endometrial veins and capillaries following exposure to levonorgestrel. This study shows that low-dose levonorgestrel has an effect on the endometrial vasculature and on its hemostatic response to endometrial bleeding.

Introduction

Following menstruation, four possible mechanisms are thought to play roles in uterine hemostasis: myometrial contraction, vasoconstriction, tissue regeneration and hemostatic plug formation. Bartelmez (1941) found that the intimal arteries at the endometrial/myometrial junction were surrounded by contracting longitudinal muscle fibres which he claimed played a role in reducing or even stopping bleeding. Meyer-Rüegg (1928) believed that vasoconstriction was responsible for the control of hemostasis during menstruation. Although it is known that vasoconstriction is important for the arrest of bleeding in larger vessels, the role it plays in controlling bleeding from smaller vessels is far from clear (Christiaens, 1983). It has also been suggested that tissue regeneration plays a role in the arrest of menstrual bleeding as re-epithelialization coincides with the cessation of menstrual flow (Beller, 1971). However, hemostatic plug formation is now thought to be one of the most important factors in hemostasis of endometrial blood vessels: studies have shown that fibrin and intravascular thrombi play a role in the very early stages of menstruation (Sixma *et al.*, 1979; Christiaens *et al.*, 1980).

Uterine fibrinolysis during the menstrual cycle

Fibrinolytic activity results from the balance between plasminogen activators and their inhibitors and those of plasmin. Plasminogen activators are present in blood and body fluids; they are produced by endothelial cells, by migratory cells and by cells involved in tissue remodelling such as activated macrophages (Unkeless *et al.*, 1974) and granulocytes (Granelli-Piperno *et al.*, 1977). The best known mammalian activators are urokinase and tissue plasminogen activator, both found in the endometrium where they are thought to be responsible for the fluidity of menstrual blood. Increased menstrual blood loss has been correlated with an increase in fibrinolytic activity (Rybo, 1966), and inhibitors of plasminogen activators have been shown to decrease menstrual blood loss (Nilsson & Rybo, 1965, 1967).

Casslén (1981) found that fibrinolytic activity paralleled activator content in uterine fluid during the menstrual cycle. The fibrinolytic activity of myometrial extracts was found always to be higher than that of endometrial extracts, with levels of activity of the endometrium and myometrium running parallel during the menstrual cycle (Shaw *et al.*, 1980). Using the fibrin slide technique, it has been demonstrated that fibrinolytic activity during the proliferative phase of the menstrual cycle is confined mainly to small blood vessels and during the luteal phase additional superficial lysis is present (Luginbuhl & Picoff, 1966; Weiss & Beller, 1969).

Fibrinolytic activity, endometrial levels of plasminogen activators and their release have been found to vary throughout the menstrual cycle. Albrechtsen (1956) and Rybo (1966) found higher levels of fibrinolytic activity in the luteal phase than in the follicular phase in endometrial extracts. Tauber (1979) found that the highest levels of diffusible plasminogen activators were released from endometrial biopsies during the periovulatory phase. Later studies have shown that plasminogen activator levels and activity in endometrial extracts and uterine fluid rise during the follicular phase, reach a maximum at midcycle, decline during the luteal phase and rise again premenstrually (Shaw *et al.*, 1980; Casslén & Åstedt, 1981).

Fibrinolytic activity and steroid hormones

Studies investigating the effects of various synthetic estrogens and progestogens show that these preparations have varying effects on fibrinolytic activity and the release of plasminogen activators from endometrial tissue. Casslén (1982) found that fibrinolytic activity of uterine fluid gradually increased during the menstrual cycle in oral contraceptive users; it is suggested that this increase contributed an additional contraceptive effect. Casslén and Åstedt (1983) found that treatment of postmenopausal women with ethinyl estradiol resulted in a higher release of tissue plasminogen activator (tPA) and urokinase from endometrial explants, whereas treatment with oral contraceptives containing both ethinyl estradiol and a progestogen resulted in a lower level of release of both activators. The authors conclude that estradiol had a stimulatory effect and progestogens depressed the release of plasminogen activators. Changes in the levels of release of both activators from endometrial explants were found to follow the same pattern during the menstrual cycle.

The effect of hormonal preparations on the release of plasminogen activators from human blood vessels has also been investigated. Åstedt (1972) found that the fibrinolytic activity of veins was not significantly altered following treatment with medroxyprogesterone acetate; d-norgestrel was shown to stimulate the release of tPA from incubated specimens of human veins, whereas ethinyl estradiol was found to have no effect on tissue activator release or on fibrinolytic activity (Kjaeldgaard *et al.*, 1984). Significantly decreased activator activity has been found in veins isolated from women using oral contraceptives for more than 5 years; however, no effect was found following periods of less than 5 years usage (Kjaeldgaard & Larsson, 1986).

Recent studies have used cultured melanoma cells as a model for testing the effect of natural and synthetic steroids on the release of tPA (Kjaeldgaard *et al.*, 1986, 1988). These studies showed that estrogens, particularly ethinyl estradiol and 17β-estradiol, had an inhibitory effect on the production of tPA; progestogens, particularly norethisterone and levonorgestrel, also had an inhibitory effect on tPA release.

Fibrinolytic activity and IUDs

Increased menstrual blood loss is often associated with the use of intrauterine devices (IUDs) (Rybo, 1978). The pathogenesis of bleeding disturbances associated with IUDs is probably multifactorial but the increase in bleeding has been attributed to a higher level of endometrial fibrinolytic activity in the presence of an IUD (Liedholm *et al.*, 1978). Extensive morphological changes are found in endometrium exposed to non-medicated and medicated IUDs (Sheppard, 1987, 1988). Vascular defects consisting of gaps between adjacent endothelial cells and apparent breaks in such cells have been found in endometrium from women using IUDs (Hohman *et al.*, 1977, 1978; Shaw *et al.*, 1979; Sheppard & Bonnar, 1980a, 1980b, 1983). It has been suggested that these defects are caused by trauma to the endometrium which is compressed between a contracting myometrium and the hard surface of a rigid IUD (Shaw, 1982; Sheppard & Bonnar, 1983). A frequent feature of these vascular defects is that they show little or no hemostatic response (Hohman *et al.*, 1978). This lack of response could be due to an increase in fibrinolytic activity as plasminogen activator activity has been shown to be higher in the endometrium of IUD users than non-users (Kasonde & Bonnar, 1976). It has been shown that plasminogen activator activity is higher in tissue surrounding a device than in tissue from areas of endometrium away from a device (Liedholm *et al.*, 1983; Shaw *et al.*, 1983). The fibrinolytic activity of uterine fluid from IUD users was found to be mainly due to plasminogen activator activity; this activity was found to follow the same cyclic pattern in IUD users and non-users and was similar to that found in endometrial tissue extracts (Casslén, 1981).

A possible source of the increased fibrinolytic activity in IUD-exposed endometrium may be leukocytes. Both granulocytes and macrophages produce plasminogen activators (Unkeless *et al.*, 1974; Granelli-Piperno *et al.*, 1977; Foley *et al.*, 1978a). These cells have been found in increased numbers in the endometrium of IUD users (Gupta *et al.*, 1971; Moyer & Mishell, 1971; Sheppard & Bonnar, 1980a).

In contrast to non-medicated and copper-releasing IUDs, the progesterone-releasing IUD is associated with a reduction in menstrual blood loss, and both quantitative and qualitative studies have shown no change in fibrinolytic activity in endometrium exposed to progesterone-releasing IUDs (Liedholm *et al.*, 1978; Bonnar & Sheppard, 1985). This lack of change has been attributed to the increased decidual reaction seen in endometrium following exposure to progesterone-releasing devices (Liedholm *et al.*, 1978). It has been shown that decidua lacks fibrinolytic activity (Owers & Blandau, 1971) and contains high levels of fibrinolytic inhibitors (Liedholm & Åstedt, 1976).

Coagulation in the endometrium

Although fibrinolytic changes in endometrial tissue have been investigated for many years, coagulation factors have received little attention. Quantitative studies have been carried out on the levels of various coagulation factors in menstrual blood and in peripheral blood throughout the menstrual cycle (for review see Hahn, 1980).

Johannisson (1986) found that the synthesis of Factor VIII in human endometrial endothelial cells *in vitro* increased following exposure to estradiol whereas progesterone was found to have no effect. In a recent study Zhu and Gu (1988) looked at Factor VIII activity throughout the cycle. No activity was found in the endometrial glands and stroma; activity was found in the endothelial cells, with cyclic changes being seen which could suggest that

Factor VIII activity responds to ovarian hormone stimulation. A gradual increase in activity was seen from the early to the late proliferative phase, with a decreased activity being seen during the secretory phase of the menstrual cycle. No activity was found during the late secretory and menstrual phase of the cycle.

Mast cells in the endometrium

Mast cells contain preformed heparin, histamine and eosinophil chemotactic factors. The majority of mast cells are present in the myometrium of the uterine wall; their numbers are low in the endometrium and their function in this tissue is not clear. As in other types of tissue they are often found adjacent to capillaries and small venules and this would seem to suggest that they have a secretory role.

Significantly higher levels of histamine are found in menstrual fluid than in peripheral blood (Drudy & Sheppard, unpublished observations). Cyclical changes in histamine concentrations have been reported in the human endometrium/myometrium throughout the menstrual cycle. The highest levels of histamine are found in the uterine wall in the late secretory phase of the cycle but there are no differences in histamine concentrations between women with normal menstrual loss and patients with dysfunctional uterine bleeding (Drudy, 1987).

Recent studies have shown low levels of histamine (<10 μmol) to stimulate the release of the tPA and Factor VIII from cultured human endothelial cells (Hanss & Collen, 1987; Hamilton & Sims, 1987). Mast cells release histamine as part of the acute inflammatory response or the foreign body response. Mehra *et al.* (1970) suggested that the metabolic products of mast cells may be responsible for the excessive bleeding seen in patients following the insertion of an IUD, as mast cells were found to be increased during bleeding episodes. A reduction in the level of IUD-induced bleeding has been reported following treatment with antihistamines (Bedi *et al.*, 1968). The heparin content of mast cells may also play a role in the hemostatic events of the endometrium as Foley *et al.* (1978b) found higher levels of heparin-like activity present in the uterine fluid of women with menorrhagia and following the insertion of an IUD.

A study of the effects of levonorgestrel on endometrial tissue plasminogen activator and morphologic and morphometric features of endometrial blood vessels

A study of the endometrial vasculature prior to and following exposure to low-dose levonorgestrel administered via a vaginal ring was undertaken. Vessel numbers of the functional endometrium were quantitated by light microscopy as were mast cell numbers and the level of fibrin deposition. Vascular features such as the presence of contracted endothelial cells, endothelial gaps and hemostatic plugs were quantitated by electron microscopy. The levels of endometrial tissue plasminogen activator prior to and following treatment were also measured.

This study was part of a multicentre clinical trial on the effect of levonorgestrel on endometrial function. Other parts, following the same clinical protocol, investigated the effect of levonorgestrel on endometrial prostaglandin metabolism, protein synthesis and lysosomal enzymes; the preliminary reports of these studies are published in this volume (respectively, Elder *et al.*, 1990; White *et al.*, 1990; Cornillie *et al.*, 1990).

Patients and methods

Thirty-nine women with regular menstrual cycles and without any gynecological disorder or hormonal therapy were selected. Their ages ranged from 29 to 42 years with a mean of 34 years. They were followed during a control cycle with basal body temperature and three times weekly blood sampling for estradiol and progesterone and they were requested to fill in a menstrual diary. On the second day of the next menstrual cycle, a vaginal ring, releasing 20 μg levonorgestrel/day, was inserted and left for 90 days.

In the third treatment month, from day 60 after the ring insertion onwards, blood samples were drawn three times weekly for measurements of estradiol and progesterone and once weekly for levonorgestrel and sex hormone-binding globulin (SHBG). Two endometrial biopsies were scheduled on day 24–26 of the control cycle and day 84–87 of the study period. Biopsies were performed with a Masterson aspiration curette and yielded about 50–100 mg of wet weight tissue in control cycles and 20–50 mg in study cycles.

Tissue plasminogen activator was extracted from the endometrial tissue by homogenizing in 2 mol/l NaSCN (pH 7.75); the homogenate was agitated for 1 hour at room temperature. Following centrifugation at 2400 rpm for 10 minutes, the supernatant was removed and dialyzed against 0.04 mol/l phosphate buffer (pH 7.4) containing 0.14 mol/l NaCl (PBS). Immunoreactive levels of tPA were measured using an enzyme-linked immunosorbent assay (Holvoet *et al.*, 1985).

A second section of the biopsy was immersed in cold fixative – 2.5 % glutaraldehyde in 0.1 mol/l phosphate buffer (pH 7.2) at 4°C – dissected into small blocks and post-fixed in 1% osmium tetroxide in 0.1 mol/l phosphate buffer (pH 7.2) at 4°C. This was followed by dehydration in a graded series of alcohol and embedded in epon. Semithin sections (1 μm) were cut and stained by the PAS/toluidine blue method (Humphrey & Pittman, 1974). These sections were used to quantitate vessel numbers by light microscopy (x 400), with 15–20 fields being examined in sections from each biopsy. Ultrathin sections were stained with uranyl acetate and lead citrate; ultrastructural vascular features were quantitated in veins and capillaries from each biopsy.

Table 1. *Immunoreactive levels of tPA in the endometrium during the luteal phase of the menstrual cycle*

Cycle stage	n	Mean (SEM) ng/mg protein
Mid/late secretory	16	1.98 (0.3)
Premenstrual	9	3.94 (1.0)

Note:
p⟨0.05.

Table 2. *Immunoreactive levels of tPA prior to and following exposure to levonorgestrel*

Group	n	Mean (SEM) ng/mg protein
Control	12	2.41 (0.83)
Levonorgestrel	12	4.36 (0.94)

A separate block of tissue was fixed in Bouins fluid for 24 hours, dehydrated and embedded in paraffin. Sections (5 μm) were cut and stained by the uranyl nitrate metachromatic method for mast cells, the Martius scarlet blue method for fibrin, and hematoxylin and eosin for routine examination of endometrial blood vessels. Quantitative work was carried out on 15–20 fields in sections from each biopsy.

Data were compared using Student's 't' test, except in the case of dilated veins and mast cells when the Wilcoxon Signed Rank and Wilcoxon Rank Sum tests were used.

Results

Immunoreactive levels of tPA

Immunoreactive levels of tPA in control endometrial samples ranged from 0.5 ng/mg to 9.5 ng/mg protein. A significant increase (p⟨0.05) was found in tPA during the premenstrual phase when compared with the mid to late secretory phase of the cycle (Table 1).

Immunoreactive levels of tPA in endometrium ranged from 0.9 ng/mg to 11.1 ng/mg protein following exposure to levonorgestrel. The difference in the levels between the treatment group and the control group was not significant (Table 2). The difference in the levels of endometrial tPA between treatment patients with normal bleeding when compared with those having longer bleeding episodes was found not to be significant.

Table 3. *Endometrial blood vessel numbers, mean (SEM)*

Group	n	Arterioles	Veins	Capillaries	Dilated veins
Control	23	1.75 (0.13)	1.48 (0.06)	3.07 (0.25)	0
Levonorgestrel	23	0.99 (0.11)*	1.52 (0.13)	2.96 (0.16)	0.009 (0.02)

Note:
*p⟨0.001.

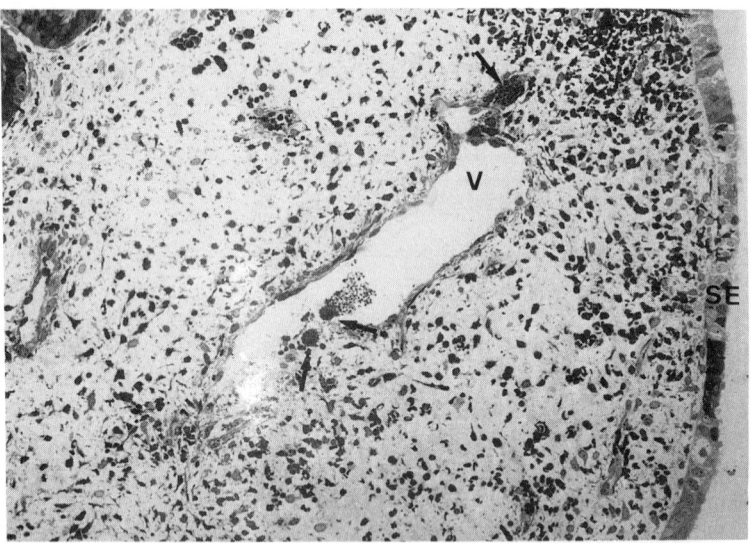

Fig. 1 A section of endometrium following exposure to levonorgestrel. A large dilated vein (V) is present just below the surface epithelium (SE). Thrombi (arrows) are present in the vessel lumen and adhering to the vessel wall (x 500).

Morphometric measurements of endometrial blood vessels

The numbers of arterioles, veins, capillaries and dilated veins in the endometrium prior to and following exposure to levonorgestrel can be seen in Table 3. A significant decrease (p⟨0.001) was found in the number of arterioles in the treatment group; these vessels did not differ significantly in ultrastructure when compared with corresponding vessels of the control group. No difference was found in the numbers of veins and capillaries between the two groups. Endometrial vessel numbers did not correlate with endometrial levels of tPA. A low incidence of dilated vessels (Fig. 1) was seen in a small number of treatment samples; however, the number of this type of vessel was found not to

Table 4. *Endometrial mast cell numbers*

Group	n	Mean (SEM)/mm²
Control	21	1.19 (0.5)
Levonorgestrel	21	3.56 (0.9)

Table 5. *Endometrial mast cell numbers following exposure to levonorgestrel*

Group	n	Mean (SEM)/mm²
Non-bleeders	14	4.62 (1.2)
Bleeders	14	1.03 (0.2)

Note:
$p < 0.002$.

be statistically significant. No difference was seen in the numbers of dilated vessels between the treatment group who had normal bleeding patterns and those who experienced longer bleeding episodes.

Morphometric measurement of endometrial mast cells
No significant variation was found in mast cell numbers of the functional endometrium throughout the secretory phase of the cycle. Mast cell numbers prior to and following exposure to levonorgestrel can be seen in Table 4. The increased number of mast cells seen in the treatment group was found not to be statistically significant. Mast cell numbers in endometrium from treatment patients who had normal bleeding patterns were found to be significantly higher ($p < 0.002$) than those of treatment patients who experienced longer or irregular bleeding episodes (Table 5).

Fibrin deposition in the endometrium
Fibrin, extra- or intravascular deposits were not seen in the majority of biopsies of both groups; the difference in the levels of deposition between the two groups was not significant. Intravascular fibrin, when present, was usually found in the spiral arterioles, though it was also seen in a small number of veins in both groups. Small extravascular deposits of fibrin were seen in the majority of late secretory and premenstrual biopsies by electron microscopy. These deposits were too small to be seen by light microscopy.

Table 6. *Ultrastructural features of endometrial veins and capillaries, mean (SEM)%*

Group	n	Contracted endothelial cells	Gaps in the endothelium	Hemostatic plugs
Control	25	63.3 (3.3)	10.7(1.3)	1.16 (0.35)
Levonorgestrel	25	66.5 (2.8)	13.6 (1.7)	4.21 (0.77)*

Note:
*$p < 0.001$.

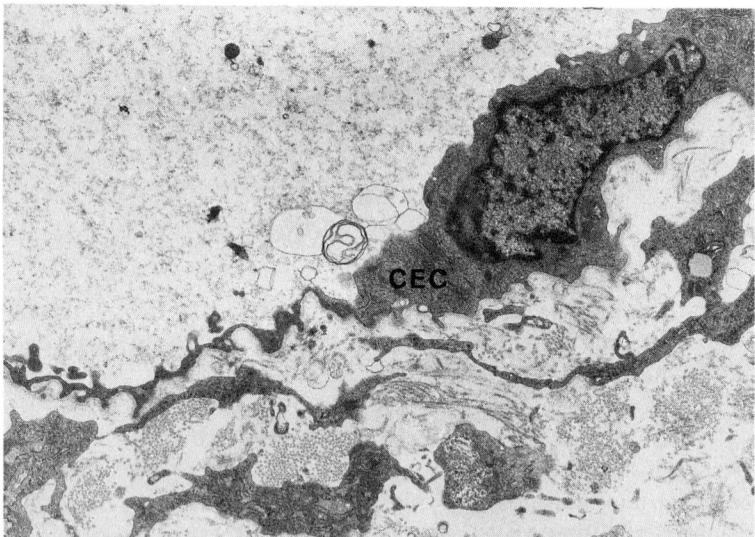

Fig. 2 Section of a vein with a contracted endothelial cell (CEC) from a control endometrial biopsy ($\times$ 5600).

Morphometric measurement of ultrastructural features of endometrial blood vessels

Forty endometrial veins and capillaries were examined in each biopsy. The percentages of vessels possessing contracted endothelial cells, endothelial gaps and hemostatic plugs can be seen in Table 6. The majority of veins and capillaries of both control and treatment specimens were found to have at least one contracted endothelial cell per vessel profile (Fig. 2). No difference was seen between the levels of contracted endothelial cells of the two groups. Gaps in the endothelial lining of veins and capillaries were almost always bordered

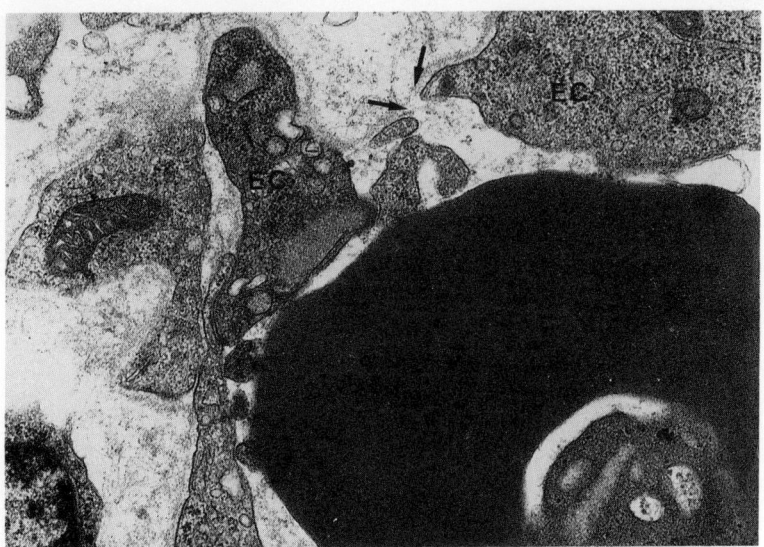

Fig. 3 Section of an endometrial capillary following exposure to levonorgestrel. A gap (arrows) can be seen between the endothelial cells (EC). An erythrocyte (E) is present in the vessel lumen (× 19000).

by at least one contracted endothelial cell (Fig. 3). A higher number of vessels with gaps in their endothelial lining was found in the treatment group, though the difference between the two groups was found not to be statistically significant. Following exposure to levonorgestrel, there was a significant increase (p⟨0.001) in the number of thrombi or hemostatic plugs (Fig. 4) occluding gaps in the vessel walls. Thrombi varied in composition from single platelet plugs to large platelet aggregates, with a small number of platelet and fibrin thrombi also being seen in specimens from both groups.

Comments

The levels of immunoreactive tPA in the endometrium were found to vary throughout the secretory phase of the menstrual cycle; a significant increase was found in the premenstrual phase when compared to the mid and late secretory phase of the cycle. Similar findings have been reported for the levels of plasminogen activators in the endometrium and in the fibrinolytic activity of uterine fluid (Shaw *et al.*, 1980; Casslén & Åstedt, 1981).

No correlation was found between the levels of tPA and the vessel numbers of the endometrium, which suggests that as well as endothelial cells, other cells may be producing significant amounts of tPA in the endometrium. Higher

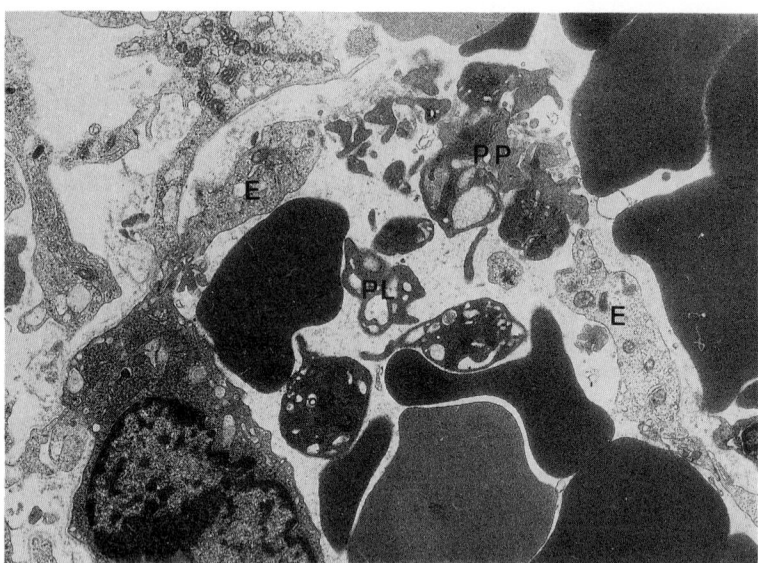

Fig. 4 Section of an endometrial venule from a biopsy following exposure to levonorgestrel. Platelets (PL) are present in the vessel lumen and a platelet plug (PP) can be seen completing the endothelial lining (E) of the vessel (× 6600).

levels of tPA were found in endometrium which had been exposed to levonorgestrel. This increase, although not significant, could be due to the difference in biopsy material as, following exposure to levonorgestrel, the tissue in the majority of cases was found to contain a higher proportion of basal endometrium whereas control samples contained more functional endometrium. Myometrium has been shown to have consistently higher levels of plasminogen activators (Shaw *et al.*, 1980); levels in the basal endometrium may also be higher than those of the stratum functionale. The difference in the tissue levels of immunoreactive tPA of post-treatment patients with longer bleeding episodes when compared with those of post-treatment patients with normal bleeding episodes was not significant; this suggests that tissue levels of tPA do not play a role in increased bleeding incidence. However, changes may occur in the level of tPA activity or in total fibrinolytic activity and in the levels of fibrinolytic inhibitors. Further research is needed in this area.

Changes in vessel number of the functional endometrium are likely to influence the hemostatic events of the endometrium. Increased numbers of vessels have been found in endometrium exposed to IUDs (Hsu *et al.*, 1976; Aparicio *et al.*, 1979). Shaw *et al.* (1979) were the first to quantitate vessel numbers in IUD-exposed endometrium and they suggest that vessel prolife-ration occurs as a result of vessel damage. In contrast, blood vessel numbers have been found to be significantly lower in endometrium exposed to progesterone-releasing IUDs (Shaw *et al.*, 1981). In the present study, levonorgestrel resulted in a significant decrease in the number of arterioles in the endometrium. Low doses of the progestogens norethisterone and levonorgestrel administered orally have also been found to decrease the number of arteries in the endometrium (Hourihan *et al.*, 1986). The decrease in arteries is probably due to the suppression of the development of spiral arteries as progestogen, both in combined regimens and when administered on its own, gives rise to underdeveloped arterioles (Ober, 1970; Kühne *et al.*, 1972; Maqueo, 1980).

Following exposure to levonorgestrel, arterioles did not differ significantly in ultrastructural appearance from those of the control group; they were found to be smaller in size and showed a lack of spiralling when compared with those of the control group. However, none of the ultrastructural changes found following treatment with low-dose oral norethisterone and levonorgestrel (Hourihan, 1985), such as distended endoplasmic reticulum and increased cytoplasmic organelles in endothelial cells and a lack of tonofilaments in the smooth muscle cells, were seen. In the present study no change was found in the numbers of veins and capillaries of the endometrium following exposure to levonorgestrel. Patients taking norethisterone were found to have increased numbers of veins and dilated veins in the functional endometrium (Hourihan *et al.*, 1986). A small number of dilated vessels were found in a minority of treatment biopsies. The presence of this type of vessel in the endometrium has been associated with the use of progestogenic preparations (Grant, 1969). Ludwig (1982) found dilated veins adjacent to the surface epithelium in patients with intermenstrual spotting or irregular bleeding during progestatio-nal steroid treatment. No difference was seen in the number of dilated vessels between the treatment group who had normal bleeding patterns and those who experienced longer or irregular bleeding episodes. This would indicate that dilated vessels in the functional endometrium did not contribute to the increased bleeding found in a large number of treatment patients.

Endometrial mast cell numbers did not vary significantly throughout the secretory phase of the cycle; a higher though not significant increase was found following exposure to levonorgestrel. Mast cell numbers in endometrium from treatment patients with normal bleeding patterns were found to be higher than those in endometrium from patients who had longer bleeding episodes. The lower numbers of mast cells in endometrium of patients with increased bleeding may be due to increased mast cell degranulation as, following degranulation, endometrial mast cells cannot be detected by light microscopy.

Increased numbers of contracted endothelial cells have been found in the endometrium following treatment with norethisterone (Johannisson *et al.*,

1982). In the present study, large numbers of veins and capillaries were found to have at least one contracted endothelial cell per vessel profile, with no difference found between the levels of contracted endothelial cells in control and treatment samples. Histamine or other inflammatory mediators, when applied topically, have been shown to give rise to endothelial cell contraction (Majno *et al.*, 1969). It has been suggested that histamine released by endometrial mast cells had an effect on endometrial endothelial cells. In the present study, no correlation was found between the number of vessels with contracted endothelial cells and mast cell numbers of the endometrium in either the control or treatment group. However, this does not imply that mast cell histamine does not play a role in endothelial cell contraction. In a recent study, Drudy and Sheppard (unpublished observations) found the highest levels of histamine in the uterine wall to occur in the late secretory phase of the menstrual cycle. The present quantitative study used a method which was possibly too coarse to establish a direct relationship between endothelial cell contraction and histamine release from mast cells: it has been shown that histamine in micromolar concentrations can influence various events in endothelial cells (Hamilton & Sims, 1987; Hanss & Collen, 1987).

Gaps in the endothelial lining of endometrial blood vessels were first reported by Hohman *et al.* (1978) in uteri removed at hysterectomy with an IUD *in situ*. A low incidence of microvascular gaps was present in the normal intermenstrual endometrium and the existence of these defects has been attributed to a defective hemostatic system which exists in the endometrium (Shaw *et al.*, 1981). Similar gaps were found up to 5 days prior to menstruation when it is thought that they play a part in the initiation of menstrual bleeding (Christiaens *et al.*, 1980). A small, but not statistically significant, increase in the number of vessel gaps was found following administration of levonorgestrel via a vaginal ring. Increased numbers of vessels with endothelial gaps have also been found following treatment with norethisterone and levonorgestrel (Hourihan, 1985). Gaps between adjacent endothelial cells occur during histamine-mediated contraction of endothelial cells (Majno *et al.*, 1969); in the present study no relationship was found between endometrial mast cells and the level of vessels possessing endothelial gaps.

In both control and treatment samples, at least one of the endothelial cells adjacent to a gap was found to be contracted, but we cannot conclude from this that endothelial contraction always results in gaps in the endothelium, as in the vast majority of cases when contracted endothelial cells were seen, vessels were found to be intact. Endometrial leukocytes may also play a role in the gaps seen between endothelial cells as, when leukocytes adhere to the endothelial surface, the intercellular junctions are opened by active contraction of endothelial actin and myosin filaments in response to mediators released by the leukocytes (Shepro, 1988).

An increase in the number of vessels with hemostatic plugs was found following exposure to levonorgestrel. Although no study of endometrial vasculature in endometrium exposed to the levonorgestrel-releasing IUD has been undertaken, a decrease in the amount of menstrual bleeding which is associated with progestogen-releasing IUDs may also be explained by an increase in the incidence of hemostatic plugs in endometrial blood vessels.

Conclusions and suggestions for further research

In recent years advances have been made in our understanding of the hemostatic events which occur in endometrium during normal menstruation and in increased (dysfunctional) uterine bleeding and bleeding disturbances associated with IUDs. Blood vessels, platelets, mast cells, histamine concentrations, eicosanoids, fibrinolytic activity and changes in coagulation factors have all been implicated as local uterine physiological and pathological processes. However, presently available evidence suggests that intermenstrual bleeding and breakthrough bleeding associated with progestogens may be of a different mechanism to bleeding which occurs during menstruation. Further studies are required which may increase our knowledge in this area; these studies may include the following.

1. Biochemical and morphological comparison of hemorrhagic and non-hemorrhagic areas of endometrium, obtained by hysteroscopy, during intermenstrual bleeding episodes in patients receiving progestogens.
2. Comparison of the effect of high- and low-dose progestogens on endometrial hemostatic mechanisms during menstruation and during intermenstrual bleeding episodes. Of particular interest would be changes in local uterine tissue plasminogen activators and inhibitors in these two different mechanisms.
3. Mast cells, histamine and leukotrienes in the endometrium compared during intermenstrual (breakthrough) bleeding, and the premenstrual and menstrual phases of the cycle.
4. Biochemical and morphological evaluation of endometrial hemostasis in ovular and anovular cycles in patients with normal and excessive, frequent menstrual bleeding.

Acknowledgement

This study received financial support from the Special Programme of Research, Development and Research Training in Human Reproduction, World Health Organization.

References

Albrechtsen, O.K. (1956). The fibrinolytic activity of the human endometrium. *Acta Endocrinologica*, **23**:207–218.

Aparicio, S.R., Bradbury, K., Bird, C.C., Foley, M.E., Jenkins, D.M., Clayton, J.K., Scott, J.S., Rajah, S.M. & McNicol, G.P. (1979). Effect of intrauterine contraceptive device on uterine haemostasis: a morphological study. *British Journal of Obstetrics and Gynaecology*, **86**:314–324.

Åstedt, B. (1972). Fibrinolytic activity of veins during treatment with medroxyprogesterone acetate. *Acta Obstetricia et Gynecologica Scandinavica*, **51**:283–286.

Bartelmez, G.W. (1941). Menstruation. *Journal of the American Medical Association*, **116**:702–704.

Bedi, P., Devi, P.K. & Chaudhury, R.R. (1968). Preliminary report of a trial of a long acting antihistaminic buclizine hydrochloride in patients with bleeding after insertion of an intrauterine device. *Indian Journal of Medical Research*, **56**:884.

Beller, F.K. (1971). Observations on the clotting of menstrual blood and clot formation. *American Journal of Obstetrics and Gynecology*, **111**:535–546.

Bonnar, J. & Sheppard, B.L. (1985). Fibrinolytic activity and intrauterine contraceptive devices. (In) *Intrauterine Contraception. Advances and Future Prospects* (Zatuchni, G.I., Goldsmith, A. & Sciarra, J.J., eds.), pp.307–318. Philadelphia, Harper & Row.

Casslén, B. (1981). Proteinases and proteinase inhibitors in uterine fluid with special reference to IUD-users. *Acta Obstetricia et Gynecologica Scandinavica*, Supplement, **98**:1–38

Casslén, B. (1981). Proteinases and proteinase inhibitors in uterine fluid with special reference to IUD-users. *Acta Obstetricia et Gynecologica Scandinavica*, Supplement, **98**:1–38.

Obstetricia et Gynecologica Scandinavica, **60**:55–58.

Casslén, B. & Åstedt, B. (1983). Reduced plasminogen activator content of the endometrium in oral contraceptive users. *Contraception*, **28**:181–188.

Christiaens, G.C.M.L. (1983). Morphology of haemostasis. *Research and Clinical Forums*, **53**:21–24.

Christiaens, G.C.M.L., Sixma, J.J. & Haspels, A.A. (1980). Morphology of haemostasis in menstrual endometrium. *British Journal of Obstetrics and Gynaecology*, **87**:425–439.

Cornillie, F.J., Brosens, I.A., Marbaix, E., Vael, T., Baudhuin, P. & Courtoy, P.J. (1990). A biochemical study of lysosomal enzymes in control and levonorgestrel-treated human endometria: analysis of total activity and evidence for secretion. (In) *Contraception and Mechanisms of Endometrial Bleeding* (d'Arcangues, C., Fraser, I.S., Newton, J.R. & Odlind, V., eds.), pp.383–406. Cambridge, England, Cambridge University Press.

Drudy, L. (1987). The mast cell and histamine concentration of the human uterus with special reference to dysfunctional uterine bleeding. PhD Thesis, University of Dublin.

Elder, M.G., Patel, L. & White, J.O. (1990). Effects of contraceptive progestogens on prostaglandins. (In) *Contraception and Mechanisms of Endometrial Bleeding* (d'Arcangues, C., Fraser, I.S., Newton, J.R. & Odlind, V., eds.), pp.279–286. Cambridge, England, Cambridge University Press.

Foley, M.E., Griffin, B.D., Zuzel, M., Aparicio, S.R., Bradbury, K., Bird, C.C., Clayton, J.K., Jenkins, D.M., Scott, J.S., Rajah, S.M. & McNicol, G.P. (1978b). Heparin-like activity in uterine fluid. *British Medical Journal*, **2**:322–324.

Foley, M.E., Jenkins, D.M. & McNicol, G.P. (1978a). Production of fibrinolytic enzymes by macrophages on intrauterine contraceptive devices. *British Journal of Obstetrics and Gynaecology*, **85**:551–556.

Granelli-Piperno, A., Vassalli, J.D. & Reich, E. (1977). Secretion of plasminogen activator by human polymorphonuclear leukocytes. Modulation by glucocorticoids and other effectors. *Journal of Experimental Medicine*, **146**:1693–1706.

Grant, E.C.G. (1969). Venous effects of oral contraceptives. *British Medical Journal*, **4**:73–77.

Gupta, P.K., Malkani, P.K. & Bhasin, K. (1971). Cellular response in the uterine cavity after IUD insertion and structural changes of the IUD. *Contraception*, **4**:375–384.

Hahn, L. (1980). Composition of menstrual blood. (In) *Endometrial Bleeding and Steroidal Contraception* (Diczfalusy, E., Fraser, I.S. & Webb, F.T.G., eds.), pp.107–137. Bath, England, Pitman Press.

Hamilton, K.K. & Sims, P.J. (1987). Changes in cytosolic Ca^{2+} associated with von Willebrand factor release in human endothelial cells exposed to histamine. Study of microcarrier cell monolayers using the fluorescent probe indo-1. *Journal of Clinical Investigation*, **79**:600–608.

Hanss, M. & Collen, D. (1987). Secretion of tissue-type plasminogen activator and plasminogen activator inhibitor by cultured human endothelial cells: modulation by thrombin, endotoxin and histamine. *Journal of Laboratory and Clinical Medicine*, **109**:97–104.

Hohman, W.R., Shaw, S.T., Macaulay, L. & Moyer, D.L. (1977). Vascular defects in human endometrium caused by intrauterine contraceptive devices: an electron microscope study. *Contraception*, **16**:507–522.

Hohman, W.R., Shaw, S.T., Macaulay, L. & Moyer, D.L. (1978). Ultrastructural haemostasis in response to vascular injury induced by intrauterine devices in human endometrium. *Thrombosis Research*, **12**:1037–1050.

Holvoet, P., Cleemput, H. & Collen, D. (1985). Assay of human tissue-type plasminogen activator (tPA) with an enzyme-linked immunosorbent assay based on three murine monoclonal antibodies to tPA. *Thrombosis and Haemostasis*, **54**:684–687.

Hourihan, H.M. (1985). The human endometrial vasculature: the normal menstrual cycle, dysfunctional bleeding and the effect of noresthisterone and levonorgestrel. PhD Thesis, University of Dublin.

Hourihan, H.M. (1985). The human endometrial vasculature: the normal menstrual cycle, dysfunctional bleeding and the effect of norethisterone and levonorgestrel. PhD Thesis, University of Dublin.

Hsu, C., Ferenczy, A., Richart, R.M. & Darabi, K. (1976). Endometrial morphology with copper-bearing intrauterine devices. *Contraception*, **14**:243–260.

Humphrey, C.D. & Pittman, F.E. (1974). A simple methylene blue-azure II basic fuchsin stain for epoxy-embedded tissue sections. *Stain Technology*, **49**:9–14.

Johannisson, E. (1986). Effects of oestradiol and progesterone on the synthesis of DNA and the anti-haemophilic Factor VIII antigen in human endometrial endothelial cells *in vitro*: a pilot study. *Human Reproduction*, **1**:207–212.

Johannisson, E., Landgren, B.M. & Diczfalusy, E. (1982). Endometrial morphology and peripheral steroid levels in women with and without intermenstrual bleeding during contraception with the 300 microgram norethisterone (NET) minipill. *Contraception*, **25**:13–30.

Kasonde, J.M. & Bonnar, J. (1976). Plasminogen activators in the endometrium of women using intrauterine contraceptive devices. *British Journal of Obstetrics and Gynaecology*, **83**:315–319.

Kjaeldgaard, A., Ahlesteen, I., Larsson, B. & Åstedt, B. (1988). Progestogen regulation of tissue plasminogen activator in a human melanoma cell line. *Thrombosis Research*, **49**:287–297.

Kjaeldgaard, A. & Larsson, B. (1986). Long-term treatment with combined oral contraceptives and cigarette smoking associated with impaired activity of tissue plasminogen activator. *Acta Obstetricia et Gynecologica Scandinavica*, **65**:219–222.

Kjaeldgaard, A., Larsson, B. & Åstedt, B. (1984). Regulatory effect of contraceptive steroids on the release of tissue-type plasminogen activator *in vitro*. *Contraception*, **30**:355–362.

Kjaeldgaard, A., Larsson, B. & Åstedt, B. (1986). Estrogen regulation of tissue plasminogen activator in a human melanoma cell line. *Thrombosis Research*, **42**:397–406.

Kühne, D., Seidl, S. & Göretzlehner, G. (1972). Contraceptive treatment with chlormadinone and its effect on the endometrium. A histological investigation. *Endokrinologie*, **59**:295–306.

Liedholm, P. & Åstedt, B. (1976). Intrauterine device increases fibrinolytic activity of the rat endometrium at deciduation, a new aspect of its contraceptive effect. *Experientia*, **32**:226–227.

Liedholm, P., Sjöberg, N.-O., Srivastava, K. & Åstedt, B. (1978). No increase of the fibrinolytic activity of the human endometrium by progesterone-releasing IUD (Progestasert^R). *Contraception*, **17**:531–536.

Liedholm, P., Srivastava, K., Wingerup, L. & Åstedt, B. (1983). Higher fibrinolytic activity in human endometrium in direct contact with an IUD. *Acta Obstetricia et Gynecologica Scandinavica*, **62**:169–170.

Ludwig, H. (1982). The morphologic response of the human endometrium to long-term treatment with progestational agents. *American Journal of Obstetrics and Gynecology*, **142**:796–808.

Luginbuhl, W.H. & Picoff, R.C. (1966). The localization and characteristics of endometrial fibrinolysis. *American Journal of Obstetrics and Gynecology*, **95**:462–467.

Majno, G., Shea, S.M. & Leventhal, M. (1969). Endothelial contraction induced by histamine-type mediators: an electron microscopic study. *Journal of Cell Biology*, **42**:647–672.

Maqueo, M. (1980). Vascular and perivascular changes in the endometrium of women using steroidal contraceptives. (In) *Endometrial Bleeding and Steroidal Contraception* (Diczfalusy, E., Fraser, I.S. & Webb, F.T.G., eds.), pp.138–152. Bath, England, Pitman Press.

Mehra, U., Devi, P.K., Chakravarti, R.N. & Chaudhury, R.R. (1970). The relationship between endometrial mast cell count and bleeding in women following insertion of an intrauterine device. *American Journal of Obstetrics and Gynecology*, **107**:852–856.

Meyer-Rüegg, H. (1928). Zur anatomie der menstruierenden uterusschleimhaut. *Archiv für Gynäkologie*, **133**:747–756.

Moyer, D. & Mishell, D.R. (1971). Reactions of human endometrium to the intrauterine foreign body. II. Long-term effects on the endometrial histology and cytology. *American Journal of Obstetrics and Gynecology*, 111:66–80.

Nilsson, L. & Rybo, G. (1965). Treatment of menorrhagia with epsilon aminocaproic acid. A double blind investigation. *Acta Obstetricia et Gynecologica Scandinavica*, 44:467–473.

Nilsson, L. & Rybo, G. (1967). Treatment of menorrhagia with an antifibrinolytic, tranexamic acid (AMCA). A double blind investigation. *Acta Obstetricia et Gynecologica Scandinavica*, 46:572–580.

Ober, W.B. (1970). Morphologic change in the uterus associated with steroid contraceptive and intrauterine contraceptive devices. *Acta Cytologica (Baltimore)*, 14:156.

Owers, N.O. & Blandau, R.J. (1971). Proteolytic activity of the rat and guinea pig blastocyst *in vitro*. (In) *The Biology of the Blastocyst* (Blandau, R.J., ed.), pp.207–223. Chicago, University of Chicago Press.

Rybo, G. (1966). Plasminogen activators in the endometrium. II. Clinical aspects. Variation in the concentration of plasminogen activators during the menstrual cycle and its relation to menstrual blood loss. *Acta Obstetricia et Gynecologica Scandinavica*, 45:429–450.

Rybo, G. (1978). The IUD and endometrial bleeding. *Journal of Reproductive Medicine*, 20:175–182.

Shaw, S.T. (1982). Endometrial blood vessels, haemostasis and bleeding: effects of non-medicated and progesterone-releasing IUDs. *Research and Clinical Forums*, 4:57–65.

Shaw, S.T., Macaulay, L.K., Aznar, R,, Gonzalez-Angulo, A. & Roy, S. (1981). Effects of a progesterone-releasing intrauterine contraceptive device on endometrial blood vessels: a morphometric study. *American Journal of Obstetrics and Gynecology*, 141:821–827.

Shaw, S.T., Macaulay, L.K. & Hohman, W.R. (1979). Vessel density in endometrium of women with and without intrauterine contraceptive devices: a morphometric evaluation. *American Journal of Obstetrics and Gynecology*, 135:202–206.

Shaw, S.T., Macaulay, L.K., Sun, N.C., Tanaka, M.S. & Roche, P.C. (1983). Changes of plasminogen activator in human uterine tissue induced by intrauterine contraceptive devices. *Contraception*, 27:131–140.

Shaw, S.T., Macaulay, L.K., Tanaka, M.S., Hohman, W.R., Moyer, D.L. & Sun, N.C. (1980). Plasminogen activator in human uterine tissue – relationship to location of sampling and time in ovarian cycle. *Biochemical Medicine*, 24:170–178.

Sheppard, B.L. (1987). Endometrial morphological changes in IUD users: a review. *Contraception*, 36:1–10.

Sheppard, B.L. (1988). The intrauterine contraceptive device. *Clinical Materials*, 3:1–13.

Sheppard, B.L. & Bonnar, J. (1980a). The response of endometrial blood vessels to intrauterine contraceptive devices: an electron microscopic study. *British Journal of Obstetrics and Gynaecology*, 87:143–154.

Sheppard, B.L. & Bonnar, J. (1980b). Scanning and transmission electron microscopy of material adherent to intrauterine contraceptive devices. *British Journal of Obstetrics and Gynaecology*, 87:155–162.

Sheppard, B.L. & Bonnar, J. (1983). The effects of intrauterine contraceptive devices on the ultrastructure of the endometrium in relation to bleeding complications. *American Journal of Obstetrics and Gynecology*, 146:829–839.

Shepro, D. (1988). The American Microcirculatory Society Landis Award lecture. Endothelial cells, inflammatory edema and the microvascular barrier: comments by a 'free radical'. *Microvascular Research*, **35**:246–264.

Sixma, J.J., Christiaens, G.C.M.L. & Haspels, A.A. (1979). Morphological aspects of haemostasis in the uterus during menstruation. *Thrombosis and Haemostasis*, **42**:239.

Tauber, P.F. (1979). Biochemical components of the human endometrium. (In) *The Biology of the Fluids of the Female Genital Tract* (Beller, F.K. & Schumacher, G.F.B., eds.), pp.131–150. New York, Elsevier/North-Holland.

Unkeless, J.C., Gordon, S. & Reich, E. (1974). Secretion of plasminogen activator by stimulated macrophages. *Journal of Experimental Medicine*, **139**:834–850.

Weiss, G. & Beller, F.K. (1969). Tissue activator of the fibrinolytic enzyme in the female reproductive system. *Obstetrics and Gynecology*, **34**:809–819.

White, J.O., Croxtall, J.D. & Elder, M.G. (1990). Effects of contraceptive progestogens on endometrial proteins. (In) *Contraception and Mechanisms of Endometrial Bleeding* (d'Arcangues, C., Fraser, I.S., Newton, J.R. & Odlind, V., eds.), pp.233–239. Cambridge, England, Cambridge University Press.

Zhu, P.D. & Gu, Z. (1988). Observation of the activity of Factor VIII in the endometrium of women with regular menstrual cycles. *Human Reproduction*, **3**:273–275.

Discussion

Clark. If your hypothesis is correct, that degranulation of mast cells is associated with uterine bleeding, would you not have expected to have seen a higher level of histamine in the uterine blood from bleeders? Secondly, would not consumption of a simple combination of antihistamines such as diphenhydramine hydrochloride (H1 blocker) or an antiacid (H2 blocker), be expected to correct the problem produced by histamine release?

Hourihan. Antihistamines have been shown to decrease menstrual blood loss (Bedi *et al.*, 1968), but because they have drastic side-effects they cannot be used to reduce bleeding. I think the reason that we found lower numbers of mast cells is probably because the method we used only measures granulated mast cells. With light microscopy we can only see mast cells by staining the granules.

Clark. But if they degranulated, why did you not find more histamine in the menstrual blood from the women with excessive loss?

Hourihan. In a study that Dr Sheppard and Dr Drudy carried out (unpublished data), no relationship was found between histamine and dysfunctional uterine bleeding. But then dysfunctional uterine bleeding and bleeding due to progestogens are different.

Sheppard. The studies which inspired the mast cell/histamine theory used very old methodology. It has not yet been possible to examine some of the newer antihistamines to study the relationship of histamine to menstrual bleeding. Another point I would like to make is that mast cell numbers and prostacyclin levels are higher in the myometrium. It is also quite evident from a study that we are undertaking that tissue plasminogen activator antigen levels are far higher in the myometrium than they are in the endometrium, and there is quite a dramatic drop in levels during menstruation, when the levels in the endometrium are increased. So it is possible that the tissue plasminogen activator, similarly to the histamine and the mast cells, is being released at the myometrial level, but having its effect on the endometrium.

Bischof. I wonder how the tPA antigen levels correlate with activity? Because you might be measuring two different things.

Hourihan. I agree with you. To get a complete picture you need to study tPA activity, inhibitor levels and inhibitor activity; tPA is only one side of the story. Unfortunately, in this study, we just did not have enough material to measure tPA and inhibitor activities.

Bischof. But do you know if they run in parallel? I mean, it is known, for instance, for antithrombin III that its biological activity is not parallel to its immunoreactivity.

Sheppard. I realize that the high levels of tPA antigen levels could be due to high levels of inhibitor, because this particular technique does measure activator that is bound to inhibitor. We are measuring the inhibitor levels, but I do not have those results to hand at the moment.

King. How do these results fit into the general concept of how progestogens might be influencing the blood vessel changes through the cycle? Could you interpret for us the changes you see, say, in the total fibrinolytic activity and mast cell numbers, with respect to how progestogens are influencing blood changes? What would you see from your data as the sequence of events happening by which progestogens can alter the bleeding pattern?

Hourihan. Well, you are getting an increase in vessel defects, and an altered hemostatic response with progestogens. This altered response may be due to changes in the levels of fibrinolytic activity and progestogens have been shown to decrease fibrinolytic activity.

Sheppard. I do not think we clearly understand if progestogens are having an effect of inhibiting fibrinolytic activity, whether it is suppressing the production of activators or is increasing the production of inhibitors. We know that this occurs during the normal process of menstruation, but we do not understand how this works in relation to progestogen-induced breakthrough bleeding.

Bischof. I am surprised to hear that progesterone is decreasing fibrinolytic activity. We made a different observation. When we tried to culture decidual cells, which are induced by progesterone, in a fibrin matrix, we could not get them for a long time, because the matrix was digested. So, do you know if decidual cells can produce plasminogen instead of the activator, which might change the whole picture?

Hourihan. I know very little about plasminogen activators in decidual cells except that they are supposed to be present in low levels and there are supposed to be high levels of inhibitors. I do not know about plasminogen levels in decidual cells.

Cornillie. Dr Sheppard, in your data on tPA localization by monoclonal antibody in the endometrium and myometrium, there was a very striking difference between the myometrium and the endometrium, but I was not convinced that in the endometrium there was no localization at all. Several cell types may synthesize and present the antigen such as epithelial cells, macrophages and leukocytes. May I ask you at what stage of the cycle the endometrium was taken? Could it be that the main source of tPA before menstruation is the migratory cells which come in, and it is known that at that stage many leukocytes and even macrophages are infiltrating the endometrium?

Sheppard. The data shown (unpublished) in fact comprised a frozen section of the mid to late secretory phase of the cycle. It was not late secretory, when there is the influx of polymorphonuclear leukocytes, but it still showed that the majority of tPA-positive reaction was in the myometrial blood vessels. Only at the late secretory phase of the cycle, when there is quite a large number of blood vessels in the functional endometrium, do we get a positive staining of the blood vessels using the immunohistochemical technique.

References

Bedi, P., Devi, P.K. & Chaudhury, R.R. (1968). Preliminary report of a trial of a long acting antihistaminic buclizine hydrochloride in patients with bleeding after insertion of an intrauterine device. *Indian Journal of Medical Research*, **56**:884.

Factors controlling menstrual blood volume

MARGARET C.P. REES

Nuffield Department of Obstetrics and Gynaecology, John Radcliffe Hospital, Oxford, UK.

Abstract

The control of menstrual blood volume is important since excessive bleeding may lead to iron deficiency anemia and ultimately necessitate hysterectomy. Although menorrhagia may be due to systemic or pelvic pathology, in 50% of cases no abnormality is found and therefore local uterine mechanisms appear to play a significant part in the regulation of menstrual bleeding. The factors which are discussed are prostaglandins, coagulation, fibrinolysis, platelets, and systemic and pelvic pathology.

Introduction

The volume of menstrual blood lost is important to women's well-being since excessive bleeding may lead to iron deficiency anemia and may ultimately necessitate hysterectomy. In 1985, 18600 hysterectomies were performed for menstrual disorders in England (Hospital Inpatient Enquiry, 1985). It is an important reason for consultation to general practitioners in that 30 per 1000 consultations are for excessive menstrual bleeding (Morbidity Statistics from General Practice, 1981–1982).

Menstrual blood loss (MBL) has a skewed distribution, with the mean of 35 ml and the 90th percentile of 80 ml, as found in the classic study of Hallberg *et al.* (1966). It is considered excessive if greater than 80 ml; without treatment such a loss leads to iron deficiency anemia and constitutes objective menorrhagia. Blood losses up to 1500 ml have been measured in some women (Rees, unpublished observations).

Any examination of MBL control must include objective blood loss measurement. It is a vital assessment since women are unreliable judges of their menstrual blood loss (Chimbira *et al.*, 1980). Only 38% of women complaining of menorrhagia have measured losses greater than 80 ml (Fraser *et al.*, 1984). MBL can be easily measured by the alkaline hematin method of Hallberg and Nilsson (1964).

The only major study in which menstruation has been directly observed *in vivo* was the classical work of Markee (1940) using intraocular endometrial implants in the monkey. He described tissue growth, degeneration and regression prior to menstruation, and bleeding from endometrial blood vessels, especially the spiral arterioles. He proposed that the factors which controlled menstrual bleeding were those which regulated hemostasis and tissue growth. Although menorrhagia may be due to systemic or pelvic pathology, no abnormality is found in 50% of cases, and most women with menorrhagia have normal ovulatory cycles (Haynes *et al.*, 1979; Chimbira *et al.*, 1980). Therefore local uterine mechanisms appear to be important in the regulation of menstrual blood loss (Rees, 1987). The factors controlling MBL which will be discussed are prostaglandins, coagulation, fibrinolysis, platelets, systemic and pelvic pathology.

Prostaglandins

Abnormal prostaglandin (PG) levels have been implicated in menorrhagia since the mid 1970s when Willman and colleagues (1976) reported elevated endometrial concentrations of both $PGF_{2\alpha}$ and PGE_2 during the menstrual cycle in women complaining of heavy periods. The structure, biosynthesis and role of PGs in menorrhagia will be discussed. The use of prostaglandin synthase inhibitors to reduce MBL will also be described. Recently, leukotrienes, like PGs also synthesized from arachidonic acid, have been found in uterine tissues. Their role in MBL control will also be examined.

Prostaglandins were first isolated by Goldblatt and von Euler in the 1930s from accessory genital glands and human semen (von Euler, 1935). The association of PGs with menstruation was first reported by Pickles *et al.* (1965), who found high concentrations of $PGF_{2\alpha}$ and PGE_2 in endometrium and menstrual fluid. Later, Wiqvist and colleagues (1971) demonstrated that administration of $PGF_{2\alpha}$ to women during the luteal phase resulted in menstrual bleeding.

Structure

Prostaglandins are 20-carbon polyunsaturated fatty acids containing a 5-membered ring with two 7- and 8-membered carbon side-chains. They are designated prostaglandin A through I, depending on the ring structure. The designations $PGF_{2\alpha}$ and PGF_β differentiate alternate stereochemistries of the hydroxyl group at C9. Prostaglandins belong to the 1, 2, or 3 series depending on whether they contain 1, 2 or 3 double bonds in their side-chains. The principal series in mammalian tissues is the 2 series. The name thromboxane A_2 (TXA_2) was given to the unstable vasoconstrictor substance formed from prostaglandin endoperoxides by platelets. This does not have the basic prostaglandin structure.

Biosynthesis

Prostaglandin synthetic pathways have been extensively reviewed and the short description presented here is based on previous work (Green, 1986) (Fig. 1). PGs are not stored in cells but are rapidly synthesized once the substrate fatty acid precursor, arachidonic acid, becomes available to the appropriate

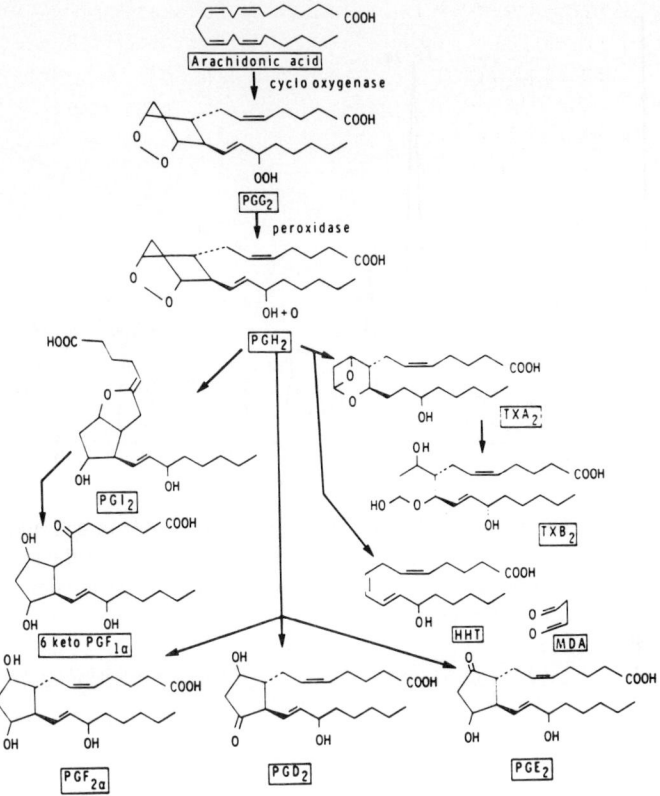

Fig. 1 Prostaglandin biosynthetic pathways.

synthetic enzymes. Arachidonic acid is not present in the free state within cells but is bound in ester linkage to phospholipids. Before PG biosynthesis can begin, free arachidonic acid must be liberated from cellular phospholipids by the action of phospholipases released from lysosomes. Once released, free arachidonic acid is metabolized either through a cyclo-oxygenase-mediated pathway to prostaglandins or by a lipoxygenase pathway to leukotrienes. Both enzyme systems have been identified in human uterine tissues (Demers *et al.*, 1984; Rees *et al.*, 1987) (Figs. 2 and 3).

In PG synthesis, arachidonic acid is converted to the endoperoxide intermediates PGG_2 and PGH_2 through the action of the cyclo-oxygenase and peroxidase enzymes. Cyclo-oxygenase is present mainly in the superficial and glandular epithelium of the endometrium (Rees *et al.*, 1982). PGH_2 and PGG_2 are rapidly converted to the primary prostaglandins $PGF_{2\alpha}$, PGE_2 and PGD_2. PGH_2 is also converted to either TXA_2 or prostacyclin (PGI_2) through the action of thromboxane and prostacyclin synthetase respectively. Human

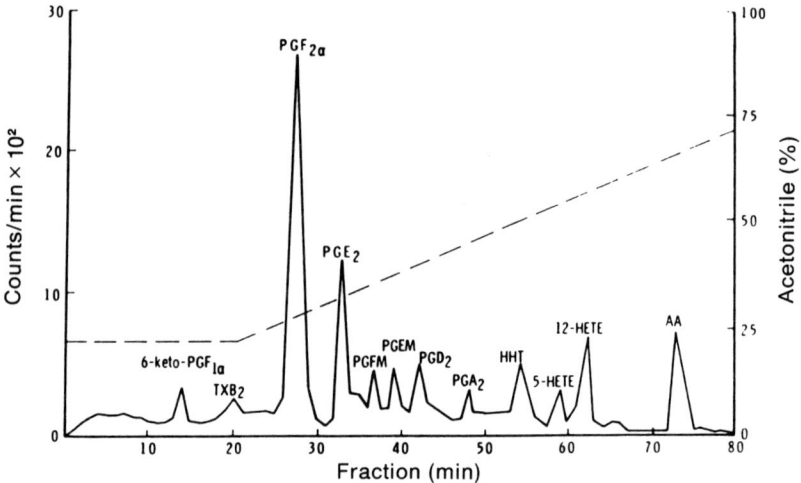

Fig. 2 High-pressure liquid chromatography profile of endometrial arachidonic acid products. PGs are produced as well as the lipoxygenase products 5-HETE and 12-HETE. (Reproduced by permission of Longman Group Ltd. from Demers *et al.*, 1984.)

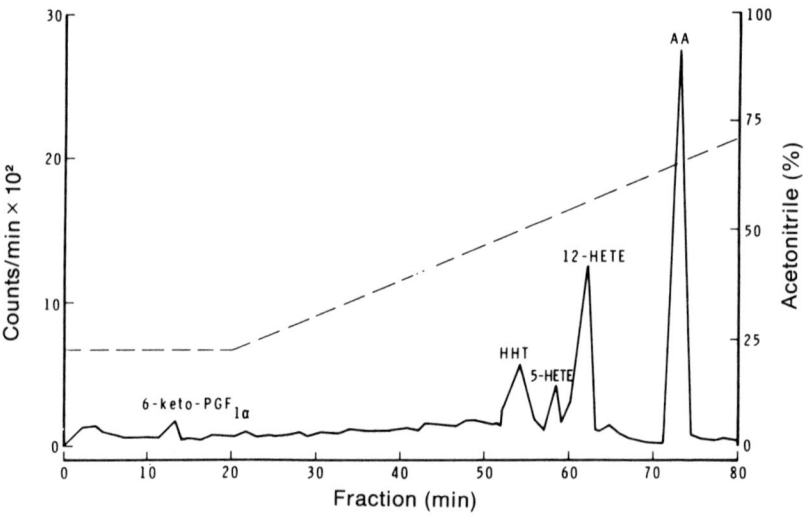

Fig. 3 High-pressure chromatography profile of myometrial arachidonic acid products showing PGs as well as 5-HETE and 12-HETE. (Reproduced by permission of Longman Group Ltd. from Demers *et al.*, 1984.)

uterine tissue has the capacity to produce all these substances (Demers *et al.*, 1984; Rees *et al.*, 1984b).

The first step in leukotriene synthesis is oxygenation at C5 by the 5-lipoxygenase enzyme to form 5-hydroperoxy-eicosatetraenoic acid. It is then converted to leukotriene A_4 by dehydration. This unstable allelic epoxide (LTA_4) is either hydrolyzed forming leukotriene B_4 (LTB_4), or conjugated with glutathione to form leukotriene C_4 (LTC_4). In turn, LTC_4 is metabolized by γ-glutamyl transpeptidase to leukotriene D_4 (LTD_4) and then by cysteinyl glycinase to LTE_4. Release of LTC_4, D_4 and E_4 has been detected in human uterine tissues (Rees *et al.*, 1987).

Prostaglandins and the control of menstrual blood loss volume

Individual PGs have differing effects on hemostasis and thus are involved in the control of menstrual blood loss volume. PGE_2, PGD_2 and PGI_2 cause vasodilatation, while $PGF_{2\alpha}$ and TXA_2 cause vasoconstriction. Platelet aggregation is promoted by TXA_2 and inhibited by PGD_2 and PGI_2 (Smith, 1980; Lundström, 1986; Wiqvist *et al.*, 1983).

Studies in relation to MBL control have examined PGs both in menstrual fluid collected during menstruation and in endometrium and myometrium collected throughout the menstrual cycle. Most include objective MBL measurement.

The levels of PGs in menstrual fluid suggest increased uterine $PGF_{2\alpha}$ and PGE_2 production in menorrhagia, at least during menstruation (Rees *et al.*, 1984a) (Fig. 4). Studies of endometrial and myometrial PGs have principally focused on tissues collected at other times during the menstrual cycle using a variety of in-vitro systems (tissue concentration, incubation, superfusion), each of which has its own limitations (Granström & Samuelsson, 1978; Peek *et al.*, 1985). In general, PG production by uterine tissues collected throughout the menstrual cycle from menorrhagic women is not increased and does not correlate with MBL (Rees *et al.*, 1984b). However, in a limited number of samples obtained during the first 2 days of menstruation when the largest volume of menstrual flow occurs, the data are suggestive of a possible relationship between the volume of menstrual blood loss and $PGF_{2\alpha}$, PGE_2 and 6-keto-$PGF_{1\alpha}$ release by endometrium and myometrium (Rees *et al.*, 1984b).

A shift in endometrial synthesizing capacity towards PGE_2 in menorrhagic women was originally suggested by Smith *et al.* (1981a) but has not been subsequently confirmed (Rees *et al.*, 1984b; Cameron *et al.*, 1987). However, PG receptor studies suggest an altered responsiveness to the vasodilator PGE_2 in menorrhagia. In human uterine tissues, PGE_2 receptors predominate over $PGF_{2\alpha}$ receptors and are found mainly in the myometrium rather than the endometrium (Hofmann *et al.*, 1983; Adelantado *et al.*, 1988). Increased concentrations of PGE receptors are present in myometrial specimens

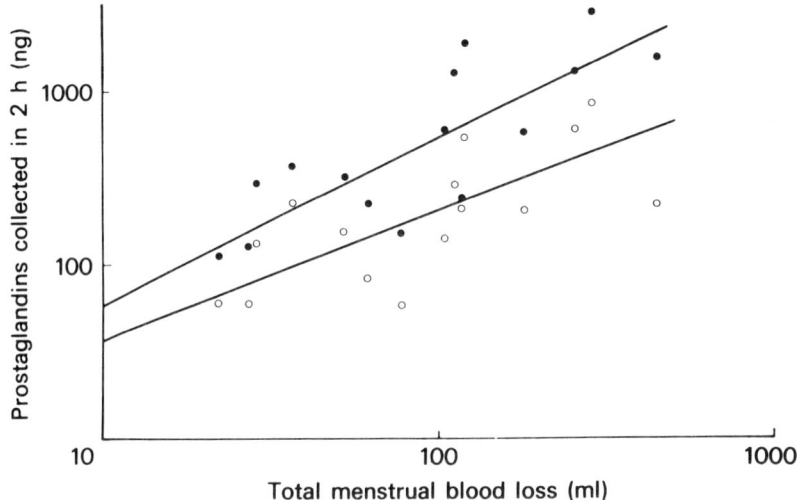

Fig. 4 Correlation between the total amount of $PGF_{2\alpha}$ (closed circles) and PGE_2 (open circles) in menstrual serum collected in 2 hours on day 1 and total MBL for that menstruation. A similar correlation was found on day 2. (Reproduced from Rees *et al.*, 1984a.)

obtained from menorrhagic women and there is a direct correlation between PGE receptor concentration and MBL (Adelantado *et al.*, 1988).

Prostacyclin, the principal myometrial PG product (Abel & Kelly, 1979; Demers *et al.*, 1984; Rees *et al.*, 1984b), has also been examined in menorrhagia. Endometrium from women with menorrhagia is more effective than endometrium from women with normal MBL in enhancing production of the prostacyclin metabolite 6-keto-$PGF_{1\alpha}$ in control preparations of myometrium (Smith *et al.*, 1981b). However, increased 6-keto-$PGF_{1\alpha}$ production by endometrium and myometrium *per se* in menorrhagia has not been found in other studies except during menstruation (Rees *et al.*, 1984b; Makarainen & Ylikorkala, 1986). The suggestion that there may be increased availability of arachidonic acid in uterine tissues obtained from menorrhagic women has led to the study of phospholipase enzymes (Kelly *et al.*, 1984; Bonney & Franks, 1987). Phospholipase C activity was increased in endometrium from menorrhagic women but MBL was not measured.

The leukotrienes have been recently identified in endometrium and myometrium and examined in relation to menorrhagia. However, no correlation was found between leukotriene release in either endometrium or myometrium and menstrual blood loss.

The implication of excessive PG levels in menorrhagia has led to the use of PG synthetase inhibitors in the treatment of this disorder (Turnbull & Rees, 1987). The effectiveness of these agents was first demonstrated by Anderson *et*

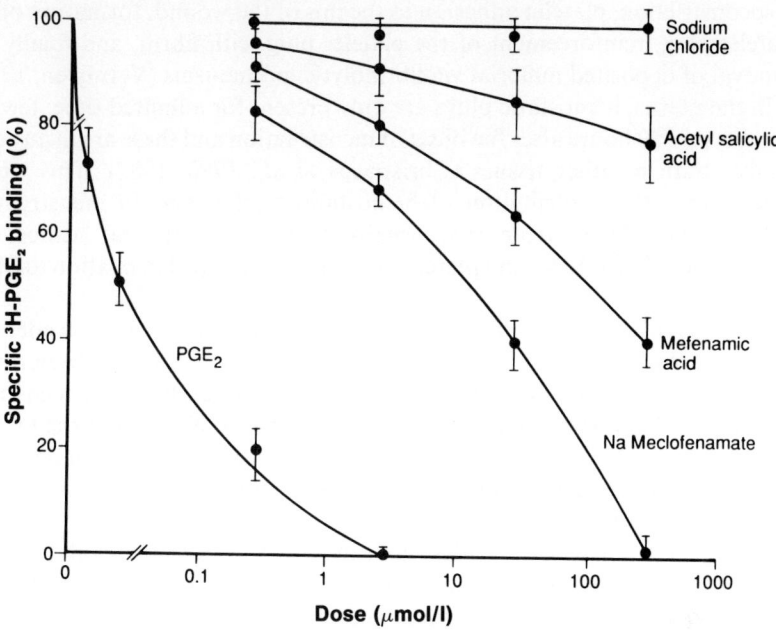

Fig. 5 Inhibition of ^{3}H-PGE$_2$ binding to membrane preparations of human myometrium. (Reproduced by permission from Rees *et al.*, 1988.)

al. (1976). In this study, it was observed that mefenamic acid reduced MBL from a pretreatment mean of 119 ml to 60 ml. These findings have been confirmed in other studies (Fraser *et al.*, 1983). Follow-up 12–15 months after commencing treatment showed that mefenamic acid continued to be effective in reducing MBL (Fraser *et al.*, 1983). Other PG synthetase inhibitors, e.g. ibuprofen, also reduce MBL (Makarainen & Ylikorkala, 1986). Mefenamic acid has been shown to reduce endometrial concentrations of PGF$_{2\alpha}$ and PGE$_2$ (Fraser, 1983). Recently, a dual mode of action has been demonstrated for fenamates: as well as reducing PG synthesis, they also inhibit binding of PGE to its receptor and this additional effect may contribute to their efficacy in the treatment of menorrhagia (Rees *et al.*, 1988) (Fig. 5).

Hemostasis and the control of menstrual blood volume

It has been apparent for many years that the mechanisms by which uterine hemostasis is achieved differ from those found in other tissue systems. Schickele (1912) was the first to observe that menstrual fluid could be kept for several weeks without detecting any obvious clotting. In most tissue systems, hemostasis consists of five somewhat overlapping phenomena: localized vasoconstriction, platelet adhesion to the lips of the wound, formation of the platelet plug, reinforcement of the platelet plug with fibrin, and finally the removal of deposited material via fibrinolytic mechanisms (Vermylen, 1978).

In the uterus, hemostatic plugs are only present for a limited time: few are seen beyond 20 hours after the onset of menstruation and these are in any case smaller than in other tissues (Christiaens *et al.*, 1980, 1982). This would suggest that the contribution of hemostatic mechanisms in menstruating endometrium differs from that usually found in peripheral hemostasis. Coagulation, fibrinolysis and platelets have been examined in relation to MBL control.

The coagulation and fibrinolytic systems have received considerable attention. With regard to fibrinolysis, plasminogen activator has been found in menstrual fluid and endometrium, with increased levels during menstruation (Rybo, 1966; Rees *et al.*, 1985). It is perhaps significant that the human uterus contains the highest level of extractable tissue plasminogen activator (200–400 μg/kg) of any organ examined: peripheral blood contains 2–4 μg/l (Wallen *et al.*, 1977).

Examination of menstrual fluid indicates that both the coagulation and fibrinolytic enzyme systems are activated during menstruation; thrombin-generating activity is virtually absent and there are high levels of fibrinogen-related antigen, plasmin and plasminogen activator, differing markedly from serum obtained from the clotting of peripheral venous blood (Rees *et al.*, 1985). In addition, heparin-like activity has been found in uterine fluid (Foley *et al.*, 1978).

Increased fibrinolytic activity in menorrhagia was originally suggested by the demonstration in the late 1960s of higher concentrations of endometrial plasminogen activator in patients with excessive menstrual bleeding (Rybo, 1966). Recent studies with present-day assays have examined fibrinolytic activity in menstrual fluid with conflicting results. Increased levels in menorrhagia were shown by Dockeray *et al.* (1987) but MBL was not measured. Studies where MBL was estimated show no difference between menstrual fluid fibrinolytic activity in women with menorrhagia compared with controls (Rees *et al.*, 1985). In both groups fibrinolytic activity was similarly high. But menstrual fluid is unlikely to provide an accurate reflection of events in the endometrium or myometrium.

The suggestion that fibrinolytic activity may be abnormal in menorrhagia has led to use of antifibrinolytic agents such as tranexamic acid and ϵ-aminocaproic acid. Taken during menstruation, they have been found to be effective in reducing MBL (Nilsson & Rybo, 1967). The average reduction of MBL is 50%. However, there have been some recent reservations regarding their use since systemic fibrinolytic activity is slightly reduced and intracranial thromboses have been reported (Agnelli *et al.*, 1982).

With regard to platelet function, menstrual fluid platelets appear to be 'spent' (Rees *et al.*, 1984c). They are unable to aggregate and metabolize arachidonic acid via the cyclo-oxygenase pathway. Furthermore, ultrastructural studies of menstrual fluid platelets have shown them to be degranulated (Sheppard *et al.*, 1983). Since degranulated platelets have also been found in endometrial hemostatic plugs, it appears that menstrual fluid platelets have already been involved in uterine hemostasis before being shed (Christiaens *et al.*, 1982). The fact that β-thromboglobulin, a protein specific to human platelets which is released during thrombus formation (Ludlam & Anderton, 1978), has been found in high concentrations in menstrual fluid also supports this observation (Paton *et al.*, 1980).

Platelets obtained from the uterine vein during menstruation do not appear to be 'spent' since they aggregate normally and metabolize arachidonic acid. Therefore 'spent' platelets that would have participated in endometrial hemostasis do not seem to be returned to the systemic circulation in significant numbers (Rees *et al.*, 1984c). On the other hand, there is some evidence that platelets which have passed through the uterus have lost their ability to adhere to glass beads (Paton *et al.*, 1980; Goodfellow *et al.*, 1982).

A relationship between measured MBL and platelet function has been explored. No differences were noted between venous and menstrual platelet samples obtained from women with either a light or a heavy loss (Rees *et al.*, 1984c). Platelet abnormalities are therefore an unlikely primary factor in the etiology of menorrhagia.

Systemic and pelvic pathology

Menorrhagia is often said to occur in the presence of systemic and pelvic pathology. However, this widespread view perpetrated by many gynecological textbooks is based on clinical impression without essential objective MBL measurement. Disorders of hemostasis are thought to increase MBL, but MBL was not measured in the cases originally reported (Quick, 1966). When it has been measured, platelet disorders (thrombocytopenia) rather than coagulation disorders have been implicated in menorrhagia (Fraser *et al.*, 1986).

With regard to pelvic pathology, leiomyomas, endometriosis, pelvic inflammatory disease, and endometrial polyps are thought to cause menorrhagia. Again there is a paucity of data with objective MBL measurement. Rybo (1982) and Fraser *et al.* (1986) have shown that most women with leiomyomas have objective menorrhagia. However, menstrual blood loss is not related to the size of the leiomyomas present (Rees, unpublished observation): women with large leiomyomas may have normal blood losses. The mechanism by which leiomyomas affect MBL may involve prostacyclin since 6-keto-PGF$_{1\alpha}$ is the principal product of these tissues (Rees & Turnbull, 1985). About 40% of women with endometriosis and adenomyosis have objective menorrhagia

(Fraser *et al.*, 1986). However the same authors found that chronic pelvic inflammatory disease and endometrial polyps were not associated with menorrhagia.

Finally, it must be noted that 50% of women with menorrhagia have no systemic or pelvic pathology and have ovulatory cycles (Haynes *et al.*, 1979; Chimbira *et al.*, 1980). The uterus in these women is not enlarged and the endometrial surface area is not increased compared to women with normal MBL (Chimbira *et al.*, 1980). Furthermore, morphometric analysis of uterine spiral arteriole density shows no correlation with MBL (Rees *et al.*, 1984d). Therefore unexplained menorrhagia is not related to the number of arteries supplying the endometrium.

Conclusion

Several factors have been identified which play a part in MBL control. It is essential that studies examining MBL should have objective measurement of blood loss. While abnormalities of prostaglandins and fibrinolysis have been detected in menorrhagia, little is known regarding their control mechanisms and future research should be directed to their examination.

Acknowledgements

Dr Rees is a Parke Davis Lecturer.

References

Abel, M.H. & Kelly, R.W. (1979). Differential production of prostaglandins within the human uterus. *Prostaglandins*, **18**:821–828.

Adelantado, J.M., Rees, M.C.P., Lopez Bernal, A. & Turnbull, A.C. (1988). Increased uterine prostaglandin E receptors in menorrhagic women. *British Journal of Obstetrics and Gynaecology*, **95**:162–165.

Agnelli, G., Gresele, P., De Cunto, M., Gallai, V. & Nenci, G.G. (1982). Tranexamic acid, intrauterine contraceptive devices and fatal cerebral arterial thrombosis. Case report. *British Journal of Obstetrics and Gynaecology*, **89**:681–682.

Anderson, A.B.M., Haynes, P.J., Guillebaud, J. & Turnbull, A.C. (1976). Reduction of menstrual blood-loss by prostaglandin synthetase inhibitors. *Lancet*, **i**:774–776.

Bonney, R.C. & Franks, S. (1987). Phospholipase C activity in human endometrium: its significance in endometrial pathology. *Clinical Endocrinology*, **27**:307–320.

Cameron, I.T., Leask, R., Kelly, R.W. & Baird, D.T. (1987). Endometrial prostaglandins in women with abnormal menstrual bleeding. *Prostaglandins, Leukotrienes and Medicine*, **29**:249–257.

Chimbira, T.H., Anderson, A.B.M. & Turnbull, A.C. (1980). Relation between measured menstrual blood loss and the patient's subjective assessment of loss, duration of bleeding, number of sanitary towels used, uterine weight and endometrial surface area. *British Journal of Obstetrics and Gynaecology*, **87**:603–609.

Christiaens, G.C.M.L., Sixma, J.J. & Haspels, A.A. (1980). Morphology of haemostasis in menstrual endometrium. *British Journal of Obstetrics and Gynaecology*, **87**:425–439.

Christiaens, G.C.M.L., Sixma, J.J. & Haspels, A.A. (1982). Haemostasis in menstrual endometrium: a review. *Obstetrical and Gynaecological Survey*, **37**:281–303.

Demers, L.M., Rees, M.C.P. & Turnbull, A.C. (1984). Arachidonic acid metabolism by the non-pregnant human uterus. *Prostaglandins, Leukotrienes and Medicine*, **14**:175–180.

Dockeray, C.J., Sheppard, B.L., Daly, L. & Bonnar, J. (1987). The fibrinolytic enzyme system in normal menstruation and excessive uterine bleeding and the effect of tranexamic acid. *European Journal of Obstetrics, Gynecology and Reproductive Biology*, **24**:309–318.

Foley, M.E., Griffin, M.D., Zuzel, M., Aparicio, S.R., Bradbury, K., Bird, C.C., Clayton, J.K., Jenkins, D.M., Scott, J.S., Rajah, S.M. & McNicol, G.P. (1978). Heparin-like activity in uterine fluid. *British Medical Journal*, **2**:322–324.

Fraser, I.S. (1983). The treatment of menorrhagia with mefenamic acid. *Research and Clinical Forums*, **5**(3):93–99.

Fraser, I.S., McCarron, G. & Markham, R. (1984). A preliminary study of factors influencing perception of menstrual blood loss volume. *American Journal of Obstetrics and Gynecology*, **149**:788–793.

Fraser, I.S., McCarron, G., Markham, R., Resta, T. & Watts, A. (1986). Measured menstrual blood loss in women with menorrhagia associated with pelvic disease or coagulation disorder. *Obstetrics and Gynecology*, **68**:630–633.

Fraser, I.S., McCarron, G., Markham, R., Robinson, M. & Smyth, E. (1983). Long-term treatment of menorrhagia with mefenamic acid. *Obstetrics and Gynecology*, **61**:109–112.

Goodfellow, C.F., Paton, R.C., Salmon, J.A., Moncada, S.,. Clayton, J.K., Davies, J.A. & McNicol, G.P. (1982). 6-oxo-prostaglandin F1α and thromboxane B2 in uterine vein blood: a possible role in menstrual bleeding. *Thrombosis and Haemostasis*, **48**:9–12.

Granström, E. & Samuelsson, B. (1978). Quantitative measurement of prostaglandins and thromboxanes: general considerations. *Advances in Prostaglandin and Thromboxane Research*, **5**:1–13.

Green, K. (1986). Structure, biosynthesis and metabolism. (In) *Prostaglandins and their Inhibitors in Clinical Obstetrics and Gynaecology* (Bygdeman, M., Berger, G.S. & Keith, L.G., eds.), pp.13–28. Lancaster, MTP Press.

Hallberg, L.,. Högdahl, A.M., Nilsson, L. & Rybo, G. (1966). Menstrual blood loss, a population study. Variation at different ages and attempts to define normality. *Acta Obstetricia et Gynecologica Scandinavica*, **45**:320–351.

Hallberg, L. & Nilsson, L. (1964). Determination of menstrual blood loss. *Scandinavian Journal of Clinical and Laboratory Investigation*, **16**:244–248.

Haynes, P.J., Anderson, A.B.M. & Turnbull, A.C. (1979). Patterns of menstrual blood-loss in menorrhagia. *Research and Clinical Forums*, **1**(2):73–78.

Hofmann, G.E., Rao₂ C.V., Barrows, G.H. & Sanfilippo, J.S. (1983). Topography of human uterine prostaglandin E and F2α receptors and their profiles during pathological states. *Journal of Clinical Endocrinology and Metabolism*, **57**:360–366.

Hospital In-patient Enquiry, Series MB4 (1985). Based on a one in ten sample of NHS patients in hospitals in England and Wales. UK Office of Population Censuses and Surveys. Table P1. London, HMSO.

Kelly, R.W., Lumsden, M.A., Abel, M.H. & Baird, D.T. (1984). The relationship between menstrual blood loss and prostaglandin production in the human: evidence for increased availability of arachidonic acid in women suffering from menorrhagia. *Prostaglandins, Leukotrienes and Medicine*, **16**:69–78.

Ludlam, C.A. & Anderton, J.L. (1978). Platelet β thromboglobulin. (In) *Platelet Function Testing* (Day, H.J., Holmsen, H. & Zucher, M.B., eds.), p.267. Washington, US Department of Health, Education and Welfare, Publication No. (NIH)78-1087.

Lundström, V. (1986). The uterus. (In) *Prostaglandins and their Inhibitors in Clinical Obstetrics and Gynaecology* (Bygdeman, M., Berger, G.S. & Keith, L.G., eds.), pp.59–82. Lancaster, MTP Press.

Makarainen, L. & Ylikorkala, O. (1986). Primary and myoma-associated menorrhagia: role of prostaglandins and effect of ibuprofen. *British Journal of Obstetrics and Gynaecology*, **93**:974–978.

Markee, J.E. (1940). Menstruation in intraocular endometrial transplants in the rhesus monkey. *Contributions to Embryology*. Carnegie Institution of Washington Publication No. 518, **28** (No. 177):219–308.

Morbidity Statistics from General Practice 1981–1982 (1981–1982). Series MB5. UK Office of Population Censuses and Surveys, Table 13. London, HMSO.

Nilsson, L. & Rybo, G. (1967). Treatment of menorrhagia with an antifibrinolytic agent: tranexamic acid (AMCA). A double blind investigation. *Acta Obstetricia et Gynecologica Scandinavica*, **46**:572–580.

Paton, R.C., Tindall, H., Zuzel, M. & McNicol, G.P. (1980). Haemostatic mechanisms in the normal endometrium and endometrium exposed to contraceptive steroids. (In) *Endometrial Bleeding and Steroidal Contraception* (Diczfalusy, E., Fraser, I.S. & Webb, F.T.G., eds.), pp.325–346. Bath, England, Pitman Press.

Peek, M.J., Fraser, I.S., Phillips, C.A., Resta, T.M., Blackwell, P.M. & Markham, R. (1985). The measurement of human endometrial prostaglandin production. A comparison of two in-vitro methods. *Prostaglandins*, **29**:3–18.

Pickles, V.R., Hall, W.J., Best, F.A. & Smith, G.N. (1965). Prostaglandins in endometrium and menstrual fluid from normal and dysmenorrhoeic subjects. *Journal of Obstetrics and Gynaecology of the British Commonwealth*, **72**:185–192.

Quick, A.J. (1966). Menstruation in hereditary bleeding disorders. *Obstetrics and Gynecology*, **28**:37–48.

Rees, M.C.P. (1987). Menorrhagia an algorithm. *British Medical Journal*, **294**:759–762.

Rees, M.C.P., Anderson, A.B.M., Demers, L.M. & Turnbull, A.C. (1984a). Prostaglandins in menstrual fluid in menorrhagia and dysmenorrhoea. *British Journal of Obstetrics and Gynaecology*, **91**:673–680.

Rees, M.C.P., Anderson, A.B.M., Demers, L.M. & Turnbull, A.C. (1984b). Endometrial and myometrial prostaglandin release during the menstrual cycle in relation to menstrual blood loss. *Journal of Clinical Endocrinology and Metabolism*, **58**:813–818.

Rees, M.C.P., Canete-Soler, R., Lopez Bernal, A. & Turnbull, A.C. (1988). Effect of fenamates on prostaglandin E receptor binding. *Lancet*, **ii**:541–542.

Rees, M.C.P., Cederholm-Williams, S.A. & Turnbull, A.C. (1985). Coagulation factors and fibrinolytic proteins in menstrual fluid collected from normal and menorrhagic women. *British Journal of Obstetrics and Gynaecology*, **92**:1164–1168.

Rees, M.C.P., Demers, L.M., Anderson, A.B.M. & Turnbull, A.C. (1984c). A functional study of platelets in menstrual fluid. *British Journal of Obstetrics and Gynaecology*, **91**:667–672.

Rees, M.C.P., Di Marzo, V., Tippins, J.R., Morris, H.R. & Turnbull, A.C. (1987). Leukotriene release by endometrium and myometrium throughout the menstrual cycle in dysmenorrhoea and menorrhagia. *Journal of Endocrinology*, **113**:291–295.

Rees, M.C.P., Dunnill, M.S., Anderson, A.B.M. & Turnbull, A.C. (1984d). Quantitative uterine histology during the menstrual cycle in relation to measured menstrual blood loss. *British Journal of Obstetrics and Gynaecology*, **91**:662–666.

Rees, M.C.P., Parry, D.M., Anderson, A.B.M. & Turnbull, A.C. (1982). Immunohistochemical localisation of cyclooxygenase in the human uterus. *Prostaglandins*, **23**:207–214.

Rees, M.C.P. & Turnbull, A.C. (1985). Leiomyomas release prostaglandins. *Prostaglandins, Leukotrienes and Medicine*, **18**:65–68.

Rybo, G. (1966). Plasminogen activators in the endometrium. II. Clinical aspects. Variation in the concentration of plasminogen activators during the menstrual cycle and its relation to menstrual blood loss. *Acta Obstetricia et Gynecologica Scandinavica*, **45**:429–450.

Rybo, G. (1982). Variations of menstrual blood loss. *Research and Clinical Forums*, **4**:81–88.

Schickele, G. (1912). Untersuchungen über die innere sekretion der ovarien. *Biochemische Zeitschrift*, **38**:169–172.

Sheppard, B.L., Dockeray, C.J. & Bonnar, J. (1983). An ultrastructural study of menstrual blood in normal menstruation and dysfunctional uterine bleeding. *British Journal of Obstetrics and Gynaecology*, **90**:259–265.

Smith, J.B. (1980). The prostanoids in haemostasis and thrombosis. A review. *American Journal of Pathology*, **99**:743–804.

Smith, S.K., Abel, M.H., Kelly, R.W. & Baird, D.T. (1981a). Prostaglandin synthesis in the endometrium of women with ovular dysfunctional uterine bleeding. *British Journal of Obstetrics and Gynaecology*, **88**:434–442.

Smith, S.K., Kelly, R.W., Abel, M.H. & Baird, D.T. (1981b). A role for prostacyclin (PGI2) in excessive menstrual bleeding. *Lancet*, **i**:522–524.

Turnbull, A.C. & Rees, M.C.P. (1987). Mefenamic acid in the treatment of gynecologic disorders. (In) *A Retrospective Review of Clinical Experience* (Turnbull, A.C., ed.), pp.1–17. Amsterdam, Excerpta Medica.

Vermylen, J. (1978). Physiology of haemostasis. (In) *Platelets: A Multidisciplinary Approach* (de Gaetano, G. & Garattini, S., eds.), pp.3–15. New York, Raven Press.

Von Euler, U.S. (1935). Uber die spezifische blut drucksenkende substanz des menschlichen prostata- und samenblasensekretes. *Klinische Wochenschrift*, **14**:1182–1183.

Wallen, P., Kok, P. & Ranby, M. (1977). The tissue activator of plasminogen. (In) *FEBS Symposium: Regulatory Proteolytic Enzymes and their Inhibitors* (Magnusson, S., Ottensen, M., Foltman, B., Dano, K. & Neureath, H., eds.), Vol. 47, pp.127–135.

Willman, E.A., Collins, W.P. & Clayton, S.G. (1976). Studies in the involvement of prostaglandins in uterine symptomatology and pathology. *British Journal of Obstetrics and Gynaecology*, **83**:337–341.

Wiqvist, N., Bygdeman, M. & Kirton, K.T. (1971). Non-steroidal antifertility agents in the female. (In) *Nobel Symposium 15: Control of Human Fertility* (Diczfalusy, E. & Borell, U., eds.), pp.137–149. Stockholm, Almqvist and Wiksell.

Wiqvist, N., Lindblom, B., Wikland, M. & Wilhelmsson, L. (1983). Prostaglandins and uterine contractility. *Acta Obstetricia et Gynecologica Scandinavica*, Supplement, **113**:23–29.

Discussion

Naftolin. How do you suppose the fenamates affect receptors?

Rees. We think that fenamates bind to the receptors, and inhibit binding of already formed prostaglandins to the receptors. Dr Fraser (1983) showed that fenamates reduced, but did not abolish, levels of prostaglandins in endometrium. So fenamates have a dual mode of action.

Naftolin. You think that the same place on the molecule binds the receptor and the enzyme?

Rees. We do not know; these studies are in progress.

Smith. Am I right in assuming that you showed that in the superfused tissue in the initial response you had a reduction in the amount of PGF produced at menstruation compared to the late luteal phase, and that in fact your apparent levels of PGE and PGF in that presumably initial superfusate were closer to unity than in the late luteal phase? This, if it was true, would go at least some way towards confirming the increased $PGE_2:PGF_{2a}$ ratio which we have argued about for 10 years.

Rees. I looked for a correlation between the $PGE_2:PGF_{2a}$ ratio and menstrual blood loss and couldn't find one.

Findlay. I just wanted to check about Figure 4 in your manuscript, relating prostaglandins collected over 2 hours versus total menstrual blood loss. If you express that as a concentration, there doesn't seem to be any change.

Rees. The concentrations of prostaglandins F_{2a} and E_2 were not significantly increased between normal women and menorrhagic subjects who had no pain, but there was a shift towards F_{2a} in the women with menorrhagia in terms of concentration. The problem about looking at PG levels in menstrual blood is: how do you compare the same PG levels, say in a woman who has passed 20 ml in 2 hours and another who has passed 2 ml in 2 hours? But in terms of absolute concentrations, there was a shift towards prostaglandin F_{2a} in that there was increased F to E ratio in women with menorrhagia.

Findlay. Well, the only thing would be then whether the prostaglandins that are actually in the menstrual fluid are important in terms of an action back on the endometrium. Because if they are, concentration is important in terms of interaction with the receptor, not the total content. Another point in relation to fenamate interaction: in Figure 5 of your manuscript, slopes of the inhibition curves were interesting; they were not actually parallel to the PGE_2. Do you have an explanation for that?

Rees. No, I have no explanation at the moment and work is in progress to look at the mechanism.

Casey. I was interested in your immunohistochemical localization of cyclo-oxygenase (Rees *et al.*, 1982) and I wonder if you might comment further. It is clear from the findings of many investigators that the endometrial stromal cell does in fact produce prostaglandins and yet you find little or no cyclo-oxygenase by this method in that cell type. Were the tissues that you evaluated permeabilized? It appeared that the cyclo-oxygenase in the glandular epithelium was at the cell periphery. Have you evaluated cyclo-oxygenase immunohistochemically in endometrium from women at various stages of the ovarian cycle?

Rees. These were hysterectomy specimens obtained throughout the menstrual cycle in women who were not taking any hormones and the tissue was frozen immediately after collection. In fact, Dr Bryant-Greenwood has used the same antibodies with endometrium and has found the same results (unpublished observations). I would have expected also to have seen staining in the stroma and in the endothelium of the spiral arterioles. But the staining is not quantitative and we may not be able to stain enzyme that is compartmentalized in a certain way.

Fraser. You have talked extensively about aspects of menstrual blood loss and I believe it is worth emphasizing that this is in fact very dilute blood and that whole blood probably only accounts for about 40% of the total menstrual volume, even in women with menorrhagia. So perhaps women who are losing 100 ml of blood are probably losing between 200–300 ml of fluid altogether. We believe there is probably an endometrial transudate accounting for a major part of the remaining fluid which does suggest that, in addition to damage and rupture of the capillaries resulting in blood loss, there probably is a substantial increase in capillary permeability at the onset of menstruation.

Rees. Unfortunately it is very difficult actually to measure the total amount of fluid lost because you have to prevent the pads from drying out, so that is why it is more convenient to express it in terms of venous blood loss. Then, what is the nature of this transudate? Is it really a transudate or more like plasma because the concentration of IgG and albumin in menstrual blood is the same as that in peripheral blood.

Harper. Have you attempted to measure platelet-activating factor (PAF) in the menstrual fluid in which you measured PGs, because platelets exposed to PAF can become desensitized, and I wondered if there might be an interaction? Also in your incubate you said you used a calcium-free medium. In some experiments we examined the conversion of exogenous arachidonic acid in rabbit blastocysts and we found that the presence or absence of calcium did not make a difference; but if we added EDTA, irrespective of whether calcium was there or not, we could get conversion of the arachidonic acid. In its absence we could not. EGTA was not as effective. We do not know what the mechanism is, unless it involves a stabilization of the membrane.

Rees. In our system, we just collected the menstrual blood without anything in the vaginal cup; we found that if we incubated peripheral venous blood with EDTA, this abolished aggregation. This is why we did not use any anticoagulant. We tried the presence and absence of citrate and it did not alter anything. We also wanted to see if perhaps blood staying in a cup for 2 hours affected platelets, so we added citrated peripheral venous blood so that the platelets would not coagulate in the cup. After 2 hours the platelets functioned as well as they had done in the beginning. So the method of collection does not seem to affect the results that we obtain. With regard to PAF, we have had problems with the measurements and we are continuing our investigations.

Clark. With respect to the relationship between the increase in PGE_2 receptors and menstrual blood loss, can you tell us which cells have the increased PGE_2 receptors; is this a generalized phenomenon or is it confined to the uterus of these women?

Rees. We have not looked at other tissues.

Åkerlund. You showed some very nice results where mefenamic acid inhibited myometrial receptor binding of PGE_2. Did you have any similar results with $PGF_{2\alpha}$?

Rees. The $PGF_{2\alpha}$ receptors are of low affinity and are in lower concentration in human uterine tissues, and in fact they bind mainly E_2 rather than $F_{2\alpha}$, which is why we have looked at PGE_2 receptors since these are specific receptors; the $PGF_{2\alpha}$ receptors are non-specific, and we are not the only group to have found the same results.

Healy. My question is a clinical one relating to women's perception of their menstrual health. When you were checking those people in the clinic, did you actually find any differences in terms of psychological or psycho-social characteristics between the people who complained of menorrhagia and yet bled only 20 ml a month and those who complained of menorrhagia and bled 500 ml per month? And did the treatments in fact have equal efficacy in at least the patient's perception of the menstrual disease?

Rees. All those women were having hysterectomies and there was nothing obvious at the time I was doing the study. Since then, we have been doing a prospective study with our psychiatric colleagues with Dr D. Gath and have been assessing women psychologically pre- and post-hysterectomy. The study is not yet finished. We need to see if the women who do well after hysterectomy are the ones who really had menorrhagia and the ones who do badly after hysterectomy are the ones who never had a problem. But all these women give equally convincing stories of social problems with excessive bleeding. We will know in about a year's time.

Cornillie. I have some small questions about the superfusion technique for doing short-term incubations. You mention that you express your results in amounts of wet weight of tissue. Can you tell us about the amount you get in your superfusion.

Rees. The average was around 50 mg of dry weight of tissue, which makes it about 500–600 mg wet weight of tissue since the ratio between wet and dry weight is about 1 to 10.

Cornillie. That is a lot. Another technical aspect of your technique is 95% oxygen. Is that not a little unphysiological?

Rees. It was a technique that worked and we knew that the tissue was viable because at the end of the superfusion, we checked trypan blue uptake, histology, the ability to respond to stimuli such as oxytocin, the inhibitory action of indomethacin and glucose uptake.

Clark. I would like to come back to the question posed by Dr Baird, concerning whether uterine bleeding occurring in various forms represented a single phenomenon or rather distinct entities. I recall Dr Baird made a fairly strong statement concerning his belief that prostaglandins played a central role in the initiation and progression of uterine blood loss. Dr Odlind also presented some evidence that non-steroidal anti-inflammatory drugs (NSAIDs) might decrease blood loss associated with the use of progestogens, similar to the decrease in blood loss with IUDs and in the so-called dysfunctional uterine bleeding condition. If NSAIDs are effective in reducing blood loss from the uterus under all conditions where it occurs, would that not then suggest that there is a central theme to this problem of bleeding and that Dr Baird's belief is indeed a correct one?

Odlind. Well, I think perhaps management may be a clue to answer Dr Baird's question. If you remember Dr Diaz' study using NSAIDs to treat bleeding problems in progestogen-only users (unpublished observations), she found much more of an effect by giving estrogens than with NSAID, although there were some effects with NSAIDs. So, maybe the answer is again that there are different mechanisms.

Baird. We need to define the terminology clearly. For example, Dr Hourihan showed us some beautiful pictures of gaps in the capillaries in women who are on the progestogen-only pill. Does this ever occur physiologically? So, we have to say under what circumstances we are defining bleeding. I suggest as the gold standard the mechanism of menstruation which – I think it is non-negotiable – is due to a withdrawal of estrogen and progestogen. And that for anything else, other than that, we define the circumstances in which the bleeding is occurring.

Johannisson. I agree entirely with you and I think that the mechanism responsible for menstruation as such is not fully known. Most of the evidence that we have points to the fact that the levels of progestogen and estradiol fall, and because of that we have the onset of menstrual bleeding. But perhaps we should also think about the receptors and how the estradiol and progesterone receptors are involved in the mechanism of onset of physiological menstruation.

Diaz. There are so many kinds of bleeding. Just to add a little more to the confusion, what would be a possible mechanism to explain why women who are fully breastfeeding by day 60 postpartum, with very low estrogen levels, start bleeding when a continuous progestogen is administered such as Norplant[R] or a progesterone-releasing vaginal ring? They bleed in a non-estrogen-primed endometrium and with no withdrawal of progesterone.

Harper. Well, it is clear that there are all sorts of different hormonal conditions which may give rise to different types of bleeding, but, surely, the key question is: is there a final common pathway at the cellular level which causes initiation of bleeding? If there is a final common pathway, then a study of physiological menstruation is going to be very helpful. If there is not, then we should forget about studying it altogether.

Perhaps we need to concentrate on what cellular mechanism causes the initiation of bleeding rather than these peripheral considerations, which are so far removed from the actual process itself.

Cornillie. I think there are at least two different types of bleeding. First of all there is the clinical evidence of bleeding at menses, say day 1 of the cycle. There is leakage of blood and debris, but also viable cells. On the other hand, when you look at the endometrium during the late secretory phase, from day 25 onwards, you will see something like microbleeding. This means extravasation or diapedesis of red cells within the stroma without tissue degradation and shedding. So there are some predisposing factors which, in menses, lead to tissue degradation and are not present in other types of bleeding. We should study these factors in tissue which is still viable at the end of the cycle.

Rees. I would agree that you can culture endometrial cells from menstrual blood and that they are viable – and you can get them into culture and they will produce substances, such as tissue plasminogen activator, as in cells taken at other phases of the cycle. I would also agree that the process of menstruation appears to differ from the bleeding that occurs in women on the progestogen-only method of contraception. So, I think there must be different mechanisms in these two entities.

Johannisson. I would like to emphasize that there is a statistically significant difference between the morphology of the endometrium of women using progestogen as contraception and the morphology of the endometrium obtained during a normal physiological cycle. I think that perhaps we could consider the modification introduced by progestogen as one of the factors predisposing for intermenstrual bleeding.

Baird. Perhaps another way of looking at this is to try to define the changes which normally do occur in the normal cycle in relation to withdrawal of estrogen and progesterone, not only morphologically but functionally. There are well-characterized changes in the pattern of uterine contractility in relation to the different phases of the menstrual cycle, which, presumably, not only represent changes in receptor concentration in the myometrium in relation to oxytocin and perhaps vasopressin and, even possibly, in receptors, but also represent the response of that myometrium to prostaglandins and other factors which cause the myometrium to contract. I wonder, Dr Åkerlund, whether you would like to be confident enough to say that there is a certain characteristic of intrauterine pressure recording which is diagnostic of a withdrawal of estrogen and progestogen at the end of the cycle?

Åkerlund. Dr Baird, your group has also shown statistically that the uterine contractility pattern varies throughout the menstrual period both in dysmenorrheic and in healthy women. However, there are individual differences between women, presumably due to variations in anatomy and in steroid hormone patterns throughout the cycle and probably in receptor concentrations. The contractility varies with the hormones, and exogenous hormones change the contractility pattern.

Baird. I was not suggesting that the pattern of myometrial contractility was necessary for normal menstruation. I was suggesting that it was an index of the changes which normally occur within the uterus parameter, which was normally associated with the endocrine changes which occur during menstruation.

Clark. One of the reasons why we know so much about normal menstruation is that Markee was able directly to observe the behaviour of endometrial tissue in the anterior chamber of the rabbit eye. From this he was able to see that there was vascular spasm, for example. It seems unfortunate, in retrospect, that he did not have the long-acting progestational contraceptive agents to see how these might affect the endometrium. Then we would be able to answer at least one question: are there common mechanisms such as vascular spasm in spite of differing histology? Dr Baird may be able to provide some information on what happens with treatment with a progestogen from his system that tests explants in the hamster cheek pouch (Abel *et al.*, 1982). Perhaps these observations might tell us if the process that leads to bleeding in a progestogen-only treated animal is the same as the type of bleeding that occurs with combined estrogen–progesterone withdrawal that causes menstruation?

Baird. We have never given progestogens to the hamsters. But we were never able to produce breakthrough bleeding by continuing progesterone. It may be a question of length of exposure: we never treated the hamsters for longer than 14 days, which was the length of the luteal phase. It might be instructive to continue low-dose progestogen for several months, though I think you would begin to have a problem with the rejection of the explants.

King. What strikes me is (a) that you have the biological system as described in the rabbit eye, and (b) Dr Baird's line of arguing, that prostaglandins are involved somehow between the progesterone withdrawal and heavy bleeding. I would strongly endorse what Dr Harper has just said, that one has to get down to some cellular aspects. One has got to devise systems in which we study the way in which different cell types talk to each other.

Ludwig. As we are talking about bleeding, we have to look at the vessels. Therefore, we have to ask why, under what circumstances, does the vessel continue to bleed, why is the bleeding time locally prolonged? This question has to do with the various components around the vessel and endometrial cells, e.g. prostaglandins. The starting point of bleeding is always the degradation of the vessel integrity. But the question is what stops the bleeding in the event of menstruation and what makes the uterus sometimes continue to bleed. I think we have to divide our question into two parts: (a) the initiation of bleeding, and (b) the cessation of bleeding. In the latter part, there are some different tissue components involved, whereas in the first part the starting point is only the degradation or destruction of the vessel wall.

Granström. Personally, I am very puzzled about the possible roles of prostaglandins or leukotrienes in these processes. Is anything known about endometrial function or menstruation or other types of bleeding in women on steroids which should inhibit the release of the precursor of fatty acids completely?

Smith. I think, from studies from Chan and Daywood (1980), in that menstrual prostaglandin levels were reduced in women who were menstruating on withdrawal of the oral contraceptive pill. Indirectly, there seems to be a correlation between menstrual bleeding associated with combined contraceptive steroid withdrawal and prostaglandin levels in menstrual fluid which is supposed to be the underlying phenomenon to the control of dysmenorrhea with the oral contraceptive.

Cornillie. I would like to comment on Dr Ludwig's remarks. I am not convinced that bleeding starts with a vessel defect. During the mid-luteal phase there is edema in the stroma of the endometrium, which is followed by rapid resorption of this edema during the fall of progesterone. One could also imagine that there is a collapse of the extracellular matrix due to dehydration.

Ludwig. Bleeding in the endometrium, as anywhere else, means that the vessel wall is no longer capable of retaining erythrocytes within the circulation. We examined the superficial layers of the terminal end of the capillaries going to the superficial endometrium and never saw an intact vessel wall in a premenstrual endometrium (28th day of the cycle). The vessels studied have larger or smaller defects, but all the defects can let erythrocytes go through into the perivascular space. In the beginning there might only be a disintegrity of a vessel wall. Erythrocytes cannot migrate like leukocytes, they have to find holes to go through. As the degradation process in the endometrium develops further, we are no longer able to identify the vessel wall integrity. I think you all will agree that bleeding means a vessel wall defect. So, I disagree that bleeding can be present with intact vessels.

Rees. I would like to continue answering Dr Granström's question about the pill and prostaglandins. There was a study done many years ago by Maathuis and Kelly (1978), when they looked at endometrial concentrations of PGs in women on the pill and found them to be elevated. Chan and Hill (1978) found that the total amount of PGs was reduced in menstrual blood in women on the pill, which is not surprising, since they are bleeding less. But the concentrations were the same and there were doubts about the validity of the assays.

Granström. What I meant were the phospholipase inhibitors, which inhibit the release of all precursor fatty acids. I do not think they influence menstrual periods or any kind of bleeding at all. People with asthma or rheumatic diseases who take NSAIDs menstruate normally.

Rees. They do have menstrual periods, but nobody has done a population study to see if all these women on NSAIDs have, in fact, much lower blood losses than women not on NSAIDs. That population study needs to be done and would have to be carefully controlled for the dose and type of NSAID.

Findlay. I wonder if it might help our conceptualizing this if we think about what is actually happening at the end of the cycle in terms of other events occurring besides bleeding. It is a time when decidual tissue is being shed, and maybe that is the primary event. You could produce that in one of several ways: an obvious one is to cut off the blood supply to that tissue, and when you do that you get some bleeding. So, in terms of a final common pathway, which I am very attracted to for developing some sort of approach, maybe we should be thinking back from bleeding and get back into cell–cell interactions.

Brosens. But would decidualization not be the way that the cell is able to survive for a long period?

Findlay. That is a possibility, but on the other hand it may also need some other message *in vivo* to continue surviving. You could make the other argument as well, that it is on a path of self-destruction unless it gets the right message from an implanting embryo. What we are doing by introducing contraceptive steroids is interrupting that pathway or speeding it up, or changing it in some way.

Casey. In response to Dr Granström's question, some years ago we presented evidence that the endometrial stromal cell was very unresponsive to the action of glucocorticosteroids with respect to inhibition of prostaglandin synthesis. In contrast, in myometrial smooth muscle cells, glucocorticosteroids inhibit prostaglandin production by 90% to 95%.

Harper. I just wanted to make a comment in relation to the phospholipid mobilization that Dr Granström mentioned and also the carbachol issue. Quinuclidinyl benzilate (QNB) is a ligand which binds to cholinergic–muscarinic receptors. It is known that stimulation of those receptors gives rise to phospholipid mobilization, release of arachidonic acid and an increase in prostaglandin levels. Normally you find these receptors on smooth muscle cells, but some years ago we examined glandular epithelial cells from rabbit endometrium, and found that there was specific binding for QNB to those cells. We should not forget altogether the cholinergic system.

References

Abel, M.H., Zhu, C. & Baird, D.T. (1982). An animal model to study menstrual bleeding. *Research and Clinical Forums*, **4**(4):25–34.

Chan, W.Y. & Daywood, Y.M. (1980). Prostaglandin levels in menstrual fluid of non-dysmenorrheic and of dysmenorrheic subjects with and without oral contraceptive or ibuprofen therapy. *Advances in Prostaglandin and Thromboxane Research*, **8**:1443–1447.

Chan, W.Y. & Hill, J.C. (1978). Determination of menstrual prostaglandin levels in nondysmenorrhoeic and dysmenorrhoeic subjects. *Prostaglandins*, **15**:365–375.

Fraser, I.S. (1983). Treatment of menorrhagia with mefenamic acid. *Research and Clinical Forums*, **5**(3):93–99.

Maathuis, J.B. & Kelly, R.W. (1978). Concentrations of prostaglandins $F_{2\alpha}$ and E_2 in endometrium throughout the human menstrual cycle, after the administration of clomiphene or an oestrogen-progesterone pill and in early pregnancy. *Journal of Endocrinology*, **77**:361–372.

Rees, M.C.P., Parry, D.M., Anderson, A.B.M. & Turnbull, A.C. (1982). Immunohistochemical localisation of cyclooxygenase in the human uterus. *Prostaglandins*, **23**:207–214.

An overview of estrogen receptor structure and function

R.J.B. KING

Hormone Biochemistry Laboratory, Imperial Cancer Research Fund, London, UK.

Abstract

Recent advances in our understanding of the receptor components involved in the initial events of estradiol action are reviewed. Two main features of the models have evolved:

1. The domain structure of the ligand-binding unit, with distinct parts of the molecule being concerned with estrogen binding and DNA interaction. Other parts of the molecule have important regulatory functions.
2. The regulatory regions (estrogen response elements) of estrogen-sensitive genes that specifically interact with the receptor protein.

The homologies between different proteins capable of binding ligands as diverse as estradiol, retinoic acid and thyroid hormone point to possible interactions between such ligands. Estrogen response elements can recognize estradiol receptor proteins complexed with either agonists or antagonists. Interactions with DNA may play an important role additional to those seen at the receptor level.

Some implications of these findings to changes in endometrial biology are discussed.

Introduction

The production of antibodies to the estradiol receptor (ER) together with the resultant identification of its mRNA, cDNAs and gene have led to the questioning of some and validation of other parts of the classical model of estrogen action. This chapter will assess recent advances in our understanding of how ER influences gene function.

Intracellular localization of receptors

The concept of a cytoplasmic–nuclear equilibrium in favour of the former in the absence of ligand and the latter in its presence has been questioned. The two extreme situations are illustrated in Fig. 1. Immunohistochemical evidence indicates that ER not bound to ligand is located predominantly within the nucleus (King, 1986, 1987), whilst enucleation of cultured anterior pituitary cells by cytochalasin has also produced evidence favouring a major nuclear locus for ER not bound to ligand (Welshons & Gorski, 1986). Unresolved debate about the relative merits of the models shown in Fig. 1 concerns questions of sensitivity and possible artefacts with the histochemical

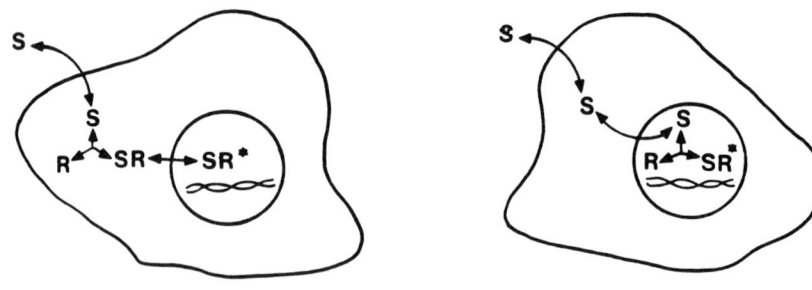

Fig. 1 Intracellular localization of steroid receptors. Steroid (S) combines with its receptor (R) as a result of which the 'activated' receptor (R*) is able to bind DNA. In the left-hand model, the initial interaction occurs in the cytoplasm; a nuclear locus is indicated in the right-hand model.

methods and how much cytoplasm accompanies the nucleus in enucleation experiments.

None of the data rules out the possibility that some cytoplasmic receptor is present but remains undetectable by current methods (King, 1986, 1987). The older autoradiographic data on ^{3}H steroid uptake (Stumpf & Sar, 1976; Sheridan *et al.*, 1979) are not helpful in resolving the question. They can be interpreted either in favour of cytosol to nuclear transfer of receptor or as non-attainment of equilibrium at the low temperatures used to demonstrate cytoplasmic localization. Given the ease with which receptor is lost from tissue sections (Penney & Hawkins, 1982), the cytoplasmic localization observed by autoradiography may be a methodological artefact. The original homogenization experiments that contributed to the evolution of the cytoplasm to nuclear transfer model could also be explained by artefactual release of ligand-free receptor.

A consensus view would be that most unliganded ER is nuclear but some extranuclear ER could also exist. From a clinical point of view, the relative truths of the two models shown in Fig. 1 matter little, although it is important to resolve the issue so that we can better understand the molecular processes involved.

Ligand-binding unit

Our knowledge about this component has been greatly enhanced by experiments with antibodies and gene probes. Monoclonal antibodies have been used to identify mRNAs and cDNAs which, in turn, have detected the appropriate genomic sequences (Green *et al.*, 1986; Greene *et al.*, 1986). Several domains can be identified in the ER protein (Kumar *et al.*, 1987; Evans, 1988), some of which are illustrated in Fig. 2. The steroid-binding

DOMAINS   **RECEPTOR**

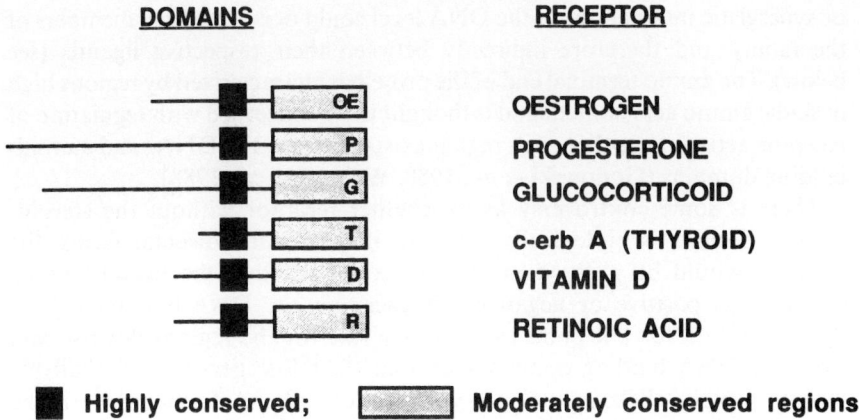

OE	**OESTROGEN**
P	**PROGESTERONE**
G	**GLUCOCORTICOID**
T	**c-erb A (THYROID)**
D	**VITAMIN D**
R	**RETINOIC ACID**

■ **Highly conserved;** ▨ **Moderately conserved regions**

Fig. 2 Domain structure of members of the soluble receptor family.

domain is at the carboxy terminal end of the protein and is separated from the DNA-binding domain by a region(s) that has been called the hinge domain. This term resulted from experiments with glucocorticoid receptor (GR) indicating that binding of ligand resulted in unmasking of the DNA-binding region (Godowski *et al.*, 1987). The relevance of this region is discussed below.

It is thought that attachment of the DNA-binding domain to the major groove of chromatin DNA is achieved via projections from the ER termed 'zinc fingers' (Kumar *et al.*, 1987). Homologies are high between the DNA-binding domains of different receptor classes but very important differences exist which are crucial in determining which gene is affected by which steroid. The essential feature is the nucleotide sequence within the genome that is capable of binding ER but not, for example, GR. Thus, genetically engineered receptor that has the DNA-binding domain of GR and the steroid-binding region of ER will elicit glucocorticoid-type responses in the presence of estradiol (Green & Chambon, 1987).

An unexpected finding arising from the computer-assisted analysis of receptor homologies is that they are related to a viral oncogene, v-erb A and its cellular counterpart c-erb A (Fig. 2). This has led to speculations about possible endogenous ligands for v-erb A and the oncogenic potential of steroid receptors (Green & Chambon, 1986; Parker, 1987). This debate has been further fuelled by the discovery that the cellular counterpart of this viral oncogene is the thyroid hormone receptor (Sap *et al.*, 1986; Weinberger *et al.*, 1986). Other members of this family of receptor proteins have been identified, the functions of most of which remain to be established, the notable exception being the retinoic acid receptor (Giguere *et al.*, 1987; Petkovich *et al.*, 1987). As the DNA-binding domains of proteins in this receptor family are similar but not identical, interest is increasing as to the possibility that either competitive or synergistic interactions at the DNA level could occur between members of the family and therefore indirectly between their respective ligands (see below). The amino terminal end of the protein is characterized by regions high in acidic amino acid content and is thought to be concerned with regulation of receptor activity; another such region exists between the DNA- and steroid-binding domains (Godowski *et al.*, 1988; Webster *et al.*, 1988).

There is some controversy as to whether receptor without the steroid-binding domain is biologically active or inactive. In molecular terms, the question would be phrased in the context of whether the ligand-binding domain has positive or negative influences on the DNA-binding region. Published data for ER point to a positive role for the regions downstream from the DNA-binding domain such that their loss generates a relatively inactive protein (Webster *et al.*, 1988). On the other hand, developments in the GR field point to both positive and negative regulatory effects such that loss of steroid-binding domain produces a constitutively active receptor (Godowski *et al.*, 1987, 1988). This conclusion about the GR system has, however, been questioned (Webster *et al.*, 1988). The basis for these divergent views possibly resides in the technical basis of the sophisticated experimental methods being utilized. It may also be a question of degree: what proportion of the original activity remains in the genetically engineered, non-ligand-binding unit?

Cytosol receptors and their activation to DNA-binding forms

When steroid-depleted cells or tissues are homogenized, most of the binding units are recovered in the cytosol fraction, usually in an approximately 8S form; after steroid treatment, a 5S nuclear form predominates, generated by dimerization of two 4S ligand-binding units (Fig. 3) (Notides, 1978; Miller *et al.*, 1985). Furthermore, in the absence of molybdate, 8S receptors are only observed under hypotonic conditions. If one accepts that *in vivo* most unliganded ER is in the nucleus, one can question the biological relevance of cytosolic forms detected after homogenization. This, in turn, leads to questions about the importance of 'activation' of cytosolic receptor to a form that will interact with nuclei or DNA (King, 1986, 1987). Steroid receptors are notoriously sticky molecules which, when placed in an unnatural environment, are capable of forming an interesting range of artefacts; homogenization may create such an environment. It is now known that the 8S form is an heterologous complex of the 68-kd estradiol-binding unit plus 90-kd heat-shock proteins (Joab *et al.*, 1984; Schuh *et al.*, 1985). It has been suggested that the attachment of estradiol to the 68-kd unit leads to dissociation of heat-shock proteins and therefore results in a DNA-binding form of ER. Such a model is compatible with in-vitro data with progesterone receptor (PR) (Bailly *et al.*, 1986) and GR (Willmann & Beato, 1986), indicating that purified, ligand-free receptor will bind specifically to DNA. An inhibitor of DNA binding (the 90-kd heat-shock protein?) may exist that is dissociated

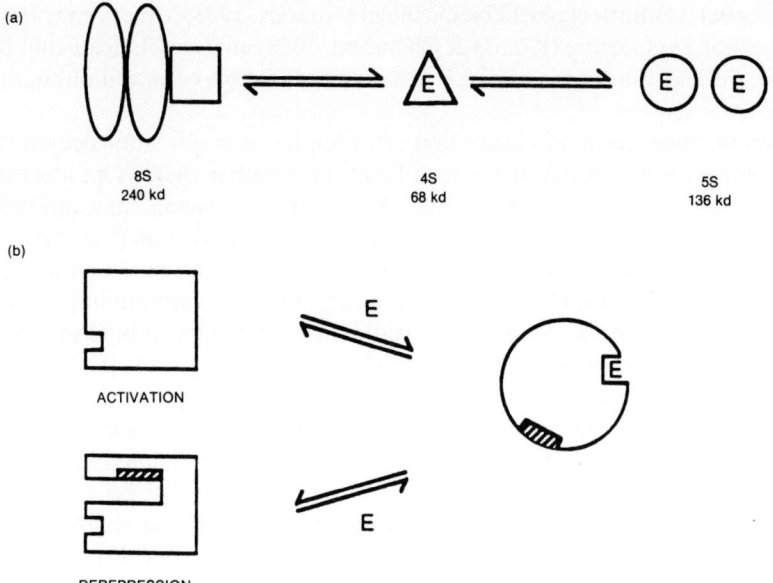

Fig. 3 Potential influences of estradiol (E) on receptor structure.
(a) Protein composition and sizes. (Ellipse = 90-kd heat-shock protein;
square = unactivated ligand-binding unit; circle = activated unit.)
(b) Alternative models of conversion to a DNA-binding form. (Adapted
from Godowski *et al.* (1987).) With the activation pathway, E binding
induces the formation of a DNA-binding site (shaded area). In the
derepression sequence, an occluded DNA-binding site is exposed as a
result of E binding.

either by steroid or during purification (Denis *et al.*, 1988). Resolution of these
enigmas must await further detailed work on the exact distributions of the
predominantly cytosolic 90-kd protein and the nuclear ER. Also, molecular
analyses to determine whether mutations in the estradiol-binding unit that
affect the attachment of the 90-kd protein influence the biological behaviour of
ER should be informative.

The debate summarized in the preceding paragraph leads to the important
question of what is the function of estradiol in these processes? The main facts
we have at present are as follows. (1) In the absence of estrogen, most ER is in
the nucleus *in vivo* but is weakly retained therein such that it is solubilized by
homogenization. (2) Addition of estradiol *in vivo* results in stronger nuclear
binding such that ER is not released by homogenization. (3) Transfection
experiments with ER cDNAs plus reporter genes (Waterman *et al.*, 1988;
Webster *et al.*, 1988) support the results of animal experiments that estradiol is
required to achieve major effects on gene function. Whether limited effects on
gene function can be achieved in the absence of ligand remains to be resolved

(see above). (4) Both classical biochemical (Notides, 1978; Miller *et al.*, 1985) and genetic engineering (Kumar & Chambon, 1988) analyses indicate that the active, nuclear-binding form of ER is a dimer of two 68-kd estradiol-binding units.

Overall, these results indicate that estradiol has a major influence on the efficiency with which ER alters gene function; whether there is an absolute requirement for estradiol is unclear. Attachment of ligand may influence several steps in the sequence of events leading to gene activation (Fig. 3a). The 8S complex does not bind to DNA so estradiol could dissociate non steroid-binding units from the 68-kd estradiol-binding units. Conformational changes in the latter unit result in both dimerization and an ability to bind to DNA. The two simplistic ways in which this might occur are illustrated in Fig. 3b. A conformational change resulting in the exposure of an occult, pre-existing DNA-binding domain (derepression) is one possibility. Alternatively, more complex changes may be required to generate the DNA-binding domain (activation). Features of both pathways may be important. The act of receptor binding to the DNA is insufficient in itself to influence gene expression. There is ample evidence that non-productive interactions can occur. For example, unliganded receptor or tamoxifen–receptor complexes can bind to specific regulatory regions of the gene without activating that gene (see below), whereas the estradiol–receptor complex will change gene activity. Additional enzymic events such as receptor phosphorylation may be involved (Auricchio *et al.*, 1987).

Nuclear acceptor sites

There is clear evidence that very specific interactions between receptor and DNA occur which are of physiological importance. It is also becoming increasingly likely that protein–protein interactions are involved. Several lines of investigation, mostly using genetic engineering techniques, point to these conclusions. Specific fragments of several hormone-sensitive genes have been isolated and their interaction with purified receptors studied. It has been part of established dogma that a major effect of steroid hormones is to increase transcription by interaction with regulatory regions 5' to the structural gene, the so-called steroid, responsive or regulatory elements (SREs; Fig. 4). These can be enhancers (Parker, 1983; Yamamoto, 1985), but other components may also be involved (Yamamoto, 1985). A common feature of the receptor-DNA experiments is that multiple binding sites have been demonstrated, some of which are within the coding region of the gene, although no such examples have yet been reported for estrogen-sensitive genes.

A second class of experiments that has greatly increased our information about DNA-binding sites involves the transfection of chimeric genes composed of SREs linked to a structural marker gene into receptor-positive cells. These provide a very powerful method for testing the biological function

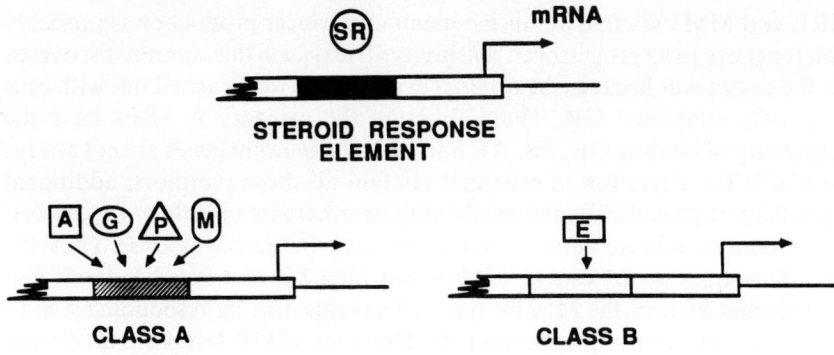

Fig. 4 Gene regulation by steroid-receptor (SR) binding to specific regulatory regions (steroid-response elements) of sensitive genes. Class A SREs bind receptors for androgen (A), glucocorticoid (G), progestogen (P) and mineralocorticoid (M). Class B regions bind estrogen (E) receptors but not those for other steroids.

of specific regions of DNA. Thus, the biological effect of modification or deletion of specific bases in an SRE can be assessed.

From data on the limited number of genes studied thus far, SREs can be divided into two categories, A and B (Fig. 4). Estrogen-responsive genes have SREs (type B) or, more specifically, estrogen-response elements (ERE) with high affinity for ER but, on currently available evidence, not other steroid receptors such as GR or PR. On the other hand, GR-sensitive genes have response elements with a wider specificity profile (type A) in which DNA binding and biological response can additionally occur with receptors for progestogens (P), androgens (A) and mineralocorticoids (M) (Arriza *et al.*, 1987; King, 1987). ER does not interact with this second category of response element although small changes in base sequence can convert a GRE to an ERE (Schütz *et al.*, 1988).

These findings raise several questions of clinical relevance, three of which will be discussed here. (1) If some genes have SREs of wide specificity, what determines the more precise specificity seen *in vivo*? (2) Efficacy of hormone response is related to receptor quantity, so how does receptor number influence gene function? (3) If more than one receptor type can bind to a given SRE, can synergistic or antagonistic interactions occur at the DNA level? This is particularly pertinent to the topic of tamoxifen action.

Questions 1 and 2 are interrelated and will be discussed together. The wide specificity of category A-type SRE was largely uncovered by the use of model systems in which specific gene activity was tested in the presence of an experimentally generated steroid receptor environment. For example, induction of mouse mammary tumour virus (MMTV) was originally said to be glucocorticoid specific, whereas we now know that it has a category A type

SRE and MMTV's role in murine mammary cancer production is probably related more to its progestogen sensitivity. The reason this was not discovered at the outset was because the original experiments were carried out with cells that only contained GR. Thus, although the category A SREs have the capability of binding GR, PR, AR and MR, the relevant genes are not always available for activation in cells that contain all those receptors; additional specificity is provided by the availability or otherwise of different receptors. Furthermore, relative numbers of receptors can influence response. Thus, the T47-D human breast cancer cell line has high PR and low GR levels and transfected SRE of the MMTV type reflects that fact by responding well to progestogens but not glucocorticoids. However, if GR levels are artificially raised, the SRE can also be efficiently activated by glucocorticoids (Parker *et al.*, 1987).

The important conclusion is that specificity and efficiency of gene activity can be determined by both receptor availability and its concentration, with the major proviso that the appropriate ligands are present (see below).

What about agonist/antagonist interaction at an ERE? It is abundantly clear that tamoxifen and analogous compounds can antagonize estradiol action by competition for available receptor (Jordan *et al.*, 1986; Watts *et al.*, 1986) and that the receptor can adopt a different conformation when bound to estradiol to that obtained with tamoxifen (Tate *et al.*, 1984). Could there be additional effects at the DNA level (Fig. 5)? Whilst this possibility has been acknowledged in the past (Jordan *et al.*, 1977), it has been impossible to resolve definitively because the presence of ER in the test systems complicates the divorcing of competitions for receptor binding from binding to DNA. Furthermore, tamoxifen can act as an agonist on some genes and not on others. Work published in a recent elegant paper has resolved these difficulties. The authors (Webster *et al.*, 1988) constructed a chimeric receptor made up of the DNA-binding domain of a yeast regulatory protein, GAL4, plus the estradiol/hydroxytamoxifen-binding domain of ER and transfected the construct into ER-negative cells containing a GAL4-sensitive gene. The normal GAL4 protein activated the gene and this was unaffected by the presence of the chimeric GAL4–ER protein provided hydroxytamoxifen was absent. Addition of hydroxytamoxifen enabled the DNA-binding form of the constructed protein to compete with normal GAL4 protein for the response element and inhibit gene function. Clearly the hydroxytamoxifen, when bound to the chimeric protein, converts the protein into a DNA-binding form. Nevertheless, this complex will not activate the gene. It will, however, block gene activation by the normal protein. In addition to showing that hydroxytamoxifen–receptor complexes can be inhibitory at the gene level, these data also support the view that receptor binding to DNA is a necessary but incomplete requirement for gene activation (see above).

Although there have been no reported examples of steroid receptors other than ER binding to EREs, it has been speculated that the product of the

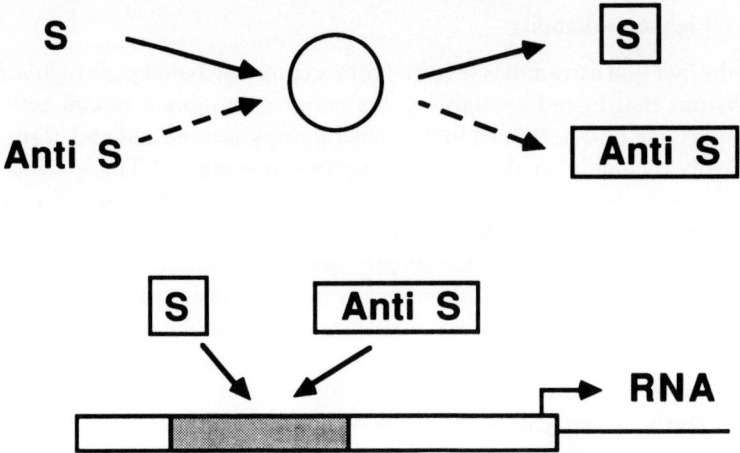

ALONE : STIMULATION / INHIBITION

TOGETHER : INTERACTION

Fig. 5 Agonist (S)–antagonist (anti S) interactions at the level of receptor (O) and the steroid response element (shaded area). The receptor adopts a different conformation when bound to agonist (estradiol) than with an antagonist (tamoxifen).

oncogene v-erb A might do so (Green & Chambon, 1986; Parker, 1987) and there is evidence that another member of the receptor family, the thyroid receptor, can indeed interact with an ERE (Glass *et al.*, 1988). This raises the fascinating possibility of apparently unrelated ligands interacting at the gene level.

Regulation of estradiol receptor numbers

Estradiol receptor numbers are regulated in normal endometrial cells through the menstrual cycle, with high values during the estrogenic (proliferative) phase and low values accompanying the secretion of progesterone during the second half of the cycle. There are only limited data on the molecular basis for this regulation, although changes in transcription are important. Thus, estradiol upregulates uterine ER mRNA (Piva *et al.*, 1988), whilst a reasonable correlation between ER numbers and ER mRNA has been demonstrated in breast tumours (Barrett-Lee *et al.*, 1987; Garcia *et al.*, 1988).

Ligand availability

Given the fact that estradiol is required for receptor-mediated gene regulation, it is obvious that ligand availability is a major determinant of cell activity. Availability can be determined in two general ways: is it present and, if so, is it biologically available to the cellular response machinery? The uterine ER machinery is present and capable of functioning prior to the onset of ovarian steroid secretion in rodents (Kaye *et al.*, 1980) so this would be an example of activity being determined by estrogen presence. However, the mere presence of estradiol in a tissue does not automatically indicate its access to the response machinery. Thus, postmenopausal uteri contain nanomolar concentrations of estradiol which would be anticipated to be biologically active; this is not the case, however, as the endometrium is atrophic (Vermeulen-Meiners *et al.*, 1984). Clearly a sequestration mechanism exists within the uterus, the identification of which would be of interest. The most likely explanation is that the inactive estradiol is extracellular and possibly bound to sex hormone-binding globulin, large amounts of which are known to be present (Wagner & Jungblut, 1976).

Estradiol receptors and cell proliferation

Overwhelming evidence indicates that estradiol-modulated cell proliferation is a receptor-mediated event but identification of the steps linking receptor activation to cell division remains elusive; current interest is largely centered on growth factors. Most data have been derived from studies with breast cancer cell lines (Dickson & Lippman, 1988) and little information is available for endometrium.

Estradiol receptors and blood vessel physiology

The changes in blood vessel function associated with menstruation are unlikely to be due to direct effects of estrogens on the blood vessels because of the temporal gap between maximal estrogen levels and arteriole constriction. Furthermore, continuous unopposed estrogen administration to postmenopausal women does not result in menstruation. However, this does not rule out a role for estrogen and its receptor in this process. The ability of estrogens to increase the efficacy of progestogen action by receptor-mediated events is one well-known way in which an estrogen effect could be mediated. Alternatively, the smooth muscle cells of the arteriole system do contain sex-steroid receptors (Shain & Lin, 1988), so additional effects are possible.

References

Arriza, J.L., Weinberger, C., Cerelli, G., Glaser, T.M., Handelin, B.L., Housman, D.E. & Evans, R.M. (1987). Cloning of human mineralocorticoid receptor complementary DNA: structural and functional kinship with the glucocorticoid receptor. *Science*, **237**:268–275.

Auricchio, F., Migliaccio, A., Di Domenico, M. & Nola, E. (1987). Oestradiol stimulates tyrosine phosphorylation and hormone binding activity of its own receptor in a cell-free system. *EMBO Journal*, **6**:2923–2929.

Bailly, A., Le Page, C., Rauch, M. & Milgrom, E. (1986). Sequence-specific DNA binding of the progesterone receptor to the uteroglobin gene: effects of hormone, antihormone and receptor phosphorylation. *EMBO Journal*, **5**:3235–3241.

Barrett-Lee, P.J., Travers, M.T., McClelland, R.A., Luqmani, Y. & Coombes, R.C. (1987). Characterization of estrogen receptor messenger RNA in human breast cancer. *Cancer Research*, **47**:6653–6659.

Denis, M., Poellinger, L., Wikstöm, A.C. & Gustaffson, J.A. (1988). Requirement of hormone for thermal conversion of the glucocorticoid receptor to a DNA-binding state. *Nature*, **333**:686–688.

Dickson, R.B. & Lippman, M.E. (1988). Control of human breast cancer by estrogen, growth factors, and oncogenes. (In) *Breast Cancer: Cellular and Molecular Biology* (Lippman, M.E. & Dickson, R.B., eds.), pp.119–165. Boston, Kluwer Academic.

Evans, R.M. (1988). The steroid and thyroid hormone receptor superfamily. *Science*, **240**:889–895.

Garcia, T., Lehrer, S., Bloomer, W.D. & Schachter, B. (1988). A variant estrogen receptor messenger ribonucleic acid is associated with reduced levels of estrogen binding in human mammary tumors. *Molecular Endocrinology*, **2**:785–791.

Giguere, V., Ong, E.S., Segui, P. & Evans, R.M. (1987). Identification of a receptor for the morphogen retinoic acid. *Nature*, **330**:624–629.

Glass, C.K., Holloway, J.M., Devary, O.V. & Rosenfeld, M.G. (1988). The thyroid hormone receptor binds with opposite transcriptional effects to a common sequence motif in thyroid hormone and estrogen response elements. *Cell*, **54**:313–323.

Godowski, P.J., Picard, D. & Yamamoto, K.R. (1988). Signal transduction and transcriptional regulation by glucocorticoid receptor-LexA fusion proteins. *Science*, **241**:812–816.

Godowski, P.J., Rusconi, S., Miesfeld, R. & Yamamoto, K.R. (1987). Glucocorticoid receptor mutants that are constitutive activators of transcriptional enhancement. *Nature*, **325**:365–368.

Green, S. & Chambon, P. (1986). A superfamily of potentially oncogenic hormone receptors. *Nature*, **324**:615–617.

Green, S. & Chambon, P. (1987). Oestradiol induction of a glucocorticoid-responsive gene by a chimeric receptor. *Nature*, **325**:75–78.

Green, S., Walter, P., Kumar, V., Krust, A., Bornert, J.M., Argos, P. & Chambon, P. (1986). Human oestrogen receptor cDNA: sequence, expression and homology to v-erb-A. *Nature*, **320**:134–139.

Greene, G.L., Gilna, P., Waterfield, M., Baker, A., Hort, Y. & Shine, J. (1986). Sequence and expression of human estrogen receptor complementary DNA. *Science*, **231**:1150–1154.

Joab, I., Radanyi, C., Renoir, M., Buchou, T., Catelli. M.-G., Binart, N., Mester, J. & Baulieu, E.-E. (1984). Common non-hormone binding component in non-transformed chick oviduct receptors of four steroid hormones. *Nature*, **308**:850–853.

Jordan, V.C., Dix, C.J., Rowsby, L. & Prestwich, G. (1977). Studies on the mechanism of action of the nonsteroidal antioestrogen tamoxifen (I.C.I.46,474) in the rat. *Molecular and Cellular Endocrinology*, **7**:177–192.

Jordan, V.C., Koch, R. & Lieberman, M.E. (1986). Structure–activity relationships of nonsteroidal estrogens and antiestrogens. (In) *Estrogen/Antiestrogen Action and Breast Cancer Therapy* (Jordan, V.C., ed.), pp.19–42. Madison, University of Wisconsin Press.

Kaye, A.M., Reiss, N. & Walker, M.D. (1980). Sequential acquisition of responsiveness to estrogen in the rat uterus. (In) *Development of Responsiveness to Steroid Hormones* (Kaye, A.M. & Kaye, M., eds.), pp.1–22. Oxford, Pergamon Press.

King, R.J.B. (1986). Receptor structure: a personal assessment of the current status. *Journal of Steroid Biochemistry*, **25**:451–454.

King, R.J.B. (1987). Structure and function of steroid receptors. *Journal of Endocrinology*, **114**:341–349.

Kumar, V. & Chambon, P. (1988). The estrogen receptor binds tightly to its responsive element as a ligand-induced homodimer. *Cell*, **55**:145–156.

Kumar, V., Green, S., Stack, G., Berry, M., Jin, J.-R. & Chambon, P. (1987). Functional domains of the human estrogen receptor. *Cell*, **51**:941–951.

Miller, M.A., Mullick, A., Greene, G.L. & Katzenellenbogen, B.S .(1985). Characterization of the subunit nature of nuclear estrogen receptors by chemical cross-linking and dense amino acid labeling. *Endocrinology*, **117**:515–522.

Notides, A.C. (1978). Conformational forms of the estrogen receptor. (In) *Receptors and Hormone Action*, Vol. 2 (O'Malley, B.W. & Birnbaumer, L., eds.), pp.33–40. New York, Academic Press.

Parker, M.G. (1983). Enhancer elements activated by steroid hormones? *Nature*, **304**:687–688.

Parker, M.G. (1987). Oncogenes from hormone receptors. *Journal of Endocrinology*, **112**:1–2.

Parker, M.G., Webb, P., Needham, M., White, R. & Ham, J. (1987). Identification of androgen response elements in mouse mammary tumour virus and the rat prostate C3 gene. *Journal of Cellular Biochemistry*, **35**:285–292.

Penney, G.C. & Hawkins, R.A. (1982). Histochemical detection of oestrogen receptors: a progress report. *British Journal of Cancer*, **45**:237–246.

Petkovich, M., Brand, N.J., Krust, A. & Chambon, P. (1987). A human retinoic acid receptor which belongs to the family of nuclear receptors. *Nature*, **330**:444–450.

Piva, R., Bianchini, E., Kumar, V.L., Chambon, P. & Del Senno, L. (1988). Estrogen induced increase of estrogen receptor RNA in human breast cancer cells. *Biochemical and Biophysical Research Communications*, **155**:943–949.

Sap, J., Munoz, A., Damm, K., Goldberg, Y., Ghysdael, J., Leutz, A., Beug, H. & Vennström, B. (1986). The C-erb-A protein is a high-affinity receptor for thyroid hormone. *Nature*, **324**:635–640.

Schuh, S., Yonemoto, W., Brugge, J., Bauer, V.J., Riehl, R.M., Sullivan, W.P. & Toft, D.O. (1985). A 90,000-dalton binding protein common to both steroid receptors and the Rous sarcoma virus transforming protein, pp60v-src. *Journal of Biological Chemistry*, **260**:14292–14296.

Schütz, G., Strähle, U., Klock, G. & Schmid, W. (1988). Similarities and differences of steroid response elements. (In) *Hormones and Cancer*, Vol. 3 (Bresciani, F., King, R.J.B., Lippman, M.E. & Raynaud, J.-P., eds.), pp.81–87. New York, Raven Press.

Shain, S.A. & Lin, A.L. (1988). Steroid receptors in the cardiovascular system. (In) *Steroid Receptors and Disease* (Sheridan, P.J., Blum, K. & Trachtenberg, M.C., eds.), pp.549–567. New York, Marcel Dekker.

Sheridan, P.J., Buchanan, J.M., Anselmo, V.C. & Martin, P.M. (1979). Equilibrium: the intracellular distribution of steroid receptors. *Nature*, **282**:579–582.

Stumpf, W.E. & Sar, M. (1976). Autoradiographic localization of estrogen, androgen, progestin, and glucocorticosteroid in 'target tissues' and 'non-target tissues'. (In) *Receptors and Mechanism of Action of Steroid Hormones*, Part I (Pasqualini, J.R., ed.), pp.41–84. New York, Marcel Dekker.

Tate, A.C., Greene, G.L., Desombre, E.R., Jensen, E.V. & Jordan, V.C. (1984). Differences between estrogen- and anti-estrogen receptor complexes from human breast tumors identified with an antibody raised against the estrogen receptor. *Cancer Research*, **44**:1012–1018.

Vermeulen-Meiners, C., Jaszmann, L.J., Haspels, A.A., Poortman, J. & Thijssen, J.H. (1984). The endogenous concentration of estradiol and estrone in normal human postmenopausal endometrium. *Journal of Steroid Biochemistry*, **21**:607–612.

Wagner, R.K. & Jungblut, P.W. (1976). Differentiation between steroid hormone receptors CBG and SHBG in human target organ extracts by a single-step assay. *Molecular and Cellular Endocrinology*, **4**:13–24.

Waterman, M.L., Adler, S., Nelson, C., Greene, G.L., Evans, R.M. & Rosenfeld, M.G. (1988). A single domain of the estrogen receptor confers deoxyribonucleic acid binding and transcriptional activation of the rat prolactin gene. *Molecular Endocrinology*, **2**:14–21.

Watts, C.K.W., Murphy, L.C. & Sutherland, R.L. (1986). Properties of high affinity intracellular binding sites for antiestrogens. (In) *Estrogen/Antiestrogen Action and Breast Cancer Therapy* (Jordan, V.C., ed.), pp.93–114. Madison, University of Wisconsin Press.

Webster, N.J.G., Green, S., Jin, J.R. & Chambon, P. (1988). The hormone-binding domains of the estrogen and glucocorticoid receptors contain an inducible transcription activation function. *Cell*, **54**:199–207.

Weinberger, C., Thompson, C.C., Ong, E.S., Lebo, R., Gruol, D.J. & Evans, R.M. (1986). The C-erb-A gene encodes a thyroid hormone receptor. *Nature*, **324**:641–646.

Welshons, W.V. & Gorski, J. (1986). Nuclear location of estrogen receptors. (In) *The Receptors*, Vol. IV (Conn, P.M., ed.), pp.97–147. New York, Academic Press.

Willmann, T. & Beato, M. (1986). Steroid-free glucocorticoid receptor binds specifically to mouse mammary tumour virus DNA. *Nature*, **324**:688–691.

Yamamoto, K.R. (1985). Steroid receptor regulated transcription of specific genes and gene networks. *Annual Review of Genetics*, **19**:209–252.

Discussion

Rees. In your presentation you stated that unopposed estrogen administration to postmenopausal women does not result in menstruation. If you give postmenopausal women unopposed estrogen for 2 weeks out of 4, many will have withdrawal bleeding the week after estrogen administration.

King. Yes, but I was talking about continuous unopposed estrogen.

Rees. But some of them will also bleed irregularly on continuous unopposed estrogen.

King. Some of them do but they are a minority.

Baird. This discussion illustrates the point I tried to make yesterday. You are saying that the estrogen treatment causes menstruation. This is vaginal bleeding, which is not necessarily the same as 'normal' menstruation.

King. If you cause unopposed proliferation of the endometrium by unopposed estrogen, then at some stage, the endometrium will break away, possibly by a completely different mechanism than by the influence on blood vessels. That is certainly true with estrogen implants in the postmenopausal period where they cause a higher degree of hyperplasia and endometrial thickening than straightforward oral hormone replacement therapy.

Findlay. We should not forget that it is possible to have peripheral production of estrogen occurring in the human, for example by fat cells, even though the ovary may be turned off. The concentrations of estrogen produced from extragonadal sources could be sufficient to maintain a significant level of progesterone receptor. It is also interesting to note that the concentration of estrogen receptors in the endometrium of the ovariectomized sheep is relatively high, although not as high as in an intact animal. With respect to the effect of steroids, estrogen in particular, on blood vessels, I think we should separate effects of steroids on angiogenesis from effects on control of flow. In some cases it may well be by a paracrine action from stromal cells or epithelial cells. On the other hand, it might be by an effect of the steroids acting through smooth muscle cells which would be an obvious candidate for effects on flow.

Baird. I would like to back up what Dr Findlay has said about distinguishing between a receptor-mediated event such as angiogenesis induced by products following estrogen stimulation and effects on blood flow. Tiny amounts of estrogens infused into the uterine arteries have an immediate and profound effect on uterine blood flow (Greiss & Anderson, 1970). Because these effects occur within a matter of minutes, it seems unlikely that they depend on the synthesis of new proteins following interaction of the steroid–receptor complex with the nucleus.

King. I would remind you of two pieces of data. Estrogen effects on blood flow, just alluded to, were rapid and could be prevented by beta blockers. The second example is taken from the atherosclerosis field. It is my understanding of that literature that there is now evidence in favour of a direct end-organ effect on the endothelial cells of the arteries as well as via lipoproteins. What those effects are I think still has to be elucidated.

Bouchard. I think we should be very careful about the non-receptor-mediated effect of steroids, because the data in the literature are not very impressive and I think you can count the well-demonstrated models on one hand. One is the electrophysiological effect of progesterone on the myometrium, but the mediation of this mechanism is completely unknown; the second model is the effect of progesterone on cAMP production in the Xenopus oocyte. We know very little about these non-receptor-mediated effects. Where do we go from now? I think we should use simple models with fixed regimens of hormonal treatments and study several hormone-dependent markers with the aim of obtaining a complete time-sequence analysis of every hormonally induced element during the menstrual cycle.

Johannisson. I would like to endorse what Dr King said about what we can learn from research on atherosclerosis. I think Colburn and Buonassisi (1978) demonstrated that estradiol receptors were present in the endothelial cells of aortic tissue, when analyzed *in vitro*.

Cornillie. I would like to recall an old hypothesis on the 'fragility' of lysosomes which may be relevant to the non-receptor-mediated actions of steroids. There has been a series of experiments done by de Duve's group in Leuven (de Duve *et al.*, 1962). They showed, at least in test-tubes, that rat liver lysosomes become permeable after the addition of steroids including β-estradiol and progesterone. That hypothesis was abandoned later because concentrations of steroids 20 to 50 times above the physiological ones were required. Having heard that inside the tissue the concentrations are much higher than those we measure in serum, and that steroids bound to proteins can have such effects, I think it would be wise at least to reconsider this hypothesis with isolated lysosomes from the human endometrium.

Healy. Regarding tamoxifen, is it still believed that, in addition to those agents acting on the estrogen receptor, there is a specific antiestrogen receptor? And if so what is known about its gene regulation and the regulatory elements?

King. There is no evidence that I am aware of for a specific antiestrogen receptor. There is a lot of evidence for the existence of a protein that will specifically bind the antiestrogen, but the whole concept of receptors implies a biological response, and the debate is currently centering around whether the specific tamoxifen-binding protein elicits a specific biological response. The data from Rob Sutherland in Sydney are the best (Watts *et al.*, 1986). They indicate that at the usual active concentrations of tamoxifen, antiestrogen binding is probably not involved in the biological response, but if you get up to enormous concentrations, then it may start to become important.

Gurpide. What is the influence of acceptor proteins around the DNA regions where the receptor is going to interact in the regulation of the gene?

King. It is an area that I only touched on, in the sense that I said that other proteins were involved. The reason I did not elaborate is that there is so little information about them that one cannot really make a clear picture from it. What one can say is that to get receptor influence on gene function you need the receptor binding to DNA, but you clearly need additional interaction with other proteins that are in the chromosomes. These could be in the category of acceptor proteins, but what they are and how they interact is far from clear. It is an area of great research activity at the moment.

Vihko. You presented the different models for the activation of the receptors to DNA-binding form. Do you think they are basically similar for the major processes of all steroids? You also presented a model for the mechanism of action of monohydroxytamoxifen. Do you think that can be generalized for other types of steroids and receptors, for example progesterone and antiprogesterones?

King. A quick generalization of action. I think possibly not, but the great desire for simplicity may have misled us in certain respects. So whether the mechanisms are identical for the estrogen action and for glucocorticoid action is still open to quite considerable doubt. My own feeling, and this is a feeling rather than based on data, is that it would not be unreasonable for a class of steroids that are essential for life, like the glucocorticoids, to have different mechanisms from classes of steroids like the estrogens that are not essential for adult life, except for propagation of the species. The second question was whether the mechanism proposed for the mechanisms of action of antagonists for the estrogen series is generally applicable. We have most data for the antagonists for estrogens. The data for antagonists for progestogens or glucocorticoids are certainly compatible with those sorts of models, but because of the paucity of data it is still possible that some differences exist.

White. What do you think of the concept that domains of the receptor may specify transcription factors that can be brought into the gene in a specific manner? That would be a level at which you could get regulation, that would accommodate the ability of different receptors to bind to the same hormone response element.

King. Are you suggesting that part of the receptor itself has regions that can recognize other proteins that regulate the transcription? I think that is true because the two domains that I hardly mentioned at all, that is other than the DNA-binding and the steroid-binding domain, are clearly important regions that influence the magnitude of the response. Those regions that influence the magnitude of the response do reflect interactions between the receptor and other proteins within the chromatin and they influence gene function.

Findlay. I would like some clarification about the influence of estrogen on the receptor with the two models that you had – activation and derepression. I was not clear about the activation model, given that the DNA-binding domain must be in the sequence. Exactly what do you mean by activation? The derepression model seems to be reasonable.

King. The idea that the actual structure that recognizes the DNA is not present in the absence of steroids comes from experiments studying activity after removal of only the part that binds steroids. If the structure is there all the time, then with the removal of the steroid-binding domain, you would expect to have a fully functional protein that did not need steroids to bind it. Now, for estrogen that is not the case. If you remove the steroid-binding domain, you decrease the biological activity of that receptor dramatically. So, therefore, there must be more required than simply exposing that region of the DNA. There must be some other changes within that DNA-binding region that the steroid can influence. On the other hand, experiments with glucocorticoid and progesterone receptors come to a different conclusion: removal of the steroid-binding domain produces a constitutively active protein.

Findlay. But that could surely be just the same as, in effect, derepression. It may be that it is still a conformational change, and it is something peculiar to the estrogen receptor.

Åkerlund. Could you tell us about how other antihormones, the competitive inhibitors of surface receptor-acting hormones such as peptides, work?

King. It is mainly outside of my normal sphere of influence. It seems that it can happen at different levels: you can get competition for binding in much the same way as I have shown for steroids, e.g. you can get competition between the binding EGF to its receptor and the monoclonal antibodies to that receptor. But the whole story of how things like LHRH superagonists act points to another way in which you can get antagonism at the receptor level, namely the whole question of down-regulation of receptor numbers.

Baird. You mentioned that in certain target organs tamoxifen acted as an antagonist by competitive inhibition and indeed in the absence of estrogen will act as an agonist. So does this mean that the Lipmann model for antagonists is not a general one for target organs, it only applies to, for example, the specific breast tumour cell line in which the induction of TGFβ by tamoxifen is able to be demonstrated.

King. No, I think it does have more generality than that. I think those data, partly from differences in the ligand, show that the mono-hydroxytamoxifen is a partial agonist and a partial antagonist. This is obviously a complex situation. There is now a new generation of antagonists which are really pure antagonists with no agonist activity and yet they are also capable of switching on certain genes. I think there are also data for RU486 that show it will switch on the production of certain proteins. So I would see that antagonists can act in more than one way. They can antagonize the effect of an agonist by all the classical mechanisms, but there are examples like the one I showed you in which an antagonist can specifically switch on a gene, and the product of that gene is actually a negative regulator.

Fraser. How good is the technology for looking at estrogen receptor or other receptor concentrations in very small amounts of tissue, for example in small endometrial biopsies that could be obtained from patients on long-term progestogen therapy?

King. I will only address part of that question. At the biochemical level the technology of measuring small amounts of receptor probably has not improved over and above that of the ligand binding, in terms of how much tissue you actually need to get a reliable result. The immunoassays for receptor that are now available have about the same level of sensitivity as the radio ligand-binding assays. They are probably a little more reliable at very low levels and therefore you would have a better chance of being more correct with small amounts of tissue with the immunoassays than with the ligand-binding assays, but at the histochemical level it is a different matter altogether.

Clark. You mention that when tamoxifen is bound to the estrogen receptor, the conformation of the complex differed from that produced when estrogen is bound with the receptor. I was wondering if you knew whether a similar difference might exist when synthetic progestogens, for example, bind to the progesterone receptor? Are there analogues of steroid hormones that produce complexes that, in one cell, will produce the effect that would occur with a naturally occurring complex, and yet in another cell will produce quite different effects? Do we know anything about differences in the shape and action of the active complex when we change the steroid structure slightly?

King. I am not aware of any data for proving that there is a difference in shape with the other complexes. The data that I showed you for the antiestrogen are based almost entirely on the ability of different antibodies to react with the steroid–receptor complex. Again, maybe the people who have the biggest battery of antibodies to the progesterone receptors have some information on that, but I am not aware of any of it.

Gurpide. We can see disassociation of the actions of estradiol and hydroxytamoxifen, working with an endometrial cell line (Ishikawa) under serum-free conditions. Estradiol increases cell number, and hydroxytamoxifen is even more effective in increasing cell density. In the presence of serum, the effects of estradiol and hydroxytamoxifen depends on the culture medium: in MEM only, estradiol increases cell number and hydroxytamoxifen is antiestrogenic, whereas in DMEM + Ham's F12, both are stimulatory. What may be happening is that the positive action of hydroxytamoxifen may take place by interaction with a binding site different from that used by estradiol. Furthermore, hydroxytamoxifen increases cell density in a variant of Ishikawa cells unresponsive to estradiol.

King. I think it is true to say that from the data, at concentrations of tamoxifen or hydroxytamoxifen of 10^{-7} mol or lower, there is really no evidence of any other binding sites that are functionally important from the receptor side.

Harper. It has been suggested that tamoxifen may bind to a site that has been identified as a histamine H_3 site.

King. There have been many suggestions, and I have seen publications of similar claims for things like protein kinases. However, these experiments are done at such astronomical levels of compound that I personally do not think they have any relationship to physiology.

Hirata. I think that there is some confusion about the binding of the antisteroid and the steroid and the conformational changes of these receptors. I would just like to point out some consensus mechanism of the glucocorticoid system. Usually the glucocorticoid receptor makes a complex with the heat-shock protein, so-called Hsp 90, and when glucocorticoid binds to the receptor complex, the conformation is changed to disassociate the receptor from heat-shock protein, that is the activated form. The group of anticorticoids can also bind to corticoidal receptor but somehow the conformational changes are a little different from those induced by the corticoid. Thus, anticorticoid receptor cannot be disassociated from heat-shock protein and, interestingly, corticoid receptors separated from the heat-shock protein can bind anticorticoid and corticoid and these complexes can bind to the DNA-binding site. Therefore, researchers in the field of corticoid receptors believe that the disassociation of corticoidal receptor from the heat-shock protein is the most important part relating to the activation of steroid receptor.

King. What you say is true, the 90-kd heat-shock protein is a component of the large 8S receptor identified in cell homogenates. What is less clear is whether the 8S receptor is a biologically important entity or an homogenization artefact.

Bischof. In your presentation you were saying that receptors are either in the nucleus or in the cytosol. You seem to exclude membrane receptors for steroids. Is that so?

King. The classical steroid receptors have not been detected in cell membranes, the vast majority are either in the cytosol or in the nucleus. I specifically excluded a small proportion of receptors that probably are associated with the endoplasmic reticulum. There are immunohistochemical data indicating a small proportion being in the endoplasmic reticulum; this is where the receptors are made in the first place. It would not be unreasonable to think that there are some there, but they are there in very small amounts.

Vihko. How do you explain, if you think of this class of response elements, what are the mechanisms that lead to the rather high degree of specificity in response? I am thinking of these different ligands. What do you think are the mechanisms?

King. It is a fascinating question: why should one gene have the ability to recognize four different classes of steroid receptor and yet you clearly do have a good degree of specificity. The answer will be complex and depend on several features: it depends on which ligand is available and the relative concentrations of different receptors. If there is only progesterone in the cell, then the ability of the gene to recognize glucocorticoid receptor is irrelevant. So, the relative concentration of those two components is important.

References .

Colburn, P. & Buonassisi, V. (1978). Estrogen binding sites in endothelial cell cultures. *Science*, **210**:817–819.

Greiss, F.C. & Anderson, S.G. (1970). Uterine blood flow during early ovine pregnancy. *American Journal of Obstetrics and Gynecology*, **106**:30–38.

De Duve, C., Wattiaux, R. & Wibo, M. (1962). Effects of fat soluble compounds on lysosomes *in vitro*. *Biochemical Pharmacology*, **9**:97–116.

Watts, C.K.W., Murphy, L.C. & Sutherland, R.L. (1986). Properties of high affinity intracellular binding sites for antiestrogens. (In) *Estrogen/Antiestrogen Action and Breast Cancer Therapy* (Craig Jordan, V, ed.), pp.93–114. Wisconsin, University of Wisconsin Press.

Evaluation of endometrial maturation with the immunocytolocalization of estradiol and progesterone receptors

P. BOUCHARD, G. SCHAISON, J. MARRAOUI, R. FRYDMAN,
E. GARCIA, E. MILGROM AND M. PERROT-APPLANAT

Service d'Endocrinologie et des Maladies de la Reproduction, Hôpital Bicêtre et Unité de Recherches 'Hormones et Reproduction' INSERM U135, Le Kremlin-Bicêtre, France.

Abstract

Endometrial progesterone (PR) and estrogen (ER) receptors were studied by immunocytochemistry using monoclonal antibodies in several circumstances: during the menstrual cycle in normal women, in anovulatory women, in women with ovarian failure treated with estrogens and progesterone.

Immunocytochemical studies showed that the concentrations and distribution of receptors change markedly during the normal menstrual cycle. During the mid-follicular period, a small proportion of stromal and glandular cells stain positively for PR, while staining for ER is more intense and more frequent. During the late follicular phase and early luteal period the staining for PR increases markedly in glandular cells. During the mid and late luteal phase, ER and PR staining disappears in glandular cells. These variations of PR, especially the disappearance of PR under the effect of progesterone, are potentially useful for studying the cumulative effect of progesterone on endometrial maturation. This was confirmed in anovulatory women, where a late luteal phase aspect was observed, i.e. the absence of PR and ER decrease in glandular cells. In women with ovarian failure, the disappearance of PR in glandular cells is correlated with the duration of progesterone therapy.

In addition, we observed a staining for PR in muscular cells of human uterine arteries, suggesting a role for steroid hormones in uterine vascular changes during the menstrual cycle.

Introduction

The appreciation of endometrial status is mandatory in order to assess infertile women and to determine the quality of the endometrium after therapeutic induction of ovulation or during hormonal therapy. Since their publication, the classic histological changes described by Noyes *et al.* (1950) have been widely used for histologic dating of human endometrium. Such criteria have generated some controversy, especially with regard to the assessment of luteal phase defects. On the basis of these criteria, luteal phase defects have been reported in as many as 4–65 % of infertile women (Li *et al.*, 1988). Endometrial estrogen (ER) and progesterone (PR) receptor measurements may help to define the state of endometrial maturation, since uterine hormone receptors are subject to fine hormonal control by estradiol and progesterone (Bayard *et al.*, 1978). Variations in these receptor levels during the menstrual cycle have been described in animals and humans by the binding technique which does not take into account the differences in receptor content of various cell types and is prone to errors due to receptor occupancy (Vu Hai *et al.*, 1977; Savouret *et al.*, 1989).

In order to evaluate the potential role of ER and PR immunocytochemistry in assessing endometrial maturation, we studied the distribution of endometrial ER and PR during the normal menstrual cycle as well as in endometrial samples obtained from anovulatory women or women receiving an hormonal treatment for oocyte donation, using monoclonal antibodies against ER and PR.

Methods

Biopsies were performed with Novak's cannula, and some of them with both Novak's cannula and Cornier's aspiration pipette (Laboratoire CCD, Paris, France). Each sample was divided in two parts: one part was frozen in isopentane, precooled in liquid nitrogen and stored in liquid nitrogen until processing; the second half was fixed in Bouin's solution and processed for histology.

Endometrial samples were sectioned (4 μm thick) at $-24°C$ and thaw-mounted on gelatin-coated glass slides. The peroxidase–antiperoxidase method was used on frozen sections after fixation with picric acid formaldehyde. The slides were blocked with normal goat or rabbit serum for 10 minutes before exposure to the first antibody. The antiprogesterone antibody LET 126 (25 μg/ml) was used (Perrot-Applanat *et al.*, 1987; Lorenzo *et al.*, 1988); ER immunostaining was performed with a kit from Abbott laboratories (North Chicago, Ill., USA). Details of the procedure have been described elsewhere (Perrot-Applanat *et al* 1987; Garcia *et al.*, 1988).

Controls included immunostaining with mouse receptors unrelated monoclonal antibody and rat normal immunoglobulins. In addition, monoclonal anti-PR antibody was presaturated with highly purified PR (Logeat *et al.*, 1985). The staining patterns were similar when other monoclonal anti PR antibodies directed against different epitopes of the receptor were used (Lorenzo *et al.*, 1988).

The intensity of specific staining was characterized as absent (0), $+$, $+ +$ or $+ + +$, and the number of stained cells was estimated as absent (0), 25%, 50% or 75%.

Immunostaining of normal endometrial samples during the menstrual cycle   (Table 1, Fig. 1.)

Endometrial tissue samples were obtained from 28 normal women (18–40 years old) participating in an in-vitro fertilization program for male infertility.

Table 1. *Immunocytochemical staining for progesterone and estrogen receptors in endometrial biopsies from normal women*

Subject no.	Chronological day	Progesterone Receptors				Estrogen Receptors			
		Stroma		Gland		Stroma		Gland	
		a*	b**	a	b	a	b	a	b
1	07	+	25	+	25	+	50	+ +	50
2	07	+	25	+	25	+	50	+	50
3	08	+	25	+	25	+ +	50	+	25
4	08	+	25	+	25	+	50	+	50
5	08	+	50	+	50	+ +	50	+	50
6	09	+ +	50	+ + +	75	+	50	+ +	75
7	12	+	25	+ + +	75	+	50	+ +	75
8	14	+ +	75	+ + +	75	+	50	+ +	75
9	14	+ +	50	+ + +	75	+	25	+	25
10	14	+ +	50	+ + +	75	+	25	+ +	25
11	15	+	50	+ + +	75	+ +	75	+ +	75
12	16	+ +	50	+ + +	75	+	25	+	25
13	17	+ +	25	+ +	50	+ +	50	+ +	50
14	18	+	25	+ + +	75	+	25	+	50
15	18	+ +	50	+ + +	75	+	25	+ +	50
16	18	+ +	75	+ + +	75	+ +	50	+ +	50
17	19	+ +	50	+ + +	75	+ +	50	+ +	50
18	19	+ +	50	+ + +	75	+ +	50	+ + +	75
19	21	+ +	50	+ +	25	+	25	+	50
20	21	+ +	75	+	25	+ +	50	+	25
21	22	+ +	50	+	25	+	50	0	
22	22	+ +	50	+	25	+	25	0	
23	22	+	25	0		+	25	0	
24	22	+	25	0		+	25	0	
25	24	+	25	0		0		0	
26	26	+	25	0		0		0	
27	27	+ +	25	0		+	25	0	
28	27	+ +	50	0		+	25	0	

*a = Intensity of staining, characterized as absent (0), +, + + or + + +.
**b = Number of stained cells, estimated as absent (0), 25%, 50%, 75%.

All women had a regular cycle, and were devoid of any hormonal therapy for the preceding 6 months.

The immunostaining patterns of endometrial fragments obtained with Novak's cannula or the aspiration technique were similar. The specific staining was always localized in cell nuclei throughout the menstrual cycle.

Follicular phase

In the midfollicular phase, stromal and glandular cells were equally marked (+ to + +) for ER and PR. The staining was slightly more intense and more frequent for ER. During the late follicular phase, glandular cells were more heavily stained and ER staining was less intense than PR staining.

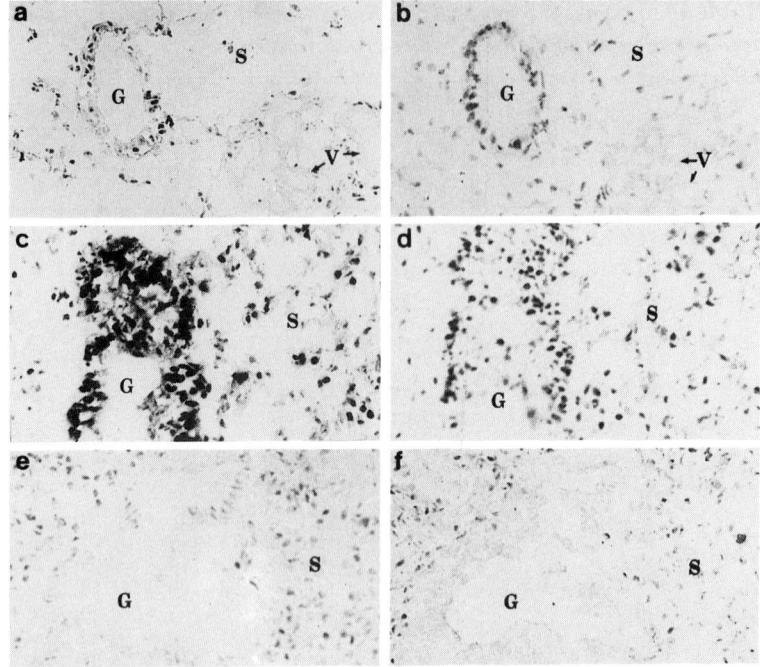

Fig. 1 Immunostaining of PR and ER during the normal menstrual cycle. Glands (G) and stroma (S) are visible in all sections:

a, c, e: staining for PR.
b, d, f: staining for ER.
a, b: day 7.
c, d: day 14.
e, f: day 22.

Luteal phase

ER In the early luteal phase (days 15–19), the stromal and glandular cell-staining patterns were similar to that during the late follicular phase. Glandular cell staining decreased on day 21 and disappeared thereafter.

PR In the early luteal phase (days 15–19), the endometrium showed a pattern and intensity of nuclear staining similar to that in the late follicular phase. In the mid and late luteal phase, the intensity of staining and percentage of stained glandular cells decreased markedly, although PR staining in glandular cells persisted longer than that of ER (day 22 versus day 21). After day 22, stained glandular cells were absent in nearly all the women. Staining of stromal cells remained quasi-identical to the late follicular phase pattern.

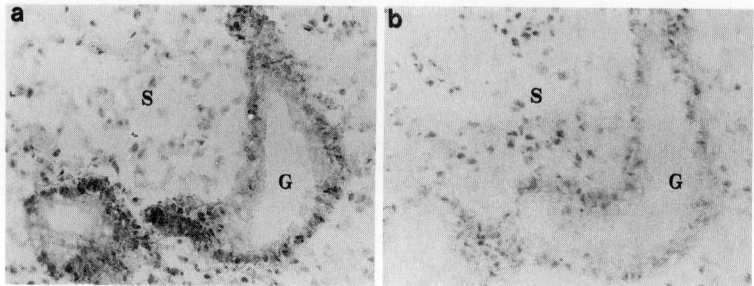

Fig. 2 Immunocytochemical staining for PR (a) and ER (b) in an anovulatory woman.

Immunostaining of endometria from anovulatory women (Fig. 2)

Immunostaining of endometrial biopsies obtained in six women with anovulation due to polycystic ovary syndrome was studied. All biopsies showed a typical midcycle pattern with a moderate staining for ER and a strong staining for PR.

Effect of estrogen and progesterone therapy on the endometrium of women with ovarian failure

In patients with ovarian failure, endometrial tissue can be receptive to embryonic implantation after substitution therapy with estrogens and progesterone, and Lutjen *et al.* (1986) reported the first pregnancy after such treatment.

We studied the effect of exogenous estradiol and progesterone replacement therapy in 16 women undergoing an oocyte donation program. Immunocyto-chemical analysis showed a typical late luteal phase aspect on day 6 after the beginning of the treatment by progesterone and not on day 2 and 4. This information suggests that transfer of the embryo should not be performed later than day 6 after the initiation of progesterone therapy.

ER and PR in human uterine arteries (Fig. 3)

The presence of ER and PR in spiral arteries of the human uterus was observed in endometrial biopsies (functionalis endometrium) (Perrot-Applanat *et al.*, 1988). Specific staining occurred in smooth muscle cells. Immunostaining was clearly observed in these cells at the end of the luteal phase, in contrast with stromal and glandular epithelial cells which at this period of the cycle contain low levels of receptors (Garcia *et al.*, 1988). We found no evidence of receptor staining in the endothelial cells lining blood vessels.

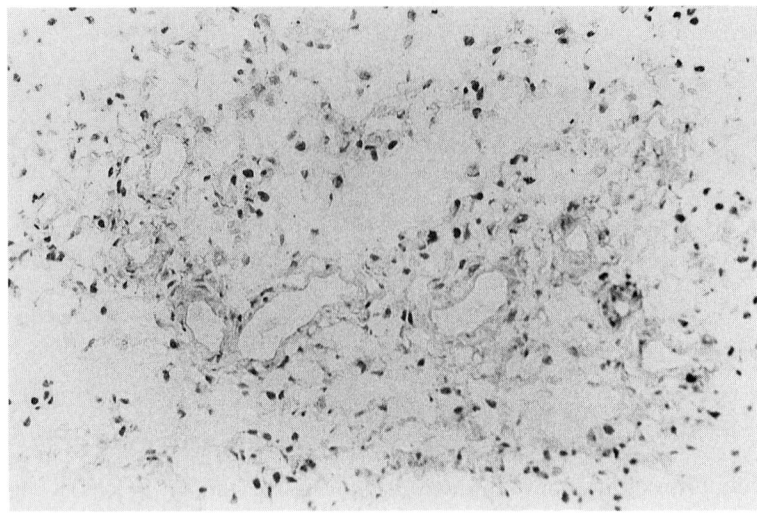

Fig. 3 PR immunostaining of human uterine arteries (day 27 of a normal cycle).

Comments

Estradiol and progesterone regulate endometrial growth. Studies of labelled estradiol and progesterone binding to endometrial samples indicate that receptor concentrations are highest in the late follicular phase and decrease thereafter. Such a decrease of ER and PR in the luteal phase is due to progesterone secretion (Kreitmann *et al.*, 1979). The development of immunocytochemical methods for detecting steroid receptors using monoclonal antibodies allowed us to analyze the presence and the relative abundance of ER and PR in stromal and glandular cells. The intense ER and PR staining during the midcycle period is probably correlated with the increased estradiol secretion at this time. The decrease and disappearance of ER and PR from glandular cells during the late luteal phase are probably due to the effect of progesterone. Our observations in anovulatory women confirm this hypothesis by showing a moderate labelling of glandular cells for ER and PR. Further, endometrial fragments obtained from women with ovarian failure, treated with high doses of estrogens and progesterone, show a typical late luteal phase aspect, i.e. a disappearance of ER and PR in glandular cells following progesterone therapy.

The results obtained in normal endometrium as well as the data collected in anovulatory women and women treated for oocyte donation suggest that receptor immunocytochemistry is useful for evaluating endometrial maturation by showing receptor increase due to the effect of estradiol, while receptor disappearance in glandular cells is an index of the cumulative activity of progesterone. Further, ER and PR are present in rabbit and human uterine arteries, which therefore suggests that physiological uterine vascular changes, such as those observed during the menstrual cycle or during pregnancy, may be modulated by steroid hormones through a direct effect on arterial muscle cells (Perrot-Applanat *et al.*, 1988).

Altogether, our data suggest that endometrial fragments, easily obtained by the aspiration technique, can be used for steroid receptor immunocyto-chemistry, and that such studies provide useful information concerning endometrial maturation. Such analysis may be important in assessing infertile women, especially women with luteal function defects.

References

Bayard, F., Damilano, S., Robel, P. & Baulieu, E.E. (1978). Cytoplasmic and nuclear estradiol and progesterone receptors in human endometrium. *Journal of Clinical Endocrinology and Metabolism*, **46**:635–648.

Garcia, E., Bouchard, P., De Brux, J., Berdah, J., Frydman, R., Schaison, G., Milgrom, E. & Perrot-Applanat, M. (1988). Use of immunocytochemistry of progesterone and estrogen receptors for endometrial dating. *Journal of Clinical Endocrinology and Metabolism*, **67**:80–87.

Kreitmann, B., Bugat, R. & Bayard, F. (1979). Estrogen and progestin regulation of the progesterone receptor concentration in human endometrium. *Journal of Clinical Endocrinology and Metabolism*, **49**:926–929.

Li, T.-C., Rogers, A.W., Dockery, P., Lenton, E.A. & Cooke, I.D. (1988). A new method of histologic dating of human endometrium in the luteal phase. *Fertility and Sterility*, **50**:52–60.

Logeat, F., Pamphile, R., Loosfelt, H., Jolivet, A., Fournier, A. & Milgrom, E. (1985). One step immunoaffinity purification of active progesterone receptor. Further evidence in favor of the existence of a single steroid binding subunit. *Biochemistry*, **24**:1029–1035.

Lorenzo, F., Jolivet, A., Loosfelt, H., Vu Hai, M.T., Brailly, S., Perrot-Applanat, M. & Milgrom, E.(1988). A rapid method of epitope mapping. Application to the study of immunogenic domains and to the characterization of various forms of rabbit progesterone receptor. *European Journal of Biochemistry*, **176**:53–60.

Lutjen, P.J., Findlay, J.K., Trounson, A.O., Leeton, J.F. & Chan, L.K. (1986). Effect on plasma gonadotrophins of cyclic steroid replacement in women with premature ovarian failure. *Journal of Clinical Endocrinology and Metabolism*, **62**:419–423.

Noyes, R.W., Hertig, A.T. & Rock, J. (1950). Dating the endometrial biopsy. *Fertility and Sterility*, **1**:3–25.

Perrot-Applanat, M., Groyer-Picard, M.T., Garcia, E., Lorenzo, F. & Milgrom, E. (1988). Immunocytochemical demonstration of estrogen and progesterone receptors in muscle cells of uterine arteries in rabbits and humans. *Endocrinology*, **123**:1511–1519.

Perrot-Applanat, M., Groyer-Picard, M.T., Lorenzo, F., Jolivet, A., Vu Hai, M.T., Pallud, C., Spyratos, F. & Milgrom, E. (1987). Immunocytochemical study with monoclonal antibodies to progesterone receptor in human breast tumors. *Cancer Research*, **47**:2652–2661.

Savouret, J.F., Misrahi, M., Loosfelt, H., Atger, M., Bailly, A., Perrot-Applanat, M., Vu Hai, M.T., Guiochon-Mantel, A., Jolivet, A., Lorenzo, F., Logeat, F., Pichon, M.F., Bouchard, P. & Milgrom, E. (1989). Molecular and cellular biology of mammalian progesterone receptors. *Recent Progress in Hormone Research*, **45**:65–116.

Vu Hai, M.T., Logeat, F., Warembourg, M. & Milgrom, E. (1977). Hormonal control of progesterone receptors. *Annals of the New York Academy of Sciences*, **286**:199.

Discussion

Cornillie. Is there any significance in the intensity of the labelling?

Bouchard. It is much more difficult to have a quantitative evaluation of immunocytochemical staining than with the binding technique. But there are some people who specialize in the quantification of this labelling and they can certainly differentiate zero from + + +. There is some work that at least one of us has done in breast cancer cells which has already been published (Perrot-Applanat *et al.*, 1987). There is a straight correlation between the intensity of labelling and the amount of receptor measured by binding techniques. But again, immunocytochemistry is not designed to be an accurate quantitative technique.

Cornillie. What is the biological significance of the difference in intensity?

Bouchard. Well, if you are asking me why the receptors disappear from the gland, the answer is 'I do not know'. All I can tell you is that at the beginning I thought it was due to a change in the receptor structure, but we have checked that with different antibodies and could not see any other pattern of staining. In addition, this work has been confirmed since we published these data, by several authors (Press *et al.*, 1984; Clarke *et al.*, 1987; Press & Greene, 1988; Lessey *et al.*, 1988), and they all observed the disappearance of estradiol and progesterone receptors in glands. What this phenomenon means, I am not sure.

King. What information do you have about the staining of decidual cells?

Bouchard. We have not studied that extensively, so I cannot answer you.

King. Is there a correlation between the sort of pictures that you are showing about the regulation in the glands and the stroma with the biochemical data from several groups who have separated epithelium and stroma and shown that you do get regulation in both cell types as you go through the cycle?

Bouchard. Well, it is obvious that although there is no labelling for steroid receptors in the glands in the luteal phase, the glandular cells are still working under the effect of progesterone.

Johannisson. Just a small question, regarding the sensitivity of the method. Have you tried yourself, or are you aware of any similar studies on the localization of steroid receptors using immunofluorescence (e.g. FITC) which is a highly sensitive method?

Bouchard. No.

Smith. Do you know specifically when the receptor is there? What happens to that estrogen/progesterone receptor, which you were able to demonstrate at midcycle, when it goes away? You might not know this specifically in the progesterone case but is it known with any other type of steroid receptor, where or how that receptor is altered so it is unable to bind with the ligand?

Bouchard. What we know is that at the time of the disappearance of receptors in the glands a uteroglobin gene is still being transcribed. I knew we were going to find some discrepancy by using different antireceptor antibodies, but all I can say is that obviously the change does not occur in that part of the receptor molecule which binds DNA. But I cannot say more than that.

Cravioto. Cerbón and co-workers have also studied uteroglobin. To assess whether NET and its metabolites have a direct effect on the uteroglobin gene expression they undertook a number of experiments in prepubertal female rabbits. The baseline concentrations of immunoreactive uteroglobin in uterine flushings from oil-treated prepuberal rabbits were within the assay limits of sensitivity, as indicated in Fig. 4. When progesterone was administered subcutaneously (1 mg/kg body weight per day) for 5 consecutive days, a significant rise of uteroglobin was noticed in both uterine flushings and endometrial cytosol. Similar results were observed when unchanged NET was administered at the same dose level (Fig. 4). The amount of uteroglobin induced by both progesterone and

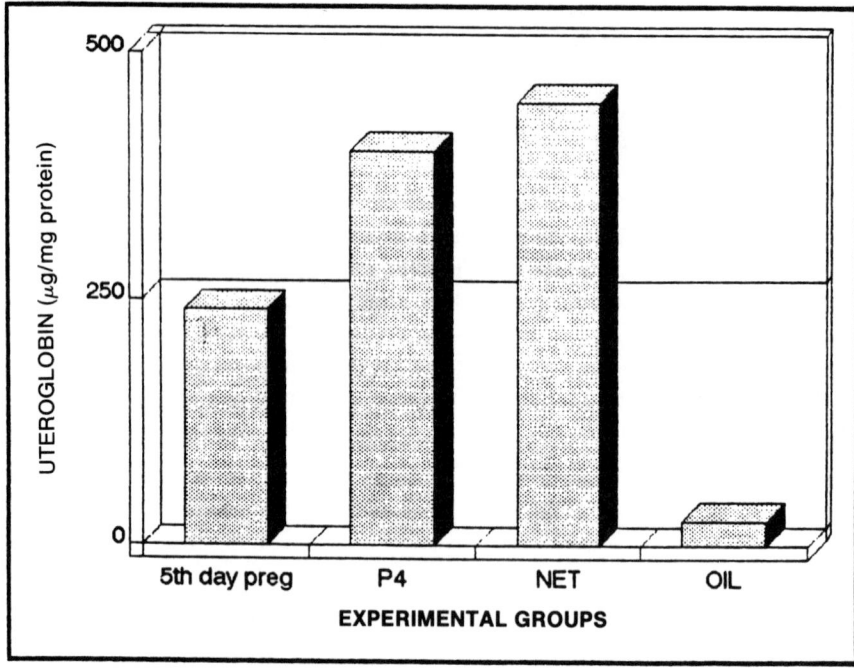

Fig. 4 Induction of endometrial uteroglobin synthesis by progesterone (P4) and norethisterone (NET) in prepubertal rabbits. Uteroglobin was measured by a specific double antibody radioimmunoassay and the results are expressed as µg/mg protein of uterine flushings. Oil-treated prepubertal rabbits (OIL) and pregnant animals on the fifth day (5th day preg) were used as controls.

NET represents ⟩40% of the total protein content of the uterine flushings. The natural progesterone-induced synthesis of uteroglobin as determined in uterine flushings from fifth day pregnant rabbits is also depicted in Fig. 4.

When the effects of progesterone and NET upon the uteroglobin gene transcription were examined by using a Northern blot method (Fig. 5), it was found that both the natural hormone and the synthetic progestin were potent inductors of the uteroglobin mRNA synthesis. This finding correlates appropriately with the endometrial synthesis of the corresponding protein (Cerbón, 1988). Interestingly, it was found that A-ring reduction of the NET molecule resulted in a significant diminution of its potency to induce uteroglobin synthesis. Indeed, 5α-DHNET given at an equivalent dose induces very little uteroglobin. Whereas the 3β, 5α-tetrahydro derivative of NET was totally ineffective. The low potency to induce uteroglobin synthesis of these reduced metabolites of NET

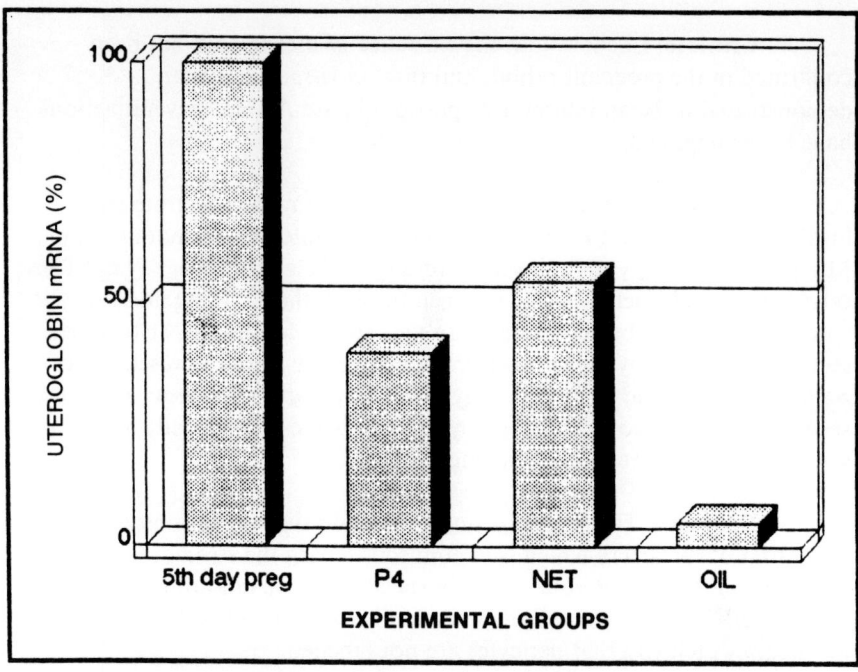

Fig. 5 Induction of endometrial uteroglobin mRNA synthesis by
progesterone (P4) and norethisterone (NET) in prepubertal rabbits.
Specific uteroglobin mRNA was measured by the use of Northern blots
and the results were expressed as the percentage of induction (as assessed
by densitometric analysis), taking the uteroglobin mRNA content of the
endometrium of pregnant animals (5th day preg) as 100%. Oil-treated
rabbits (OIL) were used as controls.

correlated with a concomitant decrease in uteroglobin mRNA synthesis
observed following their administration. The finding that 5α-DHNET
exhibited a rather low effect on the uteroglobin gene expression did not
correlate with the high-affinity binding of this metabolite to the
endometrial progesterone receptor (Chávez *et al.*, 1985). Since 5α-DHNET
exhibits anti-implantation properties in several mammalian species (Reel *et
al.*, 1979), the data presented suggest that it may display an antihormonal
effect at the endometrial level. Whether this 5α-reduced metabolite of NET
has intrinsic antiprogestational activity cannot be ascertained, and still
requires further experimental work.

Ludwig. What do we know about the physiological role of
uteroglobin?

Cravioto. I believe that the existence of uteroglobin has been confirmed in the pregnant rabbit, and that, *in vitro*, it has been demonstrated to be an inhibitor of phospholipase A2, and several actions have been suggested.

Cornillie. Dr Bouchard, you were unable to demonstrate any localization of ER and PR in capillaries and venules in the endometrium. My question is: did you look very carefully at the so-called pericytes? These cells are not endothelial but lie between the endothelial lining and the connective tissue. They are difficult to find and to localize on histological sections because they are so scanty. They resemble smooth muscle cells both in function and in morphology. They have active filaments and they seem to be able to contract, so can you look at these specifically and can you be sure that there is no labelling of these cells?

Bouchard. The answer is no. I must add that in the tunica adventitia of the artery which is in connection with the stroma, there is staining. But to answer your question specifically, we did not look for this kind of cell. What I can assure you is that smooth muscle cells are labelled but I cannot tell you that pericytes are not labelled.

Bell. I was surprised at your results in the late luteal phase of the cycle. One might expect to see areas of predecidualization, particularly in the superficial layers of the endometrial biopsies. This relates to what Dr King was saying, about the presence of these receptors in decidual cells, and also relates to your data showing that the intensity of receptor staining actually in the stroma appeared to be stronger than in those cells around the arteries. I wonder if you could make a comment on that. And also, it is perhaps not that surprising, considering the findings in other epithelial mesenchymal differentiation systems, where the product of steroid hormone action produced by epithelial cells is dependent on the action of hormones on the mesenchyme rather than directly on the epithelium. What you are seeing here is actually differentiation of the glandular epithelium and that is associated with loss of receptors and the steroid hormones are operating through the mesenchyme. I am particularly thinking of the results with the glandular epithelial protein α_2-PEG (α_2 pregnancy-associated endometrial globulin or placental protein 14), which appears to be the result of the action of steroid hormones in the luteal phase on the glandular epithelium. This protein appears at the time when your receptors disappear in glandular epithelium (day 19–21).

Bouchard. It is obvious that progesterone action persists during the luteal phase and that the disappearance of the receptors in the glands cannot explain this phenomenon. I cannot comment further. On the first point, I must acknowledge that although there is a consensus in showing receptor disappearance in glandular cells during the luteal phase in the stroma, the results are more controversial and, using different antibodies, other investigators have shown that stromal cell staining increases during the luteal phase. I must add that all these antibodies are commercially available, including the one we used.

Ludwig. Dr Bouchard, you have clearly shown the prime sequence, the disappearance of staining in the glands and an appearance of staining in the media of the vessel wall. Have you any information on how long the staining of receptors in the vessel walls remains in comparison to the menstrual shedding? And do you have any explanation about the unequal distribution of the staining of stromal cells, and, again, how long this staining of stromal cells remains visible in relation to menstrual shedding?

Bouchard. Regarding the labelling of arteries, I must say that the receptor staining is fairly easy to see in rabbit endometrium if you use good hormonal conditions, which again require low estrogen treatment to see estradiol receptors and large estrogen doses to see progesterone receptors. In the human, it is much more difficult, and, of course, these arteries are only visible during certain parts of the cycle. So far, we could only see these arteries labelled very briefly at the end of the cycle (day 27). Now, whether this is relevant to physiology or whether this is due to the low sensitivity of the technique, I cannot answer you. Regarding the stroma labelling, I think it is very difficult for me to give you firm data for this cellular compartment, because there is controversy on the labelling. According to our experience using different antibodies against human and rabbit progesterone receptors, the labelling of the stroma persists until the very end of the cycle, but it does decrease significantly from day 23 or 24. Again, I must be very cautious in saying that, because other people find very intense labelling until the end of the cycle.

Bischof. I would like to interpret your data in my personal view. I would say that what you have shown is the presence of the AB region of your receptor during the cycle, and that the disappearance you are showing from the glands is, in fact, the disappearance of the A and B region. Have you tried to localize and do the same sort of work with a monoclonal antibody which would recognize the epitopes on the DNA binding or the progesterone binding sites, and would you get the same sort of picture?

Bouchard. First of all, it is impossible to obtain antibodies against these regions, because, as I mentioned before, they are so highly conserved between species that it has not been possible to raise any single antibody, recognizing these regions of the receptor molecule (regions binding to DNA or to steroid ligand). We have other chemical methods to study receptors and other investigators duplicated these studies with autoradiographic or binding techniques but, again, these chemical studies are only visible on cell homogenates. So, if you do not want to destroy receptor structures, you have to use very careful homogenizing techniques. But I agree with you – our antibodies recognize the A and B region.

Cooke. Do you notice any heterogeneity in deposition within an individual sample, and do you see much heterogeneity between samples, that is, between patients? We have noted that about 20% of endometrial biopsy samples, when they are dated, show a substantial retardation in the degree of development that one might expect for a particular dating. Have you any experience of examining your monoclonal antibody deposition under those circumstances and is it substantially reduced?

Bouchard. The answer to the first question is: yes, all people who have worked with immunocytochemistry know that the labelling is heterogeneous. What I have shown today are the more representative modifications that you can statistically extract from the raw data. But the disappearance of the receptor of the glandular cells is indeed highly reproducible. Now, regarding your second question, are you discussing pathology?

Cooke. Well, I am not sure what you would call it – these are allegedly normal individuals; I do not know whether it represents pathology or not. And I was wondering whether you could show some pathological instance of reduced stain deposition.

Bouchard. We have been studying extensively the so-called inadequate luteal phase with so-called normal hormonal levels. And all I can say is that if this syndrome exists, it is probably extremely rare. Because, by performing biopsies on day LH + 11, we always found a normal disappearance of receptor in the glands. So, whether or not the absence of progesterone at the molecular level is a cause of infertility, I have no data to support this hypothesis.

Cooke. Dr T.C. Li, working with us, has looked at day LH + 10 and it is more difficult to demonstrate retardation at that time because histological features are more variable (Li *et al.*, 1988), although overall you will find the 20% frequency that I instanced. There seems to be much tighter biological control around the time of implantation and a much slacker level of control later on as you come towards menstruation.

Bouchard. I think this topic would deserve an entire symposium because there are many hypotheses.

Johannisson. In your human biopsy material, how well was the architecture of the endometrium preserved, and how deep do you think you could go into the functional layer to study the localization of the receptors? For instance, did you clearly identify the spiral arteries?

Bouchard. We divided all the samples in two. One was for classical histology and the other one for immunocytochemistry. I must acknowledge that on the samples which have been cut with a cryostat, the architecture is not very well conserved. You can recognize the glands and the stroma very well; in some of them you can see arteries, but the structure is damaged. We are experimenting with other antibodies and paraffin embedding to avoid this problem.

Archer. Do you have any feeling for the least amount of progesterone necessary to reduce this glandular estradiol receptor? You speak about 200 mg of vaginal progesterone. I wondered what minimum quantity and duration might be necessary.

Bouchard. There is a lot we do not know. We do not even know how many steroid receptors we need to have a biological effect, whereas this is known for peptide hormone receptors. To give an example, we know that 1–10% of occupation of gonadotrophin-binding sites is enough to achieve the complete hormonal response. With steroids, we do not know exactly.

King. I agree with Dr Bouchard, but I will just remind you of some data that are relevant to the specific question you raise about minimum doses of progestogens to affect progesterone-receptor levels. And these are from a series of studies that we carried out with Dr Whitehead (King & Whitehead, 1986; Whitehead *et al.*, 1987), looking at different doses of different progestogens added to hormone replacement therapy; progesterone receptor assays were included in all of those studies. The data that we generated indicate that 0.35 mg of norethisterone are capable of lowering progesterone-receptor levels, as is 17 μg of levonorgestrel, 2 mg of medroxyprogesterone acetate and 100 mg of progesterone. These are all daily oral doses and the analyses were done after 6 days of treatment. All of these concentrations are capable of lowering progesterone-receptor levels and eliciting biological responses.

Gurpide. A theoretical question about this. The amount of receptor you need to elicit a response depends on the end-point. We were surprised when making the correlation between progesterone and endometrial glycogen accumulation *in vitro*. We needed at least 300 femtomoles (fm) of receptor per milligram of protein, which is an extremely high level. But maybe for another end-point, for another response, you may need lower levels of receptors. How can this be seen theoretically?

King. It is a complex point. I think to a large extent it is a methodological problem of the sensitivity of the assay that you are using to detect the response that you are interested in. And, as evidence for that, I would quote the data for estrogen effect on bone. People have looked intensively for steroid receptors in bone, because they should be there. Recently, some investigators have been successful with more sophisticated methodology – you can find estrogen receptors in bone at very low levels (Komm *et al.*, 1988; Eriksen *et al.*, 1988). In the usually accepted terms, it is around about 5–10 fm/mg of protein. The problem was the sensitivity of the assay and also the sensitivity of the response procedure in that the response of bone is very difficult to quantitate. So, for glycogen, which is fairly easy to measure, I think one would come up with different answers. Methodological difficulties come into it. I would strongly suspect that with a different gene product you will get a different answer for one parameter compared to another. If you are looking at biochemical changes induced by different progestogens in the endometrium, you can get much quicker and bigger effects on cell proliferation than you can on some of the secretory responses.

Bouchard. To come back to breakthrough bleeding, I do not think it is feasible to explain its physiology at the present time. Everybody is bringing a different stone in the construction of the building. First of all, I think the presence of receptors in arteries in the endometrium and myometrium is something important and means that sex steroids can act on arteries. But they may also have a direct effect. Receptors in arteries are not regulated in the same way as the rest of the endometrium or myometrium. During pregnancy, for instance, these receptors in arterial walls are present during the entire pregnancy. They are not down-regulated. Which means that blood flow in pregnancy is, at least in part, probably regulated by steroid hormones. If SHBG or other binding proteins are present in the endometrium, they could be an alternative to receptors for tissue steroid binding.

References

Cerbón, M.A., Gutierrez, R., Pasapera, A.M. & Pérez-Palacios, G. (1988). A variable expression of the uteroglobin gene (UG) following the administration of norethisterone and its ring-A reduced metabolites. *Biological Reproduction*, **38**, Suppl. 1, Abstract 419.

Chavez, B.A., Vilchis, F., Perez, A.E., Garcia, G.A., Grillasca, I. & Pérez-Palacios, G. (1985). Stereospecificity of the intracellular binding of norethisterone and its A-ring reduced metabolites. *Journal of Steroid Biochemistry*, **22**:121–126.

Clarke, C.L., Zaino, R.J., Feil, P.D., Miller, J.V., Steck, M.E., Ohlsson-Wilhelm, B.M. & Satyaswaroop, P.G. (1987). Monoclonal antibodies to human progesterone receptor: characterization by biochemical and immunohistochemical techniques. *Endocrinology*, **121**:1123–1132.

Eriksen, E.F., Colvard, D.S., Berg, N.J., Graham, M.L., Mann, K.G., Spelsberg, T.C. & Riggs, B.L. (1988). Evidence of estrogen receptors in normal human osteoblast-like cells. *Science*, **241**:84–86.

King, R.J.B. & Whitehead, M.I. (1986). Assessment of the potency of orally administered progestins in women. *Fertility and Sterility*, **46**:1062–1066.

Komm, B.S., Terpening, C.M., Benz, D.J., Graeme, K.A., Gallegos, A., Korc, M., Greene, G.L., O'Malley, B.W. & Haussler, M.R. (1988). Estrogen binding, receptor mRNA and biologic response in osteoblast-like osteosarcoma cells. *Science*, **241**:81–84.

Lessey, B.A., Killam, A.P., Metzger, D.A., Haney, A.F., Greene, G.L. & McCarty, K.S. Jr (1988). Immunohistochemical analysis of human uterine estrogen and progesterone receptors throughout the menstrual cycle. *Journal of Clinical Endocrinology and Metabolism*, **67**:334–340.

Li, T.C., Rogers, A.W., Dockery, P., Lenton, E.A. & Cooke, I.D. (1988). A new method of histologic dating of human endometrium in the luteal phase. *Fertility and Sterility*, **50**:52–60.

Perrot-Applanat, M., Groyer-Picard, M.T., Lorenzo, F., Jolivet, A., Vu Hai. M.T., Pallud, C., Spyratos, F. & Milgrom, E. (1987). Immunocytochemical study with monoclonal antibodies to progesterone receptor in human breast tumors. *Cancer Research*, **47**:2652–2661.

Press, M.F. & Greene, G.L. (1988). Localization of progesterone receptor with monoclonal antibodies to the human progestin receptor. *Endocrinology*, **122**:1165–1175.

Press, M.F., Nousek-Goebl, N., King, W.J., Herbst, A.L. & Greene, G.L. (1984). Immunohistochemical assessment of estrogen receptor distribution in the human endometrium throughout the menstrual cycle. *Laboratory Investigation*, **51**:495–503.

Reel, J.R., Humphrey, R.R., Shih, Y.H., Windsor, B.L., Sakowski, R., Creger, P.L. & Edgren, R.A. (1979). Competitive progesterone antagonists: receptor binding and biologic activity of testosterone and 19-nortestosterone derivatives. *Fertility and Sterility*, **31**:552–561.

Whitehead, M.I., Siddle, N., Lane, G., Padwick, M., Ryder, T.A., Pryse-Davies, J. & King, R.J.B. (1987). The pharmacology of progestogens. (In) *Menopause: Physiology and Pharmacology* (Mishell, D.R., ed.), pp.317–334. Chicago, Year Book Medical.

Concentrations of levonorgestrel in endometrium and myometrium after oral and intrauterine administration

TAPANI LUUKKAINEN AND MAIJA HAUKKAMAA

Steroid Research Laboratory, Department of Medical Chemistry, University of Helsinki, Helsinki, Finland.

Abstract

Endometrial levonorgestrel (LNG) concentrations were measured in eight women who underwent hysterectomy for benign disease. Prior to surgery, two had used a levonorgestrel-releasing IUD (LNG-IUD) for 10 months and 6.5 years, respectively, and six had taken a combined oral contraceptive (OC) (levonorgestrel 150 μg and ethinyl estradiol 30 μg) for the 10 days preceding the operation.

Concentrations of LNG (expressed as ng/g protein) were higher in LNG-IUD users than in OC users, reflecting the low protein content in endometrial atrophy induced by the LNG-IUD. Expressed as ng/g tissue wet weight, the concentrations were similar. The highest myometrial concentrations were measured in OC users, while cervical and tubal concentrations were similar in both groups. Serum LNG levels were higher in OC users.

Introduction

The duration of treatment with the levonorgestrel-releasing IUD (LNG-IUD) (Nilsson & Luukkainen, 1977) is reflected in the histological appearance of the endometrium (Silverberg *et al.*, 1986). During the first 2 months after insertion of the LNG-IUD, the mucosa is 1–3 mm thick, the stroma is swollen and cells are enlarged with pseudodecidual change. Later, as early as 3 and as late as 84 months after insertion of the LNG-IUD, the endometrial glands become atrophic and the stroma decidualized (Silverberg *et al.*, 1986).

During the first 2 months of LNG-IUD use, the concentrations of levonorgestrel in the endometrium have been found to be relatively high, as expected (Nilsson *et al.*, 1982). Reliable determination of levonorgestrel concentrations in biopsies collected from long-term users of LNG-IUD has been impossible because of the atrophic and very scanty endometrium.

Indications for hysterectomy are rare in the population of LNG-IUD users. Therefore only two hysterectomies were found necessary, and the concentrations of levonorgestrel were determined in endometrium, myometrium and fallopian tubes. The control group consisted of six women ingesting levonorgestrel-containing oral contraceptives (OCs) prior to operation.

Materials and methods

Patients. Tissue samples were obtained from eight women (aged 36–55 years) undergoing hysterectomy because of uterine fibroids (seven patients) and dysmenorrhea due to endometriosis (one patient). Two women had used the LNG-IUD (Luukkainen *et al.*, 1986), which had been in place for 10 months and 6.5 years, respectively. Six women took OCs containing 150 μg of levonorgestrel and 30 μg of ethinyl estradiol during 10 days preceding the operation. The last tablet was taken 12 hours before hysterectomy. All patients were informed of the nature of the study and gave informed consent.

Tissue samples. Before general anesthesia, a venous blood sample was taken and serum was separated by centrifugation. During the operation, routine samples for microscopical examination were taken immediately after the uterus was excised. Samples for the present study were taken as follows: the endometrial tissue was scraped off with a scalpel and put in a test tube. Pieces of myometrium and cervical tissue were excised and the isthmic part of fallopian tube was obtained when possible. All samples were stored at $-20°$C until analyzed.

Steroid analysis. The tissue samples were thawed and minced with scissors in ice-cold distilled water. The tissue slices were rinsed twice with ice-cold distilled water in order to remove any blood contamination. After tapping dry on filter paper, the tissue was weighed and homogenized by an Ultraturrax apparatus in distilled water (100 mg of tissue/1.0 ml of distilled water) at 0°C. The samples were further homogenized in a glass homogenizer with a Teflon pestle by ten strokes at 0°C. The endometrial samples were homogenized with the glass homogenizer only. Duplicate 1.0-ml samples of each homogenate were then extracted twice with 5 ml of petroleum ether (b.p. 40–60°C) and the extracts were evaporated to dryness under nitrogen. The residue was dissolved in 0.5 ml of RIA buffer containing 30% volume of methanol. Duplicate samples of 100 μl were then assayed by radioimmunoassay as described previously (Stanczyk *et al.*, 1975). The concentrations of levonorgestrel in the serum samples were analyzed by the same radioimmunoassay. To determine the method blank, samples of intact myometrium obtained from routine hysterectomy were homogenized and extracted similarly to the unknown samples in each analysis. The method was tested by adding 16, 32, 64, 125, 250 and 500 pg of levonorgestrel to 1.0 ml of myometrial homogenates, which were then processed and analyzed by RIA similarly to the unknown samples. The protein concentrations of the homogenates were determined by the method of Lowry *et al.* (1951). The results have been calculated as nanograms of levonorgestrel per gram of homogenate protein or per gram of tissue wet weight.

Table 1. *The concentration of levonorgestrel in endometrium during use of an oral contraceptive (OC) or a levonorgestrel-releasing IUD (LNG-IUD)*

Patient	Method	Levonorgestrel in endometrium	
		ng/g protein	ng/g wet weight
1	LNG-IUD	157	6.8
2	LNG-IUD	326	14.4
3	OC	34	1.9
4	OC	83	7.4
5	OC	38	2.9
6	OC	63	4.6
7	OC	30	2.8
8	OC	33	5.6

Results

The macroscopic appearances of the endometrium of women using a LNG-IUD for long periods and of women taking OCs were different. The low protein content of the atrophic endometrium in women with LNG-IUD was reflected in the high concentration of levonorgestrel when expressed as ng/g of protein. The concentrations (ng of steroid/g of tissue wet weight) in women using LNG-IUD or taking low-dose OCs were not significantly different (Table 1).

The concentrations of levonorgestrel in myometrium, cervix and fallopian tubes were expressed as ng/g of protein (Table 2). The highest myometrial levels of levonorgestrel were seen among users of OCs. In cervical tissue and fallopian tubes, levonorgestrel levels were similar in both groups. However, the serum concentrations were markedly higher in women taking OCs.

Comments

In the present study, the determination of levonorgestrel concentrations in endometrium after long-term use of LNG-IUD was possible in two women (after 10 and 78 months of use). The endometrial concentrations were only a fraction of those reported during the first 2 months of use of LNG-IUD (Nilsson *et al.*, 1982) and not significantly higher than in women taking a low-dose OC.

The levonorgestrel found in endometrium in this study was protein bound because the determination was done after careful washing of the endometrial samples. An unpublished study using highly specific monoclonal antibodies

Table 2. *The concentration of levonorgestrel in uterine tissues and serum during use of an oral contraceptive (OC) or a levonorgestrel-releasing IUD (LNG-IUD)*

		Concentration of levonorgestrel			
Patient	Method	Myometrium	Cervix	Tube	Serum
		(ng per g of protein)			(pg/ml)
1	10	7	24	64	
2	LNG-IUD	25	161	—	134
3	OC	18	23	18	343
4	OC	43	34	22	892
5	OC	12	66	—	557
6	OC	44	—	29	1023
7	OC	14	29	13	710
8	OC	7	13	6	—

against human SHBG demonstrates the presence of SHBG in normal endometrial cells and in endometrium during the use of LNG-IUD (Luukkainen and co-workers, unpublished data). The reaction is very strong in pseudodecidualized cells of thick swollen stroma in short-term users of LNG-IUD as well as in the decidua of extrauterine pregnancies. The amounts of bound levonorgestrel measured in the endometrium greatly exceed the reported capacity of progesterone receptors in endometrium (Jänne *et al.*, 1979).

The results of the study on the endometrial morphology during long-term use of LNG-IUD (Silverberg *et al.*, 1986) revealed no harmful effects on the endometrium. It is reassuring to observe that the endometrial wet weight concentrations of levonorgestrel are not significantly different to the concentrations found in endometrium of women taking low-dose OCs. The overwhelmingly large experience with high-dose OCs has not indicated any harmful effects of levonorgestrel on endometrium.

References

Jänne, O., Kauppila, A., Kontula, K., Syrjälä, P. & Vihko, R. (1979). Female sex steroid receptors in normal, hyperplastic and carcinomatous endometrium. The relationship to serum steroid hormones and gonadotropins and changes during medroxyprogesterone acetate administration. *International Journal of Cancer*, 24:545–554.

Lowry, O.H., Rosebrough, N.J., Farr, A.L. & Randall, R.J. (1951). Protein measurement with the Folin phenol reagent. *Journal of Biological Chemistry*, 193:265–275.

Luukkainen, T., Allonen, H., Haukkamaa, M., Lähteenmäki, P., Nilsson, C.G. &

Toivonen, J. (1986). Five years' experience with levonorgestrel-releasing IUDs. *Contraception*, **33**:139–148.

Nilsson, C.G., Haukkamaa, M., Vierola, H. & Luukkainen, T. (1982). Tissue concentrations of levonorgestrel in women using a levonorgestrel-releasing IUD. *Clinical Endocrinology*, **17**:529–536.

Nilsson, C.G. & Luukkainen, T. (1977). Improvement of a d-norgestrel-releasing IUD. *Contraception*, **15**:295–306.

Silverberg, S.G., Haukkamaa, M., Arko, H., Nilsson, C.G. & Luukkainen, T. (1986). Endometrial morphology during long-term use of levonorgestrel-releasing intrauterine devices. *International Journal of Gynecological Pathology*, **5**:235–241.

Stanczyk, F.Z., Hiroi, M., Goebelsmann, U., Brenner, P.F., Lumkin, M.E. & Mishell, D.R. Jr (1975). Radioimmunoassay of serum d-norgestrel in women following oral and intravaginal administration. *Contraception*, **12**:279–298.

Discussion

Luukkainen. I have been working with the levonorgestrel-releasing IUD for a long time, and it is interesting to see that the endometrium, after a while, becomes completely insensitive to estrogen. It means that a woman can have a completely normal ovarian cycle and you cannot see any change in the endometrium. We have even given 200 mg of estradiol benzoate, without effect. We thought that to have a progesterone effect on the endometrium, you need to have some estrogen receptors to be able to synthesize progesterone receptors. Dr King, how do you explain this?

King. We pay a lot of attention to receptor-mediated events. However, there are data, reinforced by the data you presented, to show that within the tissue as a whole, one does have these extraordinarily high concentrations of steroids. Where they are and whether they are biologically active, I think is a question that needs addressing. We know that high concentrations of steroids are good detergents. Is there a possibility that these high local concentrations of steroids are exerting surface active type effects, not mediated by receptors? Coming back to receptor mechanisms, at least one component of a clearly multifaceted process is that there will be indirect influences of steroids on the components of the blood vessels via cell to cell communication.

In relation to your question about refractoriness, the literature is confusing. There are good data in support of what you say about long-term hormone exposure producing a refractory state. In his original experiment with monkeys, Hisaw gave them estrogens for many months and at necropsy found an inactive endometrium (Hisaw & Hisaw, 1961). The same can be demonstrated in rodents; if you give continuous infusions of estrogens, you go through one wave of cell division and then it stops, despite the presence of estrogen. That has been interpreted on the basis of down-regulation of estrogen receptors so they are present for the initial impulse but subsequently the number of estrogen receptors goes below a critical level. Both of those pieces of data would fit with what you say. In opposition to that, from our own experience with long-term estrogen exposure in post-menopausal women receiving hormone replacement therapy, the levels of progesterone receptor in endometrium stay very high.

Archer. Did you state that women using a levonorgestrel IUD do not bleed? How does that relate to the fact that you are showing declining concentrations of levonorgestrel with time in the endometrium? Do you think that there could be a level below which this endometrium would bleed?

Luukkainen. Our experience now covers over 10 000 woman-years, and the amenorrhea is something which is quite favourable. These women have increased hemoglobin and ferritin levels. These amounts of levonorgestrel in endometrium during the use of levonorgestrel-releasing IUD are high enough that they will saturate any receptor around and will keep the endometrium suppressed.

Archer. Why is it that the concentration that is delivered by the IUD maintains this endometrium? If you could generate that same concentration of levonorgestrel systemically, do you believe that you would maintain the integrity of the endometrium?

Luukkainen. I think that we really knock-out the endometrium and we do it during the first 3 months. To see equivalent effects through oral administration, you would need to give enormously higher doses.

Reference

Hisaw, F.L. & Hisaw, F.L. (1961). Action of estrogen and progesterone on the reproductive tract of lower primates. (In) *Sex and Internal Secretions* (Young, W.C. & Corner, G.W., eds.), pp.556–589. London, Bailliere, Tindall & Cox.

Decidualization and relevance to menstruation

STEPHEN C. BELL

Departments of Biochemistry & Obstetrics and Gynaecology, Medical School, University of Leicester, Leicester, UK.

Abstract

Decidualization, the hormone-dependent transient formation of decidual tissue, involving cell proliferation, differentiation and death, subserves functions in species exhibiting placentation where trophoblast penetrates the stroma to gain access to the maternal vasculature. A key feature of decidualization is the differentiation of the stromal fibroblast to the decidual cell with associated alteration in the extracellular matrix. Differentiation of the stromal cell is characterized by the de-novo synthesis of osteonectin containing basal lamina; however, its role in interstitial matrix reorganization is unknown. This modified extracellular matrix may facilitate migration of trophoblast and maternal lymphomyeloid cells, affect their function, and allow paracrine interactions between these cell types. The secretory phenotype of the decidual cell has yet to be defined, particularly with respect to growth factor synthesis, although two products have been proposed to act as paracrine regulators of cell function within the decidua. Differentiation of the decidual cell has been suggested to induce the recruitment of, and in-situ differentiation of, the precursor of a second major decidual tissue-associated cell type, the endometrial/decidual granulated lymphocyte. Whether decidual-derived paracrine regulators are involved in this process or whether such regulators affect function of resident macrophages and promote angiogenesis to ensure tissue morphogenesis remains to be explored.

In rodents, early steroid hormone withdrawal interrupts decidualization and results in tissue necrosis and loss, considered to be analogous to menstruation; however, this is not due to hormone withdrawal *per se* since it only occurs if decidualization has been induced. Therefore, in the human, where decidualization occurs spontaneously, the phenomenon and mechanism of menstruation could be dictated by interruption of a complex set of cell–cell interactions involving a range of paracrine regulators which are involved in tissue morphogenesis. Breakdown is an inherent property of decidual tissue since in rodents this occurs after a period of steroid hormone-dependent growth and differentiation in spite of continuous steroid hormone exposure. Abnormal bleeding could arise in situations where any of these elements involved in decidualization are disrupted. Investigation of the mechanisms underlying decidual morphogenesis, particularly characterization of paracrine-mediated cell–cell interactions between the novel cell types involved, the decidual cell and granulated lymphocyte, and lymphomyeloid cells and cells of the vasculature, may provide a framework to understand the mechanisms involved in normal and abnormal bleeding.

Introduction

In a number of mammals the endometrium undergoes a complex reaction (termed decidualization) to form the decidua in response to the implanting embryo. However, it must be noted that in some species the term 'deciduate placentation' has been employed, based upon identification of isolated cells of maternal origin, but no genesis of new maternal or decidual tissue is detected (Massman, 1980). The phenomenon of decidualization occurs only in species in which placentation involves breaching of the luminal epithelium by trophoblast and its invasion into the stromal matrix. In species exhibiting hemochorial placentation, it has been considered that the extent of decidualization correlates with the degree of trophoblast invasion (Ramsey *et al.*, 1976; Finn, 1983).

It is apparent that decidualization and the collective tissue responses involved subserve functions associated with implantation and establishment of the definitive placenta, in part permitting the controlled invasion of a 'foreign' tissue without induction of a classical inflammatory and wound response, and increased blood supply to the endometrium. Most marked responses during decidualization are found in the stroma, and in rodents it is apparent that it involves periods of proliferation, differentiation and appearance of histologically defined cell populations, and programmed regression in different regions of the uterus, which occur both anatomically and temporally related to placental development (De Feo, 1967; Glasser, 1972; Finn, 1977; Glasser & McCormack, 1982; Bell, 1983, 1985).

It is relevant to note that the regression of decidualized stroma occurs even in the absence of the conceptus and without declining steroid levels, and does not compromise the feto-placental unit, suggesting that this is an inherent property of the decidua. One prominent feature of decidualization is the differentiation of the stromal fibroblast into the decidual cell, a term which will be restricted to this cell type, although there has been a confusing tendency to refer to all cells isolated from decidual tissue as decidual cells. A thesis which could now be proposed is that many functions ascribed to decidualization and decidual tissue could arise as a result of decidual cell differentiation, either as a direct effect of the decidual cell or mediated via actions on other cell populations, by inducing their localization to the decidua or affecting function of resident cells (see next section). Given that the phenomenon of menstruation is more species restricted than decidualization, i.e. occurs in humans, a few primates, the elephant shrew and the bat, there would appear to be no basis for a link. However, as argued by Finn (1987), menstruation appears to occur in species in which the decidualization process is initiated spontaneously within the cycle, although the extent of its development achieved prior to menstruation varies between species.

The evolution of spontaneous decidualization subserves and reflects the different reproductive strategies observed in species. From a teleological view, controlled tissue loss is required to remove tissue embarked upon a programme of steroid-dependent differentiation. A thesis which is therefore worthy of consideration is that processes involved in this differentiation, which subserve functions in pregnancy, when interrupted by steroid removal are in part responsible for the phenomenon of tissue loss in menstruation. It should be noted that decidual tissue breakdown is a feature of decidualization and is suggested to be associated with programmed decidual cell death, further supporting the concept that the loss of decidual cell function promotes tissue breakdown via loss of its tissue growth-promoting activities/breakdown suppressive activities or direct activation of tissue breakdown activity. Other patterns of bleeding could result from a failure of induction of full functional properties associated with decidualization.

Of direct relevance are studies on rodents where a physical stimulus, either provided by the blastocyst or artificially, is required for decidualization. A precise regimen of estradiol and progesterone is essential to produce a sensitized endometrium capable of decidualization in response to stimuli. In ovariectomized mice given exogenous hormones to mimic pregnancy, hormone withdrawal produced changes in the endometrium similar to menstruation only when decidualization had been induced (Finn & Pope, 1984, 1986).

In this contribution, decidualization will be examined in this context, placing emphasis upon the personal view of the role of the decidual cell as a central conductor, regulating activity of other cell types via paracrine mechanisms, the activity of which may mediate many decidualization-associated functions.

Decidualization-associated cell differentiation

The two major cell types whose differentiation is considered to be associated with decidualization are the decidual cell and decidual granulated lymphocyte (endometrial granulocyte, granulated metrial gland cell). However, ultra-structural studies have indicated major alterations in endothelial cells (Welsh & Enders, 1985) and whether this represents further 'differentiation' of these cells is unknown. In any discussion of the potential function and relationship between these two populations, the observation that decidualization is not always associated with their co-appearance must be considered. In rodents, in the antimesometrial decidua, which is the first region to develop, granulated lymphocytes are rarely detected whereas they are prominent in the mesome-trial decidua. In the metrial gland, the final region whose development in the mesometrial myometrium is associated with decidualization, these cells appear in the apparent absence of classical decidual cell differentiation.

Decidual cell

Until recently, the definition of the decidual cell has relied upon ultrastructural characterization and this has impeded the understanding of this cell in decidualization and placentation. It is apparent that the 'decidual cell', as strictly defined in the human (Fig. 1), is not identical to that in rodents and

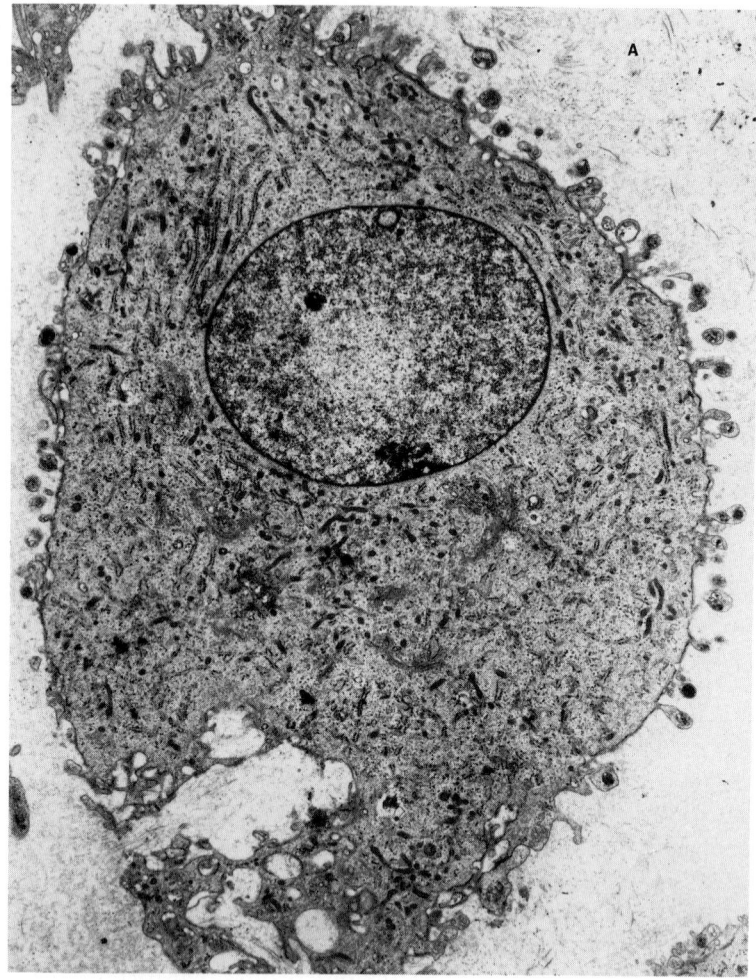

Fig. 1 (A) Transmission electron micrograph of a decidual cell in first trimester pregnancy endometrium of human (×9000). The cell possesses a large nucleus with dispersed euchromatin, prominent Golgi, moderately dilated rough endoplasmic reticulum with electron-dense matrix and long sinuous mitochondria. Through the decidual cell-associated basal lamina, lobate structures with pleiomorphic membrane-bound inclusions project into a disperse collagenous matrix. In the lower region of the cell complex,

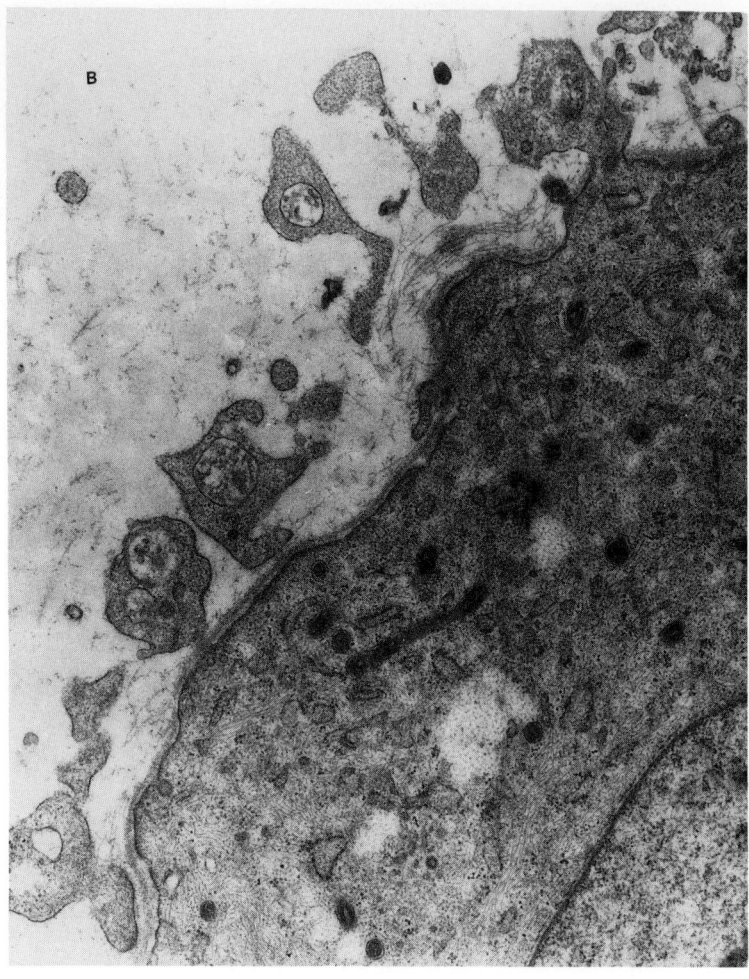

infolding is observed. (B) Higher magnification (× 54000) further illustrates those features and in addition shows extensive intermediate filaments within the cytoplasm. The cell surface exhibits a coated pit and micropinocytotic vesicles under an apparently intact basal lamina. Lobate projection, not coated with basal lamina, is observed (upper left) projecting through a narrow defect in the basal lamina. (Kindly provided by Dr D. Corcoran, Department of Pathology, University of Leicester.)

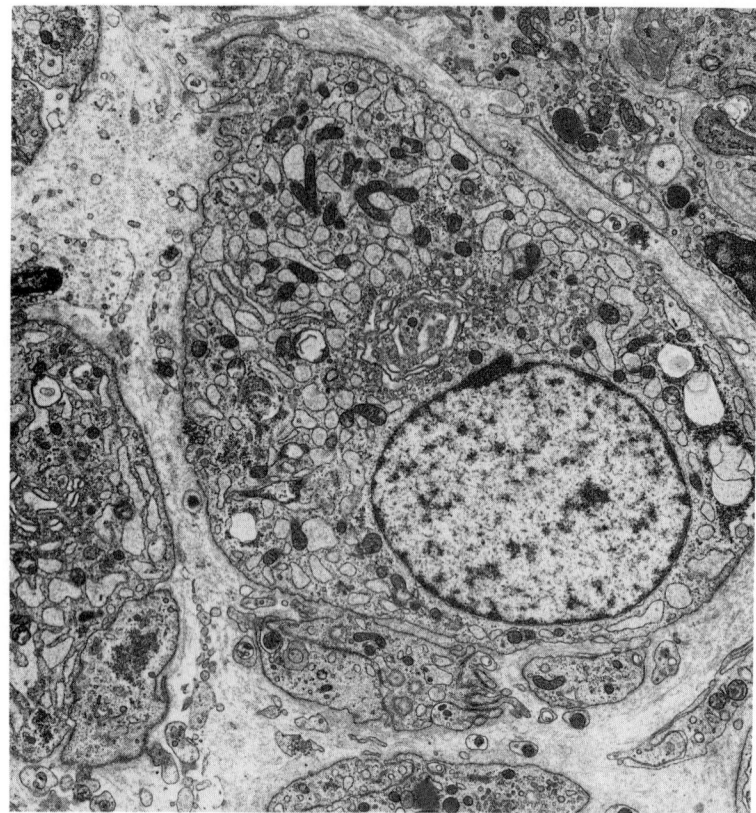

Fig. 2 Transmission electron micrograph of decidual cell in baboon
endometrium during late pregnancy ($\times$ 12000). Extensive Golgi zone,
dilated rough endoplasmic reticulum, glycogen deposits, and lobate
projections are present. (Kindly provided by A.C. Enders, University of
California School of Medicine.)

indeed in the rat the ultrastructural features of decidual cells in the
antimesometrial decidua are very different to those in the mesometrial decidua
(O'Shea *et al.*, 1983; Welsh & Enders, 1985). Such species-based definitions
have led some investigators to consider that in non-human primates decidual
cells are absent, although stromal cell hypertrophy was noted (Ramsey *et al.*,
1976). However, some authors consider that the hormone- and pregnancy-
induced stromal hypertrophy observed in these latter species represents
decidual cell differentiation (Enders *et al.*, 1985; Fig. 2). The question remains
as to whether these differences in species are reflected by different functions or
whether the concept of a common 'decidual phenotype' is tenable. Ultrastructural studies have revealed that decidual cells exhibit intimate interactions

with other cell types within the decidua such as endothelial cells, granulated lymphocytes and other lymphocytes, but the function of these associations is unknown. Recent studies on the properties of the decidual cell are now yielding information pertinent to these questions.

Intermediate filament expression

Differentiation of decidual cells *in vivo* (Tachi *et al.*, 1970; O'Shea *et al.*, 1983; Enders *et al.*, 1985) and *in vitro* (Vladimirsky *et al.*, 1977; Sananes *et al.*, 1978, 1980; Bell & Searle, 1981) is associated with a marked accumulation of intermediate filaments. Although probably not involved in basic cell function, the observed cell type-specific patterns of expression suggest their association with differentiation and functions of the differentiated cell. Characterization of the decidual cell-associated intermediate filaments may therefore provide insights into cell lineage and ultimately cell function.

In the rat, Glasser & Julian (1986) have reported that in-vitro decidualization of stromal cells is associated with an increase in vimentin expression which parallels increase in total cell protein, whereas desmin, marginally detectable in stromal cells, increases in concentration to levels equal to that of vimentin. These observations were confirmed *in vivo* where immunocytochemical analysis revealed that increase in desmin expression in cells followed the same distribution pattern characteristic for stromal cells undergoing decidual differentiation, whether induced by normal or artificial stimuli (Glasser *et al.*, 1987). These changes do not occur in stromal cells of uteri subject to the hormone regimen necessary to produce sensitivity to decidualizing stimuli. In this study, increased desmin expression was correlated with laminin deposition, suggesting that during decidual differentiation altered intermediate filament gene expression may be co-ordinated with basal lamina component gene expression. In the human, differentiated decidual cells during pregnancy have been reported to contain vimentin (Kisalus *et al.*, 1987a) and also to co-express vimentin and desmin (Khong *et al.*, 1986).

The continued expression of vimentin by the decidual cell appears to confirm that these cells arise from differentiation of mesenchymally derived stromal fibroblasts. The absence of cytokeratin expression does not support the concept that decidualization represents an 'epithelial transformation' and is limited to the cell's acquisition of basal lamina-producing ability. The production of desmin, a feature proposed to represent a marker of stromal–decidual cell differentiation (Glasser & Julian, 1986), poses many questions as to the nature of the decidual cell in terms of lineage and function. Although considered to represent a characteristic of myogenic cells (Debus *et al.*, 1983), the reports of desmin expression in endothelial cells (Fujimoto & Singer, 1986) and in actin-negative cells of the rat intestinal submucosa and testis interstitium (Skalli *et al.*, 1986) suggest that it is not muscle specific. However, Glasser *et al.* (1987) have proposed that if desmin expression is a marker of myogenesis, decidual cells may possess other myogenic properties, or alternatively if not muscle specific, may represent a characteristic of differentiation in a number of mesenchymal cells.

Interstitial components

Studies on the nature of the stromal interstitial matrix, its alterations during the menstrual cycle and associated decidualization, and the contribution of cell types within the endometrium to its synthesis and degradation, are very limited (for review see Aplin, 1988). During the menstrual cycle from the early luteal phase, a fibril-rich matrix containing collagens I, III, V and VI alters at day 21 into a more edematous matrix with loosely organized fibrillar components (Aplin, 1988). These alterations may be associated with the predecidualization process and in the interstitial matrix of decidual cells during early pregnancy these alterations are accentuated. Although the matrix still contains major collagens and fibronectin, the appearance of collagen V epitopes has suggested a reduction in interchain associations with other major collagens, and the disappearance of collagen VI, a collagen proposed to function as a cross-linking fibril between fibrils of major collagens, the production of specific protease action (Aplin, 1988). Qualitative studies would therefore suggest a major reorganization of the collagen matrix, possibly by alterations in collagen biosynthesis and enzymes involved in collagen breakdown, during differentiation of the stromal cell. Clarification of this contribution is required, together with an analysis of the role of glycosamino-glycans/proteoglycans during decidualization, since the latter would be implied by the appearance of the matrix.

Basement laminal components

Although early ultrastructural studies revealed that decidual cells were associated with a pericellular matrix resembling a pericellular basement membrane (Lawn *et al.*, 1971; Wynn, 1974; Herr *et al.*, 1978), only recently has this been characterized. In human pregnancy decidua, employing immunohistochemical techniques, the large ($>25 \mu$) decidual cells have been demonstrated to be encircled with a basal lamina containing laminin, collagen type IV, heparan sulphate proteoglycan and fibronectin (Charpin *et al.*, 1985; Wewer *et al.*, 1985; Kisalus *et al.*, 1987a). The identification of intermediate-sized decidual cells (15–25 μ), where these components were present only as pericellular punctate deposits, and small elongated cells ($<15 \mu$) which were devoid of basal lamina suggested to Wewer *et al.* (1985) that the latter represented stromal progenitor stem cells and the former an intermediate stage during decidual differentiation. Metabolic labelling studies have demonstrated synthesis of laminin and collagen type IV by human decidual tissue (Wewer *et al.*, 1985; Kisalus *et al.*, 1987a).

During the menstrual cycle no production of basal lamina components by stromal cells of proliferative endometrium has been observed (Wewer *et al.*,

1985). However, in early secretory endometrium (days 14–17), before histological evidence of predecidualization is apparent, immunoreactive laminin was detected in cytoplasm of stromal cells in periarterial and subluminal epithelial regions (Faber *et al.*, 1986). The number of stromal cells positive for laminin immunoreactivity, as well as intensity of reactivity, increased during the luteal phase until in late secretory endometrium the majority of predecidual cells were positive. In predecidual cells laminin was detected in the cytoplasm and extracellularly, as punctate deposits or discontinuous rims of material, and these were therefore similar to the intermediate decidual cells of pregnancy endometrium (Faber *et al.*, 1986; Wewer *et al.*, 1985). Laminin receptor has also been detected and its expression correlates with predecidualization (Faber *et al.*, 1986). Although not considered integral components of basal lamina, Kisalus *et al.* (1987a) have reported the localization of collagen type V and fibronectin around decidual cells corresponding with the basal lamina. Recently the de-novo synthesis and incorporation of osteonectin into the basal lamina of decidual cells have been reported (Wewer *et al.*, 1988). A similar pattern of expression to laminin with respect to the menstrual cycle and pregnancy was observed. In pregnancy decidua intermediate decidual cells possessed immunoreactivity in the cytoplasm and in punctate pericellular deposits and also high levels of mRNA. In large decidual cells pericellular staining corresponded to the basement membrane surrounding these cells. During the menstrual cycle immunoreactivity for osteonectin appeared in the cytoplasm of stromal cells in the early secretory endometrium and became prominent in predecidual cells, where osteonectin was also detected as cell surface deposits (Wewer *et al.*, 1988).

The demonstration of osteonectin synthesis and its incorporation into decidual basal lamina pose questions as to the function of osteonectin and of the decidual cell. Osteonectin is a calcium- and collagen-binding protein (Termine *et al.*, 1981a,b; Engel *et al.*, 1987; Bolander *et al.*, 1988) of bone matrix and is closely related to the proteins SPARC and BM-40. High levels of expression of osteonectin/SPARC in non-bone tissues may be related to remodelling or morphogenesis of tissues characterized by proliferation and de-novo synthesis of basement membranes. However, what function this protein serves in non-bone tissues remains to be established. In the mouse, stromal cells during in-vitro decidualization have been demonstrated to synthesize laminin, osteonectin/SPARC, entactin, collagen type IV, heparan sulphate proteoglycan and fibronectin by metabolic labelling (Wewer *et al.*, 1986, 1988). These authors have noted that production of sulphated entactin relative to laminin was higher than in other basement membrane-producing cell systems. Basal laminar components have been demonstrated associated with decidual cells in the rat (Parr *et al.*, 1986; Glasser *et al.*, 1987) in both the antimesometrial and mesometrial decidua where the decidual cells exhibit different ultrastructural features.

Soluble secretory protein products

The secretory phenotype of the decidual cell has not been fully characterized although metabolic labelling of human decidual explants has identified a limited number of śecretory protein products and these may arise from decidual cells (Bell *et al.*, 1985; Kisalus *et al.*, 1987b). Other approaches have identified the secretory enzymes diamine/polyamine oxidase and alkaline phosphatase, and prolactin and its glycosylated variant. The synthesis and secretion of prolactin by the human predecidual and decidual cell are of great significance since studies suggest that it may act as a paracrine mediator regulating osmoregulation in the amniochorion and the local activity of leukocytes (Healy *et al.*, 1989). Similarly, the identification of the quantitatively major secretory protein product of human decidualized endometrium in pregnancy as the small molecular weight insulin-like growth factor-binding protein (IGF-BP) (Bell *et al.*, 1988), also known as pregnancy-associated endometrial αl-globulin (αl-PEG) (Bell, 1988a,b) and placental protein 12 (PP12) (Seppälä *et al.*, 1988), may establish another local function of the decidual cell mediated by a paracrine regulator.

During early pregnancy, employing in-vitro precursor labelling studies, increased synthesis and secretion of IGF-BP appeared to correlate with presence of the decidualized decidua compacta region (Bell *et al.*, 1985) and at weeks 15–16 it accounted for $\rangle$90% of radiolabelled secretory proteins of the tissue. High levels of IGF-BP are detected in amniotic fluid (Rutanen *et al.*, 1982; Drop *et al.*, 1984; Povoa *et al.*, 1984; D'Ercole *et al.*, 1985; Bell *et al.*, 1986a; Hall *et al.*, 1986; Baxter *et al.*, 1987) and, as with amniotic fluid prolactin, IGF-BP is suggested to be derived from the decidua. The increased serum levels of IGF-BP observed during pregnancy have also been proposed to be derived from the decidua (Rutanen *et al.*, 1982; Bell & Smith, 1988). Immunohistological studies employing monoclonal antibodies appear to confirm the decidual cell origin of the protein; however, as well as cytoplasmic localization, immunoreactive product has been detected as a pericellular deposit and associated with the extracellular matrix (Waites *et al.*, 1989). During the menstrual cycle, synthesis and secretion by endometrial explants were elevated during the luteal phase (Bell *et al.*, 1986b). However, using polyclonal antisera to PP12, immunoreactive protein has been localized to the glandular epithelium from day 18 (Wahlstrom & Seppälä, 1984), but employing monoclonal antibodies to α1-PEG it has been localized to stromal endometrial cells in peri-spiral arterial and subluminal epithelial regions (Waites *et al.*, 1988). Predecidual cells in the endometrium during the late luteal phase were characterized by their paucity of IGF-BP immunoreactivity and they may relate to the reported progesterone induction of its synthesis by the endometrium *in vitro* (Rutanen *et al.*, 1986). That elevated IGF-BP synthesis is not an intrinsic feature of the histologically and ultrastructurally defined decidual cell is also supported by the failure to detect immunoreactive protein in decidual cells of tubal mucosa in ectopic pregnancy (Waites, Heald & Fox, unpublished observations).

The decidually derived IGF-BP represents the low molecular weight non-growth hormone-dependent IGF-binding protein, detected in its unsaturated form in sera and in media conditioned by many cell types (for review see Ooi & Herington, 1988). Since it is synthesized and secreted by fibroblast, decidual differentiation is therefore more probably associated with a dramatic increase in its synthesis rather than with new gene expression. Both inhibitory and stimulatory activities of IGF-BP upon IGF action on IGF receptor-bearing target cells have been reported, which appears paradoxical when evidence supports the existence of only one gene for this protein (Brewer *et al.*, 1988; Lee *et al.*, 1988). The stimulatory activity of IGF-BP has been reported to be dependent upon binding of the IGF-BP to the cell membrane (Clemmons *et al.*, 1986; Elgin *et al.*, 1987), and the presence of the RGD tripeptide sequence in IGF-BP, a consensus sequence for binding of intracellular proteins to the integrin family of membrane receptors (Ruoslahti & Pierschbacher, 1987), may provide a molecular basis for this membrane binding. The inhibitory action of IGF-BP could be accounted for either by absence of these integrin-type receptors on certain targets or by local proteolytic cleavage of IGF-BP yielding an IGF-BP without the C-terminal-containing RGD tripeptide region. In either case, the BP would effectively compete with the IGF receptor for IGF, preventing its action (Bell, 1989). Secretion of IGF-BP by the decidual cell at high levels into the decidual matrix may therefore affect IGF action in a paracrine manner on any IGF receptor-bearing cell type within this environment, and these include arterial smooth muscle cells, arterial endothelial cells, lymphocytes, mononuclear cells and trophoblast cells (for review see Nissley & Rechler, 1984).

Although production of IGF-BP may principally subserve functions of the decidua in association with implantation and trophoblast invasion during placental development, its action may be essential to the integrity of tissue arising during decidual morphogenesis by controlling activity of non- decidual cells, and cessation of synthesis after hormone withdrawal may have implications for cell activity within the premenstrual endometrium. If decidual cell-associated secretory proteins mediate essential functions, it would be anticipated that they would be produced in other species exhibiting decidualization and, as with prolactin, this appears to be the case with IGF-BP, since in the baboon this protein also represents the major secretory protein product of the hypertrophied stromal or decidual cell during pregnancy (Fazleabas *et al.*, 1989; Bell *et al.*, 1989). From these recent studies it appears that it may be possible to redefine the decidual cell in terms of its secretory phenotype. A number of these features bestow upon this cell the potential to affect cell activity within the decidual environment, via extracellular matrix alterations or hormone and regulatory protein secretion. Cell types in the decidua which could be potential targets for the paracrine action of prolactin

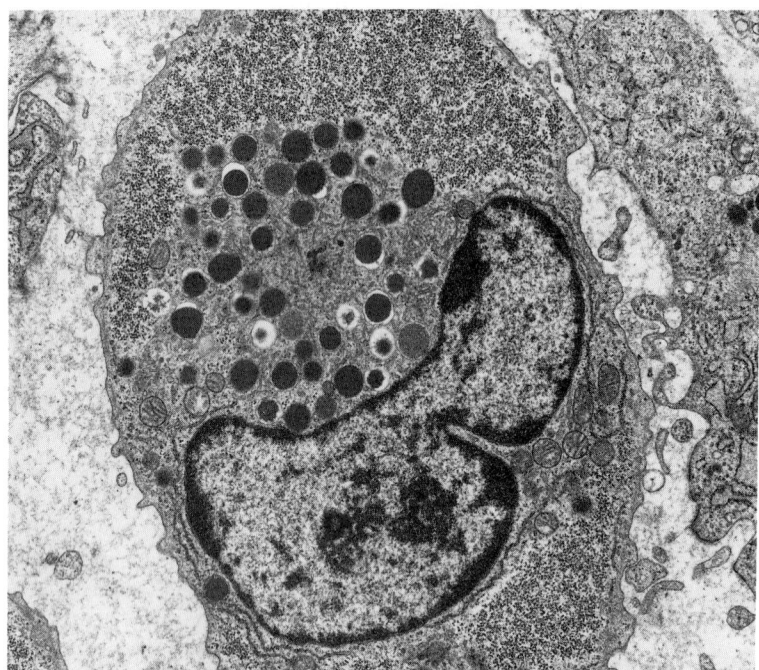

Fig. 3 Transmission electron micrograph of granulated cell in endometrium at day 29 of pregnancy in rhesus monkey ($\times 15\,900$). The cell possesses an eccentrically placed nucleus, a large Golgi region, distinctive membrane-bound granules with dense core, and often marginal vesicles, and glycogen. Cells often exhibit close associations with macrophages and decidual cells. (Reproduced with permission from Enders *et al.*, 1985.)

and IGF-BP have been listed. It is of great interest that decidual cell differentiation has also been implicated in the local control of the differentiation of the second major decidualization-associated cell type, the granulated lymphocyte.

Decidual or endometrial granulated lymphocytes (synonyms: endometrial granulocytes, granulated metrial gland cells)

Although these cells have been detected in decidualized endometrium in all species examined, and had been considered to differentiate from stromal fibroblasts (Selye & McKeown, 1935), their occurrence in non-decidualized endometrium in rodents suggests their differentiation is not uniquely associated with decidualization. These cells possess characteristic cytoplasmic granules and similar ultrastructural features in different species (Fig. 3), and although their size and uterine distribution vary in different species, this probably reflects species-specific patterns of decidual morphogenesis, and indeed recent studies suggest they may represent functionally analogous cells in all species.

In rodents, early ultrastructural studies which indicated the differentiation of these cells from lymphocyte-like precursors have been supported by 1) demonstration of leukocyte common antigen on rat cells, and 2) bone-marrow origin of precursor cells (for review see Bulmer *et al.*, 1987a). However, major questions remain concerning the factors involved in recruitment of the precursors into the uterus and their differentiation in relation to hormones and decidualization of the stroma. Peel & Stewart (1986) have demonstrated that estrogen may have a role in recruitment of precursor cells into the endometrium. Recent studies by Stewart (1987, 1988) have provided evidence for the author's thesis (Stewart, 1983) that the differentiation of precursors and maintenance of the cells are associated with activation of the stromal cells to decidual cell differentiation. However, whether this is also associated with further recruitment of precursors is uncertain. Although close associations are observed between granulated cells and stromal/decidual cells, they are also localized around blood vessels and have been observed migrating through blood vessels and detected in the vasculature of the decidua and placenta. A number of functions have been ascribed to this granulated cell population, the most recent emphasizing their role in the immunological protection of the fetal allograft (Bulmer *et al.*, 1987b). However, recent evidence could equally support the concept that the primary function of these cells lies in remodelling of the stroma and blood vessels associated with decidual morphogenesis and placental development. Pijnenborg and colleagues (1981) have indeed suggested previously that their activity was responsible for necrosis of arterial walls prior to endovascular trophoblast invasion during pregnancy.

In rodents, the cytoplasmic granules are associated with a range of hydrolytic enzymes and if this reflects their lysosomal nature, the granules may possess other lysosomal-associated proteolytic activities able to degrade basal lamina and collagen matrixes. More recently, Parr *et al.* (1987) have localized perforin, a mediator of cell target lysis, to these cells and have suggested that they represent a type of natural killer cell. This may provide a molecular basis for the observed killing of a cell population in placental cell cultures *in vitro* (Stewart & Mukhtar, 1988) and be relevant to the interaction with layer 1 of the labyrinthine trophoblast observed *in vivo* (Stewart, 1984). Whether these functions are expressed in viable decidual tissue *in vivo* and the nature of their target cells in decidual tissue remain to be determined. It is important to note that *in vitro* and *in vivo*, evidence for cell cytotoxicity has been observed for cells removed from the decidual environment, and expression of function *in vivo* may require removal of a decidual cell regulatory activity either by migration from the decidua or by death of the decidual cell, programmed or induced by falling steroid levels. As yet of undefined significance has been the report of high expression of mRNA for 2ar/osteopontin in murine decidual granulated lymphocytes (Nomura *et al.*, 1988). Osteopontin, a bone protein which contains the RGD tripeptide consensus sequence for integrin binding (Ruoslahti & Pierschbacher, 1987), is sialic acid rich and phosphorylated (Oldberg *et al.*, 1986; Prince *et al.*, 1987), has been suggested to be involved in binding of cells to the mineralized collagen matrix of bone. Although the function of secreted 2ar/osteopontin in non-bone tissue is unknown, given the suggestion that in bone the protein could be derived from osteoclasts (see Nomura *et al.*, 1988), and that these cells are derived from hematopoietic precursors and are involved in extracellular matrix degradation, the relationship between osteoclasts and decidual granulated lymphocytes is intriguing.

Studies by Bulmer and colleagues (Bulmer & Ritson, 1988) have demonstrated that 'endometrial granulocytes' of the human predecidualized endometrium and decidua are bone-marrow derived and possess certain leukocyte surface markers and have referred to these cells as endometrial/ decidual granulated lymphocytes. Although they possess both T cell and natural killer cell markers, they do not express the full spectrum of markers associated with these cells (Bulmer & Ritson, 1988). Their appearance during the period of predecidualization in the menstrual cycle and decidual tissue in early pregnancy, and close associations with blood vessels, suggest a relationship to decidualization similar to that suggested in rodents. However, the nature of their precursors and control of their migration to the endometrium is unknown. Partially purified populations of decidual granulated lymphocytes exhibit a minimal proliferative response to interleukin-2 and poor cytotoxicity against K562 cells, both assays for activity of classic natural killer cells (Bulmer & Ritson, 1988). It must therefore be considered whether activity of these cells is suppressed by the decidua or, as suggested by Bulmer & Ritson (1988), that they represent a novel or immature natural killer cell type.

Decidualization and function

A wide range of functions have been ascribed to decidualization and decidual morphogenesis. These include control of trophoblast invasion with protection of maternal tissues during this invasion, nutrition of the embryo, formation of cleavage zone at parturition, endocrine function (Amoroso, 1952), isolation of individual embryos (De Feo, 1967), immunological function (Lala *et al.*, 1987; Clark *et al.*, 1987) and vascular changes (Pijnenborg *et al.*, 1981). However, the cellular and molecular mechanisms underlying many of these proposed functions remain to be elucidated. It has already been pointed out that decidualization essentially involves the growth of a new vascularized tissue which also exhibits an inherent programme of controlled regression, and as such would be anticipated to involve mechanisms associated with other systems of tissue remodelling such as wound repair (Sporn & Roberts, 1986) and bone formation and remodelling (Vaes, 1988). The analogy between the granulation tissue reaction and decidualization has been discussed by Finn (1986). In the latter systems it is apparent that complex interactions between cells including fibroblasts, smooth muscle cells, endothelial cells and macrophages, polymorphonuclear leukocytes and lymphocytes are mediated in part by paracrine mediators such as prostaglandins, growth factors and cytokines. The relative activities of these cells and mediators may regulate the balance between tissue genesis and breakdown.

One common feature of these systems is that they involve reorganization of the extracellular matrix, and many actions of growth factors upon certain cell types involve regulation of (a) the synthesis of components of the matrix, and (b) enzymes implicated in matrix breakdown and their regulators (Sporn & Roberts, 1986). Decidual differentiation of the stromal cell is associated with the de-novo synthesis of a basal lamina rich in osteonectin/SPARC, and the alterations in interstitial matrix composition would also suggest that the decidual cell contributes to the transformation of the extracellular matrix in the endometrium. The functional significance of the decidua-associated extracellular matrix is unclear; however, studies in other systems have indicated the importance of cell–extracellular matrix interactions in cell adhesion, migration, proliferation and differentiation (Ruoslahti & Pierschbacher, 1987), and these effects may be mediated in part by the ability of the matrix to bind growth factors such as fibroblast growth factor which may be liberated upon matrix reorganization (Gordon *et al.*, 1987; Böhlen, 1989). One direct result of these alterations may be to provide a matrix which would facilitate migration of not only trophoblast cells during pregnancy, but also maternal migratory cell populations, e.g. decidual granulated lymphocytes, their precursors and macrophages. Questions remain as to whether biochemical changes in the matrix could be responsible for migration and differentiation of granulated lymphocyte precursors in the decidua, and alteration in function of these and resident cells such as macrophages, or are these latter activities the result of secretory products of the decidual cell, noting the possibility that even these could mediate activities by binding to the matrix.

The secretory phenotype of the decidual cell has yet to be fully characterized; however, the decidual cell products such as prolactin (Healy *et al.*, 1989) and insulin-like growth factor binding protein have been proposed as paracrine regulators of other cell types in the decidua. These other regulated cell types, which in this context could include cells of the vasculature, could mediate other functions ascribed to decidualization. However, function could be suppressed by the viable decidual cell, then expressed during the programmed demise of the cell, and be involved in the controlled regression of the decidual tissue. As has already been discussed precursor recruitment and differentiation of granulated lymphocytes have been suggested to be associated with stromal cell activation, and function of these cells thus becomes linked with the decidual cell. It is relevant to note that in bone, regulation of recruitment, differentiation and function of the osteoclast is closely linked with the osteoblast, and this relationship exhibits features similar to those proposed for decidual and osteopontin-positive granulated lymphocyte cells.

Decidualization would be anticipated to affect the function of resident macrophage populations since, given the range of secretory products of this cell (Nathan, 1987), particularly those products of the activated cell which are cytotoxic and lead to events associated with tissue breakdown, these latter activities would not be compatible with the tissue morphogenesis in decidualization. It is therefore possible that activities proposed as immunoregulatory agents preventing rejection of the feto-placental allograft, are instead involved in suppression of these macrophage activities to ensure tissue growth. Such a role has been proposed for transforming growth factor-β (TGF-β) which *in vitro* promotes extracellular matrix production, inhibits its breakdown, and deactivates macrophages (Heine *et al.*, 1987; Sporn *et al.*, 1987; Tsunawaki *et al.*, 1988). It may be relevant that TGF-β has been demonstrated to stimulate osteonectin/SPARC expression, a major component of the decidual cell, and injection into newborn mice produces a granulation tissue response.

Given this view, most of the functions presently ascribed to decidualization could be mediated by decidual cell activity. The decidual cell modifies the extracellular matrix, produces paracrine mediators and thus potentially affects migration, differentiation and activity of maternal cells within decidual tissue. It remains to be established which effects of the decidual cell are either involved principally in decidual tissue morphogenesis or in regulation of trophoblast activity during placental development.

Decidualization and menstruation

Although the early events of decidual induction are similar to inflammation, if decidualization represents a steroid-dependent programme of tissue morphogenesis, then elements of cell activity that promote tissue breakdown associated with inflammation and wound repair must be suppressed. Cells potentially able to mediate tissue breakdown via direct and indirect effects are present in decidualizing endometrium, e.g. macrophages (Clark & Daya, 1989), although whether their activity is inhibited directly by steroid hormones or via decidual cells remains to be determined. However, removal of steroid hormone support from predecidualized endometrium results in menstruation, and in an animal model decidual tissue breakdown upon hormone removal results in a similar phenomenon involving polymorphonuclear leukocyte infiltration. In this model, since decidualization requires an inducing stimulus, it is possible to demonstrate that the phenomenon is dependent upon prior decidualization of the stroma and not hormone removal *per se*. If this is so, then the pattern of tissue breakdown in menstruation reflects intervention in the programme of decidualization and activation of immunoinflammatory cells by cessation of decidual cell regulatory function. Another interaction that must be considered is the possible relationship between decidual cells and spiral arteries, since in the human and primates during the luteal phase, decidualization of stromal cells occurs in periarteriolar regions (Brenner & Maslar, 1988). Given this view, abnormal endometrial bleeding patterns may result from any deviation from the programme of decidualization initiated in the normal luteal phase. This may involve functional aspects of any cell type and associated paracrine interaction between these cells.

Future research

The phenomena of decidualization and menstruation would be anticipated to be as complex as other systems of tissue remodelling, e.g. bone remodelling, wound resolution and repair, where functional changes in cell–cell interactions occur involving a range of mediators such as cytokines and growth factors. It is apparent that further progress in the understanding of these mechanisms will be obtained only via two independent experimental approaches. The exact nature of the complexity of cell function and cell–cell interactions will be facilitated by isolation of the component cell types, characterization of their secretory phenotypes, and potential reactivity to paracrine and endocrine hormones. These studies must be interpreted with caution since in-vivo activity of cells may be affected differentially according to localization and anatomical relationship to other cell types. Therefore their in-vitro properties and function, both anatomically and temporally, could be assessed employing immunohistochemical methods and in-situ hybridization methods with tissue sections. It is to be anticipated that with the application of such techniques, elucidation of the mechanisms of decidualization and menstruation will define what alterations in these mechanisms can lead to abnormal bleeding patterns.

Acknowledgements

The author wishes to thank the Medical Research Council and the Wellcome Trust for financial support and Ms S. Freer for secretarial assistance.

References

Amoroso, E.C. (1952). Placentation. (In) *Marshall's Physiology of Reproduction*, Vol. 2 (Parkes, A.S., ed.), pp.127–297. London, Longman.

Aplin, J.D. (1988). Cellular biology of the endometrium. (In) *Biology of the Uterus*, 3rd edition (Wynn, R.M. & Jollie, W.P., eds.). New York, Plenum Press.

Baxter, R.C., Martin, J.L. & Wood, M.H. (1987). Two immunoreactive binding proteins for insulin-like growth factors in human amniotic fluid: relationship to fetal maturity. *Journal of Clinical Endocrinology and Metabolism*, **65**:423–431.

Bell, S.C. (1983). Decidualization: regional differentiation and associated function. *Oxford Reviews of Reproductive Biology*, **5**:220–271.

Bell, S.C. (1985). Comparative aspects of decidualization in rodents and human cell types: secreted products and associated function. (In) *Implantation of the Human Embryo* (Edwards, R.G., Purdy, J.M. & Steptoe, P.C., eds.), pp.71–122. London, Academic Press.

Bell, S.C. (1988a). Synthesis and secretion of proteins by the endometrium and decidua. (In) *Implantation: Biological and Clinical Aspects* (Chapman, M., Grudzinskas, G. & Chard, T., eds.), pp.85–118. Berlin, Springer-Verlag.

Bell, S.C. (1988b). Secretory endometrial/decidual proteins and their function in early pregnancy. *Journal of Reproduction and Fertility*, Supplement **36**:109–125.

Bell, S.C. (1989). Decidualization and insulin-like growth factor (IGF) binding protein: implications for its role in stromal cell differentiation and the decidual cell in haemochorial placentation. *Human Reproduction*, **4**:125–130.

Bell, S.C., Fazleabas, A.T. & Verhage, H.G. (1989). Comparative aspects of secretory proteins of the endometrium and decidua in the human and non-human primates – primate models for the study of the function of the endometrium and decidua. (In) *Blastocyst Implantation* (Yoshinaga, K., ed.), pp.151–162. New York, Plenum Press.

Bell, S.C., Hales, M.W., Patel, S., Kirwan, P.H. & Drife, J.O. (1985). Protein synthesis and secretion by the human endometrium and decidua during early pregnancy. *British Journal of Obstetrics and Gynaecology*, **92**:793–803.

Bell, S.C., Hales, M.W., Patel, S.R., Kirwan, P.H., Drife, J.O. & Milford-Ward, A. (1986a). Amniotic fluid concentrations of secreted pregnancy-associated endometrial alpha 1- and alpha 2-globulins (alpha 1- and alpha 2-PEG). *British Journal of Obstetrics and Gynaecology*, **93**:909–915.

Bell, S.C., Patel, S.R., Kirwan, P.H. & Drife, J.O. (1986b). Protein synthesis and secretion by the human endometrium during the menstrual cycle and the effect of progesterone *in vitro*. *Journal of Reproduction and Fertility*, **77**:221–231.

Bell, S.C., Patel, S.R., Jackson, J.A. & Waites, G.T. (1988). Major secretory protein of human decidualized endometrium in pregnancy is an insulin-like growth factor-binding protein. *Journal of Endocrinology*, **118**:317–328.

Bell, S.C. & Searle, R.F. (1981). Differentiation of decidual cells in mouse endometrial cell cultures. *Journal of Reproduction and Fertility*, **49**:425–433.

Bell, S.C. & Smith, S. (1988). The endometrium as a paracrine organ. (In) *Contemporary Obstetrics and Gynaecology* (Chamberlain, G.V.P., ed.), pp.273–298. Cambridge, Butterworths Scientific.

Böhlen, P. (1990). Angiogenic factors. (In) *Contraception and Mechanisms of Endometrial Bleeding* (d'Arcangues, C., Fraser, I.S., Newton, J.R. & Odlind, V., eds.), pp.467–486. Cambridge, England, Cambridge University Press.

Bolander, M.E., Young, M.F., Fisher, L.W., Yamada, Y. & Termine, J.D. (1988). Osteonectin cDNA sequencing reveals potential binding regions for calcium and hydroxyapatite, and shows homologies with both a basement membrane protein (SPARC) and a serine proteinase inhibitor (ovomucoid). *Proceedings of National Academy of Sciences USA*, **85**:2919–2923.

Brenner, R.M. & Maslar, I.A. (1988). The primate oviduct and endometrium. (In) *The Physiology of Reproduction* (Knobil, E., Neill, J. *et al*, eds.), pp.303–329. New York, Raven Press.

Brewer, M.T., Stetler, G.L., Squires, C.H., Thompson, R.C., Busby, W.H. &

Clemmons, D.R. (1988). Cloning, characterization and expression of a human insulin-like growth factor binding protein. *Biochemical and Biophysical Research Communications*, **152**:1289–1297.

Bulmer, D., Peel, S. & Stewart, I. (1987a). The metrial gland. *Cell Differentiation*, **20**:77–86.

Bulmer, J.N., Johnson, P.M. & Bulmer, D. (1987b). Leukocyte populations in human decidua and endometrium. (In) *Immunoregulation and Fetal Survival* (Gill, T.J. & Wegmann, T.J., eds.), pp.111–134. Oxford, Oxford University Press.

Bulmer, J.N. & Ritson, A. (1988). The decidua in early pregnancy. (In) *Early Pregnancy Loss: Mechanisms and Treatment* (Beard, R.W. & Sharp, F., eds.), pp.171–180. Ashton-under-Lyne, Peacock Press.

Charpin, C., Kopp, F., Pourreau-Schneider, N., Lissitzky, J.C., Lavaut, M.N.. Martin, P.M. & Toga, M. (1985). Laminin distribution in human decidua and immature placenta: An immunoelectron microscopic study (avidin–biotin–peroxidase complex method). *American Journal of Obstetrics and Gynecology*, **151**:822–826.

Clark, D.A., Damji, N., Chaput, A., Daya, S., Rosenthal, K.L. & Brierley, J. (1987). Decidua-associated suppressor cells and suppressor factors regulating interleukin 2: their role in the survival of the 'fetal allograft'. (In) *Progress in Immunology, VI* (Cinader, B. & Miller, R.G., eds.), pp.1089–1099. New York, Academic Press.

Clark, D.A. & Daya, S. (1990). Macrophages and other migratory cells in endometrium: relevance to endometrial bleeding. (In) *Contraception and Mechanisms of Endometrial Bleeding* (d'Arcangues, C., Fraser, I.S., Newton, J.R. & Odlind, V., eds.), pp.363–379. Cambridge, England, Cambridge University Press.

Clemmons, D.R., Elgin, R.G., Han, V.K.M., Casella, S.J., D'Ercole, A.J. & Van Wyk, J.J. (1986). Cultured fibroblast monolayers secrete a protein that alters the cellular binding of somatomedin-C/insulin like growth factor 1. *Journal of Clinical Investigation*, **77**:1548–1556.

Debus, E., Weber, K. & Osborn, M. (1983). Monoclonal antibodies to desmin, the muscle-specific intermediate filament protein. *EMBO*, **2**:2305–2312.

De Feo, V.J. (1967). Decidualization. (In) *Cellular Biology of the Uterus* (Wynn, R.M., ed.), pp.191–290. Amsterdam, North-Holland.

D'Ercole, A.J., Drop, S.L.S. & Kortleve, D.J. (1985). Somatomedin-C/insulin-like growth factor 1-binding proteins in human amniotic fluid and in fetal and postnatal blood: evidence of immunological homology. *Journal of Clinical Endocrinology and Metabolism*, **61**:612–617.

Drop, S.L.S., Kortleve, D.J., Guyda, H.J. & Posner, B.I. (1984). Immunoassay of a somatomedin-binding protein from human amniotic fluid: levels in fetal, neonatal and adult sera. *Journal of Clinical Endocrinology and Metabolism*, **59**:908–915.

Elgin, R.G., Busby, W.H. Clemmons, D.R. (1987). An insulin-like growth factor (IGF) binding protein enhances the biologic response to IGF-1. *Proceedings of the National Academy of Sciences USA*, **84**:3254–3258.

Enders, A.C., Welsh, A.O. & Schlafke, S. (1985). Implantation in the rhesus monkey: endometrial responses. *American Journal of Anatomy*, **173**:147–169.

Engel, J., Taylor, W., Paulsson, M., Sage, H. & Hogan, B. (1987). Calcium binding domains and calcium-induced conformational transition of SPARC/BM-40/ osteonectin, an extracellular glycoprotein expressed in mineralized and nonmineralized tissues. *Biochemistry*, **26**:6958–6965.

Faber, M., Wewer, U.M., Berthelsen, J.G., Liotta, L.A. & Albrechtsen, R. (1986).

Laminin production by human endometrial stromal cells relates to the cyclic and pathologic state of the endometrium. *American Journal of Pathology*, **124**:384–391.

Fazleabas, A.T., Verhage, H.G., Waites, G. & Bell, S.C. (1989). Characterization of an insulin-like growth factor binding protein (IGF-BP), analogous to human pregnancy-associated secreted endometrial αl-globulin (αl-PEG) in decidua of the baboon (Papio Anubis) placenta. *Biology of Reproduction*, **40**:873–885.

Finn, C.A. (1977). The implantation reaction. (In) *Biology of the Uterus* (Wynn, R.M., ed.), pp.245–308. New York, Plenum Press.

Finn, C.A. (1983). Implantation of ova – assessment of the value of laboratory animals as models for the study of implantation in women. *Oxford Reviews of Reproductive Biology*, **5**:272–289.

Finn, C.A. (1986). Implantation, menstruation and inflammation. *Biological Reviews*, Cambridge Philosophical Society, **61**:313–328.

Finn, C.A. (1987). Why do women and some other primates menstruate. *Perspectives in Biology and Medicine*, **30**:566–574.

Finn, C.A. & Pope, M. (1984). Vascular and cellular changes in the decidualized endometrium of the ovariectomized mouse following cessation of hormone treatment: a possible model for menstruation. *Journal of Endocrinology*, **100**:295–300.

Finn, C.A. & Pope, M. (1986). Control of leucocyte infiltration into the decidualized mouse uterus. *Journal of Endocrinology*, **110**:93–96.

Fujimoto, T. & Singer, S.J. (1986). Immunocytochemical studies of endothelial cells *in vivo*. I. The presence of desmin only, or of desmin plus vimentin or vimentin only, in the endothelial cells of different capillaries of the adult chicken. *Journal of Cell Biology*, **103**:2775–2786.

Glasser, S.R. (1972). The uterine environment in implantation and decidualization. (In) *Reproductive Biology* (Balin, H.A. & Glasser, S.R., eds.), pp.776–883. Amsterdam, Excerpta Medica.

Glasser, S.R. & Julian, J. (1986). Intermediate filament protein as a marker of uterine stromal cell decidualization. *Biology of Reproduction*, **35**:463–474.

Glasser, S.R., Lampelo, S., Munir, M.I. & Julian, J. (1987). Expression of desmin, laminin and fibronectin during *in situ* differentiation (decidualization) of rat uterine stromal cells. *Differentiation*, **35**:132–142.

Glasser, S.R. & McCormack, S.A. (1982). Cellular and molecular aspects of decidualization and implantation. (In) *Proteins and Steroids in Early Pregnancy* (Beier, H.M. & Karlson, P., eds.), pp.245–310. New York, Springer-Verlag.

Gordon, M.Y., Riley, G.P., Watt, S.M. & Greaves, M.F. (1987). Compartmentalization of a haematopoietic growth factor (GM-CSF) by glycosaminoglycans in the bone marrow microenvironment. *Nature*, **326**:403–405.

Hall, K., Hansson, U., Lundin, G., Luthman, M., Persson, B., Povoa, G., Stangenberg, M. & Ofverholm, U. (1986). Serum levels of somatomedins and somatomedin-binding protein in pregnant women with type 1 or gestational diabetes and their infants. *Journal of Clinical Endocrinology and Metabolism*, **63**:1300–1306.

Healy, D., Salamonsen, L., Moon, J., Cameron, I.T. & Findlay, J.K. (1990). Human endometrial prolactin. (In) *Contraception and Mechanisms of Endometrial Bleeding* (d'Arcangues, C., Fraser, I.S., Newton, J.R. & Odlind, V., eds.), pp.213–219. Cambridge, England, Cambridge University Press.

Heine, U.I., Munoz, E.F., Flanders, K.C., Ellingsworth, L.R., Lam, H.Y.P.,

Thomspon, N.L., Roberts, A.B. & Sporn, M.B. (1987). Role of transforming growth factor-β in the development of the mouse embryo. *Journal of Cell Biology*, **105**:2861–2876.

Herr, J.C., Heidger, P.M., Scott, J.R., Anderson, J.W., Curet, L.B. & Mossman, H.W. (1978). Decidual cells in the human ovary at term. I. Incidence, gross anatomy and ultrastructural features of merocrine secretion. *American Journal of Anatomy*, **152**:7–27.

Khong, T.Y., Lane, E.B. & Robertson, W.B. (1986). An immunocytochemical study of fetal cells at the maternal–placental interface using monoclonal antibodies to keratins, vimentin and desmin. *Cell and Tissue Research*, **246**:189–195.

Kisalus, L.L., Herr, J.C. & Little, C.D. (1987a). Immunolocalization of extracellular matrix proteins and collagen synthesis in first-trimester human decidua. *Anatomical Record*, **218**:402–415.

Kisalus, L.L., Nunley, W.C. & Herr, J.C. (1987b). Protein synthesis and secretion in human decidua of early pregnancy. *Biology of Reproduction*, **36**:785–798.

Lala, P.K., Kearns, M. & Parha, R.S. (1987). Immunology of the decidual tissue. (In) *Immunoregulation and Fetal Survival* (Gill, T.J. & Wagmann, T.G., eds.), pp.78–95. Oxford, Oxford University Press.

Lawn, A.M., Wilson, E.W. & Finn, C.A. (1971). The ultrastructure of human decidual and predecidual cells. *Journal of Reproduction and Fertility*, **26**:85–90.

Lee, Y.L., Hintz, R.L., James, P.M., Lee, P.D.K., Shively. J.E. & Powell, D.R. (1988). Insulin-like growth factor (IGF) binding protein complementary deoxyribonucleic acid from human HEP G2 hepatoma cells: predicted protein sequence suggests an IGF binding domain different from those of the IGF-I and IGF-II receptors. *Molecular Endocrinology*, **2**:404–411.

Massman, H.W. (1980). Comparative morphology of the endometrium. (In) *The Endometrium* (Kimball, F.A., ed.), pp.3–21. New York, MTP Press.

Nathan, C.F. (1987). Secretory products of macrophages. *Journal of Clinical Investigation*, **79**:319–326.

Nissley, S.P. & Rechler, M.M. (1984). Insulin-like growth factors: Biosynthesis, receptors and carrier proteins. (In) *Hormonal Proteins and Peptides*, Vol. XII (Hoa Li, C., ed.), pp.127–203. New York, Academic Press.

Nomura, S., Wills, A.J., Edwards, D.R., Heath, J.K. & Hogan, B.L.M. (1988). Developmental expression of 2ar (oesteopontin) and SPARC (oesteonectin) RNA as revealed by *in situ* hybridization. *Journal of Cell Biology*, **106**:441–450.

Oldberg, Å., Franzén, A. & Heinegård, D. (1986). Cloning and sequence analysis of rat bone sialoprotein (oesteopontin) cDNA reveals an Arg-Gly-Asp cell-binding sequence. *Proceedings of the National Academy of Sciences USA*, **83**:8819–8823.

Ooi, G.T. & Herington, A.C. (1988). The biological and structural characterization of specific serum binding proteins for the insulin-like growth factors. *Journal of Endocrinology*, **118**:7–18.

O'Shea, J.D., Kleinfeld, R.G. & Marrow, H.A. (1983). Ultrastructure of decidualization in the pseudopregnant rat. *American Journal of Anatomy*, **166**:271–298.

Parr, E.L., Parr, M.B. & Young, J.D. (1987). Localization of a pore-forming protein (perforin) in granulated metrial gland cells. *Biology of Reproduction*, **37**:1327–1335.

Parr, M.B., Tung, H.N. & Parr, E.L. (1986). The ultrastructure of the rat primary decidual zone. *American Journal of Anatomy*, **176**:423–436.

Peel, S. & Stewart, I. (1986). Oestrogen and the differentiation of granulated metrial gland cells in chimeric mice. *Journal of Anatomy*, **144**:181–187.

Pijnenborg, R., Robertson, W.B., Brosens, I. & Dixon, G. (1981). Trophoblast invasion and the establishment of haemochorial placentation in man and laboratory animals. *Placenta*, **2**:71–91.

Povoa, G., Enberg, G., Jornvall, H. & Hall, K. (1984). Isolation and characterization of a somatomedin-binding protein from mid-term human amniotic fluid. *European Journal of Biochemistry*, **144**:199–204.

Prince, C.W., Oosawa, T., Butler, W.T., Tomana, M., Bhown, A.S., Bhown, M. & Schrohenloher, R.E. (1987). Isolation, characterization and biosynthesis of a phosphorylated glycoprotein from rat bone. *Journal of Biological Chemistry*, **262**:2900–2907.

Ramsey, E.M., Houston, M.L. & Harris, J.W. (1976). Interactions of the trophoblast and maternal tissues in three closely related primate species. *American Journal of Obstetrics and Gynecology*, **124**:647–652.

Ruoslahti, E. & Pierschbacher, M.D. (1987). New perspectives in cell adhesion: RGD and integrins. *Science*, **238**:491–497.

Rutanen, E.M., Bohn, H. & Seppälä, M. (1982). Radioimmunoassay of placental protein 12: levels in amniotic fluid, cord blood, and serum of healthy adults, pregnant women and patients with trophoblastic disease. *American Journal of Obstetrics and Gynecology*, **144**:460–463.

Rutanen, E.M., Koistinen, R., Sjoberg, J., Julkunen, M., Wahlstrom, T., Bohn, H. & Seppälä, M. (1986). Synthesis of placental protein 12 by human endometrium. *Endocrinology*, **118**:1067–1071.

Sananes, N., Weiller, S., Baulieu, E.E. & Le Goascogne, C. (1978). *In vitro* decidualization of rat endometrial cells. *Endocrinology*, **103**:86–95.

Sananes, N., Weiller, S., Baulieu, E.E. & Le Goascogne, C. (1980). Decidualization in vitro: effects of progesterone and indomethacin. *Progress in Reproductive Biology*, **7**:125–134.

Selye, H. & McKeown, I. (1935). Studies on the physiology of the maternal placenta in the rat. *Proceedings of the Royal Society B*, **119**:1–31.

Seppälä, M., Riittinen, L., Julkunen, M., Koistinen, R., Wahlstrom, T., Iino, K., Alfthan, H., Stenman, U.H. & Huhtala, M.L. (1988). Structural studies, localization in tissue and clinical aspects of human endometrial proteins. *Journal of Reproduction and Fertility*, Supplement **36**:127–141.

Skalli, O., Ropraz, P., Trzeciak, A., Benzonana, G., Gillessen, D. & Gabbiani, G. (1986). A monoclonal antibody against alpha-smooth muscle actin: a new probe for smooth muscle differentiation. *Journal of Cell Biology*, **103**:2787–2796.

Sporn, M.B. & Roberts, A.B. (1986). Peptide growth factors and inflammation, tissue repair, and cancer. *Journal of Clinical Investigation*, **78**:329–332.

Sporn, M.B., Roberts, A.B., Wakefield, L.M. & De Crombrugghe, B. (1987). Some recent advances in the chemistry and biology of transforming growth factor-beta. *Journal of Cell Biology*, **105**:1039–1045.

Stewart, I. (1983). An investigation into the differentiation of granulated metrial gland cells in the early pregnant mouse uterus. *Journal of Anatomy*, **137**:85–93.

Stewart, I. (1984). A morphological study of granulated metrial gland cells and trophoblast cells in the labyrinthine placenta of the mouse. *Journal of Anatomy*, **139**:627–638.

Stewart, I. (1987). Differentiation of granulated metrial gland cells in ovariectomized mice given ovarian hormones. *Journal of Endocrinology*, **112**:23–26.

Stewart, I. (1988). Granulated metrial gland cells in the non-traumatized regions of the uterus of ovariectomized mice with deciduomata maintained on progesterone. *Journal of Endocrinology*, **116**:11–15.

Stewart, I. & Mukhtar, D.D.Y. (1988). The killing of mouse trophoblast cells by granulated metrial gland cells *in vitro. Placenta*, **9**:417–425.

Tachi, S., Tachi, C. & Lindner, H.R. (1970). Ultrastructural features of blastocyst attachment and trophoblastic invasion in the rat. *Journal of Reproduction and Fertility*, **21**:37–56.

Termine, J.D., Belcourt, A.B., Conn, K.M. & Kleinman, H.K. (1981a). Mineral and collagen-binding proteins of fetal calf bone. *Journal of Biological Chemistry*, **256**:10403–10408.

Termine, J.D., Kleinman, H.K., Whitson, S.W., Conn, K.M., McGarvey, M.L. & Martin, G.R. (1981b). Osteonectin, a bone-specific protein linking mineral to collagen. *Cell*, **26**:99–105.

Tsunawaki, S., Sporn, M., Ding, A. & Nathan, C. (1988). Deactivation of macrophages by transforming growth factor-beta. *Nature*, **334**:260–262.

Vaes, G. (1988). Cellular biology and biochemical mechanisms of bone resorption. A review of recent developments on the formation, activation and mode of action of oesteoclasts. *Clinical Orthopaedics and Related Research*, **231**:239–271.

Vladimirsky, F., Chen, L., Amsterdam, A., Zor, L.L. & Linder, H.R. (1977). Differentiation of decidual cells in cultures of rat endometrium. *Journal of Reproduction and Fertility*, **49**:61–68.

Wahlstrom, T. & Seppälä, M. (1984). Placental protein 12 (PP12) is induced in the endometrium by progesterone. *Fertility and Sterility*, **41**:781–784.

Waites, G.T., James, R.F.L. & Bell, S.C. (1988). Immunohistological localization of the human endometrial secretory protein pregnancy-associated endometrial alpha 1-globulin, an insulin-like growth factor-binding protein, during the menstrual cycle. *Journal of Clinical Endocrinology and Metabolism*, **67**:1100–1104.

Waites, G.T., James, R.F.L. & Bell, S.C. (1989). Human pregnancy associated endometrial α-globulin, an insulin-like growth factor binding protein – immunohistological localization in the decidua and placenta during pregnancy employing monoclonal antibodies. *Journal of Endocrinology*, **120**:351–357.

Welsh, A.O. & Enders, A.C. (1985). Light and electron microscopic examination of the mature decidual cells of the rat with emphasis on the antimesometrial decidua and its degeneration. *American Journal of Anatomy*, **172**:1–29.

Wewer, U.M., Albrechtsen, R., Fisher, L.W., Young, M.F. & Termine, J.D. (1988). Osteonectin/SPARC/BM-40 in human decidua and carcinoma, tissues characterized by *de novo* formation of basement membrane. *American Journal of Pathology*, **132**:345–355.

Wewer, U.M., Damjanov, A., Weiss, J., Liotta, L.A. & Damjanov, I. (1986). Mouse endometrial stromal cells produce basement-membrane components. *Differentiation*, **32**:49–58.

Wewer, U.M., Faber, M., Liotta, L.A. & Albrechtsen, R. (1985). Immunochemical and ultrastructural assessment of the nature of the pericellular basement membrane of human decidual cells. *Laboratory Investigation*, **53**:624–633.

Wynn, R.M. (1974). Ultrastructural development of the human decidua. *American Journal of Obstetrics and Gynecology*, **118**:652–670.

Discussion

Rice-Evans. Can you make a biochemical connection for us between the withdrawal of progesterone and the influx of neutrophils?

Bell. No, I cannot. High doses of progesterone are anti-inflammatory and I suppose the simplest suggestion is that the steroid is not acting on the decidual tissue but may act to prevent the recruitment of other cell types into the area. Certainly, in animals with subcutaneous implants containing progesterone, you can prevent inflammatory responses. There are a number of links between growth factors and cell activity, particularly in the regulation of the activity of the migratory cell populations in the endometrium. There are reports that will appear in the literature that the decidual tissue does produce these factors. If these are actually progesterone-dependent products of decidual cells, these factors could either directly or indirectly suppress activity of the migratory cell populations. Then withdrawal of progesterone may result in decrease of the production of factors that actually suppress the activity of migratory cells, thus allowing their activation.

Brosens. Do you have any explanation for the decrease in elasticity of spiral arteries?

Bell. There is very little information concerning the contribution of the decidual cell to extracellular matrix synthesis and degradation apart from collagen and basement membrane synthesis. This is one area that needs investigating with respect to its importance in tissue growth and breakdown.

Cornillie. We often find the endometrial granulocyte in the luminal epithelium of human and rodent endometria, together with lymphocytes and neutrophils. Can you comment on the function of decidualized cells migrating from the stroma into the epithelium?

Bell. In rodents the hypothesis that mature granulated lymphocyte cells arise from differentiation of small lymphocytes is supported by assay studies (see review by Bulmer *et al.*, 1987). Although decidualization of the stroma is required for this differentiation, once differentiated they may not require the environment of the decidual cell for their support. The cells appear to migrate into blood vessels in the labyrinthine placenta and are detected in the lung during pregnancy (Bulmer *et al.*, 1987). As far as specific interaction with the epithelium is concerned, I think these cells are probably different and are related to intraepithelial granulated lymphocytes noted in other sites.

Clark. I agree that the granulated lymphocytes which appear in epithelium are different from the large metrial gland cells that develop during pregnancy. You can find these intra-epithelial lymphocytes in other mucosal organs, such as the intestine. They represent a heterogeneous population. A proportion of the cells have natural killer activity, and it is proposed that they may play a special role in defence against parasites that may appear on that surface epithelium. I would like to add an editorial point which is provoked by the use of the term 'granulocyte'. In North America, granulocytes are polymorphonuclear leukocytes, and the confusion produced by using the term 'granulocyte' for endometrial granulated lymphocyte is considerable. I think we should strike from our memory banks the term 'endometrial granulocyte' and use instead 'endometrial granulated lymphocytes'.

Findlay. It has been suggested that extracellular matrix is also a place where growth factors can be stored (Baird *et al.*, 1986). Is there any evidence that the decidual extracellular matrix is also storing growth factors, and that when you get breakdown, you might get release of some of these growth factors, which could be important for subsequent re-epithelization?

Bell. I have no information concerning the decidua. However, it has been reported that fibroblast-derived growth factors are stored in extracellular matrices which may be liberated after tissue injury.

Sheppard. Have you any information on the presence of renin in endometrium? I remember a study by Johnson and co-workers who found a positive reaction of monoclonal antibodies to renin only in cases where the patients had hysterectomies for menorrhagia (Johnson *et al.*, 1984).

Bell. I cannot make any comment on the renin site. However, I can comment on studies referring to a relaxin site. The endometrial granulated lymphocytes were suggested to be a source of relaxin. I think that has been disproven and the original observation was based upon use of non-specific polyclonal antibodies. There are reports of relaxin being localized to decidual cells (Koay *et al.*, 1985). I do not know whether that has been verified by in-situ hybridization, but they have employed an antibody for the connecting peptide of relaxin. It is fairly good evidence that perhaps relaxin is produced.

Cornillie. What happens with these granulated endometrial lymphocytes in culture? Mitosis?

Bell. There has been some debate concerning the observation of mitosis in these cells. Dr Bulmer at Leeds has informed me (personal communication) that only rarely is mitosis observed in these cells. As far as culture is concerned, there is very limited information. Employing a tissue explant system, these cells are observed to migrate out of the explant (Stewart & Mukhtar, 1988). If one of the early events associated with decidualization is the influx of precursors of these cells, you will observe in-situ differentiation of these cells, and such observations cannot be used to support the concept of their differentiation from stromal fibroblasts.

Böhlen. With respect to Dr Findlay's question on growth factors in endometrial extracellular matrix, to my knowledge there is nothing known specifically about growth factors located in the endometrial extracellular matrix. The experiment done by Dr Baird in San Diego (Baird *et al.*, 1986), demonstrated that FGF is localized to the extracellular matrix of cultured vascular endothelial cells. It is also known that extracellular matrices in eye tissues contain FGF. It is highly suspected that other extracellular matrices contain FGF as well, but this is not really known.

Healy. A point about relaxin. We have done some work in collaboration with the Howard Florey Institute in Melbourne, and that group has cloned the H1 and H2 human relaxin gene and developed specific antibodies to human relaxin. We cannot demonstrate relaxin within human decidua, or, indeed, in other pregnancy tissues at all (Healy, Tregear & Eddie, unpublished observations). And until proven otherwise, we do not believe a separate uterine relaxin as opposed to ovarian relaxin does exist in the human.

References

Baird, A., Esch, F., Mormede, P., Ueno, N., Ling, N., Böhlen, P., Ying, S.Y., Wehrenberg, W.B. & Guillemin, R. (1986). Molecular characterization of fibroblast growth factor: distribution and biological activities in various tissues. *Recent Progress in Hormone Research*, **42**:143–205.

Bulmer, D., Peel, S. & Stewart, I. (1987). The metrial gland. *Cell Differentiation*, **20**:77–86.

Johnson, J., Johnson, I.R., Ronan, J.E. & Craven, D.J. (1984). The site of renin in the human uterus. *Histopathology*, **8**:273–278.

Koay, E.S.C., Bagnell, C.A., Bryant-Greenwood, G.D., Lord, S.B., Cruz, A.C. & Larkin, L.H. (1985). Immunocytochemical localization of relaxin in human decidua and placenta. *Journal of Clinical Endocrinology and Metabolism*, **60**:859–863.

Stewart, I. & Mukhtar, D.D.Y. (1988). The killing of mouse trophoblast cells by granulated metrial gland cells *in vitro*. *Placenta*, **9**:417–425.

Human endometrial prolactin

D.L. HEALY, L. SALAMONSEN, J. MOON, I.T. CAMERON AND
J.K. FINDLAY

Medical Research Centre, Prince Henry's Hospital, Melbourne, Australia.

Abstract

An homologous human prolactin (PRL) radioimmunoassay was reported in 1971 and endometrial and decidual synthesis of PRL was demonstrated in 1977. Secretion of immuno- and bioactive PRL into amniotic fluid was subsequently shown and the 25 N-terminal amino acid sequence of endometrial prolactin was found to be identical to pituitary PRL. PRL mRNA isolation from term decidua subsequently confirmed expression of the PRL gene in human endometrium. More recently, a glycosylated form of PRL was isolated from both human pituitary and endometrium. Glycosylated PRL is identical in amino acid sequence to the major form of PRL but has a carbohydrate unit of 2 kd molecular weight on an asparagine residue and accounts for 10–15% of pituitary PRL. Decidual explants secrete 33–50% less glycosylated PRL than non-glycosylated PRL. It appears that predominantly glycosylated PRL is secreted in the late luteal phase of the menstrual cycle while increasingly greater amounts of non-glycosylated PRL are secreted as pregnancy advances. The biological significance and regulation of PRL glycosylation are uncertain, although glycosylated ovine PRL has only 20–33% of the lactogenic activity of ovine PRL. Pituitary lactotropes, of ectodermal origin, are regulated by dopamine, estradiol and thyrotrophin-releasing hormone. Decidual cells, of mesodermal origin, are not influenced by these pituitary secretogogues. Progesterone and calcium appear to stimulate both pituitary and decidual PRL secretion, while arachidonic acid inhibits decidual PRL release. More recently, insulin-like growth factor 1 (IGF-1), a polypeptide growth factor implicated in the estrogen-promoted growth of reproductive tissues, has been found in high concentration in the pig uterus, and IGF-1 has been shown to stimulate the synthesis and secretion of PRL from human decidua.

PRL receptors have not been reported on endothelium or blood vessels and no direct effect of endometrial PRL on menstruation has been substantiated. A further putative function for endometrial PRL is as an immunoregulatory hormone. PRL appears necessary for the normal production of macrophage activating factors including interferon. Human interferon-α_2 has sequence homology to ovine trophoblast protein 1 and is found in high concentration in human pregnancy and fetal tissues. Interferon-α modestly reduces human endometrial PRL secretion to $69.0 \pm 10.2\%$ of control over a dose range of 0.5–50.0 units/ml. Whether endometrial or decidual PRL is critical in normal or abnormal uterine bleeding or in the human immunoregulatory response to pregnancy awaits further study.

Introduction

Valid and sensitive radioimmunoassays for human prolactin (PRL) were initially reported in 1971 (Hwang *et al.*, 1971). Application of this assay found

PRL concentrations in human amniotic fluid up to 100-fold higher than in maternal blood. The major source of amniotic fluid PRL was initially thought to be either the maternal or the fetal pituitary. But no other maternal hormone with a molecular weight of approximately 20 kd was known to cross the placenta to amniotic fluid in such concentrations. Furthermore, bromocriptine administration to pregnant women lowered maternal serum PRL values, but left amniotic fluid PRL values undisturbed. Whereas these data suggested the maternal pituitary was not the major source of amniotic fluid PRL, a major fetal source for amniotic fluid PRL was also inconsistent with data that radiolabelled PRL injected into rhesus monkeys did not reach amniotic fluid. Moreover, fetal death *in utero* failed to lower amniotic fluid PRL values. It was therefore possible that amniotic fluid PRL was locally produced.

Human endometrial and decidual prolactin synthesis

The placenta was the most obvious local source for high amniotic fluid PRL concentrations. However, placenta did not release PRL in organ culture and did not stain with anti-PRL antiserum when examined by immunofluorescence. Several groups then reported the identification of immunoreactive material identical to pituitary PRL in chorion laeve freed from the amnion, but containing cells from the subjacent decidua parietalis (Golander *et al.*, 1978; Healy *et al.*, 1979). Active peptide synthesis of PRL was indicated in that cyclohexamide and puromycin suppressed PRL secretion from this tissue. Moreover, labelled amino acid incorporation into a protein which behaved identically to human pituitary PRL in bioassay was demonstrated. Nevertheless, the precise tissue origin of this decidual chorionic PRL remained uncertain until Riddick and co-workers identified PRL, not only in the endometrium of women carrying an ectopic pregnancy, but also in normal secretory endometrium from day 22 of the menstrual cycle (Maslar & Riddick, 1979; Maslar *et al.*, 1980).

The conclusion that endometrial decidua, a mesodermal tissue, normally synthesized and released PRL was heretical when first presented in 1977. Although PRL secretion had been reported from non-pituitary neoplasms, identification and release of classic pituitary hormones within a normal non-pituitary tissue were novel. More recently, other data along similar lines have considerably broadened our concepts of hormonal secretion and function and generated many new hypotheses of the evolutionary origins of chemical messengers. Corroboratory evidence for endometrial secretion of a functional PRL molecule came from interaction of milligram amounts of this protein from amniotic fluid and purification by affinity chromatography which revealed that the 25 N-terminal amino acid sequence was identical to pituitary PRL. Moreover, decidual and amniotic fluid PRL molecules had potent bioactivities *in vitro*. In addition, expression of the PRL gene by identification of PRL messenger RNA in decidua reinforced the view that decidual PRL was a functional molecule of endometrial origin. More recently, PRL synthesis and secretion have also been identified in myometrium.

Glycosylated prolactin

Glycosylated PRL is identical in aminoacid sequence to the major form of PRL but has a carbohydrate unit of 2 kd molecular weight on an asparagine residue and accounts for 10–15% of pituitary PRL (Lewis *et al.*, 1984). Glycosylated PRL (G-PRL) has been identified in amniotic fluid, as a secretory product of luteal phase endometrium and in term decidual tissue. It appears that G-PRL is the predominant form of PRL secreted in the late luteal phase of the menstrual cycle (Markoff & Lee, 1987). It can be identified in the peripheral circulation at this time. The biological significance of G-PRL at this time is uncertain, although ovine G-PRL has been reported to have reduced lactogenic bioactivity compared with ovine PRL, while porcine G-PRL has been claimed to have enhanced activity compared with the non-glycosylated form of porcine PRL. These differences may relate to the differences in carbohydrate composition.

In pregnancy, decidual explants secrete less G-PRL than non-glycosylated PRL. As pregnancy advances, less and less G-PRL is secreted as determined by sodium dodecyl sulphate polyacrylamide gel electrophoresis. Before pregnancy, serum G-PRL was the predominant PRL form in the peripheral circulation, and as pregnancy progressed, increasing amounts of PRL, compared to G-PRL, appeared in serum, reaching a maximum by the third trimester (Markoff *et al.*, 1988).

Regulation of endometrial and decidual prolactin secretion

Although dopamine inhibits and thyrotropin-releasing hormone (TRH) stimulates the synthesis and release of pituitary PRL, neither dopamine nor TRH affects the synthesis or release of decidual PRL. Furthermore, the intracellular localization of PRL in decidual tissue is different from that in the pituitary. Pituitary PRL is localized in typical cytoplasmic secretory granules while decidual PRL is localized in the post-microsomal supernatant and not in granules at all. Anterior pituitary cells, which are of ectodermal origin, share common cell surface antigens such as chromogranin, a major soluble protein in secretory vesicles. Decidual cells do not contain chromogranin, consistent with their mesodermal origin, suggesting there are major differences in the cell surface antigens of these two PRL-producing tissues.

Despite these differences between pituitary and uterine PRL, calcium and progesterone appear capable of stimulating PRL secretion from both tissues (Table 1). While progesterone stimulation of decidual PRL secretion presumably acts via the decidual progesterone receptor, which is itself estrogen dependent, the addition of estradiol to the progesterone diminishes

Table 1. *Regulation of human endometrial/decidual PRL secretion*

Effect	Agent	Concentration
Stimulation	Progesterone	1–100 ng/ml
	IGF-1	100 ng/ml
	Calcium	10^{-3} mol/l
Inhibition	Arachidonic acid	10^{-4}–10^{-5} mol/l
No effect	TRH	10^{-3}–10^{-9} mol/l
	Dopamine	10^{-5}–10^{-9} mol/l
	Bromocriptine	10^{-7}–10^{-10} mol/l
	Estradiol	10^{-6} mol/l
	$PGF_{2\alpha}$, PGE_2	10^{-5}–10^{-12} mol/l
	Dibutyryl cyclic AMP	10^{-3} mol/l
	Indomethacin	10^{-4} mol/l

decidual PRL synthesis. Surprisingly, the reverse appears to be true for myometrial PRL secretion. Such an estrogen–progesterone interdependence is similar to the estrogen–progesterone synergy previously demonstrated to stimulate pituitary PRL secretion and this stimulatory mechanism appears common at both sites of PRL secretion in women (Williams *et al.*, 1981).

Calcium also appears to stimulate both pituitary and decidual PRL secretion, whereas arachidonic acid has been reported to inhibit decidual PRL release. More recently, insulin-like growth factor 1 (IGF-1), a polypeptide growth factor implicated in the estrogen-promoted growth of reproductive tissues, has been found in high concentration in the pig uterus, and IGF-1 has been shown to stimulate the release and secretion of PRL from human decidua (Thrailkill *et al.*, 1988).

Prolactin receptors in pregnancy tissues

A mandatory prerequisite for any biological action of endometrial or decidual PRL upon human endometrium would be the demonstration of PRL receptors, since interaction with receptors is assumed to be the first step in the mechanism of action of protein hormones. No PRL receptors have been identified in human endometrium.

We have identified a PRL binding site in human chorion laeve. The binding affinity (0.47×10^9 l/pmol) and capacity (175 fmol/ml) in this tissue are similar to those described for PRL receptors in liver and mammary gland. Small amounts of this receptor also appeared within placental preparations, in keeping with the identical origin of the chorion laeve and chorion frondosum. No PRL-binding sites were identified in decidua, amnion or umbilical cord. However, others have suggested the presence of PRL receptors in human amnion after studying water transport before and after in-vitro exposure of amnion to an antibody directed towards a partially purified rabbit PRL receptor (Tyson *et al.*, 1985). A reduced number of PRL receptors has been reported in patients with chronic polyhydramnios and may be responsible for the excess amniotic fluid in these women (Healy *et al.*, 1985).

Prolactin and prostaglandins

Prolactin stimulates prostaglandins E and F_{2a} (PGE and PGF_{2a}) secretion from rat granulosa cells at low concentrations while inhibiting their secretion at high concentrations (Knazek *et al.*, 1981). Similar results have been obtained by infusing PRL into the isolated superior mesenteric artery vascular bed of the rat. We have previously hypothesized that a function of the chorionic PRL receptor may be to modulate prostaglandin synthesis from these fetal membranes. Indeed, ovine PRL has been reported to reduce PGE output from human amniochorion by 39–59% (Tyson *et al.*, 1985), suggesting that endogenous PRL released by human decidual tissue might also inhibit the elaboration of PGE within the fetal membranes.

More recently, we examined the hypothesis that endometrial PRL may inhibit endometrial prostaglandin production. Human endometrial explants from the late luteal phase incubated on stainless steel grids in 35 mm culture dishes in medium M199 with added progesterone or prolactin (460, 46, 4.6 units/l) and maintained in culture for 3 days, with a medium change every 24 hours, were assayed for PGE and PGF_{2a}. Progesterone decreased PGE and PGF_{2a} production to within 64% of control cultures with no added treatments, as expected from earlier data. The response to PRL was variable. PRL (460 units/l) increased PGE released in three of nine subjects (mean 144% of control). At a PRL concentration of 46 units/l, PGE release was increased in tissue from only one of four subjects, decreased in one of four and not changed in the tissue from two remaining subjects tested at this concentration. By contrast, PGE was released by histamine in tissues from all subjects. It appears that PRL gives no clear dose/response changes in PGE or PGF_{2a} release and is not central in the control of human endometrial prostaglandin secretion.

Prolactin and menstruation

Prolactin has some effects on blood flow: it can lower blood pressure and increase cardiac output in intact rats. In isolated preparations, PRL concentrations up to 100 ng/ml have no direct effects themselves but have been reported to potentiate responses to pressure agents such as noradrenalin. PRL concentrations above 200 ng/ml have been claimed to inhibit vascular responses, including changes in mammary blood flow in lactating animals. These peripheral vascular effects seem to be dependent on the stimulation of prostaglandin synthesis.

PRL receptors have not been found in the heart, although PRL has been demonstrated to stimulate cardiac ornithine decarboxylase. Nor have PRL receptors been reported on endothelium or blood vessels and no direct effect of endometrial PRL on menstruation has been substantiated.

Prolactin and immunoregulation

Synthesis of various classic hormones by immunological tissues and cells are now confirmed in a number of species. Such data suggest that endocrine mechanisms may have an immunomodulatory role beyond the activation of the pituitary–adrenocortical axis as a result of stress. Several lines of evidence indicate that PRL may be an important immunoregulatory hormone. In rats, both hypophysectomy and treatment with bromocriptine inhibit the development of delayed cutaneous hypersensitivity and other immunological reactions. Treatment with exogenous PRL reverses these immunosuppressive effects. Hypopituitary mice develop impaired cellular immunity and this immunodeficiency is prevented by injections of milk, a PRL source.

Replication of cultured nb2 node rat lymphoma cells is specifically stimulated by lactogenic hormones such as PRL and has been used as a PRL bioassay. In these cells, the activity of the enzyme ornithine decarboxylase becomes undetectable when the cells are incubated in PRL-deficient media. This appears to be due to an inhibitor of this enzyme. Addition of PRL blocks synthesis of this inhibitor, increasing ornithine decarboxylase concentrations and promoting growth of these lymphoma cells. In hypoprolactinemic mice, there is suppression of macrophage activation and T-lymphocyte function (Bernton *et al.*, 1988). Of the multiple events leading to macrophage activation *in vivo*, the production by T-lymphocytes of interferon was the most impaired in bromocriptine-treated mice.

In mice, lymphocytes appear to constitute an important target tissue for PRL, which seems necessary for the normal production of macrophage-activating factors including interferon. Addition of interferon-α over a dose range 0.5–50.0 units/ml to human endometrial explants lowers PRL secretion to $69.0 \pm 10.2\%$ of control cultures. Since human interferon-α has sequence homology to ovine trophoblast protein 1 and is found in high concentration in human pregnancy and fetal tissues, it is possible that human interferon may regulate endometrial and decidual PRL secretion. However, evidence of this interaction between endometrial PRL and the immunological response to implantation is still preliminary and awaits further study.

Future directions

Bioactive PRL is synthesized and released in increasing amounts by decidualized human endometrium as pregnancy advances. A clear function of endometrial PRL still awaits proof, although a paracrine immunomodulatory role is feasible. Glycosylated human PRL may have different biological activities to non-glycosylated PRL but the physiological significance of these chemical changes awaits study. It seems unlikely that endometrial PRL has any major role in menstruation or breakthrough bleeding.

References

Bernton, E.W., Meltzer, M.S. & Holaday, J.W. (1988). Suppression of macrophage activation and T-lymphocyte function in hypoprolactinemic mice. *Science*, **239**:401–404.

Golander, A., Hurley, T., Barrett, J., Hizi, A. & Handwerger, S. (1978). Prolactin synthesis by human chorion–decidual tissue: a possible source of prolactin in the amniotic fluid. *Science*, **202**:311–313.

Healy, D.L., Herrington, A.C. & O'Herlihy, C. (1985). Chronic polyhydramnios is a syndrome with a lactogen receptor defect in the chorion laeve. *British Journal of Obstetrics and Gynaecology*, **92**:461–467.

Healy, D.L., Kimpton, W.G., Muller, H.K. & Burger, H.G. (1979). The synthesis of immunoreactive prolactin by decidua-chorion. *British Journal of Obstetrics and Gynaecology*, **86**:307–313.

Hwang, P., Guyda, H. & Friesen, H. (1971). A radioimmunoassay for human prolactin. *Proceedings of the National Academy of Sciences USA*, **68**:1902–1906.

Knazek, R.A., Cristy, R.J., Watson, K.C., Lim, M.F., Van Gorder, P.N., Dave, J.R., Richardson, L.L. & Liu, S.C. (1981). Prolactin modifies follicle-stimulating hormone-induced prostaglandin synthesis by the rat granulosa cell. *Endocrinology*, **109**:1566–1572.

Lewis, U.J., Singh, R.N., Lewis, L.J., Seavey, B.K. & Sinha, Y.N. (1984). Glycosylated ovine prolactin. *Proceedings of the National Academy of Sciences USA*, **81**:385–389.

Markoff, E. & Lee, D.W. (1987). Glycosylated prolactin is a major circulating variant in human serum. *Journal of Clinical Endocrinology and Metabolism*, **65**:1102–1106.

Markoff, E., Lee, D.W. & Hollingsworth, D.R. (1988). Glycosylated and non-glycosylated prolactin in serum during pregnancy. *Journal of Clinical Endocrinology and Metabolism*, **67**:519–523.

Maslar, I.A., Kaplan, B.M., Luciano, A.A. & Riddick, D.H. (1980). Prolactin production by the endometrium of early human pregnancy. *Journal of Clinical Endocrinology and Metabolism*, **51**:78–83.

Maslar, I.A. & Riddick, D.H. (1979). Prolactin production by human endometrium in the normal menstrual cycle. *American Journal of Obstetrics and Gynecology*, **135**:751–754.

Thrailkill, K.M., Golander, A., Underwood, L.E. & Handwerger, S.(1988). Insulin-like growth factor 1 stimulates the synthesis and release of prolactin from human decidual cells. *Endocrinology*, **123**:2930–2934.

Tyson, J.E., McCoshen, J.A. & Dubin, N.H. (1985). Inhibition of fetal membrane prostaglandin production by prolactin: relative importance in the initiation of labour. *American Journal of Obstetrics and Gynecology*, **151**:1032–1038.

Williams, R.F., Barber, D.L., Cowan, B.D., Lynch, A., Marut, E.L. & Hodgen, G.D. (1981). Hyperprolactinemia in monkeys: induction by an oestrogen–progesterone synergy. *Steroids*, **38**:321–331.

Discussion

Bouchard. You have shown that prolactin is synthesized in decidual cells. Did you have the opportunity to study hyperprolactinemic women? In hyperprolactinemic women, is there uptake of circulating prolactin into the decidual cells or uterus?

Healy. I am not exactly sure how one would study it and distinguish it from uterine prolactin secretion.

Åkerlund. You mentioned dopamine in connection with prolactin in the uterus. Dopamine is indeed interesting in late pregnancies and could be one of the factors actually responsible for the onset of labour: you can stimulate contractions very well with dopamine; you can even induce contractions. You said there was no effect of dopamine on uterine prolactin secretion. How has that been studied? How was the effect demonstrated in the pituitary?

Healy. The actions of dopamine and dopamine analogues were evaluated *in vitro* in terms of decidual prolactin secretion, by ourselves (with endometrium and with decidua) and certainly by Handwerger's group and others (Golander *et al.*, 1979; Healy & Hodgen, 1983). No dopaminergic binding sites in decidual cells were demonstrable in these in-vitro studies.

Bell. I want to refer to the paper by Heffner *et al.* (1986) which indicated that glycosylated prolactin was actually a major product of the endometrium in the luteal phase. We reported identical patterns to his, but in fact that major band represents α_2-PEG and not prolactin, and I think his data were actually dependent on one Western blot with a very weak reaction with prolactin antibody. The second point is about interpretation of the transition from glycosylated prolactin to prolactin, based on an unpublished observation. We demonstrated prolactin in secretory glandular epithelium as well as in the decidual cells. I wonder if glycosylated prolactin is expressed by the glandular epithelium and free prolactin by decidual cells. This would fit in with all the kinetic profiles that you observe because the decrease of glycosylated prolactin in the first trimester fits in with the involution of the secretory gland-containing decidua spongiosa region and the appearance of free prolactin with progressive decidualization of the decidua compacta in which the glands are non-secretory. And that would imply that the glycosylated prolactin and non-glycosylated prolactin could have two independent functions corresponding to the two regions in the endometrium and decidua. Have you had any experience in terms of histochemical localization?

Healy. We have not done that, although I know Dr Gurpide has done some work in that area. I believe you would need to investigate whether the prolactin gene was expressed in epithelial glandular cells.

References

Golander, A., Barrett, J., Hurley, T., Barry, S. & Handwerger, S. (1979). Failure of bromocriptine, dopamine and thyrotropin releasing hormone to effect prolactin secretion by human decidual tissue *in vitro*. *Journal of Clinical Endocrinology and Metabolism*, **49**:787–789.
Healy, D.L. & Hodgen, G.D. (1983). The endocrinology of human endometrium. *Obstetrical and Gynaecological Survey*, **38**:509–530.
Heffner, L.J., Iddenden, D.A. & Lyttle CR (1986). Electrophoretic analysis of secreted human endometrial proteins: identification and characterization of luteal phase prolactin. *Journal of Clinical Endocrinology and Metabolism*, **62**:1285–1295.

Endometrial protein secretion relative to endometrial function

MARKKU SEPPÄLÄ, ANNE-MARIA SUIKKARI AND MERVI JULKUNEN

Department of Obstetrics and Gynecology, University Central Hospital, Helsinki, Finland.

Abstract

Two endometrial proteins were purified from midtrimester amniotic fluid, namely 34K insulin-like growth factor-binding protein (IGFBP-1) and PP14. Both are synthesized and released by secretory endometrium, and both appear to be progesterone regulated. In addition, insulin regulates circulating IGFBP-1 levels. Both proteins have recently been cloned. While there are multiple sites of IGFBP-1 synthesis, the synthesis of PP14 is mainly confined to secretory endometrium. The serum PP14 level is low at the time of ovulation and the level starts rising 6–8 days after ovulation. In a fertile cycle the PP14 level continues to rise until weeks 8–10 of pregnancy. In an infertile ovulatory cycle, the PP14 level also rises during the last week of the luteal phase, the levels doubling every 3 days. High levels are maintained for the first 2 or 3 days of the next cycle. The same is seen in hyperstimulated cycles, but not in anovulatory cycles. In ovulatory cycles the administration of progesterone increases the serum PP14 level in the late luteal phase. The serum estradiol level in the proliferative phase is positively correlated with the PP14 level in the late luteal phase, indicating that estrogen priming is important for the subsequent protein secretion by the endometrium. Traces of PP14 can also be found in the serum of postmenopausal women. Cyclical administration of estrogen and progestogen increases this level provided the uterus is intact. Such an increase is not seen in hysterectomized postmenopausal women, indicating that the uterine contribution to circulating PP14 levels can be detected and quantified in serum. These results indicate that it is possible to obtain information on endometrial protein secretion by a blood test. This may have implications for detection of primary endometrial dysfunction and for assessment of direct uterine effects of various endocrine treatments. It is unclear whether these proteins may have any role in menstruation or disturbances of bleeding.

Introduction

Assessment of endometrial maturity is based on changes in endometrial histology. This requires endometrial biopsy which is an invasive procedure and may interfere with implantation and early embryonal development. No blood test is yet available for the assessment of endometrial function. We shall review here recent studies on two proteins produced by secretory and decidualized endometrium which appear to play a part in endometrial differentiation and can also be detected in blood.

Insulin-like growth factor-binding protein (IGFBP-1)

This protein, previously named PP12 (placental protein 12), is abundant in secretory and decidualized endometrium (Rutanen *et al.*, 1984), where its synthesis has been demonstrated by incorporation of labelled methionine (Rutanen *et al.*, 1985, 1986) and detection of messenger RNA (Julkunen *et al.*, 1988a). The mature peptide contains 259 amino-acid residues and has a molecular mass of 25.3 kd. The affinity of this protein to bind insulin-like growth factor 1 (IGF-1) is similar to that of the IGF-1 receptor (Marshall *et al.*, 1974; Koistinen *et al.*, 1987a). Its IGF-binding domain resides in the 17 kd N-terminal part of the molecule (Huhtala *et al.*, 1986). Recent studies indicate that IGFBP-1 has an important role in inhibiting the receptor binding and possible biological action of IGF-1 in the endometrium (Rutanen *et al.*, 1988). Other studies on a similar protein have revealed enhanced action of IGF-1 (Elgin *et al.*, 1987). Because IGFBP-1 appears in the endometrium only after ovulation, based on detection of its mRNA (Julkunen *et al.*, 1988a) and immunoperoxidase staining (Wahlström & Seppälä, 1984), it is possible that the presence of this protein at the endometrial site, apparently triggered by progesterone (Rutanen *et al.*, 1986), distracts IGF-1 from its endometrial receptor, thus contributing to the proliferative/secretory transition of the endometrium. IGFBP-1 appears to exert local action in the endometrium in an autocrine/paracrine manner. This protein is immunologically related to a_1-pregnancy-associated endometrial globulin (Bell & Bohn, 1985).

In addition to the endometrium, IGFBP-1 mRNA has been found in the liver (Julkunen *et al.*, 1988a). Preovulatory follicular fluid and luteinized granulosa cells also contain this protein (Seppälä *et al.*, 1984). Highly sensitive methods have been developed to measure the IGFBP-1 levels in blood (Suikkari *et al.*, 1987; Koistinen *et al.*, 1987b) where the levels are regulated by insulin (Suikkari *et al.*, 1988), not by growth hormone, as is the case with the 150 kd IGFBP-3 (Wilkins & D'Ercole, 1985). Because of its multiple sites of synthesis, the circulating levels of IGFBP-1 cannot be used to assess endometrial function.

Endometrial protein PP14

Endometrial protein PP14 (placental protein 14) is synthesized by secretory and decidualized endometrium, not by placenta (Julkunen, 1986; Julkunen *et al.*, 1986b). PP14 mRNA has been found in secretory and decidualized endometrium, not in proliferative endometrium, placenta or liver (Julkunen *et al.*, 1988b). This protein has significant homology to β-lactoglobulins of various species (Huhtala *et al.*, 1987), and it is immunologically related to progesterone-dependent endometrial protein (Julkunen *et al.*, 1986c) and a_2-pregnancy-associated endometrial globulin (Bell & Bohn, 1985).

PP14 is localized to endometrial secretory glands and thus may serve as a marker of endometrial differentiation. By immunoperoxidase staining, PP14 appears in the endometrium on day 5 postovulation and is most abundant in late secretory phase (Julkunen *et al.*, 1986b). PP14 has been detected in serum of non-pregnant women and in men; its highest levels are seen at 8–10 weeks' pregnancy (Julkunen *et al.*, 1985). In ovulatory cycles the highest levels are seen at the onset of menstruation provided the preceding cycle was ovulatory (Julkunen *et al.*, 1986a). No rise is seen unless the serum progesterone level has risen first. Postmenopausal estrogen–progestogen replacement therapy also brings about an increase in serum PP14 level provided the uterus is intact (Seppälä *et al.*, 1987a). Such an increase is not seen in hysterectomized women. Although all the sites in the body synthesizing PP14 are not yet known, the contribution of the uterus to the circulating PP14 level is significant (Seppälä *et al.*, 1988). We have observed great individual variations in the progestogen–PP14 responses of postmenopausal women taking the same estrogen–progestogen replacement therapy, indicating that their uterine responses are different. The mode of progestogen administration also makes a difference. Sustained administration of danazol brings about a decrease in serum PP14 level for as long as the therapeutic amenorrhea is maintained (Than *et al.*, 1987), whereas cyclical administration of micronized progesterone over the luteal phase enhances the normally occurring elevation of serum PP14 level (Seppälä *et al.*, 1987b).

These and other studies (Maslar & Riddick, 1979; Healy & Hodgen, 1983) indicate that the uterus is an active endocrine organ which not only responds to endocrine stimuli by bleeding but also secretes proteins which may have both local and remote actions. The biological role of these proteins is only beginning to be understood, and their messages outside the uterus are now a challenge for future investigations.

Acknowledgements

Original studies reviewed in this communication were supported by grants from the Academy of Finland, Sigrid Jusélius Foundation and the Finnish Social Insurance Institution.

References

Bell, S.C. & Bohn, H. (1985). Immunochemical and biochemical relationship between human pregnancy-associated secreted endometrial α_1 and α_2-globulins (α_1- and α_2-PEG) and the soluble placental proteins 12 and 14 (PP12 and PP14). *Placenta*, 7:283–294.
Elgin, R.G., Busby, W.H. Jr & Clemmons, D.R. (1987). An insulin-like growth factor (IGF) binding protein enhances the biologic response to IGF-I. *Proceedings of the National Academy of Sciences USA*, **84**:3254–3258.

Healy, D.L. & Hodgen, G.D. (1983). The endocrinology of human endometrium. *Obstetrical and Gynecological Survey*, **38**:509–530.

Huhtala, M.-L., Koistinen, R., Palomäki, P., Partanen, P., Bohn, H. & Seppälä, M. (1986). Biologically active domain in somatomedin-binding protein. *Biochemical and Biophysical Research Communications*, **141**:263–270.

Huhtala, M.-L., Seppälä, M., Närvänen, A., Palomäki, P., Julkunen, M. & Bohn, H. (1987). Amino acid sequence homology between human placental protein 14 and β-lactoglobulins from various species. *Endocrinology*, **120**:2620–2622.

Julkunen, M. (1986). Human decidua synthesizes placental protein 14 (PP14) *in vitro*. *Acta Endocrinologica*, **112**:271–277.

Julkunen, M., Apter, D., Seppälä, M., Stenman, U.-H. & Bohn, H. (1986a). Serum levels of placental protein 14 reflect ovulation in nonconceptional menstrual cycles. *Fertility and Sterility*, **45**:47–50.

Julkunen, M., Koistinen, R., Aalto-Setälä, K., Seppälä, M., Jänne, O.A. & Kontula, K. (1988a). Primary structure of human insulin-like growth factor-binding protein/ placental protein 12 and tissue-specific expression of its mRNA. *FEBS Letters*, **236**:295–302.

Julkunen, M., Koistinen, R., Sjöberg, J., Rutanen, E.-M., Wahlström, T. & Seppälä, M. (1986b). Secretory endometrium synthesizes placental protein 14. *Endocrinology*, **118**:1782–1786.

Julkunen, M., Raikar, R.S., Joshi, S.G., Bohn, H. & Seppälä, M. (1986c). Placental protein 14 and progestagen-dependent endometrial protein are immunologically indistinguishable. *Human Reproduction*, **1**:7–8.

Julkunen, M., Rutanen, E.-M., Koskimies, A.I., Ranta, T., Bohn, H. & Seppälä, M. (1985). Distribution of placental protein 14 in tissues and body fluids during pregnancy. *British Journal of Obstetrics and Gynaecology*, **92**:1145–1151.

Julkunen, M., Seppälä, M. & Jänne, O.A. (1988b). Complete amino acid sequence of human placental protein 14. A progesterone-regulated uterine protein homologous to β-lactoglobulins. *Proceedings of the National Academy of Sciences USA*, **85**:8845–8849.

Koistinen, R., Huhtala, M.-L., Stenman, U.-H. & Seppälä, M. (1987a). Purification of placental protein PP12 from human amniotic fluid and its comparison with PP12 from placenta by immunological, physicochemical and somatomedin-binding properties. *Clinica Chimica Acta*, **164**:293–303.

Koistinen, R., Stenman, U.-H., Alfthan, H. & Seppälä, M. (1987b). Time-resolved immunofluorometric assay of 34-kDa somatomedin-binding protein. *Clinical Chemistry*, **33**:1126–1128.

Marshall, R.N., Underwood, L.E., Voina, S.J., Foushee, D.B. & Van Wyk, J.J. (1974). Characterization of the insulin and somatomedin-C receptors in human placental cell membranes. *Journal of Clinical Endocrinology and Metabolism*, **39**:283–292.

Maslar, I.A. & Riddick, D.H. (1979). Prolactin production by human endometrium during the normal menstrual cycle. *American Journal of Obstetrics and Gynecology*, **135**:751–754.

Rutanen, E.-M., Koistinen, R., Sjöberg, J., Julkunen, M., Wahlström, T., Bohn, H. & Seppälä, M. (1986). Synthesis of placental protein 12 by human endometrium. *Endocrinology*, **118**:1067–1071.

Rutanen, E.-M., Koistinen, R., Wahlström, T., Bohn, H., Ranta, T. & Seppälä, M.

(1985). Synthesis of placental protein 12 by human decidua. *Endocrinology*, **116**:1304–1309.

Rutanen, E.-M., Koistinen, R., Wahlström, T., Sjöberg, J., Stenman, U.-H. & Seppälä, M. (1984). Placental protein 12 (PP12) in the human endometrium: Tissue concentration in relation to histology and serum levels of PP12, progesterone and oestradiol. *British Journal of Obstetrics and Gynaecology*, **91**:377–381.

Rutanen, E.-M., Pekonen, F. & Mäkinen, T. (1988). Soluble 34K binding protein inhibits the binding of insulin-like growth factor I to its cell receptors in human secretory phase endometrium: evidence for autocrine/paracrine regulation of growth factor action. *Journal of Clinical Endocrinology and Metabolism*, **66**:173–180.

Seppälä, M., Alfthan, H., Vartiainen, E. & Stenman, U.-H. (1987a). The postmenopausal uterus: the effect of hormone replacement therapy on the serum levels of secretory endometrial protein PP14/β-lactoglobulin homologue. *Human Reproduction*, **2**:741–743.

Seppälä, M., Riittinen, L., Julkunen, M., Koistinen, R., Wahlström, T., Iino, K., Alfthan, H., Stenman, U.-H. & Huhtala, M.-L. (1988). Structural studies, localization in tissue and clinical aspects of human endometrial proteins. *Journal of Reproduction and Fertility*, Supplement **36**:127–141.

Seppälä, M., Rönnberg, L., Karonen, S.-L. & Kauppila, A. (1987b). Micronized oral progesterone increases the circulating level of endometrial secretory PP14/β-lactoglobulin homologue. *Human Reproduction*, **2**:453–455.

Seppälä, M., Wahlström, T., Koskimies, A.I., Tenhunen, A., Rutanen, E.-M., Koistinen, R., Huhtaniemi, I., Bohn, H. & Stenman, U.-H. (1984). Human preovulatory follicular fluid, luteinized cells of hyperstimulated preovulatory follicles and corpus luteum contain placental protein 12 (PP12). *Journal of Clinical Endocrinology and Metabolism*, **58**:505–510.

Suikkari, A.-M., Koivisto, V.A., Rutanen, E.-M., Yki-Järvinen, H., Karonen, S.-L. & Seppälä, M. (1988). Insulin regulates the serum levels of low molecular weight insulin-like growth factor-binding protein. *Journal of Clinical Endocrinology and Metabolism*, **66**:266–272.

Suikkari, A.-M., Rutanen, E.-M. & Seppälä, M. (1987). Circulating levels of immunoreactive insulin-like growth factor-binding protein in non-pregnant women. *Human Reproduction*, **2**:297–300.

Than, G., Seppälä, M., Julkunen, M., Szabo, D., Bodis, J., Szilagyi, A. & Csaba, I. (1987). The effect of Danazol on the circulating levels of 34K insulin-like growth factor-binding protein (PP12) and endometrial secretory protein PP14. *Human Reproduction*, **2**:549–551.

Wahlström, T. & Seppälä, M. (1984). Placental protein 12 (PP12) is induced in the endometrium by progesterone. *Fertility and Sterility*, **41**:781–784.

Wilkins, J.R. & D'Ercole, A.J. (1985). Affinity-labeled plasma somatomedin-C/insulin-like growth factor I binding proteins. Evidence of growth hormone dependence and subunit structure. *Journal of Clinical Investigation*, **75**:1350–1358.

Discussion

Smith. Am I right in assuming that the peripheral levels of PP14 go up just before and during menstruation? That is presumably a time of progesterone withdrawal. How does that tie in with the progesterone analogy?

Seppälä. It takes 48 hours in tissue culture before it is secreted. So maybe it is not a direct effect, maybe it is a product of the differentiated endometrium. But we do not see it if there was no progesterone present.

Findlay. Are these proteins also made by the endometrium of human primates?

Seppälä. We have no experience.

Bell. We have two collaborative research projects, one with Professor Fazleabas in Chicago examining baboons and another with Dr Markoff examining the rhesus monkey, and we have also started to examine other species. These studies are using monoclonal antibodies; until recently, the cDNA probes for these two proteins were not available. It is fairly obvious that as far as the protein, if I can call it the human β-lactoglobulin, that is PP14 or α_2-PEG homologue, is concerned, there does not appear to be any protein in these species that shares cross-activity with the antibodies. However, I think there is a problem searching for analogous proteins in other species employing immunochemical methods. We do not know the function of this protein and in fact there may be an analogous protein which has the same function but different physicochemical properties. In the rhesus monkey and in the baboon, as in the human, IGF-binding protein is the major secretory product of the hypertrophied stromal cell which appears in the endometrium in response to pregnancy in both these species. We are suggesting that this could actually be used as a characteristic, secretory marker of the so-called decidual cell. As I mentioned earlier, the hypertrophied stromal cell in non-human primates is not considered to represent a decidual cell by some authors, although some do suggest they are analogous to decidual cells and the IGF-binding protein is certainly produced in those two species. We do not know as yet about the mouse and rat because the problem with these species is that the IGF-binding protein does not exhibit the same sequence as the IGF-binding protein of the human and non-human primates. We may need to use a specific antibody or cDNA probe for the rat binding protein.

Bischof. Both of the speakers who referred to PP14 or α_2-PEG were saying that no function is known. There is one paper by Bolton and co-workers (1987) that shows that PP14 is an immunosuppressive protein. Or is there another paper that says the contrary?

Seppälä. Yes, Dr Bischof, you are right, but I have not seen that reproduced and I guess some groups have not been able to do that.

Bell. There are now several publications from that group concerning the immunosuppressive property of this protein and this activity has been demonstrated in two *in vitro* assays (Pockley *et al.*, 1988). We have, however, had problems demonstrating any immunosuppressive activity associated with this protein. There is one aspect that should be considered. This protein has now been suggested to represent a member of the β-lactoglobulin-related secretory protein family which possess a ligand-binding calyx, such as retinol-binding protein. It is possible that α_2-PEG/PP14 binds an immunosuppressive ligand which is lost during our purification procedures and not in the method employed by Dr Bolton's group.

Seppälä. Yes, we tried the same for retinol and we had the same results as Dr Bell. We changed to a milder way of using monoclonals with low binding affinity but we have no conclusive evidence that it binds retinol.

King. Any thoughts on where the residual progestogen-induced PP14 comes from in your hysterectomized women?

Seppälä. We did not find PP14 in 19 samples of normal breast tissue from breast cancer patients who have progesterone receptor-positive breast cancer. We cannot find PP14 in the human uterus except at certain times of the cycle.

Baird. The persistence of PP14 in the process of menstruation is somewhat surprising if its major source is the decidua which at that time is being removed. In practical terms, if one is going to use this as a serum marker for decidualization, one would like to know, for example, its metabolic clearance rates? Do you have any information on this?

Seppälä. Only after pregnancy, and that was about 34 hours.

Baird. Is it not possible to get this after hysterectomy for example?

Seppälä. The levels are very low (close to the limit of the sensitivity of the assay, i.e. about 30–40 μg/l).

Clark. Regarding the possible immunosuppressive role of PP14, we wrote a paper (Clark *et al.*, 1988) demonstrating that the molecule which produces broad spectrum immunosuppression in the decidua is related to the TGF-β family of proteins which are potent inhibitors of a variety of cellular functions, including macrophage production of superoxide anion. Now, these are very sticky molecules and if you put them on an HPLC column at neutral pH, you can wait at the other end of the column for several years and nothing will come off. They bind to various carriers and these carriers may modify their function. This, of course, is relevant to the effect of proteins produced by endometrium because they bind a variety of molecules and we know in the case of TFG-β, for example, that an α-2 macroglobulin will reduce to a great extent its activity. If we therefore have these binding proteins in the uterus, and we measure the content of their ligands, we may expect to see a great deal of biological activity, and yet because of the binding, there may not be any activity. Where we have steroid-binding globulin, the steroid must dissociate to be active. Therefore, I wonder if we could not bring our attention to some extent back to the issue of carriers and the binding of active molecules within the endometrium and how this may affect their activity so as to lead to bleeding, i.e. by reducing the effective concentration of free ligand.

Bell. We have not tried TGF-β, but we should examine the possibility. I do not know whether α_2-PEG possesses a ligand-binding calyx but it has been suggested that, based upon sequence homology, it belongs to a secretory protein family related to the β-lactoglobulins, which are involved in binding a variety of small unstable hydrophobic ligands such as progesterone and retinol (Ali & Clark, 1988). This may mean that binding to growth factors is unlikely.

Clark. Dr Luukkainen showed pictures of steroid-binding globulins distributed almost as if they were in granules within the cells. Presumably, these binding globulins are binding the high level of steroids and preventing their action. Do any of the proteins that are produced during the normal developmental process of the endometrium also bind steroids and affect their possible impact on stroma or epithelium?

Seppälä. We have not tested steroids yet. It is a good idea.

Bell. We are testing substances other than steroids. I would like to mention that the normal route of secretion of α_2-PEG is towards the uterine lumen. Large quantities of this protein can be recovered by intrauterine flushes or intrauterine luminal biopsies. Only a small amount of protein produced locally is detected systemically and this is a problem that we have encountered when using serum levels as a marker for the action of progestogens on the endometrium. With certain treatments we can demonstrate local synthesis, but this is not reflected by a variation in systemic levels of this protein. I suggest that the protein functions locally in the lumen.

Another observation may be relevant to the discussion concerning hormone responsiveness of the basal endometrium. In the luteal phase of the cycle, using monoclonal antibodies in localization studies, α_2-PEG is detected in the whole length of the glands right into the basal region. You cannot distinguish any regional production of this protein along the length of the gland. Therefore, if this protein is hormone responsive, the glands appear to be responsive throughout their length. And this explains the blood levels that are observed during the proliferative phase which reflect release from the basal gland remnants. In immunohistological studies of hysterectomy specimens in the proliferative phase we have pictures of negative glands in the functionalis zone of the endometrium and positive ones in the basal regions. This may reflect the stability of the messenger RNA or the half-life of the protein.

References

Ali, S. & Clark, A.J. (1988). Characterization of the gene encoding ovine beta-lactoglobulin. Similarity to the genes for retinol binding protein and other secretory proteins. *Journal of Molecular Biology*, **199**:415–426.

Bolton, A.E., Pockley, A.G., Clough, K.J., Mowles, E.A., Stoker, R.J., Westwood, O.M.R. & Chapman, M.G. (1987). The identification of placental protein 14 (PP14) as an immunosuppressant factor involved in human reproduction. *Lancet*, i:593–595.

Clark, D.A., Falbo, M., Rowley, R.B., Banwatt, D. & Stedronska-Clark, J. (1988). Active suppression of host-vs-graft reaction in pregnant mice. IX. Soluble suppressor activity obtained from allopregnant mouse decidua that blocks the cytosolic effector response to IL-2 is related to transforming growth factor-β. *Journal of Immunology*, **141**:3833–3840.

Pockley, A.G., Mowles, E.A., Stoker, R.J., Westwood, O.M., Chapman, M.G. & Bolton, A.E. (1988). Suppression of *in vitro* lymphocyte reactivity to phytohemagglutinin by placental protein 14. *Journal of Reproductive Immunology*, **13**:31–39.

Effects of contraceptive progestogens on endometrial proteins

J.O. WHITE, J.D. CROXTALL AND M.G. ELDER

University of London, Royal Postgraduate Medical School, Institute of Obstetrics and Gynaecology, Hammersmith Hospital, London, UK.

Abstract

Disturbances of the menstrual cycle are a major reason for discontinuation of progestogen-only forms of contraception. Biochemical end-points of progesterone and progestogen action have defined the response to acute stimulation. The purpose of this study was to investigate biochemical changes in the endometrium of women before (control) and following (study) exposure to levonorgestrel delivered continuously via a vaginal ring. Subjects could be grouped into those who had normal menstrual cycles (NB) or those who had experienced an increase in the number of days of menstrual bleeding (B) following exposure to levonorgestrel. After exposure to levonorgestrel endometrial samples were obtained on days when there was no menstruation. Incorporation of radioactive methionine into cellular protein was not significantly different in the control cycles of each group. In the study cycle methionine incorporation was significantly increased compared with control in group B. Analysis of radioactive proteins by gel electrophoresis did not reveal any consistent pattern of change between control and study cycles in either group. Radioactivity in immunoprecipitable actin and tubulin was increased in the study cycle compared with control, suggesting effects on components that determine cellular cytoarchitecture.

Introduction

The response of normal endometrium to acute progestogenic stimulation is well characterized at the histological and biochemical level (Warren & Crist, 1973; King *et al.*, 1981). Detailed histological investigation of the response of endometrium to long-acting progestogens has been undertaken (Maqueo *et al.*, 1970; Bonnar & Sheppard, 1980) but there is a lack of information concerning changes in endometrial biochemistry. This information is necessary in order to begin to understand the underlying causes of disturbances of the menstrual cycle which are a major reason for discontinuation of progestogen-only methods of contraception.

Long-term exposure of the rodent uterus to physiological levels of estradiol unopposed by cyclical progesterone diminishes the uterotropic and biochemical response to estradiol (Schwartz *et al.*, 1986; Guest *et al.*, 1986). Changes in protein composition observed by gel electrophoresis indicated the potential of such an approach to studying hormone-induced changes in the human endometrium responding to chronic low-dose progestogen in the form of levonorgestrel released continuously via a vaginal ring.

The purpose of this study, therefore, was to analyze the protein synthetic products of primary cultures established from human endometrium. Tissue obtained during a normal control cycle was compared with that obtained at second biopsy 84–87 days following insertion of a vaginal ring releasing levonorgestrel (20 μg/day).

This study was part of a multicentre clinical trial on the effect of levonorgestrel on endometrial function. Other parts, following the same clinical protocol, investigated the effect of levonorgestrel on endometrial prostaglandin metabolism, lysosomal enzymes and hemostasis; the preliminary reports of these studies are published in this volume (respectively, Elder *et al.*, 1990; Cornillie *et al.*, 1990; Hourihan *et al.*, 1990).

Materials and methods

Forty subjects were recruited and 33 completed the study. All had a history of regular cycles and no gynecological disorder. They were followed during a control cycle with basal body temperature and three times weekly blood sampling for estradiol, progesterone and luteinizing hormone (LH). They were asked to fill in a menstrual diary. On the second day of the next menstrual cycle, a vaginal ring releasing 20 μg/day of levonorgestrel was inserted and left for 90 days. During the third treatment month, from day 60 after the ring insertion onwards, blood samples were drawn three times weekly for estradiol and progesterone and once a week for levonorgestrel and sex hormone-binding globulin (SHBG).

Endometrial biopsies were performed with a Masterson curette. In the control cycle, biopsies were timed to be taken on day LH + 10–LH + 12, calculated from the approximate time of ovulation as determined by estradiol and LH estimations (corresponding to cycle day 24–26). Endometrial biopsies in the third treatment month were taken at day 84–87 after ring insertion. If the subject was bleeding on that date, the biopsy was postponed until bleeding had ceased.

Tissues were digested in collagenase and primary cultures established for analysis of protein synthesis as previously described (Croxtall *et al.*, 1988). Proteins were metabolically labelled with ^{35}S-methionine during an 8-hour incubation in medium deficient in non-radioactive methionine. Cells were harvested by solubilization in lysis buffer – 9.5 mol/l urea, 2% NP40, 5% mercaptoethanol, 2% ampholine (1.6% pH 5–7; 0.4% pH 3–10) – and stored at −70°C prior to analysis by one- and two-dimensional gel electrophoresis (Guest *et al.*, 1986; Croxtall *et al.*, 1988). Incorporation of radioactive methionine into protein was determined by precipitation with trichloroacetic acid. Polyclonal rabbit antiserum to actin, tubulin and microtubule-associated protein (MAP) was used to immunoprecipitate radioactively labelled proteins as follows: 1×10^6 dpm (6.5–46.5 μl depending on specific activity of sample) of radioactively labelled protein was diluted to a final volume of 400 μl in reaction buffer (50 mmol/l Tris HCl, 5 mmol/l EDTA, 5mmol/l EGTA, 0.5% deoxycholate, pH 8.2) and preincubated with 40 μl of 10% crude suspension of protein A in buffer 1 (50 mmol/l Tris–HCl, 5 mmol/l EDTA, 0.5% NP40, 1 mg/ml BSA, 0.5 mol/l NaCl pH 8.0) at 4°C for 15 minutes. Protein A was removed by centrifugation, 5 μl of antiserum added to the recovered supernatant and incubated for 3 hours at 4°C. Protein A in buffer 1 (50 μl) was used to precipitate immune complexes at 4°C for 1 hour. Complexes were recovered by centrifugation and sequential washing in buffer 1, three times, and buffer 2 (50 mmol/l Tris–HCl, 5 mmol/l EDTA, 0.5% NP40, pH 8.0), twice.

Results

According to the pattern of bleeding experienced during the levonorgestrel phase, the subjects were divided between a group with a normal bleeding pattern (NB) and a group with an excessive number of days on which bleeding occurred (B). Incorporation of ^{35}S-methionine into cellular protein in tissue culture was not significantly different in material from the control phase of subjects subsequently classified as NB or B (see above) during the study phase. There was a significant increase in incorporation between control and study samples in group B (p$\langle$0.01) but no difference in group NB (Fig. 1). Qualitative analysis of labelled proteins by one- and two-dimensional gel electrophoresis did not reveal any consistent differences between the control and study cycle of group B and group NB (Fig. 2).

Protein analysis by gel electrophoresis is at best semiquantitative. To determine if there were quantitative changes in incorporation into cytoskeletal proteins, polyclonal antisera against actin, tubulin and microtubule-associated protein (MAP) were used in immunoprecipitation protocols. There were no apparent differences in the amount of immunoprecipitable MAP between control and study groups (Fig. 3). However, the amount of radioactivity in actin and tubulin immunoprecipitates was apparently higher in the study compared with the control cycle (p$\langle$0.05).

Comments

Incorporation of radioactive methionine into protein synthesized by tissue cultures of human endometrium is a method that reveals differences between samples obtained during the proliferative and secretory phases of the menstrual cycle (Bell *et al.*, 1986; Rutanen *et al.*, 1986). In the present study, an apparent lack of qualitative differences between late secretory endometrium and that exposed chronically to low-dose levonorgestrel was observed despite abnormalities in menstrual cycle pattern. These data may therefore indicate that changes in endometrial cellular protein synthesis do not predispose to menstrual irregularity. However, caution should be exercised as there may be

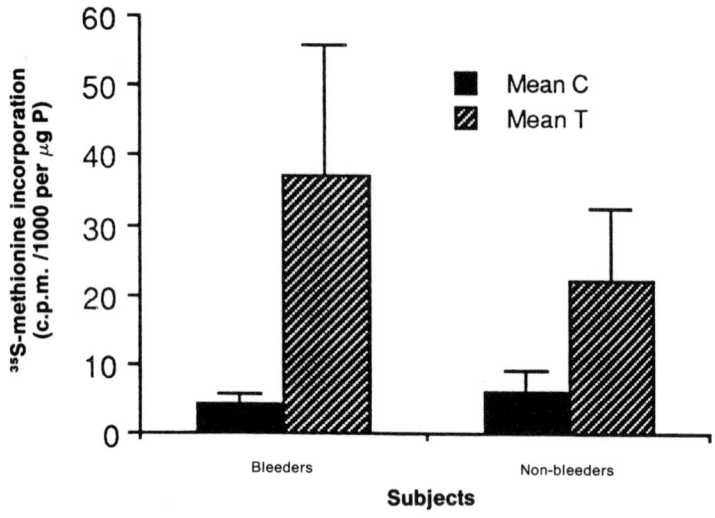

Fig. 1 ^{35}S-Methionine incorporation into cellular protein (P) in endometrial cell culture during a control cycle (C) and a treatment cycle (T) in subjects who did (bleeders) or did not (non-bleeders) have an abnormal vaginal bleeding pattern in the treatment phase of the study.

cellular parameters of importance not reflected in this study. Short-term incubation with methionine was chosen to label metabolically those proteins being synthesized at a relatively high rate. Constraints on sample size did not permit kinetic analysis which may have revealed differences in the protein profile. Secreted proteins were not analyzed due to their low specific activity. However, recent evidence implicating a progestogen-sensitive endometrial secreted protein as a growth factor binding protein (Rutanen *et al.*, 1988) may be relevant to an understanding of disturbances of uterine growth and differentiation. Finally, proteins whose cellular activities are physiologically relevant may be poorly represented when labelled to equilibrium and may escape detection by this method of analysis.

The significant increase in methionine incorporation in cultures obtained from endometrium of subjects with a history of menstrual irregularity in the study phase may indicate accelerated growth and differentiation to compensate for endometrial shedding. This is probably, therefore, a reaction to continuous progestogenic exposure but does not illuminate the primary effect underlying menstrual disorder. The apparent increase in immunoprecipitable radioactivity in actin and tubulin following exposure to levonorgestrel suggests changes in these constituents of the cytoskeleton that may be relevant to the altered end-organ response.

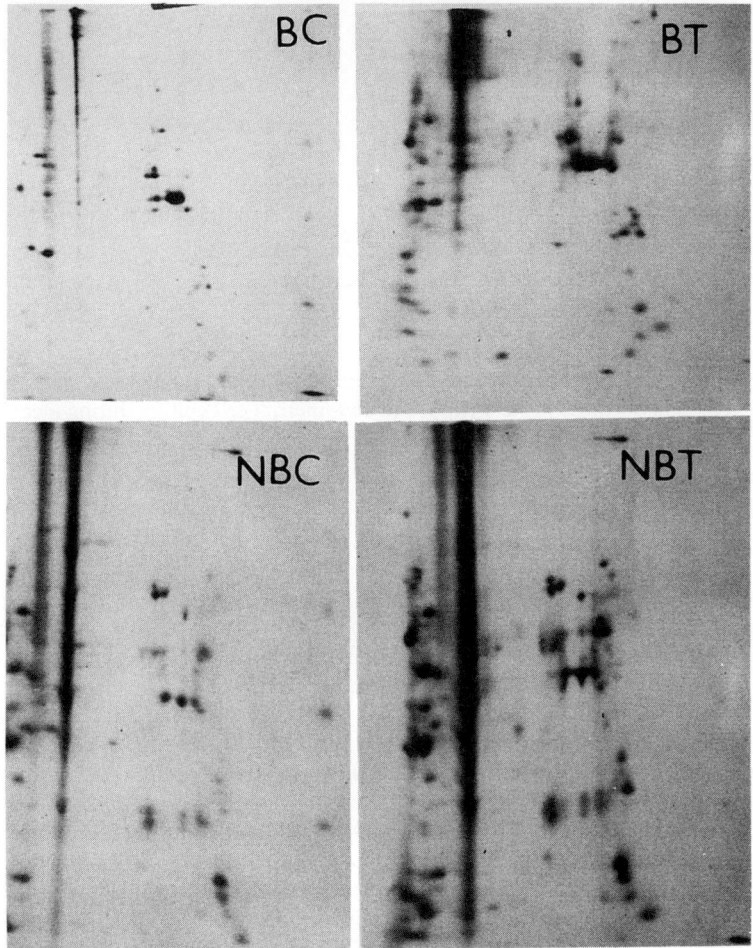

Fig. 2 Two-dimensional gel electrophoresis of endometrial proteins. Control (C) and treatment (T) cycle samples of subjects who did (B) or did not (NB) have an abnormal vaginal bleeding pattern in the treatment phase of the study.

References

Bell, S.C., Patel, S.R., Kriwan, P.H. & O'Drife, J.O. (1986). Protein synthesis and secretion by the human endometrium during the menstrual cycle and the effect of progesterone *in vitro. Journal of Reproduction and Fertility*, **77**:221–231.

Bonnar, J. & Sheppard, B.L. (1980). Endometrial changes in women using hormone-releasing intrauterine devices. (In) *Endometrial Bleeding and Steroidal Contraception*

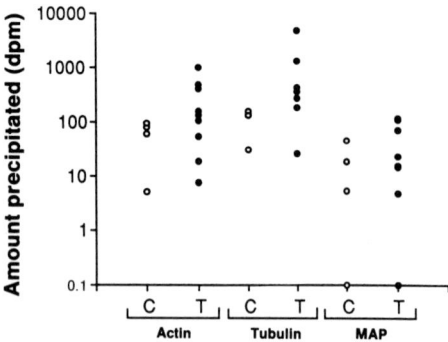

Fig. 3 Amounts of immunoprecipitable actin, tubulin and microtubule-associated protein (MAP) in endometrial cell culture during a control cycle (C) and a treatment cycle (T).

(Diczfalusy, E., Fraser, I.S. & Webb, F.T.G., eds.), pp.347–359. Bath, England, Pitman Press.

Cornillie, F.J., Brosens, I.A., Marbaix, E., Vael, T., Baudhuin, P. & Courtoy, P.J. (1990). A biochemical study of lysosomal enzymes in control and levonorgestrel-treated endometria: analysis of total activity and evidence for secretion. (In) *Contraception and Mechanisms of Endometrial Bleeding* (d'Arcangues, C., Fraser, I.S., Newton, J.R. & Odlind, V., eds.), pp.383–406. Cambridge, England, Cambridge University Press.

Croxtall, J.D., Elder, M.G. & White, J.O. (1988). Progestin regulation of protein synthesis in endometrial cancer. *Journal of Steroid Biochemistry*, **31**:207–211.

Elder, M.G., Patel, L. & White, J.O. (1990). Effect of contraceptive progestogens on prostaglandins. (In) *Contraception and Mechanisms of Endometrial Bleeding* (d'Arcangues, C., Fraser, I.S., Newton, J.R. & Odlind, V., eds.), pp.279–286. Cambridge, England, Cambridge University Press.

Guest, J.F., Elder, M.G. & White, J.O. (1986). Application of two dimensional electrophoresis to characterise hormonally sensitive proteins in the normal and abnormal uterus. *Electrophoresis*, **7**:512–518.

Hourihan, H.M., Sheppard, B.L. & Brosens, I.A. (1990). Endometrial hemostasis. (In) *Contraception and Mechanisms of Endometrial Bleeding* (d'Arcangues, C., Fraser, I.S., Newton, J.R. & Odlind, V., eds.), pp.95–114. Cambridge, England, Cambridge University Press.

King, R.J.B., Lane, G., Siddle, N., Taylor, R.W., Townsend, P.T. & Whitehead, M.I. (1981). Assessment of oestrogen and progestin effects on epithelium and stroma from pre- and post-menopausal endometria. *Journal of Steroid Biochemistry*, **15**:175–181.

Maqueo, M., Gorodovsky, J., Rice-Wray, E. & Goldzieher, J.W. (1970). Endometrial changes in women using hormonal contraceptives for periods of up to ten years. *Contraception*, **1**:115–129.

Rutanen, E.M., Koistinen, R., Sjöberg, J., Julkunen, M., Wahlström, T., Bohn, H. &

Seppälä, M. (1986). Synthesis of placental protein 12 by human endometrium. *Endocrinology*, **118**(3):1067–1071.

Rutanen, E.M., Pekonen, F. & Makinen, T. (1988). Soluble 34K binding protein inhibits the binding of insulin-like growth factor I to its cell receptors in human secretory phase endometrium: evidence for autocrine/paracrine regulation of growth factor action. *Journal of Clinical Endocrinology and Metabolism*, **66**:173–180.

Schwartz, Z., Guest, J.F., Elder, M.G. & White, J.O. (1986). Enzyme activities in the androgenized rat uterus refractory to oestrogenic stimulation. *Journal of Steroid Biochemistry*, **25**:491–496.

Warren, J.C. & Crist, R.D. (1973). Effects of ovarian steroids on uterine metabolism. (In) *Handbook of Physiology*, Section 7, Vol II, Part 2 (Greep, R.O. & Astwood, E.B., eds.), pp.49–68. Washington DC, American Physiological Society.

Discussion

Findlay. We have done similar studies as you describe using sheep tissues (Salamonsen *et al.*, 1985, 1986). The important thing which we found was that the steroid effects *in vivo* were carried over *in vitro* for up to several days in culture. We allowed the cells to settle down overnight and used a 24-hour exposure to labelled methionine so that we could analyze both cellular and secreted protein. Using that same protocol, we were able to measure prostaglandin simply by taking the medium from the first 18-hour period. I just wondered whether you had tried a similar approach with your tissue?

White. With our culture system, we found that it was best to leave them over a period of 48 hours to get attachment. But then there was no subsequent hormone treatment *in vitro*. So, it is to be hoped that the effects we were seeing were due to what had been happening *in vivo*, but we had a caveat in that we could have selected out a subpopulation of cells. And certainly, from the evidence that we have in our laboratory comparing protein synthetic products of primary cultures of endometrial cancer compared with organ cultures of endometrial cancer, you do get differences in profiles.

Bell. I wanted to make a comment concerning the comparison of secretory products of tissues, for example in an organ-type culture or short-term explant culture with dissociated cells in culture. When we were looking at the patterns of production of secretory proteins from endometrium, we went for a very short-term explant culture with high oxygen tension to try to keep it as close as possible to the physiological state. And, certainly, with the proteins that we identified, α_1-PEG (IGF-BP) and α_2-PEG, the results we got from that system seemed to reflect the in-vivo situation. But if we took pieces of tissue, from which we obtained a two-dimensional map of the secretory products, and put that into culture as dissociated cells, the two-dimensional fingerprint of the secretory products was completely different. I am always worried about actually going directly to cell culture, when we do not know, for example, what matrix to plate the cells out on. When you look at a tissue, you should always start off with the whole tissue where all the cell interactions are still as close as possible to the in-vivo situation, and use that as the reference point.

White. I think that is a valid point. Obviously we became aware of that during the course of the study, and we have got data from our own laboratory comparing normal endometrium in the way you have suggested, but not from this study.

Sheppard. Could you explain, in simple terms, what the increase in methionine incorporation signifies in the bleeders.

White. Well, my interpretation is that we have probably had some tissue loss and there may be some kind of compensation mechanism going on to regenerate tissue. But, to take that a step further, if that was the case, then we might expect to see differences in the protein profile. It is not possible to give a definitive answer yet.

Johannisson. You mentioned that you had very little material to work with and that it was difficult to differentiate between epithelium and stroma. But perhaps some kind of morphometric assessment with regard to the volume density of stroma and volume density of glands could help you to get some reference points for this estimation. I would expect from what we have seen in the normal cycle that you have a much higher percentage of glands in your control sample than you have in the treated sample.

References

Salamonsen, L.A., O, W.S., Doughton, B.W. & Findlay, J.K. (1985). The effects of estrogen and progesterone *in vivo* on protein synthesis and secretion by cultured epithelial cells from sheep endometrium. *Endocrinology*, **117**:2148–2159.

Salamonsen, L.A., Doughton, B.W. & Findlay, J.K. (1986). The effects of the preimplantation blastocyst *in vivo* and *in vitro* on protein synthesis and secretion by cultured epithelial cells from sheep endometrium. *Endocrinology*, **119**:622–628.

The cytoskeleton – a short review of current concepts

JONATHAN WEINTRAUB

Centre de Cytologie, Division de Pathologie Gynécologique, Université de Genève, Genève, Switzerland.

Abstract

The term 'cytoskeleton' refers to three intracytoplasmic protein fibre systems and their associated proteins. The fibres are classified into three groups according to ultrastructural and biochemical characteristics. They include (a) microfilaments, 7-nm diameter fibres containing actin, (b) microtubules, 25-nm diameter fibres containing tubulin, and (c) intermediate filaments, 7–11-nm diameter fibres composed of five specific classes of proteins (keratin, vimentin, desmin, glial fibrillary acidic protein (GFAP), and neurofilament proteins). The cytoskeletal elements and the structures they form participate in a wide variety of cellular processes including intracellular organization and form, cellular and subcellular movement, and intercellular contacts. While the initial description of the cytoskeleton was based on ultrastructural and biochemical observations, advances in molecular biology and immunocytochemistry now provide the means to analyze the regulation of the cytoskeletal system during differentiation and to localize precisely individual cytoskeletal elements to specific cells in tissues.

Our understanding of the role played by the cytoskeleton in the hormonally sensitive and differentiating endometrium is extremely limited. Ultrastructural studies have revealed permanent cytoskeletal structures such as cilia and microvilli, perinuclear arrays of filaments in glandular epithelium and presumed ameboid movement in regenerating epithelial cells. Biochemical studies have identified various microfilaments and intermediate filaments in endometrial cells. However, little information is available concerning the function or regulation of cytoskeletal elements. Recent studies using molecular probes have successfully analyzed the control of expression of cytoskeletal proteins in non-endometrial vascular and epithelial tissues. In a similar manner, the use of new experimental approaches may contribute to our understanding of basic endometrial physiology.

The cytoskeleton in general

Introduction

The term cytoskeleton is used to describe a diverse, complex, and interconnected network of protein fibres and accessory proteins in the cell cytoplasm. The three major protein fibre systems and the structures they form are responsible for the internal organization of cells and their shape, the movement of cells and subcellular components, and the relationship between cells and the extracellular matrix, and to other cells (Darnell *et al.*, 1986). The existence of a cytoskeleton or internal cytoplasmic structural organization was initially demonstrated by ultrastructural studies using the transmission electron microscope. Various protein fibres were observed and classified into three groups according to fibre diameter, i.e. 7-nm diameter microfilaments (MF), 8–11-nm diameter intermediate filaments (IF), and 25-nm diameter microtubules (MT). Subsequent biochemical and immunocytochemical studies showed that the MF, IF, and MT differ significantly in their biochemical and immunologic properties (Goldman *et al.*, 1985). Whereas MF and MT are linear polymers composed of one or two repeating polypeptide subunits, the IF consist of five different classes of specific proteins. In addition, the three protein fibre systems differ in their intracytoplasmic organization and in their participation in different cell processes. The structures formed by cytoskeletal protein polymers may be either temporary or permanent features of cells. They include microvilli and stress fibres (MF), cilia and flagellae (MT), muscle fibres (MF and IF), and filaments connecting spot desmosomes and other intercellular junctions (IF).

The application of recent technical advances in immunocytochemistry, immunoelectron microscopy and molecular biology to the study of the structure, function and regulation of the cytoskeleton has contributed significantly to the understanding of specific cell processes and to the more general problem of cell regulation and differentiation. While the identification and characterization of the major protein fibres have been accomplished, limited information is available concerning the way in which these fibre systems determine individual cell behavior and cell to cell interactions (Carraway *et al.*, 1987). In particular, relatively few studies have focused on the cytoskeleton of endometrial cells in normal or pathologic states. Therefore, after a brief and necessarily limited overview of the cytoskeleton in general, this review will concentrate on our current understanding of the cytoskeleton in relation to the endometrium. In addition, the possible application of new investigative techniques to the analysis of the endometrial cytoskeleton will be considered.

Microtubules

Microtubules, 24-nm diameter fibres composed of alpha and beta tubulin monomers, are present in all cells in the form of single fibres or bundles of fibres which sometimes show cross-linking (Cohen *et al.*, 1982; Cleveland & Sullivan, 1985). Microtubules play a role in the organization of the cytoplasm and appear to be linked in a specific way to a perinuclear structure called the microtubule-organizing centre which is related to the centrosome (Brinkley, 1985). Microtubules play an important role in the movement of chromosomes in mitosis and are essential for the movements of cilia and flagellae. The structure of cilia and flagellae has been elucidated and the role played by various accessory proteins in their movement defined (Goodenough & Heuser, 1985). In terms of the internal organization of the cytoplasm, microtubules appear to anchor cell organelles and determine their interrelationships. This has been demonstrated most effectively in the axon (Vale *et al.*, 1985).

Microfilaments

Microfilaments are similar in certain respects to microtubules in that they are linear polymers composed of single subunits, in this case the polypeptide monomer actin (Darnell *et al.*, 1986). Actin is the single most abundant cytoplasmic protein. Six isoforms have been defined according to variations in the amino acid sequence (Vandekerckhove & Weber, 1978). The distribution of actin isoforms varies in characteristic fashion in different organs (Vandekerckhove & Weber, 1979). The function of structures containing actin is often determined by the type and organization of the associated accessory proteins, e.g. the filamentous protein myosin, found in muscle cells. Actin in association with myosin is the major protein complex responsible for muscle contraction in all types of muscle cells. Microfilaments are present in non-muscle cells where they play a role in the structure of microvilli and stress fibres, and in the ameboid-like movement of cells (Darnell *et al.*, 1986). Recent experiments using DNA probes for actin have shown that the induction and expression of different actin isoforms are under genetic control and vary with the state of differentiation of cells (Kocher & Gabbiani, 1987). In addition, the synthesis and expression of alpha-smooth muscle actin in smooth muscle cells varied in different pathologic states.

Intermediate filaments

The study of IF proteins (8–11-nm protein fibres) has taken on increasing importance, in part as a result of their use as markers of cell lineage (Gown & Gabbiani, 1984; Corson, 1986). These markers remain stable in neoplastic states, thereby providing a means to determine the tissue of origin of poorly differentiated tumours. In addition, the expression and distribution of one class of IF proteins, the keratins, have provided valuable information concerning the state of differentiation of normal and pathologic epithelia (Bosch *et al.*, 1988; Stoler *et al.*, 1988).

The IFs are composed of five classes of proteins which include: a) desmin, a 67-kd protein present in muscle cells which appears to be a structural element which anchors the Z-discs; b) neurofilaments, present in the axons of central and peripheral nerve cells and consisting of three polypeptides with molecular weights of 68 kd, 150 kd and 200 kd; c) glial fibrillary acidic protein, found in neuroglia; d) vimentin, present in mesenchymal cells and sometimes co-expressed in normal epithelia; and e) keratin, a family of 19 polypeptides coded for by a family of 19 related genes. The polypeptides are expressed in a specific manner in different epithelia and in different states of differentiation of the same epithelia (Moll *et al.*, 1982). Two subgroups of keratins, acidic type I and basic type II, can be identified on the basis of their antigenic and biochemical properties, and gene sequences. In general, keratin filaments are composed of corresponding pairs of type I and type II proteins.

Biochemical analysis of IF proteins has revealed that they share a common structure consisting of four alpha helical regions linked by intervening sequences. The length and composition of the helical and non-helical regions vary among the classes of IF proteins. In some cell types, two classes of IF may be co-expressed, e.g. smooth muscle cells contain vimentin and desmin (Gown & Gabbiani, 1984); some epithelial cells express keratin and vimentin (Azumi & Battifora, 1986); some smooth muscle cells may express keratin and desmin (Ramaekers *et al.*, 1987; Miettinen, 1988).

In general, the functions of IFs are less well understood than those of MFs and MTs. In some cells IFs have a structural role, e.g. the desmin framework in muscle cells linking the actin–myosin contractile complex (Debus *et al.*, 1983). IFs are attached to desmosomes in muscle (Kartenbeck *et al.*, 1983) and epithelial cells and therefore may play a role in cell-to-cell communication as well as in the organization of sheets of cells (Osborn, 1984). However, in other cells the role of IFs is less clear. Furthermore, there are a large number of IF-associated proteins which appear to modify IF function and which may also be responsible for linking IFs to other fibre systems. Individual cells in which the IF network has been disrupted by the microinjection of anti-IF antibodies do not show modifications in locomotion, cell division or morphology (Gawlitta *et al.*, 1981; Lin & Feramisco, 1981). The specific role of IF proteins and of IF-associated proteins remains unclear.

Recent approaches to the understanding of IFs have focused on the regulation of their expression in normal and pathologic epithelia. This has been facilitated by the development of highly specific monoclonal antibodies (Stoler *et al.*, 1988) and molecular probes (cDNA, cRNA, oligonucleotides) (Bosch *et al.*, 1988). In the case of keratin expression, these reagents have been used to localize and precisely define the kinetics of the expression of various pairs of keratin polypeptide. Since epitopes on keratin peptides may be masked, identification by cDNA probes can verify cytologic localizations. In addition, since keratin proteins may be relatively stable in the cytoplasm, their simple presence in the cytoplasm may not necessarily mean that the cells are actively synthesizing them. Therefore, approaches using combinations of monoclonal antibodies and cDNA probes are complementary.

The cytoskeleton of endometrial cells

The endometrium is a complex tissue composed of numerous cell types including epithelial, stromal, migratory, endothelial and arterial smooth muscle. The study of the endometrial cytoskeleton is complicated by the variety of cells, by the monthly cycle of endometrial differentiation and, in some situations, by morphological alterations induced by pharmacologic concentrations of steroid hormones. Observations concerning the endometrial cytoskeleton must take into account the parameters of cell type, point in the menstrual cycle and hormonal status.

Endometrial glandular epithelial cells

At the ultrastructural level, four prominent cytoplasmic features related to the cytoskeleton have been reported. These include two relatively stable structures, cilia and microvilli, present on the epithelial cell surface (Ferenczy & Richart, 1974). The distribution and length of microvilli and cilia are modified in menopause and in hormonally altered states (Ferenczy & Richart, 1974). Thirdly, perinuclear bundles of IFs appear in the cytoplasm in the late proliferative phase but are no longer observed in the midsecretory phase (Cavazos & Lucas, 1973). These are temporary structures which may play a role in the movement of the epithelial cell secretory product to the lumen of the cell. The focal distribution of the IFs in the cytoplasm has facilitated the use of other techniques to determine their protein structure (Bolen & McNutt, 1987). Fourthly, cytoplasmic extensions similar to those seen in cells capable of migratory movements have been observed during regeneration of the epithelial cell surface following menstruation (Ferenczy, 1987). In conclusion, while ultrastructural observations suggest an important role for elements of the cytoskeletal system in endometrial glandular cells, little is known concerning the molecular mechanisms involved in the composition, synthesis, maintenance and regulation of these structures.

Most of the efforts to characterize the protein components of the normal endometrial cytoskeleton have focused on the IF proteins. This has been an offshoot of efforts in surgical pathology to develop diagnostic tissue reagents for use in the differential diagnosis of tumours (Gown & Gabbiani, 1984; Corson, 1986). Using microdissection and two-dimensional electrophoresis on polyacrylamide gels, keratin proteins number 7, 8, 18 and 19 have been identified in protein extracts of epithelial glandular cells in the proliferative phase of the cycle (Moll *et al.*, 1982; Moll *et al.*, 1983). The exact point in the proliferative phase was not identified in the three cases studied. In an immunocytochemical study, the IF proteins, keratin and vimentin were shown to be co-expressed in normal proliferative endometrium (Dabbs *et al.*, 1986). The keratin proteins were distributed throughout the cytoplasm whereas the immunostaining for vimentin was perinuclear in distribution. The specificity (in terms of the classification of keratin proteins by Moll) of the antikeratin antibodies was not precisely defined. The association of vimentin and perinuclear intermediate filaments has been confirmed (Bolen & McNutt, 1987).

Endometrial stromal cells

Ultrastructural studies of the endometrial stromal cell have been relatively unrevealing with regard to observable filament-containing structures. The non-decidualized endometrial stromal cell is characterized as relatively undifferentiated ultrastructurally, with no prominent cytoplasmic filaments or tubules (Cavazos & Lucas, 1973; Ferenczy & Richart, 1974). Decidualization has been associated with an accumulation of the IF protein, vimentin (Glasser & Julian, 1986). Attempts to characterize human stromal cells by immunocytochemistry have been descriptive and limited. In the rat, vimentin and desmin were shown to be co-expressed in decidualized cells; desmin was only present in decidualized cells while vimentin was present in both non-decidualized and decidualized cells (Glasser & Julian, 1986). Desmin may be useful as a marker of decidualization. No reports are available concerning the presence of IF proteins, including desmin, in human stromal cells.

Endometrial endothelial cells

Little is known concerning the role of the cytoskeleton in endometrial endothelial cell processes in both normal and pathologic or hormonally altered states. While ultrastructural cytoplasmic alterations have been noted in uterine endothelial cells from women treated with long-acting progestational contraceptive agents (Johannisson *et al.*, 1982), the molecular basis for these changes has not been studied. In fact, there is almost no information concerning which cytoskeletal elements may be present in endothelial cells during the normal cycle. However, the methodology is currently available to study endothelial cells *in situ*, e.g. immunocytochemistry, molecular hybridization, and *in vitro* following isolation and cultivation (Johannisson & Redard, 1984).

Studies of endothelial cells at other sites have revealed surface antigenic and biochemical differences among cells which may be related to different embryologic origins (Fujimoto & Singer, 1986; Turner *et al.*, 1987). In contrast, several features of the cytoskeletal system appear to characterize all endothelial cells, regardless of their location. Briefly, these include the role of actin filaments in: (1) direct cell-to-cell interactions mediated by adherent junctions, which are believed to maintain the integrity of the endothelial cell layer (Wong & Gotlieb, 1986); (2) points of attachment of endothelial cells to the basement membrane (Herman, 1987); and (3) cell spreading, necessary for re-endothelialization in repair processes (Dejana *et al.*, 1987; Wong & Gotlieb, 1988). Secondly, MTs linked to the centrosome are necessary for endothelial cell migration during wound repair (Wong & Gotlieb, 1988). Thirdly, while the function of IFs in endothelial cells is unknown, differences in the protein composition of IFs from endothelial cells at different sites have been described (Fujimoto & Singer, 1986). Finally, little is known concerning the effect of mediators of endothelial cell damage such as tumour necrosis factors (TNF) or interleukin 2 (IL-2) (Grau *et al.*, 1987; Aronson *et al.*, 1988) on cytoskeletal structures responsible for maintaining the integrity of the endothelial cell layer.

Structure–function and regulation of expression

The relationship between the presence of MFs and IFs and their function in endometrial cells is poorly understood. The organization of the cell cytoplasm, the way in which filament systems interact with each other, the role of accessory proteins and the regulation of cytoskeletal gene expression are all open questions. In addition, the effects of steroid hormones on cytoskeletal structures need to be defined. The hypothesis that steroid hormones may influence cells directly has been supported by observations in ovariectomized rats treated with 17β-estradiol (Szego *et al.*, 1988). Rearrangements were noted in microtubules and microvilli within 30 seconds after hormone administration. These ultrastructural modifications were no longer observed after 30 minutes. It was suggested that the reorganization of the cytoskeleton following estradiol administration may be involved in the association of the hormone with its receptor and in the propagation of the hormonal signal. In contrast to direct effects, a preliminary investigation of the genomic effect of estradiol on the regulation of actin isoforms in the whole rat uterus has shown that increased expression of MF mRNA follows estradiol administration (Hsu *et al.*, 1987). The kinetics of expression of the mRNA coding for the alpha smooth muscle isoform was different from that for beta and gamma. Myometrial tissue was shown to be the source of increased mRNA using one of the probes and in-situ hybridization.

Conclusion

What has been termed the cytoskeleton is a highly dynamic and varied system of protein fibres which play a role in numerous internal cell processes, cell movements, cell-to-cell interactions and the organization of cells with regard to the extracellular matrix. Numerous questions remain concerning the molecular mechanisms governing the structure, function and interactions of the proteins composing the cytoskeleton. The role of accessory proteins in determining the function of cytoskeletal fibres, the interactions of the fibre systems with each other and the regulation of cytoskeletal gene expression are under active investigation.

The contribution of the cytoskeleton to the cytoarchitecture of the normal endometrium is poorly understood. Even less is known about alterations in the cytoskeleton in endometrial cells in tissue subjected to long-term progesterone-only contraceptive agents. However, and on the basis of our understanding of the role played by cytoskeletal elements in the maintenance of tissue integrity in other systems, certain research approaches can be formulated to study the mechanism of endometrial bleeding in patients treated with progestational agents. The initial objectives would be as follows.

1. To obtain basic descriptive information concerning the presence and distribution of the three protein fibre systems in endometrial epithelial, stromal and vascular tissue, during the normal menstrual cycle. Technical methods would include ultrastructural studies to define cell-to-cell relationships with particular attention given to the endothelium; immunocytochemical studies to identify and localize protein antigens associated with cytoskeletal elements; and molecular hybridization studies to evaluate the modification of expression of cytoskeletal proteins.

2. To study changes in cytoskeletal fibre systems in endometrial tissues modified by treatment with long-term progestogen-only contraceptives. Putative differences in endometrial samples obtained from patients who bleed and from those who do not would be investigated. The characterization of endothelial cells in the two clinical situations would be of special interest. Technical methods would be similar to those described for objective number 1.

3. To define the pathogenetic mechanisms of alterations in the cytoskeletal systems of endometrial cells. The direct effects on cells of steroid hormones and of mediators such as tumor necrosis factor and IL-2 should be evaluated. Secondly, genomic effects manifested by alterations in the expression of cytoskeletal genes could be investigated.

References

Aronson, F.R., Libby, P., Brandon, E.P., Janicka, M.W. & Mier, J.W. (1988). IL-2 rapidly induces natural killer cell adhesion to human endothelial cells. A potential mechanism for endothelial injury. *Journal of Immunology*, **141**:158–163.

Azumi, N. & Battifora, H. (1986). The distribution of vimentin and keratin in epithelial and non-epithelial neoplasms. A comprehensive immunohistochemical study on formalin- and alcohol-fixed tumors. *American Journal of Clinical Pathology*, **88**:286–296.

Bolen, J.W. & McNutt, M.A. (1987). Cytoskeletal intermediate filaments: practical applications of intermediate filament analysis. *Ultrastructural Pathology*, **11**:175–189.

Bosch, F.X., Leube, R.E., Achtstätter, T., Moll, R. & Franke, W.W. (1988). Expression of simple epithelial type cytokeratins in stratified epithelia as detected by immunolocalization and hybridization *in situ*. *Journal of Cell Biology*, **106**:1635–1648.

Brinkley, B.R. (1985). Microtubule organizing centers. *Annual Review of Cell Biology*, **1**:145–172.

Carraway, K.L., Pratt, M.M. & Burgess, D.R. (1987). The cytoskeleton: Past, present and future. *BioEssays*, **7**:147–148.

Cavazos, F. & Lucas, F.V. (1973). Ultrastructure of the endometrium. (In) *The Uterus* (Norris, H.J., Hertig, A.T. & Abell, M.R., eds.), pp.136–174. Baltimore, Williams and Wilkins.

Cleveland, D.W. & Sullivan, K.F. (1985). Molecular biology and genetics of tubulin. *Annual Review of Biochemistry*, **54**:331–365.

Cohen, W.D., Bartlet, D., Jaeger, R., Langford, G. & Nemhauser, L. (1982). The cytoskeletal system of nucleated erythrocytes. I. Composition and function of major elements. *Journal of Cell Biology*, **93**:828.

Corson, J.M. (1986). Keratin protein immunohistochemistry in surgical pathology practice. *Pathology Annual*, **21**(2):47–81.

Dabbs, D.J., Geisinger, K.R. & Norris, H.T. (1986). Intermediate filaments in endometrial and endocervical carcinomas. The diagnostic utility of vimentin patterns. *American Journal of Surgical Pathology*, **10**:568–576.

Darnell, J., Lodish, H. & Baltimore, D. (1986). *Molecular Cell Biology*. New York, W.H. Freeman.

Debus, E., Weber, K. & Osborn, M. (1983). Monoclonal antibodies to desmin, the muscle-specific intermediate filament protein. *EMBO Journal*, **2**:2305–2312.

Dejana, E., Colella, S., Languino, L.R., Balconi, G., Corbascio, G.C. & Marchisio, P.C. (1987). Fibrinogen induces adhesion, spreading, and microfilament organization of human endothelial cells *in vitro*. *Journal of Cell Biology*, **104**:1403–1411.

Ferenczy, A. (1987). Anatomy and histology of the uterine corpus. (In) *Blaustein's Pathology of the Female Genital Tract* (Kurman, R.J., ed.), pp.257–291. New York, Springer Verlag.

Ferenczy, A. & Richart, R.M. (1974). *Female Reproductive System: Dynamics of Scan and Transmission Electron Microscopy*. New York, John Wiley and Sons.

Fujimoto, T. & Singer, S.J. (1986). Immunocytochemical studies of endothelial cells *in vivo*. I. The presence of desmin only, or of desmin plus vimentin, or vimentin only in the endothelial cells of different capillaries of the adult chicken. *Journal of Cell Biology*, **103**:2775–2786.

Gawlitta, W., Osborn, M. & Weber, K. (1981). Coiling of intermediate filaments induced by microinjection of vimentin-specific antibody does not interfere with locomotion and mitosis. *European Journal of Cell Biology*, **26**:83–90.

Glasser, S.R. & Julian, J. (1986). Intermediate filament protein as a marker of uterine stromal cell decidualization. *Biology of Reproduction*, **35**:463–474.

Goldman, R., Goldman, A., Green, K., Jones, J., Lieska, N. & Yang, H.-Y. (1985). Intermediate filaments: possible functions as cytoskeletal connecting links between the nucleus and the cell surface. *Annals of the New York Academy of Sciences*, **455**:1–17.

Goodenough, U.W. & Heuser, J.E. (1985). Substructure of inner dynein arms, radial spokes, and the central pair/projection complex of cilia and flagella. *Journal of Cell Biology*, **100**:2008–2018.

Gown, A.M. & Gabbiani, G. (1984). Intermediate-sized (10-nm) filaments in human tumors. (In) *Advances in Immunohistochemistry* (Delellis, R.A., ed.), pp.89–110. Chicago, Year Book Medical Publishers.

Grau, G.E., Fajardo, L.F., Piguet, P.F., Allet, B., Lambert, P.H. & Vassalli, P. (1987).

Tumor necrosis factor (cachectin) as an essential mediator in murine cerebral malaria. *Science*, **237**:1210–1212.

Herman, I.M. (1987). Extracellular matrix – cytoskeletal interactions in vascular cells. *Tissue and Cell*, **19**:1–19.

Hsu, C.Y.J., Fakharzadeh, S. & Frankel, F.R. (1987). Expression and regulation by estrogen of different actin isoforms in immature rat uterus. *Federation Proceedings*, **46**:2059 (Abstract No. 779).

Johannisson, E., Landgren, B.M. & Diczfalusy, E. (1982). Endometrial morphology and peripheral steroid levels in women with and without intermenstrual bleeding during contraception with the 300 μg norethisterone (NET) minipill. *Contraception*, **25**:13–30.

Johannisson, E. & Redard, M. (1984). Culture of human endothelial cells derived from capillaries of the decidual tissue. *Acta Obstetricia et Gynaecologica Scandinavica*, **63**:27–36.

Kartenbeck, J., Franke, W.W., Moser, J.G. & Stoffels, U. (1983). Specific attachment of desmin filaments to desmosomal plaques in cardiac myocytes. *European Molecular Biology Organization Journal*, **2**:735–742.

Kocher, O. & Gabbiani, G. (1987). Analysis of alpha-smooth muscle actin mRNA expression in rat aortic smooth-muscle cells using a specific cDNA probe. *Differentiation*, **34**:201–209.

Lin, J.J. & Feramisco, J.R. (1981). Disruption of the *in vivo* distribution of the intermediate filaments in fibroblasts through the microinjection of a specific monoclonal antibody. *Cell*, **24**:185–193.

Miettinen, M. (1988). Immunoreactivity for cytokeratin and epithelial membrane antigen in leiomyosarcoma. *Archives of Pathology and Laboratory Medicine*, **112**:637–640.

Moll, R., Franke, W.W., Schiller, D.L., Geiger, B. & Krepler, R. (1982). The catalog of human cytokeratins: patterns of expression in normal epithelia, tumors and cultured cells. *Cell*, **31**:11–24.

Moll, R., Levy, R., Czernobilsky, B., Hohlweg-Majert, P., Dallenbach-Hellweg, G. & Franke, W.W. (1983). Cytokeratins of normal epithelia and some neoplasms of the female genital tract. *Laboratory Investigation*, **49**:599–610.

Osborn, M. (1984). Summary: intermediate filaments 1984. *Annals of the New York Academy of Sciences*, **455**:669–681.

Ramaekers, F.C.S., Pruszczynski, M. & Smedts, F. (1987). Cytokeratins in smooth muscle cells and smooth muscle tumours. *Histopathology*, **12**:558–561.

Stoler, A., Kopan, R., Duvic, M. & Fuchs, E. (1988). Use of monospecific antisera and cRNA probes to localize the major changes in keratin expression during normal and abnormal epidermal differentiation. *Journal of Cell Biology*, **107**:427–446.

Szego, C.M., Sjostrand, B.M., Seeler, B.J., Baumer, J.W. & Sjostrand, F.S. (1988). Microtubule and plasmalemmal reorganization: acute response to estrogen. *American Journal of Physiology*, **254**:E775–E785.

Turner, R.R., Beckstead, J.H., Warnke, R.A. & Wood, G.S. (1987). Endothelial cell phenotypic diversity. *In situ* demonstration of immunologic and enzymatic heterogeneity that correlates with specific morphologic subtypes. *American Journal of Clinical Pathology*, **87**:569–575.

Vale, R.D., Schnapp, B.J., Reese, T.S. & Sheetz, M.P. (1985). Movement of organelles along filaments dissociated from the axoplasm of the squid giant axon. *Cell*, **40**:449–454.

Vandekerckhove, J. & Weber, K. (1978). At least 6 different actins are expressed in a higher mammal: an analysis based on the amino acid sequence of the amino-terminal tryptic peptide. *Journal of Molecular Biology*, **126**:783–802.

Vandekerckhove, J. & Weber, K. (1979). The complete amino acid sequence of actins from bovine aorta, bovine heart, bovine fast skeletal muscle and rabbit slow skeletal muscle. A protein–chemical analysis of muscle actin differentiation. *Differentiation*, **14**:123–133.

Wong, M.K. & Gotlieb, A.I. (1986). Endothelial cell monolayer integrity. I. Characterization of dense peripheral band of microfilaments. *Arteriosclerosis*, **6**:212–219.

Wong, M.K. & Gotlieb, A.I. (1988). The reorganization of microfilaments, centrosomes and microtubules during *in vitro* small wound re-endothelialization. *Journal of Cell Biology*, **107**:1777–1783.

Discussion

Ludwig. Do you have any information about the structural relationship of the cytoskeleton to desmosomes or to intercellular bridges?

Weintraub. There is a network of intermediate filaments within cells that are connected directly to desmosomes.

Ludwig. The reason I ask this question is that when we look at the premenstrual endometrium by scanning-electron microscopy, the overall impression is that there is a loosening of intercellular connections. I think that we should emphasize these examinations of the cytoskeleton to have an understanding of the cause and etiology of this remarkable loosening of tissue connections.

Weintraub. I agree. I think that what I tried to show here were readily observable phenomena, but I would agree that the skeleton is always there whether we see it or not.

Johannisson. I would like to mention an electron-microscopic study which we carried out some years ago in a group of women treated with norethisterone and who were bleeding following that treatment (Johannisson *et al.*, 1982). We saw a significant increase in apparently contracted endothelial cells in the treated group and it would be interesting to know if there are some biochemically contractile elements in the endothelial cells. When we look with transmission electron-microscopy at endothelial cells, we usually find many filaments in the cytoplasm. I have no information as to whether these are intermediate filaments or whether they are microfilaments. Do you have anything to say to that? Could any of these filaments be responsible for the contractility of these endothelial cells?

Weintraub. As far as microfilaments or the filament fibres in endometrial endothelial cells are concerned, we have little information. We heard Dr Bell mention the presence of desmin in endothelial cells. I think that is a provocative finding, which may speak to this problem of contraction.

Cornillie. It has been shown by Dr Lauweryns' group (Lauweryns *et al.*, 1975) in Leuven that after incubation of lymphatic capillary endothelial cells with heavy meromyosin, you can see by ultrastructural study the formation of spaced arrowheads, which means that the heavy meromyosin molecules are binding to the filaments. This is very strong evidence that these 6-nm filaments in endothelial cells are actin.

Bell. There is a family of proteins involved in anchoring the cytoskeletal framework to the membrane which includes proteins such as vinkalin. There is great interest in these proteins in the cancer field, because in cancer cells an alteration in the function of these proteins is observed with an associated disruption of the cytoskeletal matrix of the cell. I was wondering whether it would be of use to examine levels of these proteins in these cell types because alteration in those amounts may cause the phenomenon of disruption of cytoskeletal protein attachment to the cell membrane.

Luukkainen. Have you any knowledge of calcium transport or calcium activation by these microstructures, because that would be a good way to activate enzymes?

Weintraub. I do not.

References

Johannisson, E., Landgren, B.M. & Diczfalusy, E. (1982). Endometrial morphology and peripheral steroid levels in women with and without intermenstrual bleeding during contraception with the 300 μg norethisterone (NET) minipill. *Contraception*, **25**(1):13–30.

Lauweryns, J., Baert, J. & De Loecker, W. (1975). Intracytoplasmic filaments in pulmonary lymphatic endothelial cells. Fine structure and reaction after heavy meromyosin incubation. *Cell and Tissue Research*, **163**:111–124.

Paracrine interactions amongst cells of the endometrium

J.K. FINDLAY, R.A. CHERNY AND L.A. SALAMONSEN

Medical Research Centre, Prince Henry's Hospital Campus, Monash Medical Centre, Melbourne, Australia.

Abstract

The endometrium undergoes intense periods of proliferation, differentiation and then secretory activity, subsequently to degenerate and slough off in the absence of a viable blastocyst.

A major advance in our understanding of the function of the endometrium has been the realization that local or paracrine regulation operates between the constituent cells. Paracrine regulators are those which are secreted by one cell type and act on neighbouring cells, whereas autocrine regulators are those which act on the same cells which produce them. On the basis of evidence showing local production and action of a putative regulator in the endometrium, it can be concluded that the prostaglandins and possibly prolactin are acting as paracrine and/or autocrine regulators. Recent evidence suggests that the endometrial cells can produce other regulatory factors, such as fibroblast growth factor (FGF) which has angiogenic properties. The importance of paracrine regulation is that it allows different cell types within the same organ to have separate but co-ordinated growth and differentiation, while at the same time being dependent on the same peripheral endocrine stimulation. We hypothesize that this co-ordinated function under the control of local regulators is disturbed in an endometrium under the influence of contraceptive steroids, and that this leads to disturbances of menstrual rhythm. We consider angiogenesis and the degeneration of the vasculature in the endometrium to be under paracrine regulation. It is known that use of steroid contraceptives results in underdevelopment of the arterioles, degenerative changes in the venules and lesions in the vascular endothelium. We propose that cell–cell interactions related to angiogenesis and angiogenic activities should be examined in normal endometrium and endometrium from subjects taking steroidal contraceptives in order to gain further insight into the reasons for the abnormal bleeding patterns associated with long-term use of steroidal contraceptives.

Introduction

Disturbance of the normal menstrual rhythm is the major reason for women failing to continue using modern steroidal contraceptives (Gray, 1980). The disturbances range from amenorrhea to prolonged breakthrough bleeding, and are most prominent with long-acting progestogen-only contraceptives. Unfortunately our knowledge about those aspects of endometrial function which may be relevant to understanding abnormal bleeding is very inadequate. In their summary of the current status of knowledge on this subject in

1980, Fraser and Diczfalusy highlighted the need for a greater understanding of the growth and morphology of endometrial vessels and the hemostatic mechanisms in operation, particularly during endometrial breakdown. To a large extent those gaps still remain.

A major advance in our understanding of the function of the human endometrium has been the realization that local or paracrine regulation operates within that tissue, possibly involving hormones such as prostaglandins and prolactin known to be synthesized locally. We believe that this concept offers a viable approach to understanding the control of menstrual rhythm and the bleeding problems associated with steroid contraceptives.

Paracrine regulation

Cells within a tissue can communicate with each other through various types of mediators or local regulators, a concept which received particular attention from those studying malignant transformation of cells (Sporn & Todaro, 1980). Paracrine regulators are those which are secreted by one or more groups of cells and move through the interstitial spaces to act on neighbouring target cells. Autocrine regulators are those which act on the same cells which produce them. The local regulators can mediate or modulate the response of a tissue to endocrine stimulation, leading to localized differentiation and function of cells within that tissue. Local regulators can also co-ordinate other functions of cells such as growth, which may or may not be endocrine dependent.

Based on these definitions, there are three criteria which should be satisfied in order to define a substance as a paracrine or autocrine regulator. They are:

(a) evidence of local production of the regulator in a tissue, e.g. detection in the tissue, synthesis of mRNA coding for the molecule, synthesis of the molecule *in vitro* and, if possible, *in vivo*;

(b) evidence that endogenous production is hormonally and/or locally regulated, e.g. in a latent form or bound to a specific binding protein;

(c) evidence of a biological effect on cells within the same tissue at physiologically meaningful concentrations, e.g. receptors for the molecule, and time- and dose-dependent effects on cell function(s).

The importance of paracrine regulation with respect to endocrine control of a tissue is that it adds the precision and local specificity to an otherwise indiscriminate stimulation of the tissue by a peripheral hormone. It allows different cell types within the same organ to have separate but co-ordinated growth and differentiation under continued stimulation by the same peripheral hormone(s).

Our hypothesis is that the co-ordinated growth, differentiation and function of the endometrial vasculature under the control of local regulators are disturbed in an endometrium influenced by exogenous contraceptive steroids, and that this leads to disturbances of the menstrual rhythm.

Isolated cell systems to study paracrine interactions

The original descriptions of paracrine and autocrine regulators in neoplastic tissue used well-established cell lines in culture. The identification of the site(s) of production and action of paracrine regulators in normal tissues requires that the individual cell types are isolated and enriched, having minimal, and preferably no, contamination by other cell types when under study (Findlay *et al.*, 1990). The advantages of using isolated cell systems include the opportunity to study the functions and responses to stimuli of one cell type over prolonged periods, and to examine the interactions between different cells of the endometrium. The limitations of these methods include the need to isolate and identify the cell types, the effects of isolating and maintaining cells in culture which may result in cellular functions different from those *in vivo* (e.g. if the cells lack polarity in culture) and the inadvertent selection of a subpopulation of cells (e.g. luminal in preference to glandular epithelial cells or vice versa).

The published methods for isolating cell types from endometrial tissue of human, rodents and ruminants (see Findlay *et al.*, 1990) have concentrated on stromal and epithelial cells and decidual cells. Monolayer cultures of aortic endothelial cells are generally used to measure the chemotactic and mitogenic activities of putative angiogenic substances. A line of capillary endothelial cells has recently been established which responds to mitogens and forms tubes and branches *in vitro* (Folkman, 1985). Whether or not it is necessary to use endometrial endothelial cells in preference to aortic endothelial cells or endothelial cell lines to study interactions of vascular cells with other endometrial cells is not known. Cultures of endothelial cells derived from human decidual tissues have been established (Johannisson & Redard, 1984). The cells are readily identifiable by their synthesis of Factor VIII antigen (Johannisson, 1986), but they do not appear to survive in culture for long periods using this technique. The steroid dependence of development of the endometrial vasculature could be accounted for by a direct action of steroids on endothelial cells (Colburn & Buonassisi, 1978; Johannisson, 1986). These observations are in direct contrast to the lack of any immunocytochemical localization of steroid receptors in endothelial cells (McClellan *et al.*, 1986). Alternatively, steroids could act via stromal, decidual or epithelial cells, which in turn could have a paracrine influence on the endothelial cells.

An important development in culture technique has been the move to serum-free culture systems which employ defined growth factors and extracellular matrix (ECM). Cells preferring polarity in culture such as epithelial cells can now be grown on permeable membrane supports which can be adapted to dual environment chambers to study interactions with a second cell type, e.g. stromal or endothelial cells (Findlay *et al.*, 1990). Despite this limitation of knowledge about endometrial endothelial cells, there have been reports of production of paracrine factors by other endometrial cells, some of which are known to have angiogenic activity or can influence vascular function.

Cell–cell communication in the endometrium

Stromal and epithelial interactions

Morphogenetic processes are pronounced during the ovarian cycle and pregnancy in the adult female genital tract. For example, epithelial and stromal cell components may be dismantled, eliminated and later regenerated, and there is evidence to suggest that the reconstruction process is achieved via the inductive activities of non-degenerate stroma and rudimentary precursor cells (Baggish *et al.*, 1967), although this view is not shared by all (Nogales-Ortiz & Nogales, 1980). Stroma may serve in the adult to direct and maintain epithelial phenotypic expression just as it controls differentiation of epithelial cells during development (Cunha *et al.*, 1983).

In-vitro studies demonstrated that it was possible to maintain functionally differentiated epithelial cells in the absence of living stromal cells by providing a biological substrate or ECM (see Findlay *et al.*, 1990). It is now clear that part of the influence of stromal cells on epithelial cells may be mediated by components of the ECM produced by the stroma. The components of ECM from rodent stromal cells, particularly those which are decidualized, include laminin, entactin, type IV collagen, heparan sulfate proteoglycan and fibronectin (see Findlay *et al.*, 1990).

ECM has recently been demonstrated to have the capacity to bind growth factors such as fibroblast growth factor (FGF). Transforming growth factor β, a mesenchymal cell product, stimulates ECM production and stabilizes the ECM by preventing activation of collagenase (Sporn *et al.*, 1987). Growth factors, including those with angiogenic activity, could be stored in ECM and presented to adjacent vascular cells upon appropriate (hormonal?) stimulus (Roberts *et al.*, 1988).

Angiogenesis

Angiogenesis is the process of generating new capillaries and leads, therefore, to vascularization of tissues. The ovarian follicle, corpus luteum and endometrium are characterized by cyclical changes in angiogenesis which are under hormonal control (Findlay, 1986). In the endometrium, radial arteries cross the myoendometrial junction and give rise to the steroid-sensitive spiral arteries which supply the stratum functionale and the steroid-insensitive basal arteries which supply the stratum basale. Early in the proliferative phase, when estradiol levels are low, the spiral arteries extend little further than the stratum basale and are connected to the subepithelial capillary plexus by long straight precapillaries. Estradiol induces thickening and coiling of these precapillaries, with the convolution being most intense around midcycle.

Growth continues in the secretory phase under the influence of estradiol and progesterone, and is correlated with increased DNA synthesis in vascular cells. Cuffs of dense connective tissue (decidual cells) form around the arterial stems and branches in the midsecretory phase.

Angiogenesis at the cellular level is a complex process which has been shown in neoplastic tissues to involve tissue disruption and reorganization, cellular growth and changes in the composition of the fluid environment and ECM (Folkman, 1985). Assuming that the process is similar in neoplastic and non-neoplastic tissues, the events in angiogenesis are summarized as follows.

1. Local degradation of the basement membrane adjacent to the angiogenic stimulus, possibly due to increased collagenase and plasminogen activator activity.
2. Migration of endothelial cells through openings in the basement membrane.
3. Lumen formation.
4. Division of endothelial cells behind the tip of the growing capillary.
5. Canalization as sprouts join or anastomose.
6. Flow of blood in highly permeable vessels until the basement membrane forms and pericytes attach.

New capillaries originate from pre-existing microvasculature rather than large vessels with layers of smooth muscle. It is likely that a family of angiogenic agents, rather than one common substance, is responsible for the angiogenic steps of exocytosis, chemotaxis, cell division and production of ECM (Findlay, 1986).

The nature of the angiogenic stimuli in the endometrium is not known. FGF-like activity is synthesized by bovine epithelial endometrial cells (Fujii & Lee, 1987), and extracts of pig endometrium contain a polypeptide growth factor with properties similar to acidic FGF (Brigstock *et al.*, 1986). If the epithelial origin of these factors is confirmed in the human endometrium, a role for them in control of the endometrial vasculature presupposes an endothelial–epithelial cell interaction as part of the angiogenic stimulus.

Since angiogenesis in the endometrium is partly steroid dependent, it would be of interest to examine the effect of estradiol and progesterone on expression of FGF and other angiogenic activity by different endometrial cell types. Maqueo (1980) concluded that steroidal contraceptives caused underdevelopment of the arterioles, degenerative changes in the venules and even lesions in the vascular endothelium. One possibility is that the progestogens are interfering with the stimulatory action of estradiol by suppressing synthesis of steroid receptors. An examination of the distribution and concentration of estrogen and progesterone receptors in the various cell types of the endometrium under normal and exogenous steroid influences is warranted. It is of interest in this regard that McClellan *et al.* (1986) found no evidence for the presence of estrogen receptors in endometrial endothelial cells of macaques during the luteal–follicular transition. Immediately prior to progesterone withdrawal, there was evidence of estrogen receptors in stromal fibroblasts and smooth muscle cells associated with the walls of spiral arteries. Again, this suggests cell–cell communication, involving stromal–endothelial cell interactions, for the influence of estradiol on endothelial cell function in the primate endometrium.

Vascular control

Two examples of vascular control will be discussed which involve paracrine regulation in the endometrium. Prostaglandins (PGs) are well-recognized agents controlling vasoconstriction and vasodilatation, and the endometrium is a major site of production and release of PG. Bell & Smith (1988) reviewed the data supporting an interaction between different cell types and even between myometrium and endometrium to explain the mechanisms controlling PG production. It would appear that epithelial cells are the major source of endometrial PGE and $PGF_{2\alpha}$ and their metabolites, and that steroids can influence the synthesis and metabolism of PG by these cells. Progesterone withdrawal at the end of the cycle is hypothesized to allow expression by epithelial cells of PG synthesis, particularly $PGF_{2\alpha}$, which in turn has a paracrine influence on menstruation, initially by vasoconstriction of spiral arterioles. The role of stromal cells and the site(s) of action of ovarian steroids modulating PG production by epithelial cells remain subjects for further study.

The recent demonstration that interferon-related peptides (ovine trophoblast protein-1 and recombinant human interferon-α_2) attenuate the production of PGE and $PGF_{2\alpha}$ and influence protein secretion by sheep endometrial cells (Salamonsen *et al.*, 1988), raises the possible role of interferon in PG production by human endometrial cells, and more generally on endometrial function, particularly around menstruation. The origin of the interferon-like peptides could be the immune cells which infiltrate the endometrium or cells of the endometrium such as the decidua.

The vascular endothelium is now recognized as an important functional unit involved in the regulation of a vascular smooth muscle tonus. A short-lived, endothelial cell-derived relaxing factor (EDRF) made in response to vasoactive agents such as acetylcholine was recently identified as nitric oxide or a closely related substance (Palmer *et al.*, 1987). A potent vasoconstrictor peptide, endothelin, has now been isolated and purified from media conditioned by porcine aortic endothelial cells, and its cDNA cloned and sequenced (Yanagisawa *et al.*, 1988). Endothelin is a 21 amino-acid peptide, derived by two proteolytic cleavage steps via a 39 amino-acid 'big endothelin' from proendothelin. Endothelin mRNA is expressed in endothelial cells *in situ*. It does not belong to any previously known peptide family, but its sequence shows local homologies with a group of neurotoxins that act on voltage-dependent Na^+ channels. Whereas EDRF would appear to be involved in rapid local control of vascular tonus, endothelin is a very potent ($EC_{50} = 0.4$ nmol/l), long-lasting vasoconstrictor. An investigation of these paracrine activities in endometrium and the influence of steroids on their expression and action is warranted.

Conclusion

In portraying the endometrium as a paracrine organ, we aimed to focus attention on cell–cell interactions and the associated para- and autocrine agents which might be involved in the control of growth and function of blood vessels. Methods to isolate and culture stromal, epithelial (see Findlay *et al.*, 1990) and endothelial cells (Johannisson & Redard, 1984) are available, although all require improvement to increase cell yield and purity and longevity of differentiated cell function in culture. Bicameral systems to study interactions between cells and allow development of cell polarity *in vitro* should also be considered.

We recommend that these in-vitro techniques could be used to:

1. identify angiogenic activities in the endometrium and monitor isolation and identification of the active components;
2. examine the site(s) of action of estradiol and progesterone either directly on vascular endothelial cells or via stromal or epithelial cells;
3. establish whether or not endothelial-derived vasodilator and vaso-constrictor activities are an important component of the control of vascular tone in the endometrium, particularly in the presence of steroidal contraceptives;
4. compare the functions of respective cell types derived from normal endometrium and endometrium under the influence of exogenous steroids.

Acknowledgements

We thank the National Health and Medical Research Council of Australia and the Buckland Foundation for financial support, and Faye Coates for secretarial assistance.

References

Baggish, M.S., Pauerstein, C.J. & Woodruff, J.D. (1967). Role of stroma in regeneration of endometrial epithelium. *American Journal of Obstetrics and Gynecology*, **99**:459–465.

Bell, S.C. & Smith, S.K. (1988). The endometrium as a paracrine organ. (In) *Contemporary Topics in Obstetrics and Gynaecology* (Chamberlain, G.V.P., ed.), pp.273–298. Cambridge, England, Butterworth Scientific.

Brigstock, D.R., Laurie, M.S., Heap, R.B. & Brown, K.D. (1986). Characterization of an acidic, heparin-binding growth factor from pig uterus. *Biology of Reproduction*, **34**(Suppl. 1):167 Abstract.

Colburn, P. & Buonassisi, V. (1978). Estrogen-binding sites in endothelial cell cultures. *Science, New York*, **201**:817–819.

Cunha, G.R., Chung, L.W., Shannon, J.M., Taguchi, O. & Fujii, H. (1983). Hormone-induced morphogenesis and growth: role of mesenchymal–epithelial interactions. *Recent Progress in Hormone Research*, **39**:559–598.

Findlay, J.K. (1986). Angiogenesis in reproductive tissues. *Journal of Endocrinology*, **111**:357–366.

Findlay, J.K., Salamonsen, L.A. & Cherny, R.A. (1990). The use of isolated cells to study endometrial function *in vitro*. (In) *Oxford Reviews of Reproductive Biology*, Vol. 12 (Milligan, S.R., ed.), in press. Oxford, Clarendon Press.

Folkman, J. (1985). Tumour angiogenesis. *Advances in Cancer Research*, **43**:175–203.

Fraser, I.S. & Diczfalusy, E. (1980). A perspective of steroidal contraception and abnormal bleeding: what are the prospects for improvement? (In) *Endometrial Bleeding and Steroidal Contraception* (Diczfalusy, E., Fraser, I.S. & Webb, F.T.G., eds.), pp.384–413. Bath, England, Pitman Press.

Fujii, D.K. & Lee, E. (1987). Growth and hormonal responsiveness of cultured bovine uterine epithelium. *Proceedings of the Endocrine Society, USA*, **69**:127, Abstract No. 425.

Gray, R. (1980). Patterns of bleeding associated with the use of steroidal contraceptives. (In) *Endometrial Bleeding and Steroidal Contraception* (Diczfalusy, E., Fraser, I.S. & Webb, F.T.G., eds.), pp.14–49. Bath, England, Pitman Press.

Johannisson, E. (1986). Effects of oestradiol and progesterone on the synthesis of DNA and the antihaemophilic Factor VIII antigen in human endometrial endothelial cells *in vitro*: a pilot study. *Human Reproduction*, **1**:207–212.

Johannisson, E. & Redard, M. (1984). Culture of human endothelial cells derived from capillaries of the decidual tissue. *Acta Obstetricia et Gynecologica Scandinavica*, **63**:27–36.

Maqueo, M. (1980). Vascular and perivascular changes in the endometrium of women using steroidal contraceptives. (In) *Endometrial Bleeding and Steroidal Contraception* (Diczfalusy, E., Fraser, I.S. & Webb, F.T.G., eds.), pp.138–152. Bath, England, Pitman Press.

McClellan, M., West, N.B. & Brenner, R.M. (1986). Immunocytochemical localization of estrogen receptors in the macaque endometrium during the luteal–follicular transition. *Endocrinology*, **119**:2467–2475.

Nogales-Ortiz, F. & Nogales, F.F. (1980) Endometrial regeneration under physiological and pathological conditions. (In) *Endometrial Bleeding and Steroidal Contraception* (Diczfalusy, E., Fraser, I.S. & Webb, F.T.G., eds.), pp.97–106. Bath, England, Pitman Press.

Palmer, R.M.J., Ferrige, A.G. & Moncada, S. (1987). Nitric oxide release accounts for the biological activity of endothelium-derived relaxing factor. *Nature*, **327**:524–526.

Roberts, R., Gallagher, J., Spooner, E., Allen, T.D., Bloomfield, F. & Dexter, T.M. (1988). Heparan sulphate bound growth factors: a mechanism for stromal cell mediated haemopoiesis. *Nature*, **332**:376–378.

Salamonsen, L.A., Stuchbery, S.J., O'Grady, C.M., Godkin, J.D. & Findlay, J.K. (1988). Interferon-α mimics effects of ovine trophoblast protein 1 on prostaglandin and protein secretion by ovine endometrial cells *in vitro*. *Journal of Endocrinology*, **117**:R1–R4.

Sporn, M.B., Roberts, A.B., Wakefield, L.M. & de Crombrugghe, B. (1987). Some recent advances in the chemistry and biology of transforming growth factor-beta. *Journal of Cell Biology*, **105**:1039–1045.

Sporn, M.B. & Todaro, G.J. (1980). Autocrine secretion and malignant transformation of cells. *New England Journal of Medicine*, **303**:878–880.

Yanagisawa, M., Kurihara, H., Kimura, S., Tomobe, Y., Kobayashi, M., Mitsui, Y., Yazaki, Y., Goto, K. & Masaki, T. (1988). A novel potent vasoconstrictor peptide produced by vascular endothelial cells. *Nature*, **332**:411–415.

Discussion

Rice-Evans. Is there a relationship between the origins of endothelin and endothelial cell-derived relaxing factor (EDRF)? I noticed several arginine residues in the structure of the precursor molecule. Although the origins of the nitric oxide are not entirely clear, it does seem to be derived from an arginine residue, and the number of arginines in your precursor molecule was very notable.

Casey. I do not know, but I think that the potency of endothelin is such that there must be some very effective regulatory mechanism that involves a breakdown of the precursor or the factor itself. I might just add some comments on the requirements of calcium. In our very recent studies using myometrial smooth muscle cells, we are finding that endothelin will act in calcium-free medium, in the presence of EDTA, or in the presence of inhibitors of voltage-dependent calcium channels. The action of endothelin is attenuated but not abolished in the presence of those agents (which inhibit the influx of extracellular calcium).

Naftolin. Is it independent of potassium?

Casey. We have no data on that subject. In all our studies potassium is present.

Diczfalusy. Dr Brosens mentioned that endometriosis might provide an interesting model. I have some vague recollection that endometriosis cells are producing large quantities of interferon which was said to inhibit sperm motility. Do you have any information on interferon production by endometrial cells?

Findlay. No, it is an area which needs to be looked at.

Smith. Dr Findlay, in your interferon system, have you added exogenous arachidonic acid?

Findlay. We are doing those experiments now. I have no data.

King. What is the evidence that steroids influence angiogenesis?

Findlay. Very good question. If you have an ovariectomized animal, you do not get growth of blood vessels, unless you treat it with estrogen.

Naftolin. I do not think that anybody believes that steroids do not influence angiogenesis. The question, however, is whether they 'pull' angiogenesis into tissues or whether they 'push' angiogenesis into tissues.

Luukkainen. We should recall that metabolites of the steroids may have biological effects. As with angiogenesis in cancer, specific metabolites of steroids may, in the endometrium, be biologically active even when not working through the receptors.

Fraser. Dr Johannisson has a model for isolating endothelial cells from human endometrial decidua from very early pregnancy (Johannisson & Redard, 1984) and, using that model, she has shown that those endothelial cells grow in response to exposure to estradiol, to progesterone and to estradiol and progesterone together. So there is direct evidence for a response of these cells to steroids, and we have confirmed this work in Sydney with Dr Peek's experiments.

Johannisson. We used explants from decidua, particularly those which, under stereomicroscopy, contained a lot of vessels, mainly capillaries. We put them into culture medium for 4 days, after which we introduced estradiol, progesterone or nothing (controls). To find out whether we really had endothelial cells, we stained for Factor VIII, an antihemophilic factor considered specific for endothelial cells. We found that the fluorescence intensity in cells exposed to estradiol was significantly higher when compared with the controls and with those cells exposed to progesterone (Johannisson, 1986). This study was carried out at a time when methods for a cell culture system were less sophisticated than today. Nevertheless, the results raise the question as to whether we have a direct effect of ovarian steroids on the endothelial cells, which would implicate some kind of receptor mechanism in the endothelial cells. Steroid receptors have not been demonstrated as yet in the endometrial endothelial cells. We may also consider a paracrine effect, because, in addition to endothelial cells, in culture there were fibroblasts. They were not overgrowing the endothelial cells, but we cannot exclude a paracrine effect from the stromal fibroblasts. Whatever the stimulatory effect is, the results of the study suggest that an in-vitro model exists which could be further improved.

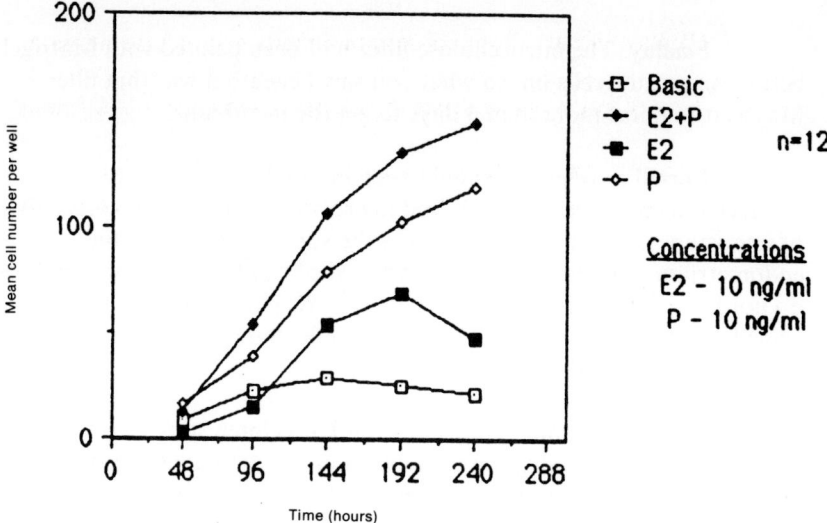

Fig. 1 Endothelial cell growth following culture of decidual explants in the presence or absence of estradiol (E2) and progesterone (P). Decidual explants were collected between the 6th and 8th week of pregnancy.

Baird. Presumably, you also have decidual cells there?

Johannisson. In the technique, we used explants from decidua, but as soon as we saw the buds growing out from the explants, we removed the decidual tissue. The buds growing most rapidly were the endothelial cells and those growing more slowly were the decidual cells. But we did not identify decidual cells.

Fraser. In Sydney, we have done the same (Peek & Fraser, unpublished observations) and removed the decidual cells. But I agree with Dr Johannisson that there are small numbers of other cells, such as fibroblasts, which could influence the outcome. Dr Johannisson has not shown the results of the relative rates of growth of the endothelial cells under exposure to different hormones. If you do not expose them to estrogen, you get relatively little growth beyond that first capillary, the first bud of cells that appears from the edge of your explant. If you expose them to estradiol and/or progesterone, you get a considerable stimulation of growth. At levels of estradiol apparently a little above the physiological range, there does appear to be some growth (Fig. 1).

Cornillie. Dr Findlay, I was a little surprised that in your system you did not see any deposition of basement membrane below the epithelial cells grown on plastic. Can you explain this?

Findlay. The nitrocellulose filter had been painted with Matrigel before we put the cells on, so what you saw beneath it was that filter. Maybe it requires more than 3 days to get the membrane.

Cornillie. While we should keep in mind that factors being produced in endometrial vessels and microcirculatory components may be of importance, the microcirculation in the superficial layer of the endometrium is at least 80–85% composed of capillaries. These capillaries do not have a muscle coat. So, if there is some paracrine activity on endothelia by endothelial cells or muscle cells, this, probably, is not of very much importance in the superficial layer.

Findlay. I would agree, but I think it is interesting to ask whether a lack of endothelin production is involved in that vasoconstriction that occurs early on in the process of menstruation and in the case of abnormal bleeding.

Gurpide. I wonder if you already have some results on polarity and secretion of prostaglandins?

Findlay. We have very preliminary data. We have completed three experiments and the major site of production of prostaglandin is the epithelial cell and not the stromal cell. The major direction of release of prostaglandin is basal.

Clark. I am having a slight anatomical problem with respect to the action of these factors that regulate vascular tone, including the release of prostaglandins by epithelial cells. Presumably, these factors have to reach the muscle in the walls of the arteriole to produce spasm. And yet, one would expect these factors would need to swim upstream in some way to reach those cells. Can you explain how factors released by capillary endothelial cells and how prostaglandins released by the glandular epithelium reach the muscle in the walls of the arterioles?

Findlay. No I cannot. It is a good point, however. I think the advantage of the systems I have been describing is that if we can get cells established, we can look at directionality and it gives us an opportunity to answer those questions. There will be limitations in the technique, but it is a way of getting further information on the problem.

Naftolin. I do not think that we should feel limited by our preconceived notions of what anatomical polarity means to cells. We must test for secretions.

Weintraub. There was a recent report by Sato and Rifkin (1988) which talked about autocrine regulation of endothelial cells and endothelial cell movement over denuded surfaces in response to fibroblast growth factor.

Bischof. I think we have to be very careful when we are studying the direction of secretion in cultures. Because what is the bottom and what is the top is relatively clear for us when we are outside the petri dish, but for cells it is not the same thing. They have to be in a three-dimensional matrix in order to see where and if there is a difference in the secretion and where the microvilli are.

Findlay. The data which I showed are from cells which showed microvilli on the luminal surface.

Bischof. Right, but you are not in a three-dimensional matrix.

Diaz. I understood that the cells from the secretory endometrium could not be cultured and I wanted to know why?

Naftolin. I do not think it is true that you cannot culture them.

Johannisson. The endothelial cells I was referring to were from biopsies obtained late in the cycle. Perhaps it would be important to · investigate the synthesis of proteins in endothelial cells during the cycle. Factor VIII is a protein synthesized by the endothelial cells and influenced by steroid function either directly or in a paracrine way. Such proteins of endothelial cells may be an important factor related to the presence or absence of intermenstrual bleeding.

References

Johannisson, E. (1986). Effects of oestradiol and progesterone on the synthesis of DNA and the antihaemophilic Factor VIII antigen in human endometrial endothelial cells *in vitro*: a pilot study. *Human Reproduction*, **1**:207–212.

Johannisson, E. & Redard, M. (1984). Culture of human endothelial cells derived from capillaries of the decidual tissue. *Acta Obstetricia et Gynecologica Scandinavica*, **63**:27–36.

Sato, Y. & Rifkin, D.B. (1988). Autocrine activities of basic fibroblast growth factor: regulation of endothelial cell movement, plasminogen activator synthesis, and DNA synthesis. *Journal of Cell Biology*, **107**:1199–1205.

Steroid effects on endometrial prostaglandin production

ERLIO GURPIDE, FREDERICK SCHATZ AND LESZEK
MARKIEWICZ

*Departments of Obstetrics, Gynecology and Reproductive Science, Mount Sinai
Medical Center, New York, USA.*

Abstract

The effects of estradiol (E_2) and progesterone (P) on prostaglandins $F_{2\alpha}$ and E_2 ($PGF_{2\alpha}$ and PGE_2) production by human endometrium were studied *in vitro*, using tissue fragments and separated epithelial and stromal cells.

Basal output of $PGF_{2\alpha}$ by proliferative endometrium was found to be higher than that of secretory tissue, both under organotypic and superfusion conditions. Estradiol (0.1–10 nmol/l) significantly increased prostaglandin production in secretory endometrium but not in proliferative tissue. Progesterone (0.1–1 μmol/l) lowered prostaglandin production and counteracted the E_2 effect. Dexamethasone (10 nmol/l–1 μmol/l) also reduced $PGF_{2\alpha}$ output, in association with an increase in lipocortin output.

Epithelial cells isolated from either proliferative or secretory endometria produced $PGF_{2\alpha}$. Basal rates were increased by E_2 and this effect was counteracted by hydroxytamoxifen and by P. Estradiol enhanced the utilization of arachidonic acid by epithelial cells and acted synergistically with the Ca^{2+} ionophore A23187 in stimulating $PGF_{2\alpha}$ output, apparently by increasing PG synthase activity. In contrast, $PGF_{2\alpha}$ production by stromal cells was not influenced by E_2, A23187 or increasing Ca^{2+} concentrations. These results indicate that the stimulatory effects of E_2 and the inhibitory effects of P on prostaglandin production by the endometrium take place mainly in the glandular epithelium.

The onset of normal menstruation follows a fall in levels of ovarian hormones and appears to be associated with an increase in endometrial prostaglandin (PG) production. The in-vitro studies described in this chapter and other investigations reviewed by Hagenfeldt (1987) examined the role of estradiol and progesterone on endometrial fragments and isolated epithelial and stromal cells.

Prostaglandin production by the endometrium

Most of the early measurements of concentrations of $PGF_{2\alpha}$ and PGE_2 in human endometrial tissue collected at different phases of the menstrual cycle (Downie *et al.*, 1974; Green & Hagenfeldt, 1975; Singh *et al.*, 1975; Maathuis & Kelly, 1978), in uterine washes (Demers *et al.*, 1975) and in uterine venous blood (Jordan & Pokoly, 1977) have indicated a progressive increase in prostaglandin levels during the luteal phase and highest values during the menstrual process.

Abel and Baird (1980) published an important article in which they showed continuous production of $PGF_{2\alpha}$ and PGE_2 by endometrial fragments kept in culture, changes in the output rates of these prostaglandins when ovarian hormones were added to the medium and, in agreement with the in-vivo data, higher basal output of prostaglandins by secretory endometria than by proliferative tissue. Other laboratories obtained similar results (Peek *et al.*, 1985).

On the basis of such observations, hypotheses on mechanisms by which progesterone might increase PG production by the endometrium during the luteal phase have been proposed. However, interpretation of the experimental data remains controversial as further information is gathered. For instance, in a series of in-vitro studies on prostaglandin production by human endometrium, we have consistently found greater prostaglandin production by proliferative than by secretory tissue under basal conditions (Schatz *et al.*, 1984; Markiewicz *et al.*, 1985a; Schatz *et al.*, 1985). In a total of 34 proliferative and 98 secretory specimens studied in our laboratory, the mean values for $PGF_{2\alpha}$ output rates, obtained using radioimmunoassays conducted in two different aliquots of medium from each of duplicate dishes, at two dilutions within the appropriate range of the standard curve, were 130 ng and 310 ng $PGF_{2\alpha}$/mg protein per day, respectively. These values are significantly different at the $p \langle 0.001$ level, as evaluated by Student's t test. Similar results were obtained using superfusion techniques (Liggins *et al.*, 1980; Markiewicz *et al.*, 1985b). Other groups have also found higher levels of in-vitro PG production by proliferative endometrium (Tsang & Ooi, 1982; Leaver & Richmond, 1984). In another extensive study, endometrial levels of $PGF_{2\alpha}$ were not significantly different in proliferative and secretory tissues (Levitt *et al.*, 1975).

The lack of agreement between different laboratories, likely to be due to differences in tissue collection and processing or other experimental conditions, has resulted in uncertainty about the phase of the cycle dependence of prostaglandin output by endometria in culture. The data considered to provide information on in-vivo changes in prostaglandin production during the menstrual cycle also require critical evaluation. Since PGs are secreted products, data on tissue levels may not reflect rates of production and can be strongly influenced, in a phase- and time-dependent manner, by levels of PG binders and by metabolism and release of PGs during the period of sample collection. A premenstrual increase in production of $PGF_{2\alpha}$ has been associated with a decline of its metabolic degradation by a progesterone-stimulated 15-hydroxyprostaglandin dehydrogenase (Casey *et al.*, 1980). Furthermore, sample collection itself can introduce traumatic stimuli that alter prostaglandin production (Peek *et al.*, 1987); values from samples obtained at the onset and during menstruation may also reflect trauma rather than hormonal control. The higher levels of prostaglandins in uterine vein plasma during the luteal phase, reported by Jordan and Pokoly (1977), may correspond to the larger mass of endometrial tissue present in the luteal phase.

Estrogen effects on endometrial tissue in culture

As described by Abel and Baird, E_2 enhances significantly $PGF_{2\alpha}$ and PGE_2 output by secretory endometrium, but not by proliferative tissue, under organ culture conditions (Abel & Baird, 1980). We have confirmed this effect of E_2, showing that it could also be obtained with estriol at equimolar (10 nmol/l) concentrations (Schatz *et al.*, 1984), and demonstrating that these effects can be antagonized by 4-hydroxytamoxifen (Schatz *et al.*, 1986). Furthermore, 2-hydroxyestradiol has also been reported to be effective (Kelly & Abel, 1980).

We interpret the lack of responsiveness of proliferative endometrium as an indication of full stimulation by endogenous hormone.

Progesterone effects on endometrial tissue in culture

Abel and Baird (1980) have shown that progesterone reduces the in-vitro PG output by both proliferative and secretory endometria and antagonizes the stimulatory effect of E_2 on secretory endometrium. We have fully confirmed their conclusions.

These results are not easily reconciled with an elevation of PG production by endometrium during the luteal phase suggested by the in-vivo data, or at least with the interpretation that progesterone is responsible for it. A priming role of progesterone on estradiol actions, reported to occur in some non-primate species (Poyser, 1980), has been proposed but there is no direct evidence for such an effect in humans. Since possible effects of blood-borne factors other than estradiol and progesterone, such as oxytocin (Roberts *et al.*, 1976), are eliminated under in-vitro conditions, further physiologic studies on uterine production of prostaglandins are needed.

Effects of dexamethasone; lipocortin production by the endometrium

We found that dexamethasone, like progesterone, reduces $PGF_{2\alpha}$ output of both proliferative and secretory endometria in culture (Gurpide *et al.*, 1986). This effect was concentration dependent and correlated with an increase in lipocortin secreted into the culture medium, measured by Dr F. Hirata, Johns Hopkins University. In contrast, progesterone decreased the output of both $PGF_{2\alpha}$ and immunoreactive lipocortin into the medium. Further work is needed to clarify these observations since both lipocortin, the active phospholipase A_2 inhibitor, and its inactive phosphorylated derivative are recognized by the antibody used for the RIA. Kelly and Smith (1987) have recently reported that they could not detect effects of dexamethasone or cortisol in a similar system, even though progesterone was strongly inhibitory; the reason for such discrepancy with our results is not evident.

Prostaglandin production by isolated endometrial epithelial cells

Endometrial glands can be isolated by filtration through small-pore stainless steel sieves of a suspension obtained after treatment of tissue fragments with collagenase to disperse stromal cells (Schatz & Gurpide, 1983). When glands resuspended in culture medium are placed in plastic dishes, the epithelial cells migrate to form monolayer colonies. Basal and hormone-modulated prostaglandin output was estimated in isolated glands and epithelial monolayer preparations.

Epithelial cells isolated from either proliferative or secretory endometrium responded markedly, and to a similar extent, to estradiol or estriol added to the medium (Schatz & Gurpide, 1983; Schatz et al., 1984). The response to estrogens of epithelial cell derived from proliferative endometrium contrasts with the unresponsiveness of the tissue of origin under culture conditions. Smith and Kelly (1987) reported estrogen effects on $PGF_{2\alpha}$ output in epithelial cells derived from secretory endometrium but not from proliferative tissue, and reported that E_2 has no effect on PGE_2 production, even in cells from secretory tissue. Progesterone does not lower the basal output of $PGF_{2\alpha}$ by epithelial cells from either proliferative or secretory endometrium but partially counteracts the stimulatory effect of estrogens (Schatz et al., 1985).

Prostaglandin production by isolated stromal cells

Stromal cells, collected with the filtrate obtained during the separation of glands described above and isolated by selective attachment to plastic culture dishes during a 30-minute period (Schatz et al., 1987), also secrete prostaglandins under basal conditions. However, in contrast to epithelial cells, they do not respond to added estrogens by increasing $PGF_{2\alpha}$ output. These results, first reported at a Serono Symposium held in 1983 (Markiewicz et al., 1985b), have been confirmed (Smith & Kelly, 1987). A recent report from Neulen et al. (1988) on stimulatory E_2 effects on stromal cells might actually reflect estrogen-induced increases in cell numbers during the week-long incubation period.

Mechanisms of estrogenic stimulation of PG production

The most likely mechanisms by which estrogens enhance PG production in endometrial tissue and endometrial epithelial cells involve activation of at least one of the phospholipases A_2 present in endometrial cells (Bonney et al., 1987), resulting in an increased availability of arachidonic acid for PG synthesis, or augmentation of PG synthase activity. Experiments in which E_2

was found to increase the utilization of excess arachidonic acid added to the medium or assumed to be generated intracellularly by addition of A23187, can be taken as evidence in favour of estrogenic stimulation of PG synthase activity (Schatz *et al.*, 1987).

Whether the action of E_2 on PG output is receptor mediated remains unclear since it can be counteracted by the antiestrogen 4-hydroxytamoxifen but does not correlate with estrogen receptor levels in endometrial tissue, experimentally modified by exposure of tissue fragments to 40°C for 2 hours, or with the presence or absence of receptor in specimens of endometrial adenocarcinoma (Markiewicz *et al.*, 1986).

Human endometrium as an in-vitro system to evaluate estrogenic, antiestrogenic and progestogenic effects of test compounds

As described above, estrogens would increase PGF_{2a} production by secretory endometrium, antiestrogens would diminish the effect of estradiol, and progesterone would reduce the basal output of prostaglandins during incubations of proliferative endometrium. Using such systems, we have demonstrated estrogenic activities of adrenal C_{19}-steroids as well as antiestrogenic and progestogenic activities of several drugs (Markiewicz & Gurpide, 1988; Markiewicz *et al.*, 1988) .

Conclusions

Although substantial basic information on production and regulation of prostaglandins in the human endometrium has been accumulated, further evaluation of prostaglandin production rates by the endometrium and their regulation under physiologic conditions, as well as biochemical information on mechanisms by which ovarian hormones exert their action on prostaglandin synthesis, are still needed. Interactions between endometrial stroma and epithelium and between myometrium and endometrium, suggested by in-vitro studies (Cameron *et al.*, 1985), regulation of PGF_{2a}:PGE_2 ratios, and production of other eicosanoids, are important basic research topics of current endometrial studies. Incubation systems in which endometrial epithelial cells can be placed on an extracellular matrix (Matrigel™, Collaborative Research, Lexington, MA) in Millicell™-CM chambers (Millipore, Bedford, MA) provide improved culture conditions allowing cell polarization and formation of tight junctions (Schatz *et al.*, 1989), and offering the possibility of studying paracrine interactions between epithelial cells and stromal cells placed below them.

Fruitful studies may be conducted not only with endometrial tissue and cells from cycling women, but with the endometrium of pregnancy. In addition to its relevance to the understanding of mechanisms involved in the onset of normal menstruation and breakthrough bleeding, knowledge in this area is required to approach fundamental problems related to fertility (e.g. implantation, endometrial dysfunction) and preterm birth.

Acknowledgements

This work was supported by Grant No. HD 07917, awarded by the National Institute of Child Health and Human Development.

References

Abel, M.H. & Baird, D.T. (1980). The effect of 17-β-estradiol and progesterone on prostaglandin production by human endometrium maintained in organ culture. *Endocrinology*, **106**:1599–1606.

Bonney, R.C., Qizilbash, S.T. & Franks, S. (1987). Endometrial phospholipase A$_2$ enzymes and their regulation by steroid hormones. *Journal of Steroid Biochemistry*, **27**:1057–1064.

Cameron, I.T., Kelly, R.W. & Baird, D.T. (1985). Prostaglandins in the human uterus: an interaction between endometrium and myometrium. *Prostaglandins, Leukotrienes and Medicine*, **17**:329–335.

Casey, M.L., Hemsell, D.L., MacDonald, P.C. & Johnston, J.M. (1980). NAD$^+$-dependent 15-hydroxy-prostaglandin dehydrogenase activity in human endometrium. *Prostaglandins*, **19**:115–122.

Demers, L.M., Halbert, D.R., Jones, D.E. & Fontana, J. (1975). Prostaglandin F levels in endometrial jet wash specimens during the normal human menstrual cycle. *Prostaglandins*, **10**:1057–1065.

Downie, J., Poyser, N.L. & Wunderlich, M. (1974). Level of prostaglandins in human endometrium during the normal menstrual cycle. *Journal of Physiology*, **236**:465–472.

Green, K. & Hagenfeldt, K. (1975). Prostaglandins in the human endometrium. Gas chromatographic–mass spectrophotometric quantitation before and after IUD insertion. *American Journal of Obstetrics and Gynecology*, **122**:611–614.

Gurpide, E., Markiewicz, L., Schatz, F. & Hirata, F. (1986). Lipocortin output by human endometrium *in vitro*. *Journal of Clinical Endocrinology and Metabolism*, **63**:162–166.

Hagenfeldt, K. (1987). The role of prostaglandins and allied substances in uterine haemostasis. *Contraception*, **36**:23–35.

Jordan, V.C. & Pokoly, T.B. (1977). Steroid and prostaglandin relations during the menstrual cycle. *Obstetrics and Gynecology*, **49**:449–453.

Kelly, R.W. & Abel, M.H. (1980). Catechol oestrogens stimulate and direct prostaglandin synthesis. *Prostaglandins*, **20**:613–626.

Kelly, R.W. & Smith, S.K. (1987). Glucocorticoids do not share with progesterone the potent inhibitory action on prostaglandin synthesis in human proliferative phase endometrium. *Prostaglandins*, **33**:919–929.

Leaver, H.A. & Richmond, D.H. (1984). The effect of oxytocin, estrogen, calcium ionophore A23187 and hydrocortisone on prostaglandin F$_{2\alpha}$ and 6-oxo-prostaglandin F$_{1\alpha}$ production by cultured human endometrial and myometrial explants. *Prostaglandins, Leukotrienes and Medicine*, **13**:179–196.

Levitt, M.J., Tobon, H. & Josimovich, J.B. (1975). Prostaglandin content of human endometrium. *Fertility and Sterility*, **26**:296–300.

Liggins, G.C., Campos, G.A., Roberts, C.M. & Skinner, S.J. (1980). Production rates of prostaglandin F, 6-keto-PGF$_{1a}$ and thromboxane B$_2$ by perifused human endometrium. *Prostaglandins*, **19**:461–477.

Maathuis, J.B. & Kelly, R.W. (1978). Concentrations of prostaglandins F$_{2a}$ and E$_2$ in the endometrium throughout the human menstrual cycle, after the administration of clomiphene or an oestrogen–progestogen pill and in early pregnancy. *Journal of Endocrinology*, **77**:361–371.

Markiewicz, L., Gravanis, A., Schatz, F., Holinka, C.F., Deligdish, L. & Gurpide, E. (1986). Prostaglandin production by human endometrial adenocarcinoma *in vitro*. (In) *Endocrinology and Malignancy* (Baulieu, E.E., Iacobelli, S. & McGuire, W.L., eds.), pp.420–427. Carnforth, UK, Parthenon.

Markiewicz, L. & Gurpide, E. (1988). C$_{19}$ adrenal steroids enhance prostaglandin F$_{2a}$ output by human endometrium *in vitro*. *American Journal of Obstetrics and Gynecology*, **159**:500–504.

Markiewicz, L., Laufer, N. & Gurpide, E. (1988). *In vitro* effects of clomiphene citrate on human endometrium. *Fertility and Sterility*, **50**:772–776.

Markiewicz, L., Schatz, F., Barg, P. & Gurpide, E. (1985a). Prostaglandin F$_{2a}$ output by human endometrium under superfusion and organ culture conditions. *Journal of Steroid Biochemistry*, **22**:231–235.

Markiewicz, L., Schatz, F., Barg, P. & Gurpide, E. (1985b). Effects of estradiol and estriol on PGF$_{2a}$ output by superfused human endometrium and isolated endometrial glands. (In) *Mechanism of Menstrual Bleeding* (Baird, D.T. & Michie, E.A., eds.), pp.129–137. New York, Raven Press.

Neulen, J., Zahradnik, H.P., Flecken, U. & Breckwoldt, M. (1988). Effects of estradiol-17-β and progesterone on the synthesis of prostaglandin F$_{2a}$, prostaglandin E$_2$ and prostaglandin I$_2$ by fibroblasts from human endometrium *in vitro*. *Prostaglandins*, **36**:17–30.

Peek, M.J., Fraser, I.S., Phillips, C.A., Resta, T.M., Blackwell, P.M. & Markham, R. (1985). The measurement of human endometrial prostaglandin production. A comparison of two *in vitro* methods. *Prostaglandins*, **29**:3–18.

Peek, M.J., Norman, T.M., Morgan, C., Fraser, I.S. & Markham, R. (1987). Trauma-induced human endometrial prostaglandin concentrations. *Prostaglandins*, **34**:919–925.

Poyser, N.L. (1980). *Prostaglandins in Reproduction*. Chichester, UK, RSP Division of John Wiley & Sons.

Roberts, J.S., McCracken, J.A., Gavagan, J.E. & Soloff, M.S.A. (1976). Oxytocin-stimulated release of prostaglandin F$_{2a}$ from ovine endometrium *in vitro*: correlation with estrous cycle and oxytocin-receptor binding. *Endocrinology*, **99**:1107–1114.

Schatz, F., Gordon, R.E., Laufer, N. & Gurpide, E. (1989). Regulation of prostaglandin F$_{2a}$ output in human endometrial epithelial cells: implications in implantation. (In) *Proceedings of the Second International Conference on Leukotrienes and Prostaglandins in Health and Disease*. Jerusalem, Israel, October 1988. Basel, S. Karger.

Schatz, F. & Gurpide, E. (1983). Effects of estradiol on prostaglandin F$_{2a}$ levels in primary monolayer cultures of epithelial cells from human proliferative endometrium. *Endocrinology*, **113**:1274–1279.

Schatz, F., Markiewicz, L., Barg, P. & Gurpide, E. (1985). *In vitro* effects of ovarian steroids on prostaglandin $F_{2\alpha}$ output by human endometrium and endometrial epithelial cells. *Journal of Clinical Endocrinology and Metabolism*, **61**:361–367.

Schatz, F., Markiewicz, L., Barg, P. & Gurpide, E. (1986). *In vitro* inhibition with antiestrogens of estradiol effects on prostaglandin $F_{2\alpha}$ production by human endometrium and endometrial epithelial cells. *Endocrinology*, **118**:408–412.

Schatz, F., Markiewicz, L. & Gurpide, E. (1984). Effects of estriol on $PGF_{2\alpha}$ output by cultures of human endometrium and endometrial cells. *Journal of Steroid Biochemistry*, **20**:999–1003.

Schatz, F., Markiewicz, L. & Gurpide, E. (1987). Differential effects of estradiol, arachidonic acid, and A23187 on prostaglandin $F_{2\alpha}$ output by epithelial and stromal cells of human endometrium. *Endocrinology*, **120**:1465–1471.

Singh, E.J., Baccarini, I.M. & Zuspan, F.P. (1975). Levels of prostaglandins $F_{2\alpha}$ and E_2 in human endometrium during the menstrual cycle. *American Journal of Obstetrics and Gynecology*, **121**:1003–1006.

Smith, S.K. & Kelly, R.W. (1987). The effect of estradiol-17β and actinomycin D on the release of PGF and PGE from separated cells of human endometrium. *Prostaglandins*, **34**:553–561.

Tsang, B.K. & Ooi, T.C. (1982). Prostaglandin secretion by human endometrium *in vitro*. *American Journal of Obstetrics and Gynecology*, **142**:626–633.

Discussion

Naftolin. What do you think is going on in those cells? Do you think they are differentiated? Are they, in fact, still proliferative cells or are they secretory cells as a result of being exposed to the steroids for several days?

Gurpide. They come from proliferative tissue. There are changes during culture and we are now looking for markers of differenciation in culture.

Harper. If you leave these stromal cell cultures long enough and expose them to progesterone for more than 2 days, prolactin production is increased in a dose-dependent manner; you get bigger increases with the larger dose of progesterone up to about 10^{-6} mol/l. My question relates to the interpretation of your results. What you are showing is prostaglandin output, and output obviously is a balance between synthesis and metabolism within the cells. The major metabolic enzyme that metabolizes the prostaglandins (15-hydroxyprostaglandin dehydrogenase) is sensitive to the action of steroids. Some years ago we were looking at rabbit uterine cytosols and at metabolism with PGF and PGE_2, and we found that in-vivo progesterone treatment increased the activity of 15-OH PG dehydrogenase. This could result in lowered PG output, which would fit with your in-vitro results. Have you looked at metabolism in these cells?

Gurpide. We looked at metabolism of secreted $PGF_{2\alpha}$ or PGE_2 by adding tritiated tracers of these compounds to the incubation medium, separating precursor and products by TLC. Although we observed the formation of some radioactive products, there were no differences between cultures with or without E_2.

Ludwig. Did you find any differences in prostaglandin production in relation to the date of the cycle within the proliferative phase? Is there any significant difference between the 4th or 6th day of the cycle and the periovulatory days?

Gurpide. No, we did not. Your question is very relevant in relation to stromal cells since we have observed under similar culture conditions, in the absence of progesterone, transitory production of prolactin by cells isolated from late proliferative but not from early proliferative endometrium.

Granström. I would like to raise a technical point related to the one Dr Harper raised, that concerns whether $PGF_{2\alpha}$ is really the best compound to measure. It is chemically stable and it is very cheap to assay. But one should perhaps keep in mind that it is not always an enzymatic product. As soon as you get formation of the prostaglandin endoperoxides, you will, to some extent, get $PGF_{2\alpha}$ non-enzymatically. The presence of reducing factors, such as thiol groups and metal ions and so on, will influence the proportions of the so-called classical prostaglandins formed. So, I think an assay of at least the three compounds, PGE_2, PGD_2 and $PGF_{2\alpha}$, together might give a more reliable picture. It can be done in a rather simple way and does not require the expensive PGE_2 radioimmunoassay kits. What you can do is simply assay the culture medium as such for $PGF_{2\alpha}$ and then, after reduction with sodium borohydride, you assay $PGF_{2\alpha}$ again plus $PGF_{2\beta}$. You get three values – $PGF_{2\alpha}$ before and after, and $PGF_{2\beta}$ after reduction – and from these three values you can quite easily calculate how much you had of the three different compounds PGE_2, PGD_2 and $PGF_{2\alpha}$ in your culture medium.

Smith. About metabolism, it does not make much difference whether it is proliferative, secretory or decidual tissue, at least in terms of the PG production. So the different prostaglandins do seem to work in conjunction.

Healy. A question about the proliferative phase, either with the explants or the isolated epithelial cells and estradiol. Have you done the experiment of actually adding IGF or EGF with estradiol?

Gurpide. No, we did not.

Findlay. I would just like to follow up Dr Naftolin's question about the possibility that the cells are changing in culture. PP14 is a product of the secretory glandular epithelium. Have you had the opportunity to measure the production of PP14, because that would, presumably, indicate whether they were changing from proliferative to secretory?

Gurpide. We did not measure PP14 in the medium.

Casey. Back to this issue of metabolism once again. Some years ago, we found that in human endometrial tissue obtained at various stages of the cycle there was an increase in the specific activity of prostaglandin dehydrogenase in the early secretory phase. We interpreted that to mean that there was a means for preventing a high prostaglandin production in the early secretory phase, and that with the withdrawal of progesterone, prostaglandin dehydrogenase declines, and, consequently, the tissue levels of prostaglandins increase.

Cornillie. What percent of calf serum did you use in your culture systems and did you treat this calf serum to get rid of the steroids that are there?

Gurpide. We used 15% of calf serum which was charcoal-treated twice under conditions that remove added radioactive estradiol and estrone sulphate.

Cornillie. Charcoal extraction is not able to get rid of all the steroid in culture medium.

Gurpide. In our case it did. We treated the serum very thoroughly, repeating the treatment twice, the second time at 56°C for 30 minutes.

Baird. Earlier, you raised the important issue as to whether, *in vivo*, the human endometrium releases more prostaglandin F or E in the proliferative or secretory endometrium. Now, my interpretation of the existing results is entirely compatible with the hypothesis that, *in vivo*, there is very little release, either in the proliferative or the secretory endometrium, of prostaglandins until the levels of progesterone fall at the time of luteal regression. I think that if one looks at the systems that have been used to study prostaglandin productions – concentration, short-term incubation or incubation in culture up to 24 hours – they demonstrate that secretory endometrium has a greater capacity when traumatized and removed from the body to produce prostaglandin than the proliferative endometrium. Virtually all the organ-culture studies, which, like yours, have waited for 24 or 48 hours for tissue trauma to be overcome, have shown that the basal production of prostaglandins is actually very little. Indeed, our original results showed that the production of prostaglandin $F_{2\alpha}$ from secretory endometrium, 48 and 72 hours after removing it, was actually less than from proliferative endometrium. Do you have data from the culture fluid you discard, on the amount of prostaglandins which are released into the medium during these first 24 hours from secretory and proliferative endometrium?

Gurpide. Prostaglandin levels were very high immediately after preparation of tissue for incubation or during the period of attachment of epithelial cells. Therefore, we allow for a period of stabilization before starting the experiments.

Baird. I think this is an extremely important issue because we have to remember the levels of endogenous progesterone *in vivo*, in the secretory phase of the cycle; although that tissue has the capacity to make prostaglandins, it releases practically nothing. At 10–20 ng/ml in your organ-culture system, progesterone wipes out PG production. So that if we are trying to reproduce the changes that normally occur *in vivo*, that is the normal hormonal environment at which that endometrium is growing.

Rees. We found that PG release was higher in tissue that had been collected when women were actually bleeding than when their bleeding had stopped, whether it was called menstruation or not. But, histologically, it is all endometrium, and the levels in menstrual endometrium were higher than when the bleeding had stopped. The PG levels in the early luteal phase were still quite low, and then started to climb in the midluteal and late luteal phase. We also found increased conversion in the luteal phase compared to the follicular phase when the tissues were collected while the women were not bleeding. We also found very little conversion of PGF to its metabolites using this system. Thus, two models have given us the same answers when we define the phase of the cycle at which we obtain the tissue.

Naftolin. I am impressed with the problems of the interpretation of Dr Gurpide's work, because one must define precisely the cells with which one is dealing before the results can be interpreted *in vitro* in terms of the in-vivo cycle. To go from those in-vitro measurements to talk about in-vivo situations which then have implications for some of the functional responses of the uterus, is difficult.

Gurpide. The in-vitro finding that epithelial but not stromal cells of the endometrium respond to estradiol may be physiologically meaningful. As I indicated during the talk, the interpretation of in-vivo studies can also be questionable. Clarification of contradictory in-vitro and in-vivo findings will, in this case, bring us closer to physiologically meaningful answers.

Effects of contraceptive progestogens on prostaglandins

M.G. ELDER, L. PATEL AND J.O. WHITE

Royal Postgraduate Medical School, Institute of Obstetrics and Gynaecology, Hammersmith Hospital, London, UK.

Abstract

Arachidonic acid is metabolized through the cyclo-oxygenase, lipoxygenase and epoxygenase enzyme systems to a range of compounds with vasoactive effect. These compounds could influence endometrial bleeding as a result of progestogen-only contraception. This study was carried out to see whether the metabolism of arachidonic acid by human endometrial cells in culture was altered by exposure *in vivo* to 3 months of a low daily dose (20 μg) of levonorgestrel. Endometrial biopsies were taken at day 24–26 (determined endocrinologically) of the control cycle and on day 84–87 after insertion of the vaginal ring releasing levonorgestrel. Levonorgestrel and sex hormone-binding globulin (SHBG) levels in plasma were determined weekly during the last month of the 90-day treatment period. Endometrial cells were cultured for 24 hours in the presence of labelled arachidonic acid and a further 24 hours in the absence of excess arachidonic acid to determine the basal production of metabolites. Thirty paired samples were suitable for analysis.

Reverse phase high performance liquid chromatography was used so that the full range of metabolites could be determined. There were no significant alterations in the proportion of arachidonic acid which was metabolized via the cyclo-oxygenase and lipoxygenase enzymes in the treatment cycle compared with the control cycle. There was a significant increase in the proportion of arachidonic acid metabolized to epoxides after progestogen exposure. When the group was divided into those who had regular bleeding compared with those who had irregular bleeding, there was no increase in epoxide formation in the former group, but a big increase in the latter group.

The possible relationship of these findings to irregular bleeding from the endometrium is not clear. Some epoxides inhibit platelet aggregation which could be important. An increase in free radicals in endometrial tissue may be a factor in the disproportionate increase in epoxygenase products compared with the other arachidonic acid metabolites. Further studies to determine the mechanism of increase in epoxide and its consequences on cellular function are necessary.

Introduction

Prostaglandin (PG) production by human endometrium is influenced by changing levels of estrogen and progesterone. The capacity of the endometrium to synthesize PGE_2 and $PGF_{2\alpha}$ increases markedly during the secretory phase of the menstrual cycle, reaching a maximum at the time of menstruation (Downie *et al.*, 1974).

In addition, there is an increased uptake of arachidonic acid into phospholipids in the cells of the endometrium during the secretory phase of the cycle compared with the proliferative phase (Downing *et al.*, 1983). The inference is that the synthetic capacity of the endometrium to produce prostaglandins is influenced by changing levels of estrogen and progesterone. There is a reduction in $PGF_{2\alpha}$ production by endometrial stroma incubated *in vitro* with progesterone, while the antiprogestational compound RU486 increases the $PGF_{2\alpha}$ production in a dose-dependent manner (Kelly *et al.*, 1986). Estradiol has been shown to increase prostaglandin production principally by endometrial glandular cells *in vitro* (Smith *et al.*, 1982). It is postulated that progesterone has a priming effect allowing maximum prostaglandin production in response to estradiol but that persistent exposure to progesterone will diminish prostaglandin production, as well as increase catabolism by increasing 15-hydroxyprostaglandin dehydrogenase (Smith *et al.*, 1981).

An interaction between prostaglandins produced by myometrium and endometrium is probably important in controlling the amount of bleeding, particularly at menstruation (Abel & Kelly, 1979). However, this interaction is probably not relevant to the etiology of progestogen-induced breakthrough bleeding. Contraceptive progestogens are administered continuously in doses ranging from high (depot-medroxyprogesterone acetate injectable 150 mg 3-monthly) to low (intravaginal ring 20 μg levonorgestrel daily). Independent of the dose used, it is well established that these compounds are associated with intermenstrual bleeding. Little is known about the effect of continuous progestogens on arachidonic acid metabolism in the endometrium.

Arachidonic acid is metabolized not only via the cyclo-oxygenase enzyme to prostaglandins but also by the lipoxygenase enzyme system to leukotrienes and mono- and di-hydroxy-eicosatetraenoic acids (HETEs) and by the cytochrome P450 epoxygenase enzymes to epoxyeicosatrienoic acids. The range and diversity of effects of these metabolites are great and one or more of them could be important mediators in progestogen-induced breakthrough bleeding as they are in menstruation.

Our own studies (unpublished) have shown not only an increase in the synthetic capacity for cyclo-oxygenase products from secretory phase endometrium, but also an increase in lipoxygenase and epoxygenase products. Leukotriene B_4 is known to cause arteriolar constriction and a subsequent increase in vascular permeability with extravasation of fluid, which is in turn potentiated by PGE_2 and PGD_2 (Bray *et al.*, 1981; Williams *et al.*, 1983).

Leukotrienes (LT) are one thousand times more potent than histamine in causing plasma leakage (Dahlén *et al.*, 1981). LTB_4 has also been shown to increase lysosomal enzyme release (Hafstrom *et al.*, 1981). The numbers of lysosomes and the release of lysosomal enzymes have been shown to be related to changes in estrogen and progesterone levels (Henzl *et al.*, 1972). Release of lysosomal phospholipase A_2 is important in liberating arachidonic acid from cell membranes and so increasing synthesis of eicosanoids.

For these reasons, the effect of low-dose progestogens on endometrial synthesis of eicosanoids was studied. This research was part of a multicentre trial on the effect of levonorgestrel on endometrial function. Other groups, following the same clinical protocol, investigated the effect of levonorgestrel on endometrial protein synthesis, lysosomal enzymes and hemostasis; the preliminary reports of these studies are published in this volume (respectively, White *et al.*, 1990; Cornillie *et al.*, 1990; Hourihan *et al.*, 1990).

Methods

Levonorgestrel was given via an intravaginal ring which released 20 μg/day over 90 days. As low-dose progestogens have a variable effect on ovarian function, endocrine profiles for each subject were monitored during the control cycle and the third treatment month. Forty subjects were recruited and 33 completed the study. All had a history of regular cycles and no gynecological disorder. They were followed during a control cycle with basal body temperature and three times weekly blood sampling for estradiol, progesterone and luteinizing hormone (LH), and they were asked to fill in a menstrual diary. On the second day of the next menstrual cycle a levonorgestrel-releasing ring was inserted and left for 90 days. During the third treatment month, from day 60 after the ring insertion onwards, blood samples were drawn three times weekly for estradiol and progesterone and once a week for levonorgestrel and sex hormone-binding globulin (SHBG).

Endometrial biopsies were performed with a Masterson aspiration curette. In the control cycle, biopsies were timed to be taken between day LH + 10 and LH + 12, calculated from the approximate time of ovulation as determined by estradiol and LH estimations (corresponding to cycle day 24–26). Endometrial biopsies in the third treatment month were taken at day 84–87 after insertion of the ring. If the patient was bleeding on that date, the biopsy was postponed and performed as soon as bleeding had stopped.

The endometrial tissue obtained was placed in phosphate buffered saline for transfer to the laboratory, minced into 1-mm cubes and dispersed using a solution of collagenase and DNAse in phosphate buffered saline. Digestion was completed within 45–60 minutes at 37°C. The cells were predominantly epithelial. Cells were grown in multi-well tissue culture plates at a density of 1×10^5 cells per well in medium 199, with Earle's modified salts, glutamine, antibiotics and 10% horse serum.

Tritiated arachidonic acid was added (0.5 μCi in 2 ml of fresh medium) to growing cells and incorporation allowed to proceed for 24 hours. Secretion of labelled eicosanoids was allowed to occur during a second 24-hour incubation period in fresh medium without added arachidonic acid. Labelled metabolites are therefore produced from arachidonic acid already incorporated in the cell membranes and without the stimulus of excess arachidonic acid in the medium and so these conditions should be closer to the in-vivo situation.

Reverse phase high performance liquid chromatography (HPLC) using an acetonitrile triethylamine formate solvent gradient was used to separate the arachidonic acid metabolites.

Because of incorporation of inadequate amounts of ^{3}H arachidonic acid, usually due to an inadequate number of cells obtained and cultured, only 30 paired biopsy samples were available for analysis.

Results

The counts incorporated into individual metabolites were expressed as a percentage of the counts incorporated into all the metabolites. Radioactivity in metabolites at 48 hours in culture (mean $\pm$ s.e.m., dpm/μg protein) was 163 ± 24 in the control cycle and 133 ± 29 in the third treatment month.

There was no difference between the production of eicosanoids by endometrial cells derived from control cycle biopsies compared to treated cycle biopsies, except for an increase in epoxide production by the endometrium exposed to progestogens ($p < 0.025$).

The subjects were divided into those who, in the third treatment month, showed endocrine evidence (LH surge and progesterone peak) of ovulation and those in whom this was lacking or equivocal. No difference in endometrial eicosanoid production could be detected between these groups. A more reliable way of quantifying the effect of steroid exposure on a tissue is by using the area under the curve of the steroid levels rather than single values. In addition, the bioavailability of levonorgestrel is influenced by SHBG levels. These data need to be analyzed in detail before firm conclusions can be drawn about the relationship of endocrine status *in vivo* to endometrial eicosanoid production.

Subjects were divided into those with 'normal' and 'abnormal' bleeding profiles during the 90 days of use of the intravaginal ring. A total of 20 days or less of bleeding or spotting during the 90-day period was taken as the arbitrary definition of a 'normal bleeding pattern', provided there were no more than four episodes of bleeding. In those women with normal bleeding patterns there was no significant increase in epoxygenase metabolite production by endometrial cells after exposure to levonorgestrel (Fig. 1). In those women with abnormal bleeding patterns as arbitrarily described, the increase in epoxygenase metabolites by endometrium produced in the third treatment month was significantly greater than that obtained in the control cycle (Fig. 2).

Comments

These data show that the major arachidonic acid metabolites in endometrium are the lipoxygenase and epoxygenase products. The cyclo-oxygenase

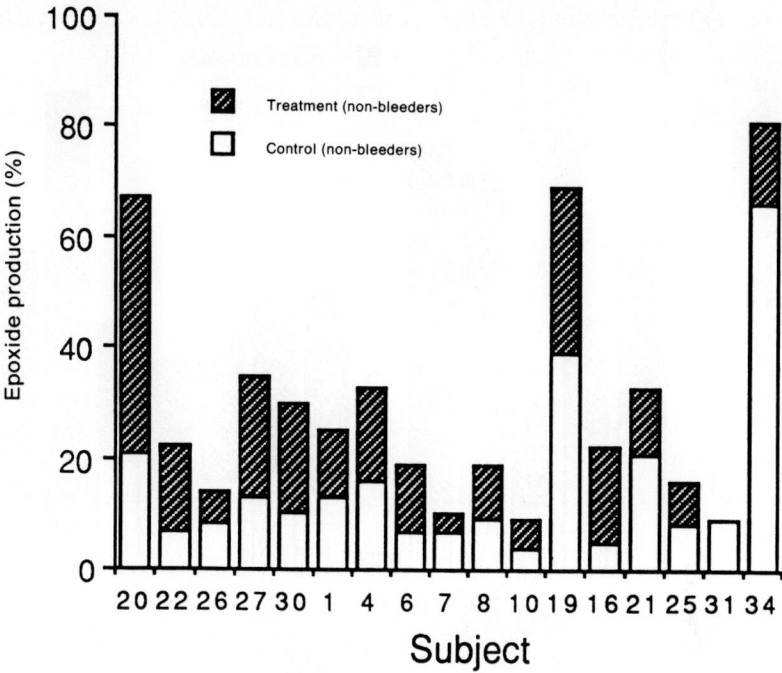

Fig. 1 Epoxide production as the percentage of all arachidonic acid metabolites produced by endometrial cells in culture. Endometrium was obtained before (unshaded) and after (shaded) 3 months exposure to 20 μg levonorgestrel daily. Subjects in this group had normal bleeding patterns during the 3 months of treatment.

products would probably have been greater if the endometrium had been biopsied closer to the time of menstruation. The methods used have the disadvantages of any primary cell culture system: the arachidonic acid metabolites are released by these cells under basal conditions and are free of the artefact of those produced by tissues recently biopsied or by cells cultured in excess of substrate, which acts as an artificial stimulus to the synthesis of metabolites.

The putative epoxide identified as an increase in peak height at a retention time of 48 minutes is not yet characterized, and this work needs to be carried out. However, we know that the peak does not elute from the HPLC column at the same time as the HETEs and it is appropriately altered by inhibitors (10^{-5} mol/l SKF525A) and stimulants (10^{-5} mol/l alpha naphoflavene) of the cyclo-oxygenase pathway.

A cytochrome P450 isoenzyme that catalyzes arachidonic acid epoxidation has been purified and it oxidizes arachidonic acid to 5,6; 8,9; 11,12 and 14,15 epoxyeicosatrienoic acids (EET) (Laniado-Schwartzman *et al.*, 1988). The

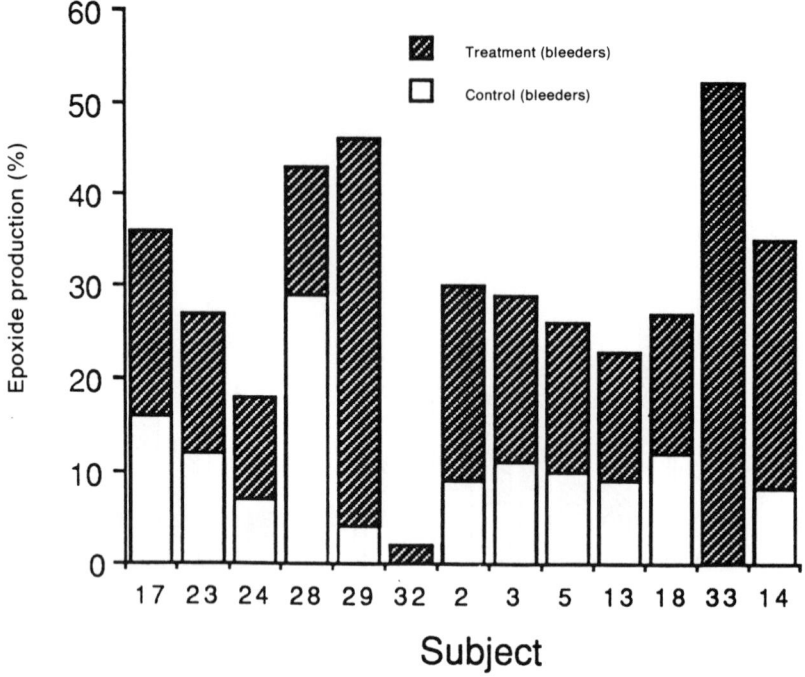

Fig. 2 Epoxide production as the percentage of all arachidonic acid metabolites produced by endometrial cells in culture. Endometrium was obtained before (unshaded) and after (shaded) 3 months exposure to 20 μg levonorgestrel daily. Subjects in this group had abnormal bleeding patterns during the 3 months of treatment.

physiological role of these compounds has not yet been determined, but preliminary work has shown that they may mediate in the release of insulin and glucagon from pancreatic islet cells in culture (Falck *et al.*, 1983) and that they may be a component of the reaction whereby luteinizing hormone-releasing hormone leads to LH production (Snyder *et al.*, 1983). A cytochrome P450-dependent mono-oxygenase system has been shown to metabolize arachidonic acid in the kidney to biologically active compounds. One of these inhibits the intracellular sodium–potassium pump while the other has vasodilatory effects.

A role for epoxygenase products in endometrial bleeding is at this stage speculative. However, we have demonstrated that progestogen exposure increases the production of arachidonic acid metabolites of the epoxygenase pathway in the endometrium of women with progestogen-induced bleeding problems. Both 14,15 EET and 8,9 EET have been shown to be inhibitors of the cyclo-oxygenase pathway and in particular can reduce platelet thromboxane production (Fitzpatrick *et al.*, 1986). Platelet aggregation induced by arachidonic acid is inhibited by all EET isomers but the most potent is 14,15 EET (Fitzpatrick *et al.*, 1986). Increased synthesis of epoxides may therefore have a direct effect on platelet function, making bleeding more likely.

Inhibition of platelet aggregation by epoxides may combine with a progestogen-induced increase in platelet-activating factor (PAF) through the phospholipase A_2 enzyme common to the synthesis of both. PAF can cause an increase in vascular permeability which may be an earlier step in the onset of irregular bleeding.

Finally, a possible reduction in vitamin E, an antioxidant, which can be brought about by contraceptive steroids could lead to an increase in free radicals within tissues, which in turn will enhance arachidonic acid metabolism, particularly via the epoxygenase enzyme system, and lead to cell damage.

Future research

1. The putative epoxide peak demonstrated on HPLC needs to be chemically characterized.
2. The physiological and biochemical roles of the characterized compound(s) require investigation.
3. The relationship of these compounds to platelet behaviour may be important in understanding the bleeding problems.
4. Assessment of vitamin E status in subjects using continuous progestogen contraception would be valuable.
5. Interaction and synergism between eicosanoid and PAF production need to be evaluated.

References

Abel, M.H. & Kelly, R.W. (1979). Differential production of prostaglandins within the human uterus. *Prostaglandins*, **18**:821–828.

Bray, M.A., Cunningham, F.M., Ford-Hutchinson, A.W. & Smith, M.J.H. (1981). Leukotriene B4: A mediator of vascular permeability. *British Journal of Pharmacology*, **72**:483–486.

Cornillie, F.J., Brosens, I.A., Marbaix, E., Vael, T., Baudhuin, P. & Courtoy, P.J. (1990). A biochemical study of lysosomal enzymes in control and levonorgestrel-treated human endometria: analysis of total activity and evidence for secretion. (In) *Contraception and Mechanisms of Endometrial Bleeding* (d'Arcangues, C., Fraser, I.S., Newton, J.R. & Odlind, V., eds.), pp.383–406. Cambridge, England, Cambridge University Press.

Dahlén, S.E., Björk, J., Hedqvist, P., Arfors, K.E., Hammarström, S., Lindgren, J.A. & Samuelsson, B. (1981). Leukotrienes promote plasma leakage and leukocyte adhesion in post-capillary venules: *in vivo* effects with relevance to the acute inflammatory response. *Proceedings of the National Academy of Sciences USA*, **78**:3887–3891.

Downie, J., Poyser, N.L. & Wunderlich, M. (1974). Levels of prostaglandins in human endometrium during the normal menstrual cycle. *Journal of Physiology*, **236**:465–472.

Downing, I., Hutchon, D.J.R. & Poyser, N.L. (1983). Uptake of [^{3}H] arachidonic acid by human endometrium. Differences between normal and menorrhagic tissue. *Prostaglandins*, **26**:55–69.

Falck, J.R., Manna, S., Moltz, J., Chacos, N. & Capdevila, J. (1983). Epoxyeicosatrienoic acids stimulate glucagon and insulin release from isolated rat pancreatic islets. *Biochemical and Biophysical Research Communications*, **114**:743–749.

Fitzpatrick, F.A., Ennis, M.D., Baze, M.E., Wynalda, M.A., McGee, J.E. & Liggett, W.F. (1986). Inhibition of cyclo-oxygenase activity and platelet aggregation by epoxyeicosatrienoic acids. Influence of stereochemistry. *Journal of Biological Chemistry*, **261**:15334–15338.

Hafstrom, I., Palmblad, J., Malmsten, C.L., Rådmark, O. & Samuelsson, B. (1981). Leukotriene B4 – a stereospecific stimulator for release of lysosomal enzymes from neutrophils. *FEBS Letters*, **130**:146–148.

Henzl, M.R., Smith, R.E., Boost, G. & Tyler, E. (1972). Lysosomal concept of menstrual bleeding in humans. *Journal of Clinical Endocrinology and Metabolism*, **34**:860–875.

Hourihan, H.M., Sheppard, B.L. & Brosens, I.A. (1990). Endometrial hemostasis. (In) *Contraception and Mechanisms of Endometrial Bleeding* (d'Arcangues, C., Fraser, I.S., Newton, J.R. & Odlind, V., eds.), pp.95–114. Cambridge, England, Cambridge University Press.

Kelly, R.W., Healy, D.L., Cameron, M.J., Cameron, I.T. & Baird, D.T. (1986). The stimulation of prostaglandin production by two anti-progesterone steroids in human endometrial cells. *Journal of Clinical Endocrinology and Metabolism*, **62**:1116–1123.

Laniado-Schwartzman, M., Davis, K.L., McGiff, J.C., Levere, R.D. & Abraham, N.G. (1988). Purification and characterization of cytochrome p-450-dependent arachidonic acid epoxygenase from human liver. *Journal of Biological Chemistry*, **263**:2536–2542.

Smith, S.K., Abel, M.H., Kelly, R.W. & Baird, D.T. (1981). Prostaglandin synthesis in the endometrium of women with ovular dysfunctional uterine bleeding. *British Journal of Obstetrics and Gynaecology*, **88**:434–442.

Smith, S.K., Abel, M.H., Kelly, R.W. & Baird, D.T. (1982). The synthesis of prostaglandins from persistent proliferative endometrium. *Journal of Clinical Endocrinology and Metabolism*, **55**:284–289.

Snyder, G.D., Capdevila, J., Chacos, N., Manna, S. & Falck, J.R. (1983). Action of luteinizing hormone-releasing hormone: involvement of novel arachidonic acid metabolites. *Proceedings of the National Academy of Sciences USA*, **80**:3504–3507.

White, J.O., Croxtall, J.D. & Elder, M.G. (1990). Effects of contraceptive progestogens on endometrial proteins. (In) *Contraception and Mechanisms of Endometrial Bleeding* (d'Arcangues, C., Fraser, I.S., Newton, J.R. & Odlind, V., eds.), pp.233–239. Cambridge, England, Cambridge University Press.

Williams, T.J., Jose, P.J., Wedmore, C.V., Peck, M.J. & Forest, M.J. (1983). Mechanisms underlying inflammatory edema: the importance of synergism between prostaglandins, leukotrienes and complement-derived peptides. *Advances in Prostaglandin, Thromboxane and Leukotriene Research*, **11**:33–37.

Discussion

Fraser. Can you tell us whether the women who were biopsied were actually bleeding at the time at which the biopsies were taken and did they show any obvious difference compared with the others?

Elder. None of them was bleeding at the time of biopsy. Some of them did, in fact, bleed on the planned biopsy day and we put it off by 2 or 3 days. But I think that the picture is obviously different in someone who has just finished bleeding compared with someone who has not bled for maybe 20 or 25 days.

Platelet-activating factor and the reproductive system

MICHAEL J.K. HARPER

Department of Obstetrics and Gynecology, The University of Texas Health Science Center, San Antonio, USA.

Abstract

Platelet-activating factor (PAF) is an acetylated glycero-phospholipid with potent biological activities, including among others increased vascular permeability and stimulation of smooth muscle activity. PAF has been found in rat and rabbit uterus and in human endometrial cell cultures; it appears to be localized in the endometrial stroma. Its concentration in the uterus is regulated by progesterone, and is increased greatly during pregnancy and pseudopregnancy. A dramatic decline in the uterine level of PAF is seen during the 24 hours prior to implantation of the blastocyst, and this decline is greatest at the site of the blastocyst attachment. The release of PAF at the implantation site correlates well with the increased capillary permeability that occurs there. It is suggested that, since endometrial bleeding occurs under progestational influence, and since PAF is increased by progesterone and can stimulate endometrial prostaglandin release, PAF may be a very significant factor in induction of endometrial bleeding. The availability of many potent PAF antagonists will permit the rapid assessment of the role of PAF in endometrial function.

Introduction

Platelet-activating factor (PAF) is a term used to describe a family of biologically active acetylated phospholipids. PAF was first reported as a factor released from leukocytes which triggered the release of histamine from platelets: this is the derivation of the name platelet-activating factor (Benveniste *et al.*, 1972) – with hindsight, as large a misnomer as that of the prostaglandins. It is now known that PAF is synthesized and released from a variety of stimulated inflammatory cells, including the neutrophil, basophil, platelet and macrophage–monocyte (Pinckard *et al.*, 1982; Pinckard, 1983). Structural characterization and synthesis of PAF were first achieved by Demopoulos *et al.* (1979). Synthetic PAF is 1-0-alkyl-2-acetyl-**sn**-glycero-3-phosphorylcholine; the most active compounds have either a 16 or 18 carbon alkyl side-chain in position 1, an acetyl group in position 2, and a phosphorylcholine side-chain in position 3 (Fig. 1). All of these features seem to be essential for biological activity (Ludwig & Pinckard, 1987). Modification of these structural elements has permitted the development of many potent antagonists, and other antagonists derived from plants, which are not structural analogues of PAF, have also been described (Braquet & Godfroid, 1986).

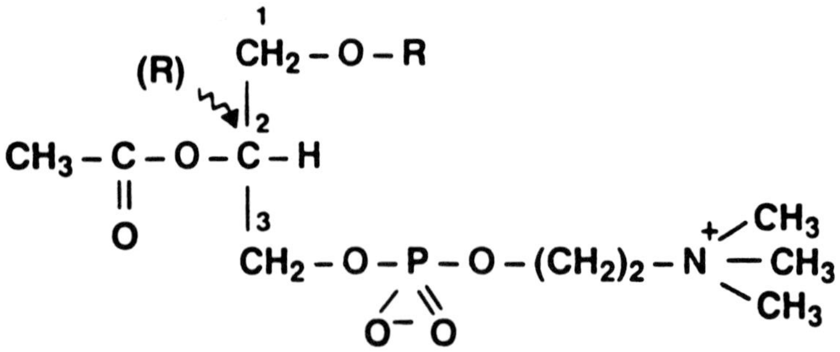

$$CH_2 - O - R$$
(R)
$$CH_3 - C - O - C - H$$
$$\underset{O}{\parallel} \quad \underset{3}{\vert}$$
$$CH_2 - O - P - O - (CH_2)_2 - \overset{+}{N} \begin{array}{l} CH_3 \\ - CH_3 \\ CH_3 \end{array}$$
$$\underset{O^- \ O}{\diagup \ \diagdown}$$

Fig. 1 Chemical structure of PAF: $R = C_{16}H_{35}$ or $C_{18}H_{37}$.

PAF has a variety of biological actions. In a recent review, Braquet *et al.* (1987) listed the effects caused following intravenous (i.v.) injection of PAF.

Hypotension in rats, baboons, guinea-pigs, dogs and rabbits.
Pulmonary hypertension in rabbits.
Bronchoconstriction in guinea-pigs and baboons.
Increased vascular permeability in rats and guinea-pigs.
Thrombocytopenia. Neutropenia. Death.

The effects of PAF are very dependent on the route of administration and the species under investigation. *In vitro*, PAF can be shown to cause other effects, such as platelet, neutrophil and monocyte activation, and alterations in cardiac, pulmonary and hepatic function (Ludwig & Pinckard, 1987). It is also thought that PAF may be involved in a variety of pathophysiological conditions, including arterial thrombosis, acute inflammation, endotoxic shock, acute allergic diseases (asthma and anaphylaxis) and gastrointestinal ulceration (see Pinckard *et al.*, 1983; Braquet *et al.*, 1987).

PAF is synthesized *in vivo* by acetylation of its precursor, lyso-PAF, which in turn is synthesized from alkylacyl-GPC by deacylation. This latter phospholipid is mobilized from cell membranes by phospholipase A_2 to release lyso-PAF and arachidonic acid, the major precursor for prostaglandin synthesis. Hence, it is not unusual to find both PAF and prostaglandins elevated by the same stimuli.

Quantitation

One of the major difficulties encountered in PAF research is the lack of a simple, robust and reliable assay for PAF. The development of an antibody to PAF that would permit development of a radioimmunoassay would be of inestimable benefit to the field*. In the interim, for large numbers of samples

---

*A radioimmunoassay kit is now available (Biotechnology Systems, NEN Research Products, Boston, MA. Cat. No. NEK-062), but prior extraction and column chromatography are still required.

inestimable benefit to the field. In the interim, for large numbers of samples one is left with a variety of bioassays, with all the flaws to which such assays are heir. At present, the most reliable method of quantitation involves: (a) lipid extraction (Folch *et al.*, 1957), (b) separation of the lipids by thin-layer chromatography (TLC) or high-pressure liquid chromatography (HPLC) (Pinckard *et al.*, 1984; Miwa *et al.*, 1987), and (c) bioassay of the various fractions by release of tritiated serotonin from preloaded rabbit platelets or aggregation of rabbit platelets (Pinckard *et al.*, 1979). The sensitivity for detecting synthetic PAF in our own studies is 11 fmol for the platelet [^{3}H]serotonin secretion assay and 6 fmol for the platelet aggregation assay (Angle *et al.*, 1988).

To increase the specificity of the aggregation assay, it is necessary to add indomethacin and creatine kinase/creatine phosphate to the assay buffer. Specificity of the bioassays is, however, mainly assured by prior lipid extraction and TLC, and by use of platelet desensitization assays (Demopoulos *et al.*, 1979). Another bioassay for PAF using the reduction in platelet count in splenectomized mice has also been described (O'Neill, 1985a). Although this assay has been used to quantitate PAF-like material, its overall specificity has not been established, since injection of Iloprost (a stable analogue of prostacyclin PGI_2) into mice produces a similar effect (Spinks & O'Neill, 1987). Furthermore, lipid extraction and TLC have not been routinely used prior to injection of the unknown samples into the splenectomized mice. However, in the one study where this was done, all the activity was found in the chloroform layer (after lipid extraction), the same as for synthetic PAF, and both the lipid-extracted embryo factor and PAF exhibited the same relative mobility on TLC (O'Neill, 1985c). The induction of thrombocytopenia in mice may, however, be an indirect effect of PAF, since PAF does not cause aggregation of mouse platelets *in vitro* (Lanara *et al.*, 1982; Namm *et al.*, 1982). Specific identification and absolute quantitation of PAF can also be done by gas chromatography/mass spectrometry, but this method is not suitable for large numbers of samples.

Biological occurrence and actions

As noted above, PAF has a large number of biological actions, many of them associated with pathophysiological conditions involving stimulation of leukocytes. It is now recognized that many, if not all, cells may have the capacity to produce PAF. For example, PAF has been found in lung, kidney, gastrointestinal tract, central nervous system, retina and reproductive system (see Braquet *et al.*, 1987; Hwang, 1987; Junier *et al.*, 1988; Kudolo & Harper, 1989). However, localization of these receptors has not yet been accomplished, for PAF have been described in the membranes of a number of different cell types, e.g. platelets, lung, retina, endothelium, hypothalamus, liver and uterus (see Braquet *et al.*, 1987; Hwang, 1987; Junier *et al.*, 1988; Kudolo & Harper, 1988). However, localization of these receptors has not yet been accomplished, so it is unknown whether the receptors are located on the outer, inner or both surfaces of cell membranes. It may be that in some situations PAF acts in a paracrine, and in others in an autocrine, manner. PAF is thought to be synthesized in the endoplasmic reticulum and then transferred to the cell membrane, where if it is to be secreted, it is removed from the cell by serum albumin (Pinckard, 1983).

One of the difficulties with localization experiments is the metabolism of PAF that occurs in physiological situations. PAF is rapidly metabolized to lyso-PAF, the biologically inactive deacetylated derivative, by an acetylhydrolase which is ubiquitous in plasma and also associated with cell cytoplasm. Lyso-PAF is also the major substrate for the formation of PAF by an acetyltransferase, and can itself be recycled to the alkylacyl-GPC via an acyltransferase (see Braquet *et al.*, 1987). Thus, the presence of silver grains, denoting tritium disintegrations on autoradiographs, cannot necessarily be assumed to represent PAF itself, but may also include tritium associated with lyso-PAF or alkylacyl-GPC. Synthetic analogues of PAF, that are not metabolized and still bind to receptors, are now becoming available (O'Flaherty *et al.*, 1987), and such compounds may significantly advance localization and binding studies.

Up to now, most of the studies on PAF have concentrated on platelets and leukocytes, and its role in allergic and cardiopulmonary disease. It is only recently that studies to examine its actions and presence in other systems has begun. Some of the actions of PAF have been referred to above, and space does not permit further discussion here of its actions on the pulmonary, cardiovascular and renal systems. However, one action that is of direct relevance to the possible role of PAF in the reproductive tract is the ability to cause increased vascular permeability at extremely low concentrations (1 pmol) (Humphrey *et al.*, 1982; Humphrey *et al.*, 1984; Angle *et al.*, 1986). As discussed above, the assays utilized can detect PAF even at these low concentrations.

PAF and the hypothalamic–pituitary system

Junier *et al.* (1988) have recently studied the effects of PAF on brain neuropeptides. PAF was found to decrease luteinizing hormone-releasing hormone (LHRH) and somatostatin release from the median eminence with a maximal inhibition at 10^{-14} mol/l for both neuropeptides, whereas growth hormone-releasing factor (GRF) release was not significantly altered. In addition, the stimulatory action of the calcium ionophore A23187 on the release of LHRH and somatostatin from median eminence and medial basal hypothalamus was strongly reduced. PAF had no effect on LH and growth hormone (GH) release from the anterior pituitary. These authors also demonstrated a specific, saturable and reversible binding of [³H]PAF to membrane preparations from rat hypothalamus. Two classes of binding sites were demonstrated with affinities (K_D) of 2.14 ± 0.32 and 61.63 ± 16.4 nmol/l for the high- and low-affinity sites respectively. The respective binding capacities (B_{max}) were 25.4 ± 3.2 and 146.2 ± 47.5 fmol/mg protein. Under the same conditions, no specific binding of [³H]PAF to pituitary membranes was seen. PAF antagonists reduced the inhibition of LHRH and somatostatin release by PAF with the same order of potency that they inhibited [³H]PAF binding to the hypothalamic membranes. Thus, it was concluded that inhibition of neuropeptide release by PAF was a receptor-mediated effect.

PAF and the zygote

The pioneering work in this area has been done by O'Neill and his associates. In 1985, they reported that in mice there was a significant reduction in platelet count on the morning of day 1 of pregnancy, continuing through day 6 of pregnancy. This response was not observed in pseudopregnant mice. Using various surgical manipulations, O'Neill was able to show that this thrombocytopenia was dependent on the presence of fertilized eggs (O'Neill, 1985a). In a second study (O'Neill, 1985b), it was found that injection into splenectomized mice of medium from cultures of mouse embryos caused a dose-dependent thrombocytopenia within 10 minutes; medium from cultures of unfertilized ova did not have the same effect. The thrombocytopenia caused by injection of the embryo culture media demonstrated a dose–response curve that was parallel to that for synthetic PAF (O'Neill, 1985b). The embryo-derived material, during lipid extraction and TLC, behaved similarly to synthetic PAF (O'Neill, 1985c). In these studies, PAF was found in the medium after 24 hours of culture of thirty 8–16-cell mouse zygotes. PAF-like material was never found in cultures of oocytes. Cultures of mouse zygotes for longer than 24 hours led to a diminution of detectable PAF-like activity. This activity was not, however, confined to early stage embryos, since four out of four 12-hour cultures of mouse blastocysts tested positive (O'Neill, 1987).

That production of PAF-like material from zygotes was not confined to the mouse was shown in a further study (O'Neill et al., 1985). Thrombocytopenia from day 1 through day 6 was seen in women receiving transferred zygotes (in an in-vitro fertilization procedure) who became pregnant, while no such effect was seen in similar women who failed to become pregnant. Furthermore, the culture media from the 10 embryos transferred to women who became pregnant caused a much greater decrease in platelet count in splenectomized mice than did that from the 10 embryos transferred to women who failed to become pregnant. These ova were cultured individually for a period of 24–36 hours after in-vitro insemination (approximately 4-cell stage), and the medium from each culture was assayed separately (O'Neill et al., 1985). This is in sharp contrast to the mouse experiments in which the medium tested was usually derived from 24-hour cultures of thirty 8–16-cell embryos (O'Neill, 1985c). Since the maximal depressions in platelet count seen after intraperitoneal (i.p.) injection of 300 μl of culture medium were 31% and 32% respectively from mouse and human zygotes (O'Neill, 1985c; O'Neill et al.,

1985), this suggests that human zygotes produce greater quantities of the PAF-like material. Experiments with marmosets were much less clear, although there was some evidence of a thrombocytopenia associated with the pre-implantation stage of pregnancy (O'Neill, 1987).

In contrast to the results obtained with mouse blastocysts, in our laboratory we were unable to find evidence of PAF in day 5 or 6 rabbit blastocysts, or in culture media derived from pools of 10 day-5 blastocysts cultured for 24 hours and subjected to lipid extraction and TLC (Angle *et al.*, 1988). The reason for this discrepancy is not known.

PAF is not essential for the survival of the pre-implantation embryo, since PAF antagonists that can inhibit implantation do not affect embryo development *in vitro* from the 2-cell to blastocyst stage (O'Neill, 1987). This suggests that PAF exerts its actions on the maternal reproductive tract rather than on the embryo *per se*.

PAF and the reproductive tract

The above supposition is strengthened by the observation that injection of estrous mice with synthetic PAF caused the appearance of early pregnancy factor (EPF) in the sera (Orozco *et al.*, 1986). EPF is otherwise only detected during pregnancy. Thus, PAF released from early stage embryos could act on oviductal cells via the presence of specific binding sites. We have preliminary evidence for specific binding of [^{3}H]PAF to day-2 rabbit oviductal membrane preparations (unpublished data), but what significance this may have for maintenance of pregnancy or control of oviduct function remains to be determined.

The presence of PAF in rat uterus has been described by Yasuda *et al.* (1986). The total content of PAF was 21.3 ng in the non-pregnant uterus. It was also reported that the rabbit uterus contained much smaller quantities. In our studies (Angle *et al.*, 1988), we found that the uterus from estrous rabbits contained 1.9 ± 1.0 pmol of PAF/g wet weight of tissue. When measurements were made on endometrium and myometrium separately, the values were 2.2 ± 1.2 and 0.4 ± 0.4 pmol/g, respectively. This clearly demonstrates that PAF is located in the endometrium rather than the myometrium.

From other studies with human luteal phase endometrial glandular and stromal cell cultures, it is apparent that PAF is synthesized in the stromal cells and not in the glands (Alecozay *et al.*, 1989). Basal levels of PAF in stromal cell cultures were low, but after stimulation with 10^{-6} mol/l of progesterone for 24 hours, PAF levels in the cells increased significantly; little PAF was found in the culture media. PAF levels were not different when 10^{-8} mol/l of estradiol was combined with the progesterone. PAF was undetectable in cultures of glandular cells from the same patients (Alecozay *et al.*, 1989).

Although the levels of PAF are low in the non-pregnant rabbit uterus, we found (Angle *et al.*, 1988) that during pregnancy or pseudopregnancy uterine levels increased dramatically. In pseudopregnant rabbits, uterine PAF levels peaked on day 4 at 30.6 ± 2.8 pmol/g, declined to 20.5 ± 2.4 pmol/g on day 5, and then remained at that level through day 7. In contrast, in pregnant animals uterine PAF was maximal on day 5 at 37.8 ± 4.9 pmol/g, and by day 7 had returned to basal levels similar to those found at estrus. Furthermore, this decline in uterine PAF levels in pregnant rabbits was greater at the implantation site than in the interimplantation areas. Since the increases in uterine PAF paralleled the increase in peripheral plasma progesterone levels, we concluded that uterine PAF synthesis was hormonally regulated. In the same animals, bladder concentrations of PAF did not vary with hormonal status.

The reduction in PAF concentrations at the implantation sites between days 6 and 7 appeared to be due to the presence of the blastocysts, since this is the major difference between pseudopregnancy and pregnancy at this stage. These results could be interpreted either as indicating that the presence of a blastocyst inhibits further production of PAF by the stromal cells, or that it triggers the release of the preformed PAF. We conclude that the latter explanation is more likely, because PAF may have an obligate role in the implantation process. Acker *et al.* (1988) showed that, in rats, the instillation of 10 nmol of the PAF antagonist BN52021 into the uterine horn on day 4 inhibited implantation; this treatment was much less effective on other days of pregnancy. It should be noted, however, that inhibitors of the prostanoid cyclo-oxygenase and lipoxygenase enzymes were equally effective in the same protocol. Systemic injections of BN52021 were not effective. In mice, i.p. injection of another PAF antagonist – SRI63-441 – on the first 4 days of pregnancy inhibited implantation. Iloprost, a stable analogue of PGI_2, similarly inhibited implantation, and its effect could be reversed by concomitant administration of PAF (Spinks & O'Neill, 1987). In view of the actions of the prostanoid synthesis inhibitors, it cannot be concluded that Iloprost is acting solely through inhibition of PAF synthesis or action. Taken together, however, the results are suggestive of the importance of endometrial PAF in the preparation for implantation.

One of the earliest events that occurs at the implantation site is an increase in capillary permeability in the stroma. In part this is due, at least in the rabbit, to the release of prostaglandin E_2 from the blastocyst (Jones & Harper, 1984; Jones *et al.*, 1985), which is transported across the epithelium to the stroma (Cao *et al.*, 1984), where receptors for this prostaglandin are located (Kennedy *et al.*, 1983). In view of the induction of vascular permeability by PAF, and its presence followed by disappearance at the critical time before implantation when capillary permeability is increased by the presence of the blastocyst (Jones *et al.*, 1986), it seems probable that PAF is an important regulator of uterine permeability. Indeed, Smith and Kelly (1988) recently showed that PAF causes a dose-dependent increase in prostaglandin E_2 by an enriched glandular cell culture of secretory human endometrium. Stromal cell cultures were not stimulated by PAF, and prostaglandin $F_{2\alpha}$ was not changed in either type of cell culture. These observations indicate a delicate interplay between these different autocoids.

In other experiments, we have found that rabbit uterine membranes exhibit specific binding sites for [^{3}H]PAF, and that these sites are located in the endometrium and not the myometrium. Two classes of binding sites have been observed, a high-affinity and a low-affinity component, in an enriched plasma cell membrane fraction from a whole uterus homogenate (Kudolo & Harper, 1989). The apparent K_D values for the type 1 and 2 sites were 3.49 ± 0.61 nmol/l and 114.26 ± 12.98 nmol/l respectively. The binding capacities (B_{max}) were 3.84 ± 0.60 and 164.33 ± 56 pmol/mg membrane protein respectively. Saturation analysis using a purified *endometrial* membrane preparation, however, gave an apparent K_D value of 0.79 ± 0.46 nmol/l, and a B_{max} of 376.82 ± 163.30 fmol/mg protein for the type 1 sites (Kudolo & Harper, 1989). These latter incubations were done at a ligand concentration of 4 nmol/l, for 150 minutes at 4°C. Kinetic analysis using the same membrane preparation gave a calculated K_D of 3.28 ± 1.14 nmol/l. Although these K_D values are similar to those reported for the hypothalamus (Junier *et al.*, 1988), the binding capacities are greater. The reason for this discrepancy is not known, but the derived values could be inflated by the metabolism of the ligand that occurs during the binding incubations. Only 40% of the [^{3}H]PAF remained unchanged after 150 minutes incubation at 25°C: 16% was recovered as lyso-PAF and 40% as alkylacyl-GPC (Kudolo & Harper, 1989). Further studies are needed to refine these values, but, nonetheless, it seems clear that the endometrium does contain abundant specific binding sites for PAF. Preliminary studies suggest that binding affinities for PAF to uterine membranes do not differ between various stages of pregnancy (unpublished data), but whether binding capacity changes remains to be determined. The presence of endogenous inhibitors of PAF has been reported in the estrous rat uterus (Nakayama *et al.*, 1987). About 10^5 times greater concentration of these compounds is necessary to inhibit the action of PAF, and their concentration in the uterus was of this required magnitude. Their function is not known, but they could act to regulate the activity of PAF in the uterus, if they are also hormonally regulated in an inverse manner to PAF.

Concluding remarks and future directions for research

At present, it is not known whether the PAF binding sites are on the stromal or glandular cell membranes, or both. Thus, the question regarding autocrine or paracrine regulation of endometrial cell function is still open. Nevertheless, it is certain that PAF is produced by the stromal cells, and that this synthesis is hormonally regulated. Furthermore, it seems that uterine PAF concentrations are reduced by the presence of a blastocyst, and presumably the released PAF could cause increased leakiness of the stroma, luminal epithelial breakdown and neovascularization. The uterus could presumably react similarly to the presence of an IUD. Whether a foreign body, in addition, stimulates PAF synthesis remains to be determined, but given the interrelationship between PAF and prostaglandins, this seems possible.

Recent studies have demonstrated that endothelial cells from diverse vascular beds both produce and accumulate PAF, and that accumulation occurs in response to soluble mediators, such as bradykinin and angiotensin II (Whatley *et al.*, 1988). The endothelial cell is strategically located to mediate hemostatic and inflammatory events. PAF accumulation in such cells is associated with release of PGI_2, and the combination of pro-inflammatory and vasoactive substances may result in increased vascular permeability, amplification of endothelial cell breakdown and vasodilatation (Whatley *et al.*, 1988). Thus, PAF is likely to be implicated in inappropriate endometrial bleeding.

In the same context, it seems probable that whenever prostaglandin levels are increased pathologically, PAF levels will also be increased, e.g. in dysmenorrhea, endometritis and abnormal uterine bleeding. Smith and Kelly (1988) have already shown that PAF stimulates endometrial glandular release of the vasodilatory prostaglandin E_2, and so there is evidence to support this speculation. The known stimulation of PAF production by stromal cells under progestational dominance (Angle *et al.*, 1988; Alecozay *et al.*, 1989), the occurrence of breakthrough endometrial bleeding in women using progestogen-only contraceptive pills or long-acting preparations (see Diczfalusy *et al.*, 1980), and the involvement of platelets in the menstrual process (Sixma *et al.*, 1980), all provide further evidence for a probable role of PAF in endometrial bleeding.

It seems essential, therefore, to investigate urgently whether PAF synthesis and release are stimulated inappropriately in such conditions, and as a practical matter to determine whether any of the potent PAF antagonists can alleviate the occurrence of inappropriate endometrial bleeding. Some of these antagonists can act systemically, but it is not certain that they can enter the uterine cavity in adequate concentration; it may therefore be necessary to examine their effect given directly into the uterine lumen, as has been done with antifibrinolytic agents (Weström & Bengtsson, 1970). In the case of the PAF antagonists, a compound such as L-659,989 [(+/-)-trans-2-(3-methoxy-5-methyl-sulfonyl-4-propoxyphenyl)-5-(3,4,5-tri–methoxyphenyl)-tetrahydrofuran] exhibits an equilibrium inhibition constant for PAF binding to rabbit platelets of 1.1 nmol/l, which is one to two orders of magnitude lower than that of other PAF antagonists. In addition, L-659,989 is orally active in rats, and has a duration of action of 12–16 hours after an oral dose of only 1 mg/kg (Ponpipom *et al.*, 1988). Thus, the need for large doses of the antagonists may be avoided. The availability of a wide variety of PAF antagonists, some of which have already been clinically tested, provides good hope for rapid progress in the elucidation of the role of PAF in endometrial bleeding. However, it should be noted that PAF has great molecular heterogeneity (Ludwig & Pinckard, 1987), and that since most PAF antagonists have been tested using inhibition of PAF activity on platelets, it is not certain that all antagonists will be equally effective in other tissues. This is certainly the case with endometrial membrane PAF binding sites, where only structural analogues will displace the [^{3}H]PAF (Kudolo & Harper, 1988).

Acknowledgements

Work described in this chapter was financially supported in part by NIH grants HD14048 and HD25224, a Lalor Foundation Fellowship to G.B. Kudolo, and a technical services agreement from the Special Programme of Research, Development and Research Training in Human Reproduction, World Health Organization.

References

Acker, G., Hecquet, F., Etienne, A., Braquet, P. & Mencia-Huerta, J.M. (1988). Role of platelet-activating factor (PAF) in the ovoimplantation in the rat: effect of the specific PAF-acether antagonist, BN52021. *Prostaglandins*, **35**:233–241.

Alecozay, A.A., Casslén, B.G., Riehl, R.M., DeLeon, F.D., Harper, M.J.K., Silva, M., Nouchi, T.A. & Hanahan, D.J. (1989). Platelet-activating factor in human luteal phase endometrium. *Biology of Reproduction*, **41**:578–586.

Angle, M.J., Jones, M.A., McManus, L.M., Pinckard, R.N. & Harper, M.J.K. (1988). Platelet-activating factor in the rabbit uterus during early pregnancy. *Journal of Reproduction and Fertility*, **83**:711–722.

Angle, M.J., McManus, L.M. & Pinckard, R.N. (1986). Age-dependent differential development of leukotactic and vasoactive responsiveness to acute inflammatory mediators. *Laboratory Investigation*, **55**:616–621.

Benveniste, J., Henson, P.M. & Cochrane, C.G. (1972). Leukocyte-dependent histamine release from rabbit platelets: the role of IgE, basophils, and a platelet-activating factor. *Journal of Experimental Medicine*, **136**:1356–1377.

Braquet, P. & Godfroid, J.J. (1986). PAF-acether specific binding sites: 2. Design of specific antagonists. *Trends in Pharmacological Sciences*, **7**:397–403.

Braquet, P., Touqui, L., Shen, T.Y. & Vargaftig, B.B. (1987). Perspectives in platelet-activating factor research. *Pharmacological Reviews*, **39**:97–145.

Cao, Z.D., Jones, M.A. & Harper, M.J.K. (1984). Prostaglandin translocation from the lumen of the rabbit uterus *in vitro* in relation to day of pregnancy or pseudopregnancy. *Biology of Reproduction*, **31**:505–519.

Demopoulos, C.A., Pinckard, R.N. & Hanahan, D.J. (1979). Platelet-activating factor. Evidence for 1-0-alkyl-2-acetyl-**sn**-glyceryl-3-phosphorylcholine as the active component (a new class of lipid chemical mediators). *Journal of Biological Chemistry*, **254**:9355–9358.

Diczfalusy, E., Fraser, I.S. & Webb, F.T.G., eds. (1980). *Endometrial Bleeding and Steroidal Contraception*. Bath, England, Pitman Press.

Folch, J., Lees, M. & Sloane-Stanley, G.H. (1957). A simple method for the isolation and purification of total lipids from animal tissues. *Journal of Biological Chemistry*, **226**:497–509.

Humphrey, D.M., McManus, L.M., Hanahan, D.J. & Pinckard, R.N. (1984). Morphologic basis of increased vascular permeability induced by acetyl glyceryl ether phosphorylcholine. *Laboratory Investigation*, **50**:16–25.

Humphrey, D.M., McManus, L.M., Satouchi, K., Hanahan, D.J. & Pinckard, R.N. (1982). Vasoactive properties of acetyl glyceryl ether phosphorylcholine and analogues. *Laboratory Investigation*, **46**:422–427.

Hwang, S.B. (1987). Specific receptor sites for platelet-activating factor on rat liver plasma membranes. *Archives of Biochemistry and Biophysics*, **257**:339–344.

Jones, M.A., Anderson, W., Turner, T.G. & Harper, M.J.K. (1985). Storage *in vivo* of [^{3}H]prostaglandins by rabbit blastocysts. *Endocrinology*, **116**:993–997.

Jones, M.A., Cao, Z.D., Anderson, W., Norris, C. & Harper, M.J.K. (1986). Capillary permeability changes in the uteri of recipient rabbits after transfer of blastocysts from indomethacin-treated donors. *Journal of Reproduction and Fertility*, **78**:261–273.

Jones, M.A. & Harper, M.J.K. (1984). Rabbit blastocysts accumulate [^{3}H]prostaglandins *in vitro*. *Endocrinology*, **115**:817–823.

Junier, M.P., Tiberghien, C., Rougeot, C., Fafeur, V. & Dray, F. (1988). Inhibitory effect of platelet-activating factor (PAF) on luteinizing hormone-releasing hormone and somatostatin release from rat median eminence *in vitro* correlated with the characterization of specific PAF receptor sites in rat hypothalamus. *Endocrinology*, **123**:72–80.

Kennedy, T.G., Martel, D. & Psychoyos, A. (1983). Endometrial prostaglandin E_2 binding: characterization in rats sensitized for the decidual cell reaction and changes during pseudopregnancy. *Biology of Reproduction*, **29**:556–564.

Kudolo, G.B. & Harper, M.J.K. (1989). Characterization of platelet-activating factor binding sites on uterine membranes from pregnant rabbits. *Biology of Reproduction*, **41**:587–603.

Lanara, E., Vakirtzi-Lemonias, C., Kritikou, L. & Demopoulos, C.A. (1982). Response of mice and mouse platelets to acetyl glyceryl ether phosphorylcholine. *Biochemical and Biophysical Research Communications*, **109**:1148–1156.

Ludwig, J.C. & Pinckard, R.N. (1987). Diversity in the chemical structures of neutrophil-derived platelet-activating factors. (In) *New Horizons in Platelet-activating Factor Research* (Winslow, C.M. & Lee, M.L., eds.), pp.59–71. New York, John Wiley & Sons.

Miwa, M., Hill, C., Kumar, R., Sugatani, J., Olson, M.S. & Hanahan, D.J. (1987). Occurrence of an endogenous inhibitor of platelet-activating factor in rat liver. *Journal of Biological Chemistry*, **262**:527–530.

Nakayama, R., Yasuda, K. & Saito, K. (1987). Existence of endogenous inhibitors of platelet-activating factor (PAF) with PAF in rat uterus. *Journal of Biological Chemistry*, **262**:13174–13179.

Namm, D.H., Tadepalli, A.S. & High, J.A. (1982). Species specificity of the platelet responses to 1-0-alkyl-2-acetyl-**sn**-glycero-3-phosphocholine. *Thrombosis Research*, **25**:341–350.

O'Flaherty, J.T., Redman, J.F. Jr, Schmitt, J.D., Ellis, J.M., Surles, J.R., Marx, M.H., Piantadosi, C. & Wykle, R.L. (1987). 1-0-alkyl-2-N-methylcarbamyl-glycerophosphocholine: a biologically potent, non-metabolizable analog of platelet-activating factor. *Biochemical and Biophysical Research Communications*, **147**:18–24.

O'Neill, C. (1985a). Thrombocytopenia is an initial maternal response to fertilization in mice. *Journal of Reproduction and Fertility*, **73**:559–566.

O'Neill, C. (1985b). Examination of the causes of early pregnancy-associated thrombocytopenia in mice. *Journal of Reproduction and Fertility*, **73**:567–577.

O'Neill, C. (1985c). Partial characterization of the embryo-derived platelet-activating factor in mice. *Journal of Reproduction and Fertility*, **75**:375–380.

O'Neill, C. (1987). Embryo-derived platelet-activating factor: a preimplantation embryo mediator of maternal recognition of pregnancy. *Domestic Animal Endocrinology*, **4**:69–86.

O'Neill, C., Gidley-Baird, A.A., Pike, I.L., Porter, R.N., Sinosich, M.J. & Saunders, D.M. (1985). Maternal blood platelet physiology and luteal-phase endocrinology as a means of monitoring pre- and post-implantation embryo viability following *in vitro* fertilization. *Journal of In Vitro Fertilization and Embryo Transfer*, **2**:87–93.

Orozco, C., Perkins, T. & Clarke, F.M. (1986). Platelet-activating factor induces the expression of early pregnancy factor activity in female mice. *Journal of Reproduction and Fertility*, **78**:549–555.

Pinckard, R.N. (1983). Platelet activating factor. *Hospital Practice*, **70**:67–76.

Pinckard, R.N., Farr, R.S. & Hanahan, D.J. (1979). Physicochemical and functional identity of platelet-activating factor (PAF) released *in vivo* during IgE anaphylaxis with PAF released *in vitro* from IgE sensitized rabbit basophils. *Journal of Immunology*, **123**:1847–1857.

Pinckard, R.N., Jackson, E.M., Hoppens, C., Weintraub, S.T., Ludwig, J.C., McManus, L.M. & Mott, G.E. (1984). Molecular heterogeneity of platelet-activating factor produced by stimulated human polymorphonuclear leukocytes. *Biochemical and Biophysical Research Communications*, **122**:325–332.

Pinckard, R.N., McManus, L.M., Halonen, M., Humphrey, D.M. & Hanahan, D.J. (1983). Acetyl glyceryl ether phosphorylcholine (AGEPC). A model anaphylactomimetic mediator. (In) *Biological Response Mediators and Modulators* (August, J.T., ed.), pp.67–82. New York, Academic Press.

Pinckard, R.N., McManus, L.M. & Hanahan, D.J. (1982). Chemistry and biology of acetyl glyceryl ether phosphorylcholine (platelet-activating factor). (In) *Advances in Inflammation Research*, Vol.4 (Weissmann, G., ed.), pp.147–180. New York, Raven Press.

Ponpipom, M.M., Hwang, S.-B., Doebber, T.W., Acton, J.J., Alberts, A.W., Biftu, T., Brooker, D.R., Bugianesi, R.L., Chabala, J.C., Gamble, N.L., Graham, D.W., Lam, M.-H. & Wu, M.S. (1988). (+/-)-Trans-2-(3-methoxy-5-methylsulfonyl-4-propoxyphenyl)-5- (3,4,5-trimethoxyphenyl) tetrahydrofuran (L-659,989), a novel, potent PAF receptor antagonist. *Biochemical and Biophysical Research Communications*, **150**:1213–1220.

Sixma, J.J., Christiaens, G.C.M.L. & Haspels, A.A. (1980). The sequence of haemostatic events in the endometrium during normal menstruation. (In) *Endometrial Bleeding and Steroidal Contraception* (Diczfalusy, E., Fraser, I.S. & Webb, F.T.G., eds.), pp.86–96. Bath, England, Pitman Press.

Smith, S.K. & Kelly, R.W. (1988). Effect of platelet-activating factor on the release of PGF-2α and PGE-2 by separated cells of human endometrium. *Journal of Reproduction and Fertility*, **82**:271–276.

Spinks, N.R. & O'Neill, C. (1987). Embryo-derived platelet-activating factor is essential for establishment of pregnancy in the mouse. *Lancet*, **1**:106–107.

Weström, L. & Bengtsson, L.P. (1970). Effect of tranexamic acid (AMCA) in menorrhagia with intrauterine contraceptive devices. A double blind study. *Journal of Reproductive Medicine*, **5**(4):41–48.

Whatley, R.E., Zimmerman, G.A., McIntyre, T.M. & Prescott, S.M. (1988). Endothelium from diverse vascular sources synthesizes platelet-activating factor. *Arteriosclerosis*, **8**:321–331.

Yasuda, K., Satouchi, K. & Saito, K. (1986). Platelet-activating factor in normal rat uterus. *Biochemical and Biophysical Research Communications*, **138**:1231–1236.

Discussion

Findlay. Dr Harper, you said that you could only find PAF in the stromal cells. The receptors are on the membranes of some cell types in the endometrium; why are you not picking it up in the media, and how is it going to act if it is intracellular? Is it metabolized in the medium? And how are PAF and prostaglandins related?

Harper. Any time that you get prostaglandins increasing, you are almost certainly going to get PAF increased. Because when alkylacyl-GPC is being produced by phospholipase A_2 and then via lyso-PAF is converted to PAF itself, you get arachidonic acid split off from that second carbon atom before the acetylation. So the two are totally interrelated. On the metabolism question, I think that if PAF gets out of the cell into the circulation, it is going to be rapidly metabolized. I did not even mention that there are also endogenous inhibitors which can block the actions of PAF as well, and we really do not know what the functions of these are.

Findlay. It is still not clear to me why you are not measuring release into the medium from the stromal cells.

Harper. Because it is not normally released from the cells. Maybe there needs to be some trigger which causes release. I do not have the answer.

Findlay. If PAF binds to a membrane receptor, does it have to get out of the cell before it gets on to the membrane?

Harper. The receptors may be on the inside, the outside or both sides of the membrane.

Hirata. Relating to the metabolism of PAF, you indicated that progesterone increased PAF formation in the stromal cells. Which receptors are stimulated by the progesterone treatment?

Harper. I do not know. We have not looked for progesterone receptors in these cells. Increased PAF can result from increased synthesis or a decrease in metabolism. This is not known, yet. All that I can tell you is that there is a higher concentration of PAF in the cell, and it is not secreted into the medium. This is very early work so there is obviously much more we need to do.

Ludwig. I am not aware of a defect of the platelet-activating factor, but in thrombocytopenic patients, platelet activation is reduced, because of the decreased number of platelets. Several times, we have observed that thrombocytopenic patients have heavy menstruation. They bleed for 7 days or more and their total blood loss is increased. Current therapy in gynecology is to put them on a combined oral contraceptive which reduces bleeding time and decreases blood loss. However, the platelet counts are still low. Their bleeding time from other sites is still prolonged, only the uterus acts with reduced bleeding time and with reduced blood loss. My question is, do you have any explanation for this? Does platelet-activating factor play a role, and is it activated by degrading tissue?

Harper. The short answer is no, but we know from O'Neill's work in Australia that early stage embryos from mouse and human do apparently secrete PAF *in vitro* (O'Neill, 1985; O'Neill *et al.*, 1987). In pregnant animals or in-vitro fertilization (IVF) patients who are going to become pregnant, there is a marked thrombocytopenia. Inside the uterus, I do not know if thrombocytopenia occurs. I do not think anyone has studied this.

Casey. In reply to Dr Findlay's question, I do not have the answer, but I believe that there is evidence that PAF is secreted from the macrophage (Elstad *et al.*, 1988), but not by certain other cell types.

Harper. We have not been able to do any localization. The lack of antibodies to PAF is a major constraint at this point. One would like to do some autoradiographic studies, but until we solve the problem of PAF metabolism, those are not going to be feasible because we do not know what metabolites are there.

References

Elstad, M.R., Prescott, S.M., McIntyre, T.M. & Zimmerman, G.A. (1988). Synthesis and release of platelet-activating factor by stimulated human mononuclear phagocytes. *Journal of Immunology*, **140**:1618–1624.

O'Neill, C. (1985). Partial characterization of the embryo-derived platelet-activating factor in mice. *Journal of Reproduction and Fertility*, **75**:375–380.

O'Neill, C., Gidley-Baird, A.A., Pike, I.L. & Saunders, D.M. (1987). Use of a bioassay for embryo-derived platelet-activating factor as a means of assessing quality and pregnancy potential of human embryos. *Fertility and Sterility*, **47**:969–975.

Biomolecular mechanisms in human parturition: activation of uterine decidua

M. LINETTE CASEY AND PAUL C. MACDONALD

The Cecil H. and Ida Green Center for Reproductive Biology Sciences, and the Departments of Biochemistry and Obstetrics–Gynecology, University of Texas Southwestern Medical Center, Dallas, Texas, USA.

Abstract

There is appreciable evidence in support of the view that the biomolecular events critical to the initiation of parturition in the human transpire in response to the action of bioactive agents (including prostaglandins) formed *in situ* in uterine decidua and myometrium and in extraembryonic fetal tissues. The parturitional process *per se* involves at least two coordinated components of uterine function: (i) uterine preparedness for labour, and (ii) the myometrial contractions that effect delivery of the fetus. The functional component of this process that serves to promote uterine preparedness for labour causes cervical ripening, increased uterine sensitivity to uterotonic agents (e.g. prostaglandins and oxytocin), an increase in the number of oxytocin receptors in myometrium, and an increase in the number of gap junctions between myometrial cells. It is extraordinarily important, we believe, to recognize that these biochemical and morphologic adaptations of the uterus, which are preparatory to labour, occur in all mammalian species irrespective of differences in endocrine physiology that precede or accompany labour. Thus, it seems likely that the basic processes involved in uterine preparedness for parturition are similar in all species. This is a satisfying concept because it enables us to set aside, temporarily, the fundamental differences between the endocrine physiology of parturition in most mammalian species (e.g. the sheep model) and that in primates, including the human – differences that sometimes appear to present an insurmountable impasse to an understanding of parturitional processes.

We suggest that, in the human, menstruation is the parturition of failed fertility. Moreover, we speculate that there is a key intermediate modulator that will link the biochemical events of parturition that occur in decidua and those of menstruation that occur in endometrium. Presently, there are three principal hypotheses concerning the mechanisms by which parturition is initiated (progesterone withdrawal, the oxytocin theory, and the fetal–maternal organ communication system postulate); but in each of these, so far as we can ascertain, there is some role envisioned for the prostaglandins, which are generated in uterine decidua, myometrium, and extraembryonic fetal tissues. Indeed, this premise (an obligatory role for prostaglandins in parturition) also is one that embraces yet another concept, namely, that parturition is regulated by way of paracrine events that involve uterine tissues and extraembryonic fetal membranes. Thus, we propose that the decidua serves a key role in the biomolecular events that lead to the initiation of parturition.

Introduction

Evidence of decidual activation during parturition has been accruing for a number of years. And today, there are a number of reasons to believe that decidual activation may be the penultimate event in the parturitional process. Teleologically, it is satisfying to believe that the events of parturition and those of menstruation in primates involve similar phenomena. If this were true, the critical role of the endometrium/decidua in the two processes is self-evident. For example, it is easy to accept the proposition that progesterone withdrawal is extraordinarily important in the induction of menstruation in primates just as it is evident that progesterone withdrawal is vitally important in parturition in many species other than primates. It also is reasonable to surmise that the bioactive uterotropins (agents that act to cause uterine preparedness for labour) and uterotonins (agents that act to cause the myometrial contractions of labour) of parturition are produced in tissues contiguous with the myometrium, namely, the decidua.

It is well known that in sheep (the species in which the physiological events of parturition are best defined), there is a precise sequence of endocrine events that seem to herald the onset of labour (for review, see Challis & Olson, 1988). Increased responsiveness of the sheep fetal adrenal to ACTH results in increased cortisol secretion; fetal cortisol acts upon trophoblasts to cause an increase in the expression of the cytochrome P-450 enzyme, steroid 17α-hydroxylase (17,20-desmolase); in consequence, there is a decrease in progesterone secretion and an increase in estrogen formation. Progesterone withdrawal and an increase in estrogen, by way of mechanisms not yet defined, promote an increase in the formation of prostaglandin $F_{2\alpha}$ ($PGF_{2\alpha}$) in decidua and the onset of labour. Progesterone withdrawal does not occur in human pregnancy (Batra *et al.*, 1976). Nonetheless, uterine preparedness for labour, as well as labour itself, does occur despite the lack of progesterone withdrawal; and it may be that the biomolecular processes that eventuate in uterine preparedness for and the contractions of labour are similar in all mammalian species.

It seems reasonable, therefore, to evaluate the possibility that uterotropins and uterotonins are produced in intrauterine or extraembryonic fetal tissues in all species, irrespective of the precise nature of the endocrine events that transpire before the time of parturition. Accepting the likelihood of the correctness of this argument, it is then crucial to identify the bioactive products of the uterine and extraembryonic fetal tissues produced during parturition and to define the metabolic function of these agents in appreciable detail.

This proposition also is important if one also assumes that the 'trigger' for the initiation of parturition may not be a uterotonin or uterotropin: namely, it is quite likely that the bioactive agents (uterotropins and uterotonins) of parturition are produced synchronously with parturition and not before. In the past, many of us have searched for a 'trigger' for the initiation of parturition among those agents known to be active to cause myometrial contractions, i.e. prostaglandins or oxytocin, or both. This was probably an unreasonable expectation. It now seems much more likely that whatever the trigger for parturition, however it is operative, the generation of uterotropins and uterotonins probably occurs with and not before the parturitional event.

Evidence in favour of some obligatory role for the prostaglandins in parturition has been reviewed on many occasions (Novy & Liggins, 1980; Bleasdale & Johnston, 1985; Casey & MacDonald, 1986). Stated briefly, the salient features of this argument are as follows. (i) Prostaglandins act to cause myometrial contractions and thence abortion or labour at any stage of gestation. (ii) The levels of prostaglandin E_2 (PGE_2) and prostaglandin $F_{2\alpha}$ ($PGF_{2\alpha}$) or metabolites thereof are increased strikingly in amniotic fluid and in blood and urine of women during labour. (iii) Inhibitors of prostaglandin synthesis delay the onset of parturition, arrest the premature onset of labour, and delay the induction–abortion interval.

The capacity to produce prostaglandins has been demonstrated in human extraembryonic fetal membranes and in the human uterine decidua and myometrium. Moreover, there is evidence that all uterine and extraembryonic fetal tissues are activated to new levels of metabolic function during parturition (cf. Casey & MacDonald, 1986). These new levels of metabolic activity include the generation of bioactive agents that are probably important in parturition – agents that may serve as uterotropins or as uterotonins, or both.

Activation of uterine tissues during parturition

Decidua

Today, there is reason to believe that decidual activation will, through the generation of bioactive agents in this tissue, bring about activation of contiguous fetal membranes as well as myometrium. But more than this, there is reason to believe that premature decidual activation by way of xenobiotics, e.g. bacterial endotoxin lipopolysaccharide (LPS), is a common cause of preterm labour.

Prostaglandins of decidual origin

One of the fundamental reasons for believing that activation of decidua to new levels of metabolic function is important in parturition is the finding of increased concentrations of $PGF_{2\alpha}$ and 13,14-dihydro-15-keto-prostaglandin $F_{2\alpha}$ (PGFM) in amniotic fluid during labour (Dray & Frydman, 1976; Ghodgaonkar *et al.*, 1979) together with the finding of increased levels of PGFM in maternal plasma during labour (Ghodgaonkar *et al.*, 1979; Satoh *et al.*, 1979). The importance of this finding is related to the fact that neither amnion nor chorion laeve produces $PGF_{2\alpha}$ in significant amounts (Kinoshita *et al.*, 1978; Okazaki *et al.*, 1981). Thus, the $PGF_{2\alpha}$ and metabolites thereof must be derived from tissue sources other than the fetal membranes or else PGE_2 produced in fetal membranes must be converted to $PGF_{2\alpha}$. This latter possibility is very unlikely. The enzyme that catalyzes the conversion of PGE_2 to $PGF_{2\alpha}$, i.e. PGE_2-9-ketoreductase, is demonstrable in decidual tissue (Schlegel *et al.*, 1984; Niesert *et al.*, 1986); but, the specific activity of this enzyme in decidua is very low and is orders of magnitude less than the specific activity of prostaglandin dehydrogenase (PGDH) (Niesert *et al.*, 1986). Thus, it is highly unlikely that PGE_2 arising in fetal membranes is converted in appreciable quantities to $PGF_{2\alpha}$.

The decidua is known to produce both $PGF_{2\alpha}$ and PGE_2 (Kinoshita *et al.*, 1978; Okazaki *et al.*, 1981). Therefore, the increase in $PGF_{2\alpha}$ formation during labour is likely to arise by way of the formation of this primary prostaglandin in decidual tissue. There seems to be an increase in the concentration of PGE_2 in amniotic fluid during labour that precedes the increase in concentration of $PGF_{2\alpha}$ or PGFM (Dray & Frydman, 1976). This may be indicative of a simultaneous increase in PGE_2 in the fetal membranes during labour and relatively greater entry of PGE_2 from membranes (which are contiguous with the amniotic fluid) into amniotic fluid during early labour. But as labour progresses, there is a greater increase in both $PGF_{2\alpha}$ and PGFM than in PGE_2, perhaps reflective of the preferential production of $PGF_{2\alpha}$ in decidua and its ultimate entry into amniotic fluid. Thus, $PGF_{2\alpha}$ and PGFM may represent markers of decidual activation during parturition.

A somewhat curious and as yet inexplicable phenomenon is the fact that the rate of $PGF_{2\alpha}$ production during labour is very low (Casey & MacDonald, 1988). There is a clear-cut increase in the concentration of PGFM in plasma during parturition and there is a striking increase in the concentration of both $PGF_{2\alpha}$ and PGFM in amniotic fluid during parturition (as long as the fetal membranes are intact), but the computed rate of formation of $PGF_{2\alpha}$ is small. Nonetheless, this is consistent with the observation that, at term, the amount of infused $PGF_{2\alpha}$ required to produce labour also is small. And, the amount of infused $PGF_{2\alpha}$ that reaches myometrium to cause labour and that produced in intrauterine tissues during labour are similar. This has prompted us to consider the likelihood that there is 'iron-handed' regulation of $PGF_{2\alpha}$ formation in decidua during pregnancy, a process that may be fundamental to the maintenance of pregnancy.

Arachidonic acid release from decidua during labour
There is no direct evidence that arachidonic acid is released from decidua during parturition. Nonetheless, there is appreciable indirect evidence in support of this probability: the concentration of arachidonic acid in amniotic fluid increases during parturition (MacDonald *et al.*, 1974; Keirse *et al.*, 1977); moreover, there is a steady increase in the concentration of this free fatty acid

in amniotic fluid as a function of the progress (duration) of labour (Keirse *et al.*, 1977). Arachidonic acid is lost from amnion and chorion laeve phosphatidylinositol and phosphatidylethanolamine during early labour (Okita *et al.*, 1982). For this reason, we originally took the view that the arachidonic acid in amniotic fluid arose by liberation of this fatty acid from glycerophospholipids in the fetal membranes during parturition. And this may be the case during early labour. But also the arachidonic acid content of amnion and chorion laeve is replenished as labour progresses (Okita, 1981). This is a very important consideration because it then becomes evident that there is a net gain in the arachidonic acid composition of the fetal membrane–amniotic fluid compartment during labour. This gain in the essential fatty acid composition of this compartment (all components of which are avascular) must have come from arachidonic acid released from another tissue site. This obtains because all of the arachidonic acid in amnion arises by way of the amniotic fluid (Okita *et al.*, 1983). This fact was established by studies of the arachidonic acid composition and distribution in glycerophospholipids in the fused and non-fused portions of amnion and chorion laeve of diamnionic–dichorionic twin placentae.

One source of amniotic fluid arachidonic acid during labour that has been suggested is fetal lung secretions. In the remodelling of surfactant phosphatidylcholine to produce the disaturated form of this lipid, arachidonic acid is probably released during the remodelling process. We reject this formulation of the source of arachidonic acid in amniotic fluid, however, for several reasons. First, there is, during labour and possibly for 1 or 2 days or more before the onset of labour, a decrease in fetal breathing movements (Castle & Turnbull, 1985). This would favour a decrease in the excretion of lung secretions into the amniotic fluid. Second, and perhaps most importantly, the increase in amniotic fluid-free arachidonic acid seems to occur after the onset of labour and is progressive during labour; i.e. there is no documented increase in free arachidonic acid in amniotic fluid before the onset of parturition. These findings, together with the likelihood of increased $PGF_{2\alpha}$ formation in decidua during parturition, are suggestive that the net gain in arachidonic acid in the fetal membrane–amniotic fluid compartment during labour is the result of transfer of liberated arachidonic (or linoleic) acid from decidua to amniotic fluid.

Platelet-activating factor (PAF) formation in decidua

The formation of PAF in decidua also has been demonstrated (Ban *et al.*, 1986). In the case of decidua, unlike that of amnion, PAF formed in this tissue is secreted into the extracellular space. Therefore, the possibility must be considered that the PAF in amniotic fluid during labour arises, at least in large measure, from activated decidua. If this were the case, the simultaneous release of arachidonic acid, the formation of $PGF_{2\alpha}$, and the secretion of PAF by a single tissue are even more reminiscent of the response of macrophages to challenge. And because of the macrophage-like properties of the decidua, this would be supportive of the likelihood that parturition involves a set of biomolecular events analogous to those known to occur in stimulated monocytes/macrophages. It is this line of reasoning that led us to evaluate the possibility that other bioactive agents of parturition may be found by examining amniotic fluid for products known to be released by macrophages in response to a variety of stimuli.

Cytokines formed in decidua during parturition

As stated, the stimulated macrophage responds to a number of challenges by way of a robust response that includes the release of free arachidonic acid and prostaglandins (Kunkel & Chensue, 1986), PAF (Albert & Snyder, 1983), and interleukin-1 (IL-1) (Gery *et al.*, 1971). IL-1 is an immunohormone and is active in a number of tissues outside the immune system in provoking a series of responses, among which is increased prostaglandin formation in responsive tissues (Bernheim & Dinarello, 1985; Wood *et al.*, 1985; Balavoine *et al.*, 1986; Chang *et al.*, 1986; Casey *et al.*, 1988b). And, IL-1β mRNA and protein are expressed in human decidual tissue (Casey *et al.*, 1988b; Romero *et al.*, 1989). Thus, we set out to ascertain whether IL-1 levels in amniotic fluid were increased during spontaneous parturition.

We found that IL-1β is not present or else is present in low or undetectable amounts in amniotic fluid obtained at any stage of gestation before the onset of labour (Cox *et al.*, 1988a). But after spontaneous labour at term, there sometimes (but not always) is a striking increase in the concentration of IL-1β to levels of approximately 1.7 ng/ml on average (Cox *et al.*, 1988a). We believe this to be an important finding for several reasons. (i) An increase in IL-1β in amniotic fluid during labour provides further support for the probability of decidual activation during parturition. (ii) IL-1β acts on amnion to cause an increase in PGE$_2$ formation (Casey *et al.*, 1988b). Thus, activation of decidua may give rise to activation of the fetal membranes at a time when the amniotic fluid concentration of arachidonic acid is too low to support EGF receptor-mediated increases in PGE$_2$ formation by an increase in the synthesis of PGH$_2$ synthase (Casey *et al.*, 1987; Casey *et al.*, 1988a). (iii) An increase in IL-1β is further support for the macrophage-like properties of the decidua. (iv) IL-1β is a bioactive immunohormone that may serve as a uterotropin and indirectly cause an increase in uterotonins by way of the stimulation of PGF$_{2\alpha}$ formation in decidua (Casey *et al.*, 1988b).

Activators of decidua during parturition

Based on the evidence cited, it seems reasonable to predict that an important clue to the physiologic and pathophysiologic bases of parturition in women lies in the identity of the bioactive agents that are characteristic of labour. Again, this bioactive agent set is comprised of arachidonic acid, prostaglandins, IL-1β, platelet-activating factor, and probably a number of other agents.

These agents also are those that are produced by stimulated macrophages, and, as stated, it is likely that activated, macrophage-like decidua is a principal site of origin of these agents. The question then arises as to the nature – or, more precisely, the identity – of the agent(s) that serves to activate uterine decidua vera.

IL-1β, also referred to in the past as lymphocyte activator, endogenous pyrogen and other names, is a potent immunomodulator–immunohormone that serves key functions in response to inflammatory and immunologic challenges. IL-1β is produced primarily in monocytes and macrophages; but, this cytokine also is produced in a number of other cell types, including decidua and endometrial stromal cells (Casey *et al.*, 1988b). It is established that one mechanism of IL-1β action in responsive cells involves the stimulation of prostaglandin (Raz *et al.*, 1988) and platelet-activating factor production (Bussolino *et al.*, 1986).

IL-1β may serve a similar role in promoting prostaglandin synthesis in uterine endometrium in the initiation of menstruation. Macrophages obtained from the peritoneal cavity of women before ovulation (Glover *et al.*, 1987) do not produce IL-1β, whereas those obtained during the luteal phase of the cycle do. Thus, progesterone may serve to modulate the rate of IL-1β formation. IL-1β is synthesized as pro-IL-1β (mol. wt approximately 31 500). This larger molecular weight form of IL-1β is not secreted from the cell but rather accumulates in the cytoplasm.

We envision the role of IL-1β as a key intermediary in the regulation of prostaglandin biosynthesis in uterine decidua, in extraembryonic fetal membranes, and possibly in myometrium to stimulate prostaglandin production.

Once again, we return to the analogy of activated macrophages and decidual tissue of women in labour. A principal 'activator' of macrophages is bacterial endotoxin lipopolysaccharide (LPS); we propose, therefore, to extend the analogy of macrophage-like decidua and macrophages further. It is well recognized and well documented that a major cause of preterm labour in women is infection (Friedman, 1973; Burkman & Friedlander, 1975; Miller *et al.*, 1980; Kass *et al.*, 1981; Gilstrap *et al.*, 1981; Bobitt *et al.*, 1981; Garite & Freeman, 1982; MacDonald *et al.*, 1983; Polk, 1984; Wahbeh *et al.*, 1984; Leveno & Cunningham, 1987). In pregnancies in which there is infection of uterine tissues, intrauterine tissues (e.g. fetal membranes, or fetal membrane–decidual interface), or extrauterine tissues (e.g. as in pyelonephritis, appendicitis, tuberculosis), preterm labour commonly occurs. The possibility exists, therefore, that LPS or other bacterial products (e.g. lipoteichoic acid (LTA) in group β streptococci and other gram-positive bacteria) may serve to activate uterine decidua in pregnancies complicated by infection.

In a recent study, we found that LPS is not normally a constituent of amniotic fluid (Cox *et al.*, 1988b) but in 50% of singleton pregnancies complicated by preterm labour with intact membranes, LPS is present (Cox *et al.*, 1988b). And in preterm labour pregnancies in which LPS is present, the IL-1β is increased to levels that may exceed by many-fold those present in amniotic fluid during normal labour. But more than that, TNF-α also was present in 40% of cases of preterm labour in which LPS was present in amniotic fluid.

Based on the findings of studies conducted *in vitro*, we conclude that this association between the presence of LPS and various cytokines may well be a cause–effect relationship. LPS acts in uterine decidual tissue explants in culture to cause an increase in the production of IL-1β as well as TNF-α (Casey *et al.*, 1988b, 1989). Other bacterial products, e.g. LTA, also cause increased production of these cytokines by decidual tissue (Casey *et al.*, 1988b). Accepting bacterial products (i.e. LPS and LTA) as potential activators of macrophage-like decidua in pregnancies complicated by infection, a question of paramount importance is the identification of 'activators' of decidua in normal pregnancies. Presently, such an agent(s) has not been identified.

Uterine preparedness for parturition

As stated in the introduction, it is reasonable to presume that the generation of uterotropins, i.e. agents that act on uterus to cause preparedness for labour, occurs in uterine or extraembryonic fetal tissues. There is no doubt that certain fundamental biochemical and morphological alterations precede successful, atraumatic labour and delivery in mammals. If these fundamental changes in uterus that occur in all species were brought about by similar biomolecular phenomena, a significant step toward a definition of parturition in all species could be taken.

Cervical ripening

Ripening of the cervix, i.e. softening and effacement preparatory to labour, is essential for atraumatic, successful parturition. Regrettably, little is known of the physiological processes that bring about this dramatic change in cervical morphology. Realignment of collagen fibres is fundamental to this process (Pritchard *et al.*, 1985); and there appears to be a role for prostaglandin, PGE$_2$ in particular (cf. Stys, 1986), in this process and possibly a role for relaxin as well (Bryant-Greenwood & Greenwood, 1988). Nonetheless, stimuli of this particular event in the uterine preparedness for labour or the mediators of this process have not been defined.

Myometrial activation

Before the onset of the vigorous contractions of the myometrium, which constitute clinically discernible labour, there are modifications in function and morphology of the myometrium and myometrial cells that favour increased contractility of this tissue. And, as in the case of cervical ripening, these changes appear to take place in all mammalian species irrespective of the endocrine physiology that accompanies the parturitional event.

Oxytocin receptors

Since the discovery of the uterotonic activity of oxytocin, a role for this peptide in the spontaneous initiation of parturition has been suspected by many investigators. Until now, the principal objection to the oxytocin theory of parturition was the failure of identification of an increase in the concentration of oxytocin in blood before or during labour. There is an increase in oxytocin levels during the second stage of labour, but not before this time (Leake, 1983).

New impetus was given to the oxytocin theory, however, with the discovery that there is a striking increase in oxytocin receptors in myometrium before or during labour in all mammalian species examined (Fuchs *et al.*, 1982). And, in addition, it has been reported that there is an increase in oxytocin receptors in decidua as well and that oxytocin acts upon decidua to cause the outpouring of prostaglandins (Roberts *et al.*, 1976). An increase in oxytocin receptors can be effected by endocrine manipulations, i.e. estrogen treatment or progesterone withdrawal (Sheldrick & Flint, 1985). But, there is an increase in oxytocin receptors in primates at the time of parturition, i.e. in species in which there is no identifiable endocrine alteration at the time of increased synthesis of oxytocin receptors. Thus, the identification of the uterotropin that acts to cause increased oxytocin receptors is a fundamental question of monumental importance.

Sensitivity to uterotonins

Increased responsiveness to uterotonins, both oxytocin and prostaglandins, is a characteristic feature of late pregnancy in a number of mammalian species, including the sheep and the human. An increase in responsiveness to oxytocin may be the consequence of an alteration in the number of myometrial or decidual receptors for this uterotonin. The cause of increased responsiveness to prostaglandins is not defined; and as in the case of an increase in oxytocin receptors, a vital question relative to the cause of labour is related to an identification of the uterotropin that brings about increased contractility of the myometrium to prostaglandins as well as to oxytocin.

Gap junctions

Near term or during early labour, there is an increase in the number of gap junctions between myometrial cells (MacKenzie & Garfield, 1985, 1986). Presumably, this physiological alteration in myometrium will favour the development of coordinated contractions of the uterus during labour. The identity of the uterotropin that causes an increase in gap junction formation is not identified. As in the case of oxytocin receptors, alterations in the hormonal milieu will serve to increase the formation of gap junctions: estrogen acts to increase as does progesterone withdrawal (Burghardt *et al.*, 1984; MacKenzie & Garfield, 1985, 1986). Nonetheless, gap junctions appear in myometrial cells in primates, in which there is no dramatic endocrine change that precedes parturition.

Summary

Parturition in all mammalian species is accompanied by an increase in the level of metabolic activity in uterine and extraembryonic fetal tissues. This increased function of these tissues probably gives rise to uterotropins, which serve to effect uterine preparedness for labour, and to uterotonins, which act to cause the myometrial contractions of parturition. Several bioactive agents that are produced in increased amounts during parturition have been identified. In fact, many of these agents accumulate in amniotic fluid during labour. Armed with this information, it may now be possible to ascertain, with considerable precision, the exact identity of the uterotropins and the uterotonins by defining the specific roles of each of these agents in the parturitional process.

Armed also with the knowledge of the response of each of the tissues, uterine and extraembryonic fetal membranes, during parturition, it should be possible to define the source and mechanism of action of processes or agents that could serve to promote premature activation of these tissues and thereby preterm labour.

Acknowledgements

This work was supported, in part, by USPHS Grant No. 5-P50-HD11149 and March of Dimes National Foundation Grant No. 6-522.

References

Albert, D.H. & Snyder, F. (1983). Biosynthesis of 1-alkyl-2-acetyl-**sn**-glycero-3-phosphocholine (platelet-activating factor) from 1-alkyl-2-acyl-**sn**-glycero-3-phosphocholine by rat alveolar macrophages. Phospholipase A_2 and acetyl transferase activities during phagocytosis and ionophore stimulation. *Journal of Biological Chemistry*, **258**:97–102.

Balavoine, J.-F., de Rochemonteix, B., Williamson, K., Seckinger, P., Cruchaud, A. & Dayer, J.M. (1986). Prostaglandin E_2 and collagenase production by fibroblasts and synovial cells is regulated by urine-derived human interleukin 1 and inhibitor(s). *Journal of Clinical Investigation*, **78**:1120–1124.

Ban, C., Billah, M.M., Truong, C.T. & Johnston, J.M. (1986). Metabolism of platelet-activating factor (1-O-alkyl-2-acetyl-**sn**-glycero-3-phosphocholine) in human fetal membranes and decidua vera. *Archives of Biochemistry and Biophysics*, **246**:9–18.

Batra, S., Bengtsson, L.P., Grundsell, H. & Sjöberg, N.O. (1976). Levels of free and protein-bound progesterone in plasma during late pregnancy. *Journal of Clinical Endocrinology and Metabolism*, **42**:1041–1047.

Bernheim, H.A. & Dinarello, C.A. (1985). Effects of purified human interleukin-1 on the release of prostaglandin E_2 from fibroblasts. *British Journal of Rheumatology*, 24(Suppl. 1):122–127.

Bleasdale, J.E. & Johnston, J.M. (1985). Prostaglandins and human parturition: Regulation of arachidonic acid mobilization. *Reviews in Perinatal Medicine*, 5:151–191.

Bobitt, J.R., Hayslip, C.C. & Damato, J.D. (1981). Amniotic fluid infection as determined by transabdominal amniocentesis in patients with intact membranes in premature labor. *American Journal of Obstetrics and Gynecology*, 140:947–952.

Bryant-Greenwood, G.D. & Greenwood, F.C. (1988). The human fetal membranes and decidua as a model for paracrine interactions. (In) *Cellular and Integrative Mechanisms in the Onset of Labor. An NICHD Workshop* (McNellis, D., Challis, J.R.G., MacDonald, P.C., Nathanielsz, P. & Roberts, J., eds.), pp.253–273. Ithaca, New York, Perinatology Press.

Burghardt, R.C., Matheson, R.L. & Gaddy, D. (1984). Gap junction modulation in rat uterus. I. Effects of estrogen on myometrial and serosal cells. *Biology of Reproduction*, 30:239–248.

Burkman, R.T. & Friedlander, R.L. (1975). Ruptured appendix in pregnancy. *American Journal of Obstetrics and Gynecology*, 122:265.

Bussolino, F., Breviario, F., Tetta, C., Aglietta, M., Mantovani, A. & Dejana, E. (1986). Interleukin 1 stimulates platelet-activating factor production in cultured human endothelial cells. *Journal of Clinical Investigation*, 77:2027–2033.

Casey, M.L., Cox, S.M., Beutler, B. & MacDonald, P.C. (1988b). The formation of cytokines in human decidua: The role of decidua in the initiation of both term and preterm labor. *Proceedings of the Society of Gynecological Investigation*, 35th Annual Meeting, Baltimore, p.219.

Casey, M.L., Cox, S.M., Beutler, B., Milewich, L. & MacDonald, P.C. (1989). Cachectin/tumor necrosis factor-α formation in human decidua: Potential role of cytokines in infection-induced preterm labor. *Journal of Clinical Investigation*, 83:430–436.

Casey, M.L., Korte, K. & MacDonald, P.C. (1988a). Epidermal growth factor stimulation of prostaglandin E_2 biosynthesis in amnion cells: Induction of prostaglandin H_2 synthase. *Journal of Biological Chemistry*, 263:7846–7854.

Casey, M.L. & MacDonald, P.C. (1986). The initiation of labor in women: regulation of phospholipid and arachidonic acid metabolism and of prostaglandin production. *Seminars in Perinatology*, 10:270–275.

Casey, M.L. & MacDonald, P.C. (1988). The role of a fetal–maternal paracrine system in the maintenance of pregnancy and the initiation of parturition. (In) *Fetal and Neonatal Development* (Jones, C.T., ed.), pp.521–532. Ithaca, New York, Perinatology Press.

Casey, M.L., Mitchell, M.D. & MacDonald, P.C. (1987). Epidermal growth factor-stimulated prostaglandin E_2 production in human amnion cells: Specificity and nonesterified arachidonic acid dependency. *Molecular and Cellular Endocrinology*, 53:169–176.

Castle, B.M. & Turnbull, A.C. (1985). The significance of preterm breathing. (In) *Research in Perinatal Medicine (III)* (Beard,R.W. & Sharp, F., eds.), pp.53–57. Ithaca, New York, Perinatology Press.

Challis, J.R.G. & Olson, D.M. (1988). Parturition. (In) *The Physiology of Reproduc-*

tion, Vol. 2 (Knobil, E. & Neill, J.D., eds.), pp.2177–2216. New York, Raven Press.

Chang, J., Gilman, S.C. & Lewis, A.J. (1986). Interleukin 1 activates phospholipase A_2 in rabbit chondrocytes: A possible signal for IL-1 action. *Journal of Immunology*, **136**:1283–1287.

Cox, S.M., MacDonald, P.C. & Casey, M.L. (1988a). Assay of bacterial endotoxin [lipopolysaccharide] in human amniotic fluid: potential usefulness in diagnosis and management of preterm labor. *American Journal of Obstetrics and Gynecology*, **159**:99–106.

Cox, S.M., MacDonald, P.C. & Casey, M.L. (1988b). Decidual activation is synchronous with spontaneous parturition and with bacterial endotoxin lipopolysaccharide (LPS)-induced preterm labor. *Proceedings of the Society of Gynecological Investigation*, p.89, 35th Annual Meeting, Baltimore.

Dray, F. & Frydman, R. (1976). Primary prostaglandins in amniotic fluid in pregnancy and spontaneous labor. *American Journal of Obstetrics and Gynecology*, **126**:13–19.

Friedman, E.A. (1973). Obstetric infections in labor. (In) *Obstetric and Perinatal Infections* (Charles, D. & Finland, M., eds.), pp.501–516. Philadelphia, Lea & Febiger.

Fuchs, A.R., Fuchs, F., Husslein, P., Soloff, M.S. & Fernström, M.J. (1982). Oxytocin receptors and human parturition: a dual role for oxytocin in the initiation of labor. *Science*, **215**:1396–1398.

Garite, T.J. & Freeman, R.K. (1982). Chorioamnionitis in the preterm gestation. *Obstetrics and Gynecology*, **59**:539–545.

Gery, I., Gershon, R.K. & Waksman, B.H. (1971). Potentiation of cultured mouse thymocyte responses by factors released by peripheral leucocytes. *Journal of Immunology*, **107**:1778–1780.

Ghodgaonkar, R.B., Dubin, N.H., Blake, D.A. & King, T.M. (1979). 13,14-dihydro-15-keto-prostaglandin $F_{2\alpha}$ concentrations in human plasma and amniotic fluid. *American Journal of Obstetrics and Gynecology*, **134**:265–269.

Gilstrap, L.C., Leveno, K.J., Cunningham, F.G., Whalley, P.J. & Roark, M.L. (1981). Renal infection and pregnancy outcome. *American Journal of Obstetrics and Gynecology*, **141**:709–716.

Glover, D.M., Brownstein, D., Burchett, S., Larsen, A. & Wilson, C.B. (1987). Expression of HLA class II antigens and secretion of interleukin-1 by monocytes and macrophages from adults and neonates. *Immunology*, **61**:195–201.

Kass, E.H., McCormack, W.M. & Lin, J.-S. (1981). Genital mycoplasmas as a cause of excess premature delivery. *Transactions of the Association of American Physicians*, **94**:262–266.

Keirse, M.J., Hicks, B.R., Mitchell, M.D. & Turnbull, A.C. (1977). Increase of the prostaglandin precursor, arachidonic acid, in amniotic fluid during spontaneous labour. *British Journal of Obstetrics and Gynaecology*, **84**:937–940.

Kinoshita, K., Satoh, K. & Sakamoto, S. (1978). Biosynthesis of prostaglandin in human decidua, amnion, chorion, and villi. *Endocrinologia Japonica*, **24**:343–350.

Kunkel, S.L. & Chensue, S.W. (1986). The role of arachidonic acid metabolites in mononuclear phagocytic cell interactions. *International Journal of Dermatology*, **25**:83–89.

Leake, R.D. (1983). Oxytocin. Initiation of parturition: prevention of prematurity. (In) *Report of the Fourth Ross Conference on Obstetric Research* (Porter, J.C. & MacDonald, P.C., eds.), pp.43–51. Columbus, Ohio, Ross Laboratories.

Leveno, K.J. & Cunningham, F.G. (1987). Dilemmas in the management of preterm birth. Part one: Pregnancies at risk. (In) *Williams Obstetrics*, Supplement 12 (Gant, N.F., MacDonald, P.C. & Pritchard, J.A., eds.). Appleton-Century-Crofts.

MacDonald, P.C., Alexander, D., Catz, C. & Edelman, R. (1983). Summary of a workshop on maternal genitourinary infections and the outcome of pregnancy. *Journal of Infectious Diseases*, 147:596–605.

MacDonald, P.C., Schultz, F.M., Duenhoelter, J.H., Gant, N.F., Jimenez, J.M., Pritchard, J.A., Porter, J.C. & Johnston, J.M. (1974). Initiation of human parturition. I. Mechanism of action of arachidonic acid. *Obstetrics and Gynecology*, 44:629–636.

MacKenzie, L.W. & Garfield, R.E. (1985). Hormonal control of gap junctions in the myometrium. *American Journal of Physiology*, 248:C296–C308.

MacKenzie, L.W. & Garfield, R.E. (1986). Effects of 17β-estradiol on myometrial gap junctions and pregnancy in the rat. *Canadian Journal of Physiology and Pharmacology*, 64:462–466.

Miller, J.M., Pupkin, M.J. & Hill, G.B. (1980). Bacterial colonization of amniotic fluid from intact fetal membranes. *American Journal of Obstetrics and Gynecology*, 136:796–804.

Niesert, S., Christopherson, W., Korte, K., Mitchell, M.D., MacDonald, P.C. & Casey, M.L. (1986). Prostaglandin E$_2$ 9-ketoreductase activity in human decidua vera tissue. *American Journal of Obstetrics and Gynecology*, 155:1348–1352.

Novy, M.J. & Liggins, G.C. (1980). Role of prostaglandins, prostacyclin, and thromboxanes in the physiologic control of the uterus and in parturition. *Seminars in Perinatology*, 4:45–66.

Okazaki, T., Casey, M.L., Okita, J.R., MacDonald, P.C. & Johnston, J.M. (1981). Initiation of human parturition. XII. Biosynthesis and metabolism of prostaglandins in human fetal membranes and uterine decidua. *American Journal of Obstetrics and Gynecology*, 139:373–381.

Okita, J.R. (1981). Alterations in arachidonic acid content of specific glycerophospholipids of amnion and chorion laeve during human parturition. Doctorate Dissertation, The University of Texas Southwestern Medical School, Dallas, Texas.

Okita, J.R., Johnston, J.M. & MacDonald, P.C. (1983). Source of prostaglandin precursor in human fetal membranes: Arachidonic acid content of amnion and chorion laeve of diamnionic–dichorionic twin placentas. *American Journal of Obstetrics and Gynecology*, 147:477–482.

Okita, J.R., MacDonald, P.C. & Johnston, J.M. (1982). Mobilization of arachidonic acid from specific glycerophospholipids of human fetal membranes during early labor. *Journal of Biological Chemistry*, 257:14029–14034.

Polk, B.F. (1984). Infectious processes and preterm birth. (In) *Preterm Birth: Causes, Prevention, and Management* (Fuchs, F. & Stubblefield, P.G., eds.), pp.86–97. New York, MacMillan.

Pritchard, J.A., MacDonald, P.C. & Gant, N.F. (1985). *Williams Obstetrics*, 17th edition. Norwalk, Connecticut, Appleton-Century-Crofts.

Raz, A., Wyche, A., Siegel, N. & Needleman, P. (1988). Regulation of fibroblast cyclooxygenase synthesis by interleukin-1. *Journal of Biological Chemistry*, 263:3022–3028.

Roberts, J.S., McCracken, J.A., Gavagan, J.E. & Soloff, M.S. (1976). Oxytocin-stimulated release of prostaglandin F$_{2\alpha}$ from ovine endometrium *in vitro*: correlation

318   *M.L. Casey and P.C. MacDonald*

with estrous cycle and oxytocin-receptor binding. *Endocrinology*, **99**:1107–1114.

Romero, R., Wu, Y.K., Brody, D.T., Oyarzun, E., Duff, G.W. & Durum, S.K. (1989). Human decidua: a source of interleukin-1. *Obstetrics and Gynecology*, **73**:31–34.

Satoh, K., Yasumizu, T., Fukuoka, H., Kinoshita, K., Kaneko, Y., Tsuchiya, M. & Sakamoto, S. (1979). Prostaglandin F$_{2\alpha}$ metabolite levels in plasma, amniotic fluid, and urine during pregnancy and labor. *American Journal of Obstetrics and Gynecology*, **133**:886–890.

Schlegel, W., Kruger, S. & Korte, K. (1984). Purification of prostaglandin E$_2$-9-oxo-reductase from human decidua vera. *FEBS Letters*, **171**:141–144.

Sheldrick, E.L. & Flint, A.P. (1985). Endocrine control of uterine oxytocin receptors in the ewe. *Journal of Endocrinology*, **106**:249–258.

Stys, S.J. (1986). Endocrine regulation of cervical functions during pregnancy and labor. (In) *The Physiology and Biochemistry of the Uterus in Pregnancy and Labor* (Huszar, G., ed.), pp.281–295. Boca Raton, Florida, CRC Press.

Wahbeh, C.J., Hill, G.B., Eden, R.D. & Gall, S.A. (1984). Intra-amniotic bacterial colonization in premature labor. *American Journal of Obstetrics and Gynecology*, **148**:739–743.

Wood, D.D., Bayne, E.K., Goldring, M.B., Gowen, M., Hamerman, D., Humes, J.L., Ihrie, E.J., Lipsky, P.E. & Staruch, M.J. (1985). The four biochemically distinct species of human interleukin-1 all exhibit similar biological activities. *Journal of Immunology*, **134**:895–903.

Discussion

Clark. Is there any evidence that women with bacterial infections are more likely to have intermenstrual bleeding on oral contraceptive agents or will have heavier menstrual periods?

Casey. Yes, I believe so.

Ludwig. Endometritis is often associated with bleeding. There is a link. My question to you is: at the site of the placenta, it is very difficult to differentiate between decidua and trophoblastic cells. Are you able to differentiate the macrophages of the placental side and those from the side opposite to the membranes, and how do you differentiate those two elements from fetal origin?

Casey. In these studies, all the decidual tissue was taken from the chorion laeve; we have not investigated the decidual tissue contiguous with the placenta. To distinguish between fetal and maternal cells, we have used the technique of quinacrine fluorescence of the Y chromosome.

Cornillie. In women with endometriosis, there are more macrophages in peritoneal fluid (Halme *et al.*, 1987). It was shown recently by Fakih *et al.* (1987) that when these macrophages are isolated and put in culture, they produce quite a lot of interleukin-1. If you take this peritoneal fluid and dilute it out in culture medium, it is impossible to grow blastocysts from mouse embryos in that system. Interleukin-1 is toxic for embryos, at least in those experimental conditions. Could you give any link between interleukin and embryo toxicity or cell toxicity?

Casey. Certainly there are a number of cytotoxic factors that are produced by macrophages such as tumour necrosis factor-α, superoxide anion, and even interleukin-1, which may well be important in the initiation of uterine bleeding.

Åkerlund. Your hypothesis, the parallel of pregnancy and menstruation was fascinating. I would, if I may, suggest that you change one word in your hypothesis and that it would be to exchange 'initiation' to 'progression'. All the factors you presented are really involved with the progression of labour. They might come very early but they do not initiate labour. With preterm labour, in at least 50%, there are no known factors. Even in cases with infection, the substances you discussed are involved in the progression, not in the initiation.

Casey. I would agree with you in part. Prostaglandins, which are produced in response to these agents (i.e. cytokines) may act to maintain the uterine contractions of labour. (Parturition and labour are not equivalent; parturition includes uterine preparation for labour).

Healy. With regard to the issue of menstruation being parturition of failed fertility, I have a conceptual problem with that. Menstruation results from a fall of estradiol and progesterone. I am not aware that human labour is being characterized as having any fall in progesterone before the onset of labour, unlike species like the sheep. Secondly, is the interleukin increase progesterone induced or is it the absence of progesterone which raises interleukin?

Casey. You are quite right that in women there is no progesterone withdrawal prior to the onset of labour. We speculate that progesterone stimulates the capacity of the tissue to produce interleukin-1β. Perhaps progesterone withdrawal in menstruation (and fetal retreat in parturition) is in fact important further in the processing of that interleukin-1β which is required for secretion and thence actions on other cell types.

King. How do you see the changes of either prostaglandins or the other intermediaries, specifically in the context of the breakthrough bleed that one gets under the influence of contraceptives? How do these supposed intermediaries fit into the scheme of things?

Findlay. I suppose, Dr King, that some prostaglandins are vasoconstrictors and others are vasodilators. If we accept the hypothesis that Dr Baird has been suggesting is the one that currently stands, the important thing is going to be the ratio between those PGs that cause vasodilatation and those that cause vasoconstriction. There is a lot of indirect evidence for both PGs being produced. The role of the myometrium in producing PGI_2 is relatively old data and we have not really moved much further than that.

Smith. The effect of antiprogestins on prostaglandin release, in my view anyway, clearly demonstrates that progesterone withdrawal is a mechanism for the release of prostaglandins from glandular cells in human endometrium. So, at the risk of grossly simplifying it, I still think that the hypothesis that there is a steroid withdrawal mechanism which can result in increased prostaglandin production is correct, and nothing so far that I have heard makes me change from that view. It also then happens that the main prostaglandin produced is PGF, which happens to be vasoconstrictor. So although there is a balance, you might get heavier bleeding if that balance gets disturbed. We do actually have quite a clear link between steroid action, steroid withdrawal, prostaglandin production and vasoconstriction.

Baird. To put forward a hypothesis to explain directly in terms of prostaglandin Dr King's question, that is, how does breakthrough bleeding occur in response to progestogen therapy, I would say if you require progesterone action in order to induce adequate prostaglandin production by synthetic capacity, then progestogens are bound to alter the concentration of steroid receptors, particularly the progesterone steroid receptors in the endometrium. I am surprised: we discussed this 10 years ago and nobody as far as I know in this audience has actually taken the trouble to measure progesterone receptors in women who are on progestogen-only pills and who are likely to get breakthrough bleeding. If we assume that this does alter the concentration of progesterone receptors, then we have an endometrium which is relatively deficient of progesterone. In fact, progesterone is unable to exert its full action on the endometrium.

Rice-Evans. What is causing the initial vasoconstriction that leads to the initiation of endometrial bleeding? The first idea that we all seem to have is that there is an increase in the ratio of $PGF_{2\alpha}:PGE_2$ on withdrawal of steroids. We heard from Dr Findlay about endothelin, a vasoconstricting substance, but also the endothelial cells release a vasodilating substance, nitric oxide. Now, what is interesting about the balance between vasoconstriction and vasodilatation of the endothelial cells, is that there is another process that seems to go on when we withdraw steroids. This is the infiltration of leukocytes and possibly also macrophages. Superoxides released from activated leukocytes will actually interact with nitric oxide, a vasodilator, and inhibit it because nitric oxide happens to be a free-radical, as superoxide is. So now we seem to have a mechanism removing the vasodilator. We also have endothelin, $PGF_{2\alpha}$, and platelet activator, I think, contributing towards the vasoconstriction. What we really need to know is the time-scale of these events and where these events are happening.

Casey. Perhaps I could offer as an example a model system based on some direct and a lot of indirect evidence that would be testable and might put into perspective some of the things that have been said. If you consider endometrial tissue with the macrophage component, you can imagine that with long-term progesterone treatment, there could be an enormous capacity in that endometrial tissue for the production of a cytokine, for example interleukin-1β. The macrophage is unique in that it will release interleukin-1β whereas other cells do not release interleukin-1β necessarily *a priori*. The interleukin could then act on endometrial stromal cells to cause further production of interleukin-1β. But that would not be released from the stromal cell until progesterone receptors decline as the consequence of the long-term progesterone action, giving rise to a decrease in effective progesterone action, which might facilitate plasminogen activator activity.

In summary, a decrease in the inhibitor, an increase in the activator, giving rise to the serine protease activity allows for the release of interleukin-1β. Interleukin-1β, acting together with a decreased progesterone action, would in turn facilitate the production of prostaglandin in a cascade type of effect. This is one possible mechanism that might then lead to progesterone withdrawal bleeding or breakthrough bleeding to long-term progesterone action.

Naftolin. Dr Casey, where, in the uterus, do you think is the key area to be which would (a) trigger bleeding, and (b) fail to stop bleeding?

Casey. I do not know. Certainly, interleukin can be made by many different cells, therefore the potential is immense. I should not limit it to interleukin, because tumour necrosis factor and TGF-β are going to be present. They can act on a whole host of different cell types to cause prostaglandin production. So I do not think that we know how to limit it to a single cell type. In fact, it might not be limited.

Rees. The idea of changes in tissue plasminogen activator levels between bleeders and non-bleeders is interesting, but Dr Hourihan showed that the difference in level of endometrial tPA between post-treatment patients with normal bleeding when compared to those with longer bleeding episodes was not significant (Hourihan *et al.*, 1990). So, while tPA was an interesting candidate, it has been measured and does not seem to be involved.

Hourihan. We have measured the tissue levels but we have not measured the levels of activity, which are completely different, and those need to be assessed, and nor have we looked at the levels of the inhibitors. So we cannot say that it is not involved.

Casey. I agree fully with what you are saying. The activity is the key and perhaps not only the tPA activity but urokinase, which is also produced in the uterus.

Gurpide. Dr Casey, you mentioned an effect of interleukin-1β on prostaglandin synthesis in stromal cells. What kind of stromal cell were you using?

Casey. The endometrial stromal cells were isolated from secretory endometrium by your method, cultured in monolayer, in Waymouth enriched culture medium in the presence of fetal bovine serum. Interleukin-1β also stimulates prostaglandin production in the decidual tissue explants.

Böhlen. Have you considered transforming growth factor-β (TGF-β) for a role as an intermediate mediator? TGF-β is made by activated macrophages and released from them. It is also likely to be made in several endometrial or decidual cell types. Does TGF-β stimulate prostaglandin synthesis?

Casey. Yes, TGF-β may have a role. It has been reported by others that TGF-β will stimulate prostaglandin synthesis in a manner somewhat similar to that of TGF-α and epidermal growth factor (EGF). We have found that, again, in another model system of an epithelial cell type, the amnion, which is very responsive to EGF or TGF-α in terms of increasing synthesis of PGE_2, TGF-β actually inhibits PGE_2 production. So there is a tissue-specific response in terms of prostaglandin production to TGF-β.

Findlay. One aspect of Dr Casey's hypothesis of the initiation is that the macrophage is the important cell type. I wonder if the morphologists in the audience can tell us whether in those subjects who are taking long-term progestogens there is increased infiltration of macrophages in the endometrium?

Johannisson. In the specimens we have seen following various treatments of progestogens, we do see decidualization, but we do not see specifically an increase in macrophages. However, when we have normal menstrual bleeding we see a lot of macrophages after, or in relation to this bleeding.

Brosens. We have not heard much about decidualization. If there is decidualization, there is usually a lot of spontaneous necrosis. If you look at a hamster pseudopregnancy, you will see necrosis all over the decidua, where in pregnancy the trophoblast will proliferate. Also in the human in the decidua you see a lot of necrosis. So I wonder whether once the endometrium is in the secretory phase and is going to be decidualized, you will end up with spontaneous necrosis and bleeding.

Naftolin. But since pregnancy continues following that necrosis, why would you assume that it always has to lead to that bleeding?

Brosens. I think that in pregnancy, with the necrosis occurring, it is being healed by the trophoblast.

References

Fakih, H., Baggett, B., Holtz, G., Tsang, K.Y., Lee, J.C. & Williamson, H.O. (1987). Interleukin-1: a possible role in the infertility associated with endometriosis. *Fertility and Sterility*, **47**:213–217.

Halme, J., Becker, S. & Haskill, S. (1987). Altered maturation and function of peritoneal macrophages: possible role in pathogenesis of endometriosis. *American Journal of Obstetrics and Gynecology*, **156**:783–789.

Hourihan, H.M., Sheppard, B.L. & Brosens, I.A. (1990). Endometrial hemostasis. (In) *Contraception and Mechanisms of Endometrial Bleeding* (d'Arcangues, C., Fraser, I.S., Newton, J.R. & Odlind, V., eds.), pp. 95–114. Cambridge, England, Cambridge University Press.

Antiprogestogens and endometrial morphology

R. SITRUK-WARE*, H. YANEVA AND I.M. SPITZ**

*Hôpital Necker, Paris, France. *Present address: Ciba-Geigy Ltd, Medical Department, Basel, Switzerland.
**The Population Council, Center for Biomedical Research, New York, USA.

Abstract

Endometrial effects of the antiprogestogen RU486 were evaluated by morphological and immunocytochemical techniques. The human endometrium was collected by biopsy from early abortion material induced by RU486 and also from normal volunteers receiving the drug during the late luteal phase or in the follicular phase. Morphological evaluation indicated that in pregnant women RU486 induced a non-complete necrosis seen in disseminated foci. In normal women RU486 induced premature involution of the endometrium with necrosis mimicking that observed with normal menstruation. The localization of the antiprogestogen RU486 binding in the human endometrium has been investigated using immunocytochemical techniques. A highly specific anti-RU486 antiserum and the indirect antibody peroxidase–antiperoxidase method were used. Specific staining was observed in the stromal and the glandular cells of the decidual tissue, mainly in the cytoplasm, and light labelling was present in the nuclei. Nuclear staining was evident in the syncithiotrophoblastic cells, attesting the progesterone dependence of human implantation in early pregnancy. In normal endometrium the staining was found mostly in the stromal cells, with predominant nuclear staining. No staining was found when RU486 was given during the follicular phase.

These findings indicate that RU486 acts on the endometrium through binding to progesterone receptors, blocks the effect of progesterone and induces premature involution and partial necrosis of the decidualized tissue.

Introduction

Under physiological conditions, progesterone (P) secreted during the luteal phase in synergy with estrogens leads to the secretory transformation of the endometrium which differentiates in preparation for implantation and gestation. On the day following ovulation, characteristic changes occur in the endometrium. Indeed, accurate dating of the luteal phase is possible based on the morphological features observed (Noyes et al., 1950; Li et al., 1988). If the ovarian output of estradiol (E_2) and P is not maintained by chorionic gonadotrophin elaborated by the implanting blastocyst, endometrial tissue regresses and sheds. On the other hand, if fertilization and implantation occur, well-described changes appear in the glands and stroma, and the secretory endometrium evolves into a decidualized endometrium.

During the past decade, biochemical studies have elucidated the antiestrogenic effect of progesterone on the endometrial cells. It has been shown that Pstimulates several enzymes, especially 17-β-estradiol dehydrogenase (E_2DH) (Tseng & Gurpide, 1975), which allows for conversion of E_2 into estrone, a less active metabolite. P also regulates E_2 receptors and decreases their level both in cytosolic and nuclear fractions of the endometrial cells (Hsueh *et al.*, 1976). Finally Gerschenson *et al.* (1974) have shown that P decreases cell multiplication, which is due to a receptor-mediated process (Horwitz *et al.*, 1985).

Recently, a promising new antiprogesterone compound, RU486 (Mifepristone, Mifegyne[R], Roussel-Uclaf, Paris, France), has been synthesized. This compound exerts a high binding affinity for the progesterone and glucocorticoid receptors and exerts potent antiprogestational and antiglucocorticoid effects (Philibert *et al.*, 1985; Okulicz, 1987). In both monkeys and humans, RU486 has been shown to induce bleeding when administered during the luteal phase, and also to terminate early pregnancy (Herrmann *et al.*, 1982; Kovacs *et al.*, 1984; Couzinet *et al.*, 1986). The mechanism of action of RU486 in the induction of bleeding and in pregnancy interruption appears to be mainly a local effect on the endometrium mediated via the P receptor (Croxatto *et al.*, 1985).

In order to evaluate the mechanism of RU486 action on the endometrium, several authors have investigated its effect from a morphological and a biochemical aspect under various conditions in animals and in women.

Animal studies

In cynomolgus monkeys, Koering *et al.* (1986) have investigated the acute effects of RU486 on the morphological characteristics of a mature secretory-type endometrium. In castrated female monkeys, Silastic[R] capsules delivering E_2 in increasing doses were implanted. This mimicked follicular phase levels of E_2, and resulted in priming of the endometrium. RU486 was administered in daily intramuscular injections of 1 mg/kg, either at the end of the 'follicular' phase from day 13 to day 16 of estrogen therapy, or at the end of a 'secretory' phase on day 29, after sequential progesterone therapy delivered from Silastic[R] capsules from day 12–32 of estrogen therapy. In both groups, laparotomy was performed. The complete uterus and endometrial tissue from four different anatomic zones were evaluated morphologically.

In all tissue samples evaluated by light microscopy, the results indicated that E_2 alone induced intracellular stromal development, while RU486 given in estrogen-primed animals exerted weak progestational activity as shown by an increase in the glandular areas. When given to animals which had received $E_2 + P$, when the endometrium showed a secretory pattern, RU486 exerted strong antiprogestational activity as shown by regression of the superficial endometrial layer within 32 hours after a single injection of RU486 (Koering *et al.*, 1986).

In another study in normal cycling cynomolgus monkeys, Chillik *et al.* (1986) demonstrated that RU486 administered from days 21 to 24 of the luteal phase induced nearly uniform sloughing of the endometrial tissue. Exogenous P addition did not prevent the menses induction; however, the depth of the endometrial sloughing was less than when RU486 was given alone.

Human studies

In postmenopausal women, Gravanis *et al.* (1985) performed biochemical studies on the endometrium treated with RU486 after estrogen replacement therapy. Seventeen postmenopausal women received injections of estradiol benzoate (0.625 mg) daily for 15 days. During the last 6 days of therapy, they received either RU486 (100–200 mg daily), or P (25 mg/day), or both together. The authors showed that RU486 exerted both agonistic and antagonistic effects on the endometrium. In the absence of P, RU486 exerted a mild progestational effect, increasing 17β-hydroxysteroid-dehydrogenase (E_2DH) activity in the endometrium and inducing secretory transformation of the tissue. On the other hand, when given together with P, RU486 counteracted the P effect and E_2DH activity remained as low as in the women treated with E_2 alone. The same dual effect of RU486 on DNA polymerase was observed by the authors.

Croxatto *et al.* (1989) studied premenopausal women. In their study they showed that during maintenance of corpus luteum function with exogenous hCG given during luteal phase (days 9–15), RU486 could induce endometrial bleeding despite high circulating progesterone and estradiol levels. With the lower doses of RU486, incomplete sloughing of the endometrium was observed which accounted for the occurrence of a second bleeding episode at the time of corpus luteum demise when hCG was stopped. With the high dose of RU486, only one bleeding episode was evident.

In order to study the localization of RU486 in the endometrium and the changes it could induce in normal women, we decided to undertake morphological and immunocytochemical studies both in normal non-pregnant and pregnant women who applied for abortion.

Morphological and immunocytochemical studies in premenopausal women

Non-pregnant women

To determine the usefulness and the safety of RU486 as a menses inducer in ovulatory women, we evaluated the morphologic and immunocytochemical changes of the endometrium when RU486 was given either during the mid or late luteal phase in fertile women. These women used barrier contraceptive methods during the trial to prevent pregnancy.

Five women received RU486 (50 mg/day) from day 22 to 25 of the luteal phase of a normal cycle (midluteal phase); another five subjects received the same dose from day 25 to 28 (late luteal phase). Three additional subjects received RU486 25 mg daily for 14 days starting on day 5 of the cycle (follicular phase).

In all subjects, an endometrial biopsy was performed at the end of the treatment, either on day 24 or day 27, according to the treatment group. The tissue was examined both morphologically and with an immunocytochemical method. In all cases, the endometrial samples were collected in saline solution. Half of the tissue was fixed in alcoholic Bouin's solution, dehydrated and embedded in paraffin. Sections of 4 μm were cut, deparaffinized and washed in water for half an hour, then rinsed with PBS. The other half of the tissue was frozen in isopenthane and cooled in liquid nitrogen at -180°C. The frozen tissue was cut in a cryostat at -20°C (4–6 μm thick), then fixed in acetone and washed for 10 minutes in 0.01 mol/l PBS, pH 7.4. Both frozen and deparaffinized sections were then immunostained with the immunoperoxidase–antiperoxidase method (PAP) of Sternberger (1979).

A rabbit antiserum of RU486 was supplied by Roussel–Uclaf (Romainville, France). The antibody was highly specific for RU486 and cross-reaction with P, cortisol, desoxycorticosterone and E_2 was $\langle 0.01\%$. After neutralization of the native peroxidase, sections were treated with a goat anti-BSA serum to minimize non-specific binding. Tissue sections were incubated with RU486 antibody, then processed with the usual PAP method (i.e. pig antirabbit antibody and rabbit PAP complex) (Sternberger, 1979). Using the same method and changing the primary antibody, we tested serial sections with antihuman albumin, antiorosomucoid (a protein known to bind RU486 in humans) (Philibert *et al.*, 1985) and antiglucocorticoid antibodies. Since the anti-RU486 antibody is also directed against albumin, these studies could evaluate non-specific staining for albumin, orosomucoid or cortisol.

Morphological studies

In the two groups who received RU486 during the luteal phase, morphological examination of the endometrial samples indicated premature involution of the endometrium. Numerous hemorrhagic lakes infiltrated the stroma. There was an increase in lipid deposit in the glands with karyorrhexis (i.e. disruption of the nuclei, apoptotic cells). These findings are usually observed at the time of the menstrual period and correspond to the decrease in action of both E_2 and P. However, at the time of menstruation other features such as necrosis, spiral arteriolar constriction and stromal infiltration with inflammatory cells are also present. These latter manifestations were not observed under RU486 therapy. Thus RU486 administered during the midluteal phase led to earlier endometrial involution but without necrosis. No signs of hyperplasia were observed.

Table 1 shows the morphological characteristics of the secretory endome-

Table 1. *Endometrial morphology during the midluteal phase and at the time of menstruation in non-treated subjects and after RU486 intake either during the midluteal or the late luteal phase*

Endometrial tissue	Characteristics	Midluteal phase[a] (RU486 day 22–25)	Midluteal phase[a]	Late luteal phase[b] (RU486 day 25–28)	Menstruation
Glands	Connective spikes (E_2)	+	++	++	++
Epithelial cells	Mitosis (E_2)	−	−	−	−
	Cubic cells (P)	+++	+++	+++	+++
	Secretion (P)	+	+	+	+
	Caryorrhexis ($E_2{\downarrow}P{\downarrow}$)	++	−	+++	+++
	Lipids ($\downarrow E_2{\downarrow}P$)	++		+++	+++
Stroma	Granulocytes (P)	+	++	+++	+++
	Lipids ($\downarrow E_2{\downarrow}P$)	++	++	+++	+++
	Hemorrhagia	+	−	+++	+++
	Necrosis ($\downarrow E_2{\downarrow}P$)	+	−	+++	+++
Vessels		N	N	N	N

Notes:
[a] endometrial biopsy performed on day 24.
[b] endometrial biopsy performed on day 27.
N = normal.
+ = low.
+ + = moderate.
+ + + = marked.
− = absent.

trium on day 24 of the cycle as well as at the time of menstruation. Also shown are the histological findings in women who received RU486 in the mid and late luteal phase. There is clear evidence of premature involution of the endometrial tissue in women treated during the midluteal phase, with increase in lipid deposit in the epithelial cells, karyorrhexis and hemorrhage in the stroma. The women treated in the late luteal phase showed no differences in the morphological aspects of the endometrium collected on day 27 after 3 days of RU486, compared to the characteristics of a normal menstruating endometrium.

Immunocytochemical aspects

Only women who received RU486 during the luteal phase demonstrated staining for RU486, which was located in the stromal cells. Within these cells, although staining was mostly heterogeneous, it was predominantly nuclear in localization. No staining was observed in the glandular epithelium. In those subjects who received RU486 during the follicular phase, no staining was observed.

Pregnant women

Pregnant women of less than 49 days amenorrhea applying for legal abortion received RU486 (either 100 mg/day for 7 days or 450 mg in a single dose). Subjects came frequently to the clinic for blood sampling and ultrasonography. In the case of induced abortion, the subjects brought back expelled products in a vial with fixative which they had received at the first visit. In the case of an unsuccessful abortion (i.e. RU486 non-responders), the products obtained after aspiration were collected under the same conditions. All subjects gave written consent for the study.

Morphological aspects

Pathological aspects of the products of conception were examined in 38 subjects who responded to RU486 with successful abortion and in 23 subjects who had undergone vacuum extraction. In contradistinction to the findings observed in normal spontaneous abortion, where complete necrosis of all layers is observed (Novak & Woodruff, 1962), only partial necrosis of the compacta was evident in both responders and non-responders to the drug. Nevertheless, in all instances the decidua compacta showed necrosis and hemorrhage in some areas (Fig. 1), while the decidua spongiosa and the trophoblastic villi were intact with minimal fibrotic areas. The decidua compacta showed larger areas of necrosis and diffuse hemorrhagic lakes in the RU486 responders, but there were small zones where the compacta was intact. In contrast, in the non-responders, both necrotic and hemorrhagic areas were minimal.

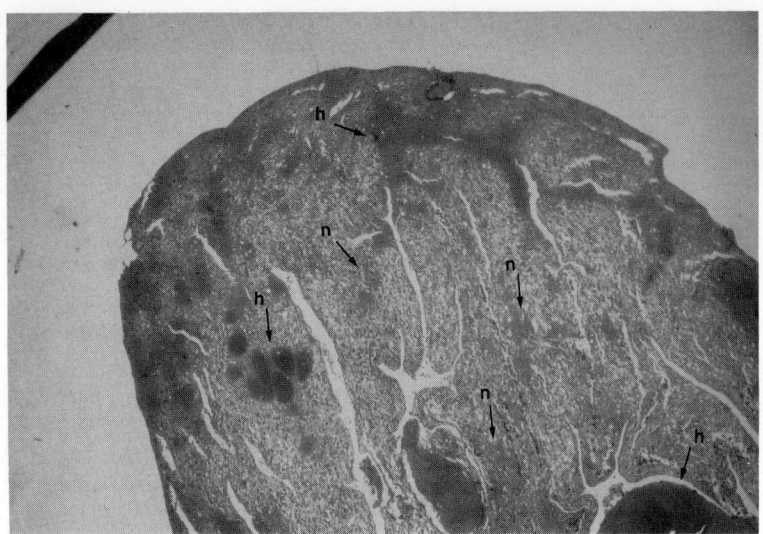

Fig. 1 Decidual histology in a patient who responded to RU486. The products of abortion were eliminated 4 days after commencement of therapy, at 46 days of amenorrhea. The decidua compacta contains numerous areas of necrosis (n) and hemorrhagic lakes (h) (× 10).

Immunocytochemical aspects

With the immunoperoxidase technique, RU486 binding was localized to the decidualized endometrium. None of the necrotic areas stained for the drug. The remaining areas stained in an heterogeneous pattern. In the decidua compacta, few nuclei retained the staining for RU486. No staining was obtained after testing the same areas with anti-orosomucoid, anti-glucocorticoid or anti-albumin antibodies. In the decidua spongiosa, the glands and the stroma were weakly stained and the nuclear staining was far less marked than in the compacta.

A marked heterogeneity of response was observed in the trophoblastic villi. In the responders, staining was evident in some areas of the syncithiotrophoblastic cells within the nuclei, while no staining was present within the cytotrophoblastic cells (Langhans cells). In the non-responders, only some syncithiotrophoblastic cells had a positive nuclear staining (Fig. 2). The localization of staining for RU486 in these cells is related to the well-known progesterone dependence of implantation in early human pregnancy. Indeed, P receptors are present within the trophoblastic villi. Careful testing of serial sections of the tissues with antibodies directed against albumin, orosomucoid and glucocorticoids did not reveal any staining. This indicates that tissue

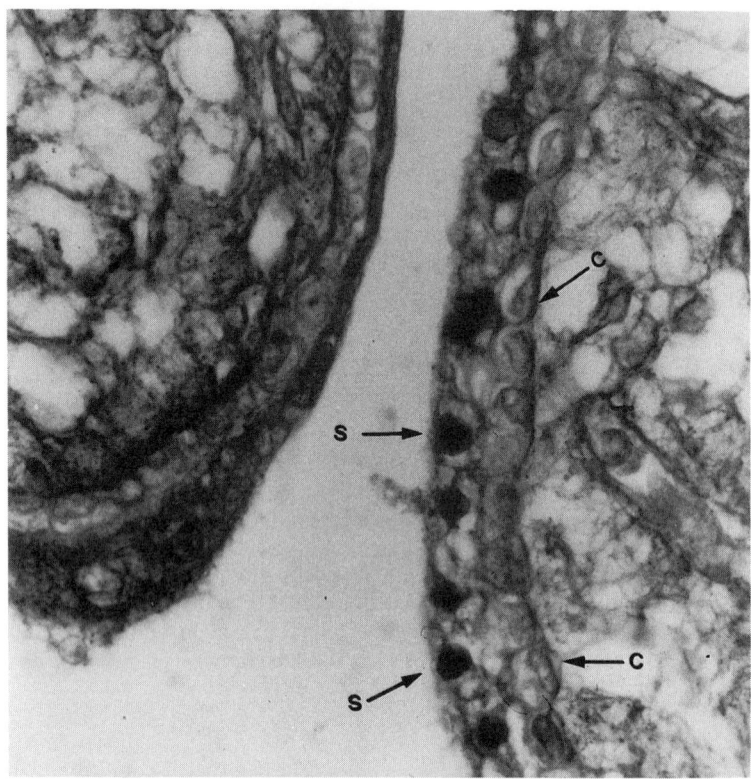

Fig. 2 Immunocytochemical localization of RU486 binding in the nuclei of syncithiotrophoblastic (s) cells. No staining is observed in the cytoplasm. The cytotrophoblastic cells (c) are not stained (× 400).

staining observed with anti-RU486 could reliably be attributed to the specific presence of RU486 in the cells.

These observations could suggest that because of its high affinity to the P receptor compared to P itself (Philibert *et al.*, 1985), RU486 binds to the P receptor only in secretory tissues. Also, in endometrial cells suffering from imminent necrosis, the cell metabolism and kinetics could be modified and affect RU486 binding.

In conclusion, there is strong evidence that RU486, through its binding to the P receptor in estrogen-primed endometrium, can block P action and lead to premature involution of the tissue and bleeding in non-pregnant women. In human decidualized tissue, its binding to the P receptor deprives the tissue from P action at the site of implantation which leads to abortion. However, it is possible that in non-responders to RU486 there was insufficient supply of the drug at the receptor level within the trophoblastic villi. Also, a separate effect on the decidualized endometrium leading to bleeding and on the trophoblastic villi leading to abortion could explain the non-responsiveness despite the presence of bleeding which occurs uniformly after RU486 administration even in the non-responders. Further trials on the exact localization of RU486 to the target cells are needed.

Acknowledgements

Original studies reviewed in this communication were supported by grants from the George J. Hecht Fund, Rockefeller Foundation and Andrew W. Mellon Foundation.
We thank C.W. Bardin, Population Council for his help and advice.

References

Chillik, C.F., Hsui, J.G., Acosta, A.A., Van Uem, J.F.H.M. & Hodgen, G.D. (1986). RU486 induced menses in cynomolgus monkeys: uniformity of endometrial sloughing. *Fertility and Sterility*, **45**:708–712.

Couzinet, B., Le Strat, N., Ulmann, A., Baulieu, E.E. & Schaison, G. (1986). Termination of early pregnancy by the progesterone antagonist RU486 (Mifepristone). *New England Journal of Medicine*, **315**:1565–1570.

Croxatto, H.B., Salvatierra, A.M., Croxatto, H.D. & Spitz, I.M. (1989). Variable effects of RU486 on endometrial maintenance in the luteal phase extended by exogenous hCG. *Clinical Endocrinology*, in press.

Croxatto, H.B., Spitz, I.M., Salvatierra, A.M. & Bardin, C.W. (1985). The demonstration of the antiprogestin effects of RU486 when administered to the human during HCG-induced pseudo-pregnancy. (In) *The Antiprogestin Steroid RU486 and Human Fertility Control* (Baulieu, E.E. & Segal, S., eds.), pp.263–269. New York, Plenum Press.

Gerschenson, L.E., Berliner, J. & Yang, J.J. (1974). Diethylstilbestrol and progesterone regulation of cultured rabbit endometrial cell growth. *Cancer Research*, **34**:2873–2880.

Gravanis, A., Schaison, G., George, M., De Brux, J., Satyaswaroop, P.G., Baulieu, E.E. & Robel, P. (1985). Endometrial and pituitary responses to the steroidal antiprogestin RU486 in postmenopausal women. *Journal of Clinical Endocrinology and Metabolism*, **60**:156–163.

Herrmann, W., Wyss, R., Riondel, A., Philibert, D., Teutsch, G., Sakiz, E. & Baulieu, E.E. (1982). Effect d'un stéroide anti-progestérone chez la femme: interruption du cycle menstruel et de la grossesse au début. *Comptes Rendus de L'Académie des Sciences*, **294**:933–938.

Horwitz, K.B., Wei, L.L., Sedlacek, S.M. & d'Arville, C.N. (1985). Progestin action and progesterone receptor structure in human breast cancer: A review. *Recent Progress in Hormone Research*, **41**:249–316.

Hsueh, A.J.W., Peck, E.J. & Clark, J.H. (1976). Control of uterine estrogen receptor levels by progesterone. *Endocrinology*, **98**:438–444.

Koering, M.J., Healy, D.L. & Hodgen, G.D. (1986). Morphologic response of endometrium to a progesterone receptor antagonist, RU486, in monkeys. *Fertility and Sterility*, **45**:280–287.

Kovacs, L., Sas, M., Resch, B.A., Ugocsai, G., Swahn, M.L., Bygdeman, M. & Rowe, P.J. (1984). Termination of very early pregnancy by RU486 – an antiprogestational compound. *Contraception*, **29**:399–410.

Li, T.C., Rogers, A.W., Dockery, P., Lenton, E.A. & Cooke, I.D. (1988). A new method of histologic dating of human endometrium in the luteal phase. *Fertility and Sterility*, **50**:52–60.

Novak, E.R. & Woodruff, J.D. (1962). *Novak's Gynecologic and Obstetric Pathology*, 5th edition. Philadelphia, Saunders.

Noyes, R.W., Hertig, A.T. & Rock, J. (1950). Dating the endometrial biopsy. *Fertility and Sterility*, **1**:3–25.

Okulicz, W.C. (1987). Effect of the antiprogestin RU-486 on progesterone inhibition of occupied nuclear estrogen receptor in the uterus. *Journal of Steroid Biochemistry*, **28**:117–122.

Philibert, D., Moguilewski, M., Mary, I., Lecaque, D., Tournemine, C., Secchi, J. & Deraedt, R. (1985). Pharmacologic profile of RU486 in animals. (In) *The Antiprogestin Steroid RU486 and Human Fertility Control* (Baulieu, E.E. & Segal, S., eds.), pp.49–68. New York, Plenum Press.

Sternberger, L.A. (1979). *Immunocytochemistry*, 2nd edition. New York, Wiley Medical.

Tseng, L. & Gurpide, E. (1975). Induction of human endometrial estradiol dehydrogenase by progestins. *Endocrinology*, **97**:825–833.

Discussion

Clark. The table in your manuscript described hemorrhage and necrosis but the blood vessels were normal in all cases. Does that mean hemorrhage and necrosis occur without the vascular spasm that we have been talking about up until this moment?

Sitruk-Ware. From the morphological point of view, there was no change in the structure of the arterial vessels.

Sheppard. After administration of RU486, near the beginning of the follicular phase, the morphology showed a tremendous amount of stromal hemorrhage but I could not see any blood vessels in that. You said that it was having little effect on the arteries but I think we have a reasonable consensus of opinion now that the bleeding is not coming from the arteries but it is coming from the vessels in the subepithelial capillary plexus. Have you looked at those, are they more dilated, or damaged in any way?

Sitruk-Ware. No, we have not looked in detail at the structure of the capillaries. We have immunocytochemical evidence of RU486 within the nucleus of cells around the vessels but no change, and no destruction. For the normal women, we had good tissue; however, with the abortions, the women bled and they collected the tissue under conditions that were not conducive to subsequent analysis. So it is difficult to assess if there were direct actions on the vessels.

Bouchard. I do not think it is fair to say that RU486 is both a progestogen and an antiprogestogen because, if you study RU486 effects with modern techniques, it is indeed a very weak progestogen and a very potent antiprogesterone.

Johannisson. I thought I should add to your presentation information on the vascular changes following the use of RU486. We did a study in Stockholm with Professor Bygdeman using a similar protocol (Johannisson *et al.*, 1989). RU486 was given for 4 days in the secretory phase and in all these patients, bleeding occurred on the fourth day of treatment. Biopsies were taken just before the onset of bleeding and we found definite vascular changes in the endometrium. We carried out a morphometric study on the diameter of the capillary vessels in the superficial layer of the endometrium and found that in treated women who had started to bleed or were bleeding, there was a significant decrease in the diameter of the capillary lumen. This indicates vasoconstriction when compared with normal biopsies taken at the same time of the cycle. So there are some vascular changes.

Healy. Was there any difference in the appearance of the endometrium between those women with a progesterone fall and those women in whom estradiol and progesterone did not fall? This may be a model of progesterone withdrawal without any estrogen withdrawal.

Sitruk-Ware. There was no difference.

Cooke. I was interested in your statement that some patients given RU486 had what appeared to be a second menstruation. We did a dose-finding study on RU486 in the early luteal phase, and there were quite a number of patients who had a second bleed at the time of the expected menstruation. Biopsies done at the time of the first bleed showed that a number of these did not have complete shedding of the endometrium and the histological features included a reduction in the glandular activity. There was also a reduction in the predecidual changes and a marked reduction in the leukocytic infiltration.

Sitruk-Ware. There have been publications showing that there is an increase in leukocyte infiltration with RU486 given during the luteal phase. I think that part of the problem is that when you give RU486 orally, the metabolism is different according to each patient, and therefore we do not know what amount reaches the endometrium. It has also been shown in anovulatory patients, that when you give RU486, you do not have bleeding – again showing that this effect exists only when there is progesterone present.

Ludwig. I would like to stress the similarity of the endometrium you described, with endometrium from women with spotting and intermenstrual bleeding, which is multifocal disseminating interstromal bleeding. I think we should use RU486 as a model to study intermenstrual bleeding and we should introduce into the histological examination, staining of capillary walls by staining elastin for example, so that one can identify the vasculature in this terminal endometrium.

Findlay. Dr Ludwig, implicit in your suggestion of using RU486 to study intermenstrual bleeding is that a withdrawal of the action of progesterone is in fact involved in intermenstrual bleeding, and I am not aware that we actually know that.

Baird. We need information from situations where intermenstrual bleeding is common, that is with continuous progestogen, as to whether these endometria are defective in progesterone receptors, in which case, one can use the withdrawal of progesterone – like the use of RU486 – as an adequate model.

Diaz. We completed a preliminary trial, using a single dose of RU486 on day 12 of the cycle in 10 Norplant[R] users after the third year of use, when they were cycling regularly. They did not bleed.

Baird. That is further evidence that you require some degree of progesterone priming with progesterone receptors in the endometrium, in order to induce a bleed. If you give RU486 immediately after ovulation, you very seldom get a menstrual bleed because a minimum degree of priming of the endometrium with progesterone is needed in order to induce it.

References

Johannisson, E., Oberholzer, M., Swahn, M.L. & Bygdeman, M. (1989). Vascular changes in the human endometrium following the administration of the progesterone antagonist RU486. *Contraception*, **39**:103–118.

Antiprogestogens and endometrial function

S.K. SMITH

Department of Obstetrics and Gynaecology, University of Cambridge, School of Clinical Medicine, The Rosie Maternity Hospital, Cambridge, UK.

Abstract

Ovarian steroids alter the synthesis of prostaglandins (PG) by endometrium. *In vivo* this is reflected in the different capacities of endometrium and decidua to release PGs. Measured in freshly removed tissue, PG release is greatest from secretory endometrium, with lowest levels being found in decidua of early pregnancy. However, *in vitro*, proliferative endometrium releases most PGs followed by secretory tissue and decidua. Separation of glandular and stromal cells reveals that these changes are reflected solely in the capacity of glandular cells, not stromal cells, to synthesize PGs. Progesterone suppresses PG release from proliferative tissue in the presence and absence of exogenous arachidonic acid. Antiprogestogens, which compete for the nuclear receptor, stimulate the synthesis of PGs from decidua only from the glandular cells not from stromal cells. This effect occurs both with and without added arachidonic acid, suggesting that part of the action of progesterone involves reduction of PG synthase activity. The increase in PG levels is not reflected by a similar increase in metabolites, indicating that a further mechanism is reduced metabolism. This stimulation of PG synthesis from decidual glandular cells induced by antiprogestogens is abolished by actinomycin, indicating that de-novo protein synthesis is required. If the predominant effect of progesterone was to stimulate the synthesis of inhibitory proteins, this would be expected to increase PG release. Calcium is required, as verapamil; the L-type calcium channel blocker also inhibits PG-stimulated release by antiprogestogens.

Prostaglandins are important second messengers whose altered synthesis is known to be associated with menstrual dysfunction, possibly because of their effects on local vasculature and endometrial proliferation. The mechanism whereby progestogens inhibit PG release and antiprogestogens stimulate its synthesis from glandular cells remains unknown, but is likely to be an important factor in understanding the mechanisms of menstrual bleeding of women taking the oral contraceptive pill.

Introduction

The investigation of the action of progesterone on endometrial function is relevant to the mechanism of normal menstruation and could be important in bleeding arising in women taking long-acting progestogens. The recent synthesis of antiprogestogens which compete with natural progesterone for the progesterone receptor provides a means for studying the effects of progesterone. The hypothesis that withdrawal of progesterone provides the trigger for natural menstruation because of an elevation of prostaglandin (PG) synthesis can be tested by the use of antiprogestogens. Before considering the effects of antiprogestogens on PG synthesis by human cells, it is important to review the action of progesterone.

Prostaglandin synthesis during the cycle and in early pregnancy

Early studies of PG synthesis measured 'basal' levels of PG in which freshly removed tissue was placed in ethanol to prevent further degradation of PGs and the amount present determined by radioimmunoassay. In these circumstances, levels of $PGF_{2\alpha}$ but not PGE_2 were raised in the secretory phase of the cycle, suggesting that progesterone increases the capacity of the tissue to synthesize PGs (Downie *et al.*, 1974; Singh *et al.*, 1975). This effect of progesterone was mimicked in postmenopausal women given estradiol and progesterone (Smith *et al.*, 1984). However, decidua which is also exposed to progesterone has grossly reduced levels of PGs compared to non-pregnant tissue (Maathuis & Kelly, 1978). This does not appear to be a direct effect of the trophoblast on endometrial function as the same pattern is observed in decidua removed from women with ectopic pregnancies (Abel *et al.*, 1980).

Incubation of endometrium *in vitro* provided conflicting results, not only between different culture systems but with the findings of 'basal' release. Abel and Baird (1980) found that secretory endometrium released more PG into culture medium than proliferative endometrium, whereas Tsang and Ooi (1982) and Schatz *et al.* (1986) found the converse to be true. However, Abel and Baird did demonstrate that progesterone suppressed PG synthesis. Gal *et al.* (1982) incubated stromal and glandular cells in culture for at least 9 days and found that stromal cells had the greater capacity to release PGs. However, shorter cultures of up to 4 days demonstrated that it was the glandular epithelial cells which released most PGs (Schatz *et al.*, 1986; Smith & Kelly, 1988a). Immunohistochemical identification of cyclo-oxygenase in the glandular cells of the endometrium supports the latter case (Rees *et al.*, 1982). Further, enriched fractions of glandular cells release most $PGF_{2\alpha}$ both in the first and second 24 hours in culture, when prepared from proliferative endometrium (Smith & Kelly, 1988a), and these cells respond to histamine in culture with a greater release of PGs than secretory cells. In the same system, the ability of enriched stromal cells to synthesize PGs did not alter throughout the cycle. In early pregnancy the capacity of enriched glandular cells to release PGs is further suppressed, as is their response to histamine (Smith & Kelly, 1988a).

Progesterone and prostaglandin synthesis and metabolism

Explants

Progesterone suppresses PG release from explants of human endometrium maintained in culture (Abel & Baird, 1980; Kelly & Smith, 1987a). This suppression occurs in the presence of exogenous arachidonic acid (AA), suggesting that progesterone acts by preventing metabolism of AA. Cell-to-cell contact appears necessary to demonstrate this effect, as progesterone alone causes a slight rise in PG release from separated epithelial cells (Smith & Kelly, 1987). However, progesterone does suppress PG release from separated cells when incubated in the presence of estradiol (Schatz *et al.*, 1986).

Antiprogestogens

The recent introduction of the antiprogestogens RU486 (Roussel-Uclaf) and ZK 98734 (Schering) has raised the possibility of investigating further the action of progesterone on PG synthesis by endometrium. Incorporation of the 11-dimethylamino-phenyl group to the steroid molecule confers antagonistic action (Hendersen, 1987). The antiprogestogen combines with the nuclear receptor and blocks the DNA binding of the activated receptor by stabilizing the complex formed by the receptor and the heat shock protein 90 (Baulieu, 1987).

Both antiprogestogens cause the release of $PGF_{2\alpha}$ to rise over the dose range of 10–1000 nmol/l from glandular cells obtained from decidua of early pregnancy. No response was obtained from stromal fractions. This picture is different from that attained with secretory endometrium (Kelly *et al.*, 1986). In this tissue, RU486 causes a slight decline in PG release from the glands. These differences could be explained by the antiprogestogen acting as an agonist in non-pregnant tissue for reasons which are not immediately apparent. Alternatively, it may reflect differences in receptor populations between glandular and stromal cells obtained from non-pregnant and pregnant endometrium. Epithelial cells contain more receptors than stromal cells (King *et al.*, 1982) but not all are occupied (Levy *et al.*, 1980). If there were more occupied receptors in the stromal cells, then displacement of progesterone by the antiprogestogen would be more pronounced in the stromal cells. Similarly, if circumstances were altered in decidual cells and epithelial cells contained the greater number of occupied receptors, antiprogestogens would be expected to cause a rise in PG synthesis by these cells.

The rise of PG release induced by antiprogestogens could occur by several mechanisms. Firstly, antiprogestogens might block accumulation of AA into membrane lipids, normally promoted by progesterone. Persistent proliferative tissue exposed to at least 2 weeks of estrogen and no progesterone, has the same capacity as secretory tissue to synthesize PGs only in the presence of added AA (Smith *et al.*, 1984). Alternatively, progesterone may act by reducing the activity of phospholipases A_2 and C (PLA_2, PLC). Wilson *et al.* (1986) failed to demonstrate such an action of progesterone, though Bonney *et al.* (1987; Bonney & Franks, 1988) found that steroids regulated PLA_2 and PLC activity but gave no indication as to the mechanisms. Glucocorticoids suppress PG synthesis in other tissues by stimulating the synthesis of a lipocortin (Blackwell *et al.*, 1980; Huang *et al.*, 1986; Wallner *et al.*, 1986) which antagonizes phospholipase activity. However, human endometrium does synthesize lipocortin 1 (Gurpide *et al.*, 1986) but dexamethasone and cortisol do not suppress PG synthesis (Kelly & Smith, 1987b).

Many of the previous studies have emphasized the importance of the availability of free AA in regulating PG synthesis. But progesterone suppresses PG release from human endometrial explants in the presence of exogenous AA (Kelly & Smith, 1987a) and RU486 and ZK 98734 stimulate PG synthesis in the presence of AA. Both of these findings suggest that progesterone and the antiprogestogens act at the level of cyclo-oxygenase, a finding confirmed by Jeremy & Dandona in the rat (1986). Finally, antiprogestogens do reduce the metabolism of PGs, at least in the presence of excess AA.

Recent studies suggest that progesterone and the antiprogestogens exert their actions by influencing genomic expression. The rise of PG release induced by ZK 98734 is abolished by incubation in the presence of actinomycin which inhibits transcription and prevents new protein formation (Smith & Kelly, 1988b). The relative importance of PLA_2, PLC, PG synthase and the lipocortins in regulating PG synthesis is unknown. However, if the most important mediator of PG synthesis in early pregnant decidua was a suppressing protein, then actinomycin would be expected to increase PG synthesis. Calcium is required for the synthesis of PGs, as ZK 98734 stimulation is abolished by the calcium channel blocker, verapamil.

Conclusion

There is convincing evidence to suggest that progesterone inhibits PG synthesis and that antiprogestogens antagonize this inhibition. However, the mechanism remains unclear. Progesterone does reduce the activity of PLA_2, PLC and cyclo-oxygenase (Bonney *et al.*, 1987; Bonney & Franks, 1988; Smith & Kelly, 1988b) but it is not known if this reflects changes in the genomic expression of the enzyme or changes in the intracellular environment such as pH or calcium levels. The suppression of PG synthesis from endometrium is required in species with epitheliochorial placentation to prevent luteolysis. In women, PG suppression is needed to prevent menstruation and the loss of the blastocyst. Several strategies have evolved to achieve these ends, including steroid suppression, inhibitory agents released by the trophoblast, e.g. interferon (Salamonsen *et al.*, 1988), or inhibitory proteins synthesized within the endometrium (Gross *et al.*, 1988). Prostaglandins subserve many modulatory functions within the cell and the effect of long-acting progestogens on their synthesis is at least likely to be an important marker of endometrial function. Further work is required to establish fully the mechanisms regulating PG release from human endometrium.

References

Abel, M.H. & Baird, D.T. (1980). The effect of 17β-estradiol and progesterone on prostaglandin production by human endometrium maintained in organ culture. *Endocrinology*, **106**:1599–1606.

Abel, M.H., Smith, S.K. & Baird, D.T. (1980). Suppression of concentration of endometrial prostaglandin in early intra-uterine and ectopic pregnancies in women. *Journal of Endocrinology*, **85**:379–386.

Baulieu, E.E. (1987). Contragestion by the progesterone antagonist RU 486: a novel approach to human fertility control. *Contraception*, **36**(Supplement):1–5.

Blackwell, G.J., Carnuccio, R., Dirosa, M., Flower, R.J., Parente, L. & Persico, P. (1980). Macrocortin: a polypeptide causing the antiphospholipase effect of glucocorticoids. *Nature*, **287**:147–149.

Bonney, R.C. & Franks, S. (1988). Hydrolysis of phosphatidylinositol by human endometrium: modulating effects of steroids on arachidonic acid and 1,2-diacylglycerol release. *Journal of Endocrinology*, **117**:309–314.

Bonney, R.C., Qizilbash, S.T. & Franks, S. (1987). Endometrial phospholipase A2 enzymes and their regulation by steroid hormones. *Journal of Steroid Biochemistry*, **27**:1057–1064.

Downie, J., Poyser, N. & Wunderlich, M. (1974). Levels of prostaglandins in human endometrium during the normal menstrual cycle. *Journal of Physiology*, **236**:465–472.

Gal, D., Casey, M.L., Johnston, J.M. & MacDonald, P.C. (1982). Mesenchyme–epithelial interactions in human endometrium. Prostaglandin synthesis in separated cell types. *Journal of Clinical Investigation*, **70**:798–805.

Gross, T.S., Thatcher, W.W., Hansen, P.J., Johnson, J.W. & Helmer, S.D. (1988). Presence of an intracellular endometrial inhibitor of prostaglandin synthesis during early pregnancy in the cow. *Prostaglandins*, **35**(3):359–378.

Gurpide, E., Markiewicz, L., Schatz, F. & Hirata, F. (1986). Lipocortin output by human endometrium *in vitro*. *Journal of Clinical Endocrinology and Metabolism*, **63**:162–166.

Hendersen, G. (1987). Antiprogestational and antiglucocorticoid activities of some novel 11 aryl substituted steroids. (In) *Pharmacology and Clinical Uses of Inhibitors of Hormone Secretion and Action* (Furr, B.J.A. & Wakeling, A.E., eds.), pp.184–211. London, Bailliere Tindall.

Huang, K.S., Wallner, B.P., Mattaliano, R.J., Tizard, R., Burne, C., Frey, A., Hession, C., McGray, P., Sinclair, L.K., Chow, E.P., Browning, J.L., Ramachandran, K.L., Tang, J., Smart, J.E. & Pepinsky, R.B. (1986). Two human 35kd inhibitors of phospholipase A2 are related to substrates of pp60 v-src and of the epidermal growth factor receptor/kinase. *Cell*, **46**:191–199.

Jeremy, J.Y. & Dandona, P. (1986). RU 486 antagonises the inhibitory action of progesterone on prostacyclin and thromboxane A2 synthesis in cultured rat myometrial explants. *Endocrinology*, **119**:655–660.

Kelly, R.W., Healy, D.L., Cameron, M.J., Cameron, I.T. & Baird, D.T. (1986). The stimulation of prostaglandin production by two antiprogesterone steroids in human endometrial cells. *Journal of Clinical Endocrinology and Metabolism*, **62**:1116–1123.

Kelly, R.W. & Smith, S.K. (1987a). Progesterone and anti-progestogens, a comparison of their effect on prostaglandin production by human secretory phase endometrium and decidua. *Prostaglandins, Leukotrienes and Medicine*, **29**:181–186.

Kelly, R.W. & Smith, S.K. (1987b). Glucocorticoids do not share with progesterone the potent inhibitory action on prostaglandin synthesis in human proliferative phase endometrium. *Prostaglandins*, **33**:919–929.

King, R.J.B., Townsend, P.T., Siddle, N., Whitehead, M.I. & Taylor, R.W. (1982). Regulation of estrogen and progesterone receptor levels in epithelium and stroma from pre- and post-menopausal endometria. *Journal of Steroid Biochemistry*, **16**:21–29.

Levy, C., Gautray, J.P., De Brux, J., Verma, U., Descomps, B., Baulieu, E.E. & Eychenne, G. (1980). Estradiol and progesterone receptors in human endometrium; normal and abnormal menstrual cycles and early pregnancy. *American Journal of Obstetrics and Gynecology*, **136**:646–651.

Maathuis, J.B. & Kelly, R.W. (1978). Concentrations of prostaglandins $F_{2\alpha}$ and E_2 in the endometrium throughout the menstrual cycle, after the administration of clomiphene or an oestrogen–progestogen pill and in early pregnancy. *Journal of Endocrinology*, **77**:361–371.

Rees, M.C.P., Parry, D.M., Anderson, A.B.M. & Turnbull, A.C. (1982). Immunohistochemical localisation of cyclo-oxygenase in the human uterus. *Prostaglandins*, **23**:207–214.

Salamonsen, L.A., Stuchbery, S.J., O'Grady, C.M., Godkin, J.D. & Findlay, J.K. (1988). Interferon-α mimics effects of ovine trophoblast protein 1 on prostaglandin and protein secretion by ovine endometrial cells *in vitro*. *Journal of Endocrinology*, **117**:1–4.

Schatz, F., Markiewicz, L., Barg, P. & Gurpide, E. (1986). *In vitro* inhibition with antiestrogens of estradiol effects on prostaglandin $F_{2\alpha}$ production by human endometrium and endometrial epithelial cells. *Endocrinology*, **118**:408–412.

Singh, E.J., Baccarini, I. & Zuspan, F.P. (1975). Levels of prostaglandins $F_{2\alpha}$ and E_2 in human endometrium during the menstrual cycle. *American Journal of Obstetrics and Gynecology*, **121**:1003–1006.

Smith, S.K., Abel, M.H. & Baird, D.T. (1984). Effects of 17beta-estradiol and progesterone on the levels of prostaglandins F2alpha and E in human endometrium. *Prostaglandins*, **27**:591–597.

Smith, S.K. & Kelly, R.W. (1987). The effect of the anti-progestins RU486 and ZK98734 on the synthesis and metabolism of $PGF_{2\alpha}$ and PGE_2 in separated cells from early human decidua. *Journal of Clinical Endocrinology and Metabolism*, **65**:527–534.

Smith, S.K. & Kelly, R.W. (1988a). The release of $PGF_{2\alpha}$ and PGE_2 from separated cells of human endometrium and decidua. *Prostaglandins, Leukotrienes and Fatty Acids*, **33**:91–96.

Smith, S.K. & Kelly, R.W. (1988b). Prostaglandin and steroid induced endometrial changes in early human pregnancy. *Journal of Reproduction and Fertility*, **36**(Supplement):143–154.

Tsang, B.K. & Ooi, T.C. (1982). Prostaglandin secretion by human endometrium *in vitro*. *American Journal of Obstetrics and Gynecology*, **142**:626–633.

Wallner, B.P., Mattaliano, R.J., Hession, C., Cate, R.L., Tizard, R., Sinclair, L.K., Foeller, C., Chow, E.P., Browning, J.L., Ramachandran, K.L. & Pepinsky, R.B.

(1986). Cloning and expression of human lipocortin, a phospholipase A2 inhibitor with potential anti-inflammatory activity. *Nature*, 320:77–81.

Wilson, T., Liggins, G.C., Aimer, G.P. & Watkins, E.J. (1986). The effect of progesterone on the release of arachidonic acid from human endometrial cells stimulated by histamine. *Prostaglandins*, 31:343–360.

Discussion

Harper. In experiments on glandular epithelium, you were able to show a stimulation of prostaglandin production by platelet-activating factor (PAF). Would you like to speculate whether you think there is a similar mechanism or a different mechanism, and have you done any experiments in combinations with the antiprogestogens?

Smith. No, I have not. What we showed with PAF is that it did not increase PGF production, it simply increased PGE_2 production. I think that your work with the idea that the stroma can influence prostaglandins is obviously attractive and this is something that we hope to look at in the next few months. I think it is true to say that in platelets PAF works principally through the phosphatidyl inositol pathway rather than through stimulation of PLA_2. In addition, PAF had no effect on proliferative tissues.

Bouchard. When you use RU486 or ZK 98734 alone they are not antiprogestogens, they are weak progestogens. So you have to test a reversal of the effect with a high dose of progesterone to demonstrate specificity.

Smith. Yes, I accept that point but those cultures were done over 24 hours. So presumably, if the cells did have progesterone bound to the nucleus, although it might be released during the 24 hours, I think they were progesterone-dominated cells.

Sitruk-Ware. My question is to Dr Baird. I think there are discrepancies in the results and the presentation as to whether progestogen stimulates or decreases the production of prostaglandins.

Baird. In the original experiments which I published with Margaret Abel (Abel & Baird, 1980), we showed that an endometrium, exposed *in vivo* to progesterone, has a greater capacity to synthesize and release prostaglandins than one which has not been exposed to progesterone. But in the presence of progesterone in the medium in concentrations which are consistent with luteal phase levels, that capacity is not expressed.

Toppozada. What is the vasospastic capacity of $PGF_{2\alpha}$ compared with other prostaglandins or other vasoconstrictive compounds that can be found in the endometrium?

Baird. I think the answer to that was reflected in Dr Åkerlund's paper in which the problems of actually measuring the effects of prostaglandins in a quantitative way on human uterine arterial samples were shown to be enormous. The other prostaglandin which is produced in very small amounts in the uterus is thromboxin A_2, but it is such a potent vasoconstrictor that it is entirely possible that it may have an effect on blood vessels within the myometrium. If I could just add a further point: $PGF_{2\alpha}$ is the dominant prostaglandin which you see if you incubate endometrium. It is the one prostaglandin that reproducibly increases menstrual bleeding if you put it in the lumen of the uterus. Of all the compounds we have talked about at this meeting, I do not know of another compound that will do that.

Casey. Clearly, in the secretory endometrium, as well as in decidua, whether it be from early or late pregnancy, there is prostaglandin dehydrogenase (PGDH) activity, in relatively high specific activity. In our experience, with organ culture or a variety of types of cell in culture, we find that within 6–12 hours of placement of that tissue within the culture media, the specific activity of PGDH declines to undetectable levels. We have tried to prevent that decline with steroid hormone treatment, prolactin treatment and a variety of potential agents, and have been unsuccessful in doing so. Noting you found relatively low amounts of metabolites, do you know if PGDH activity was demonstrable under optimal in-vitro conditions in those tissue samples?

Smith. Dr Kelly, using labelled substitute, showed relatively low amounts of PGDH activity in fresh tissue; it was not in tissue cultured for 24 hours.

Archer. What is the relationship between the initiating event and the bleeding induced by the antiprogestogens? In tissue, if you show, within 24 hours of antiprogestogen exposure, a rapid change in prostaglandin secretion, does it always take 4 days of antiprogestogen treatment before bleeding occurs?

Sitruk-Ware. No. In non-pregnant women, it is generally on the third day of administration. Women who are pregnant and who take the drug can bleed on the first day. So, there is a discrepancy between this situation and the total amount of progesterone they have.

Fraser. Dr Baird did say $PGF_{2\alpha}$ is the only known substance that causes menstrual-like bleeding when it is instilled into the uterine cavity. But I wonder how many other substances have actually been tested in that way?

Baird. The only other two substances we have tested are prostaglandin E_2 and prostacyclin, and neither induced bleeding.

Bischof. Dr Gurpide and Dr Smith said that cultured endometrial explants produce prostaglandin, but when they destroyed the cells, the production was much higher. I wondered if this is not something physiological and that there might be, in intermenstrual bleeding or in menstrual bleeding, an initial cell damage which would liberate prostaglandin. This cell damage could come perhaps from infiltrating lymphocytes.

Smith. That is highly likely. It is related to the point which we are trying to address, namely, what is it that initiates menstrual bleeding, as opposed to what happens when you get a breakthrough bleeding? I think steroid withdrawal is part of normal menstruation. Once you have got that tissue damage, there is bound to be release of prostaglandins. Now, in breakthrough bleeding there might be some other trigger which causes the cell damage, a bit like the changes that you get with the RU486 in terms of the necrosis, which then releases prostaglandins. That strikes me as a very relevant question on breakthrough bleeding.

Reference

Abel, M.H. & Baird, D.T. (1980). The effect of 17β-estradiol and progesterone on prostaglandin production by human endometrium maintained in organ culture. *Endocrinology*, **106**:1599–1606.

Protein kinases and cellular function: molecular mechanism of eicosanoid formation

FUSAO HIRATA

Department of Environmental Health Sciences, School of Hygiene and Public Health, The Johns Hopkins University, Baltimore, USA.

Abstract

Most extracellular signal molecules activate cells by binding to cell surface receptors. The receptors stimulate the production inside the cells of one or more second messengers (such as cyclic AMP, diacylglycerol and Ca^{2+}), which bind to and activate second messenger-dependent kinases. These kinases transduce extracellular signals into intracellular effects via modulation of the phosphorylation of target proteins including other kinases. This communication reviews the signal transduction and the action of steroidal hormones involved in the regulation of the arachidonic acid release by a network of cyclic AMP-dependent kinase, protein kinase C and tyrosine protein kinase.

Introduction

Several reproductive processes such as luteolysis, menstruation, implantation, parturition and ovulation are well known to be provoked by a complex network of hormones, neurotransmitters and cytokines. These compounds first bind to their specific receptors, located on cell surfaces. These signals are then amplified by the second messenger systems, including cyclic AMP, cyclic GMP, diacylglycerol and Ca^{2+} (Fig. 1). All these second messengers are modifiers (activators) of protein kinase A, G and C, respectively (Edelman *et al.*, 1987; Hunter, 1987; Shenolikar, 1988). In contrast, receptors for growth factors such as insulin, epidermal growth factor (EGF) and platelet-derived growth factor (PDGF) are well established to contain an intrinsic tyrosine kinase activity which can be directly activated by binding of ligands (Hunter, 1987). Thus, most, if not all, physiological stimuli are directly or indirectly connected to activation of various kinases.

Protein phosphorylation by protein kinases is one of the major mechanisms by which intracellular events in many cells are controlled by various stimuli (Edelman *et al.*, 1987; Hunter, 1987, Shenolikar, 1988). Most proteins are phosphorylated at serine and threonine residues to change their biological activities, while a small number of proteins are phosphorylated at tyrosine residues (Hunter, 1987). Phosphorylation of proteins is catalyzed by protein kinases, while phosphate of phosphorylated proteins is removed by protein phosphatases. Thereby, alteration of the biological activities of proteins

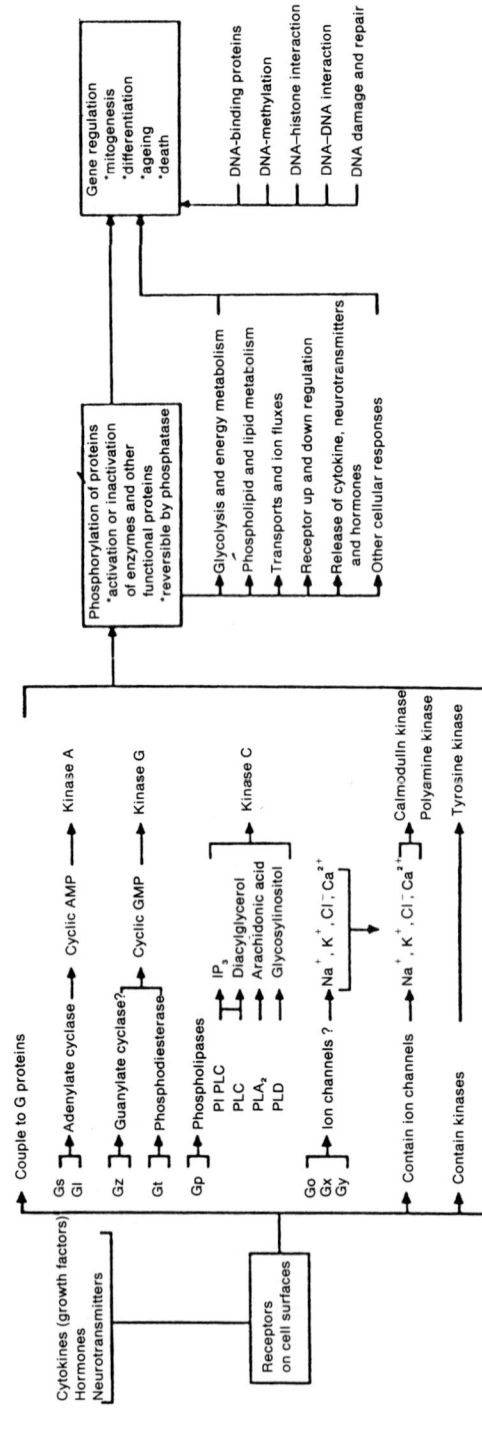

Fig. 1 Hypothetical mechanism of receptor signal transduction which leads to gene regulation.

Table 1. *Protein kinases*

Kinase	Modulator	Substrate
Cyclic nucleotide regulated		
Cyclic GMP dependent	Cyclic GMP	
Cyclic AMP dependent	Cyclic AMP	Phosphorylase kinase
		Glycogen synthetase
Diacylglycerol regulated		
Protein kinase C	Phorbol esters	p47, p82
	Diacylglycerol	
Calmodulin regulated		
Myosine light chain kinase	Calmodulin	Myosine phosphorylase
Phosphorylase kinase		Tyrosine hydroxylase
Calmodulin-dependent kinase		
Protein–tyrosine kinase		
Growth factor receptors	Growth factors	Ca^{2+}-binding proteins
EGF receptor		
Insulin receptor		Calpactins
PDGF receptor		
src gene family		
abl gene family		
fps gene family		
Others		
RNA-regulated kinase		
DNA-regulated kinase		
Polyamine-stimulated kinase		
Beta-receptor kinase		Beta-receptor
CDC 2H		Histone H
raf gene family		
Guanylate cyclase	ANF	

brought about by phosphorylation is reversible, and the activities of both kinases and phosphatases are subject to control by various stimuli. Proteins which are phosphorylated by these kinases include ion channels, Ca^{2+}-binding proteins, receptors, enzymes and DNA-binding proteins (Table 1). Hence, phosphorylation of these proteins results in alterations of cellular functions mediating through changes in ion fluxes, Ca^{2+} homeostasis, down- and up-regulation of receptors, energy production and gene transcription.

With the advent of molecular cloning followed by the discovery that many **onc** genes encode protein kinases, the number of proven or putative protein kinases has risen rapidly. This explosion in identifying new kinases mainly results from molecular cloning of protein kinase genes rather than enzyme purification. An important factor in a protein kinase family is that all protein kinases have a striking sequence similarity in their catalytic domains (Pearson *et al.*, 1988; Taylor *et al.*, 1988). In addition, they have autophosphorylation sites as well as pseudosubstrate sites.

Table 2. *Various phospholipase inhibitory proteins in cells*

Phospholipases	Lipomodulins/ lipocortins	Molecular weight
A_1	α	28000*
A_2	β	38000 ± 2000†
		11000 ± 2000*
C	γ	36000 ± 2000†
		14000 ± 2000*
D	δ	—
Phosphatidylinositol phospholipase C	ϵ	30000 ± 2000*

* Bacterial origins.
† Mammalian origins.

Autophosphorylation and phosphorylation by other kinases are also known to regulate the catalytic activity of the kinase. Various protein kinases are expected to have different biological roles, which may be attributed to some differences in their enzymatic properties and substrate specificities. However, in cell-free systems, most protein kinases can phosphorylate many proteins, only some of which are physiological substrates. Therefore, it is sometimes difficult to discuss how an individual kinase reaction induces a specific cellular function. In this chapter, the role of protein kinases in cellular functions is described, focusing on the molecular mechanism of arachidonic acid release by a network of protein kinases.

Receptor-mediated arachidonic acid release

Many, if not all, cells release arachidonic acid when they are stimulated by hormones, neurotransmitters and cytokines (Irvine, 1982; Hirata, 1988). Arachidonic acid is mostly present as an esterified form rather than as a free form. Therefore, activation of phospholipases, enzymes that cleave membrane phospholipids, is a prerequisite for the release of arachidonic acid. Phospholipases are inactive until cells are stimulated, although they are surrounded by phospholipid substrates in the membranes. It is reasonable to assume that these enzymes make a complex with their endogenous inhibitors, thus staying inactive in the membranes. In keeping with this interpretation, most purified phospholipases are active even in the absence of Ca^{2+}, an activator.

We have recently identified and characterized several naturally occurring inhibitory proteins against phospholipases (Table 2). These proteins could be purified from various sources of tissues and cells including human placenta. We have named this family of phospholipase inhibitory proteins lipomodulin/

lipocortin (Hirata, 1984, 1988). The mechanism by which these inhibitory proteins inhibit phospholipase activity remains to be elucidated. Since phospholipase-affinity chromatography was effective for the isolation of these peptides, we believe that they make a complex with phospholipases in the cells.

Calpactin/lipocortin, a major substrate in the placenta for tyrosine kinase, has been reported to inhibit phospholipase A_2 by binding phospholipid substrates, especially phosphatidylinositol (PtdIns) and phosphatidylserine (PtdSer), in the presence of Ca^{2+} (Davidson *et al.*, 1987). Initially, this protein has been purified as phospholipase A_2 inhibitory protein and two cDNA clones have been isolated. Since the biochemical properties of this protein were essentially similar, if not identical, to those we had previously reported with respect to in-vitro inhibitory effects on phospholipases, the apparent molecular weight on SDS-gel electrophoresis, and tyrosine and serine/threonine phosphorylation, the Biogen group named it lipocortin (Hirata *et al.*, 1984a; Huang *et al.*, 1986; Wallner *et al.*, 1986). The sequences deduced from the cDNAs isolated from the human placenta revealed that these proteins are identical to calpactins, calcium-binding proteins which serve as the major substrate proteins for tyrosine kinases, including EGF receptors (Kretsinger & Creutz, 1986).

To determine whether lipomodulin/lipocortin is identical with lipocortin/calpactin, we examined the kinetic properties of these inhibitory proteins. When lipomodulin was incubated with porcine pancreas phospholipase A_2, it reduced the initial rate of phospholipase A_2 reaction in a dose-dependent manner as measured by the hydrolysis of arachidonic acid from 1-stearyl-2-[1-^{14}C]arachidonyl-phosphatidylcholine (PtdCho). However, it did not change the maximal extent of the reaction. The maximal inhibition of phospholipase A_2 was always obtained, when a one-to-one stoichiometric amount of lipomodulin was added to phospholipase A_2. The inhibition of phospholipase A_2 by lipomodulin was non-competitive with respect to both PtdCho and Ca^{2+}. Lipomodulin (beta) could not inhibit rat brain PtdIns phospholipase C when measured with PtdIns as substrate. Further, it inhibits porcine pancreas phospholipase A_2 even with phosphatidylethanolamine (PtdEtn), a phospholipid which cannot bind to calpactin/lipocortin. However, apolipoprotein A_{II}, one of the major serum lipoproteins which binds phosphatidylcholine, was found to inhibit phospholipase A_2 under our assay conditions. The degrees of inhibition by apolipoprotein were inversely related to substrate concentrations but not to amounts of phospholipase A_2 present in the reaction mixture. The mode of inhibition was essentially identical to that reported with calpactin and PtdSer. In addition, monoclonal antibodies raised against our lipomodulin/lipocortin did not cross-react with either apolipoprotein or calpactin/lipocortin. These results suggest that there may be several phospholipase inhibitory proteins which inhibit phospholipases by distinct mechanisms.

Which phospholipase is a key enzyme to release arachidonic acid is still

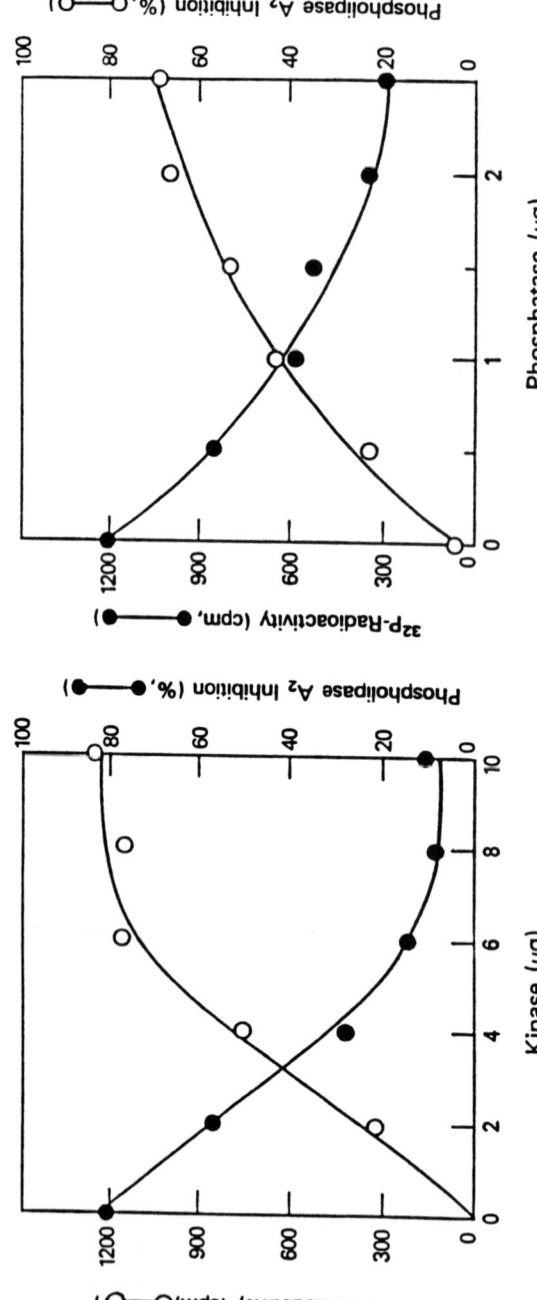

Fig. 2 Effects of phosphorylation–dephosphorylation reaction on the antiphospholipase activity of lipomodulin.

unclear. Phospholipase A_2 can directly hydrolyze arachidonic acid in the 2 position of the glycerol moiety of phospholipids. 1-Alkyl-2-acyl-glycerophosphorylcholine, a precursor of platelet-activating factor (PAF), contains predominantly arachidonic acid, because this phospholipid exchanges arachidonic acid with other phospholipids (Sugiura *et al.*, 1983). Another class of phospholipids rich in arachidonic acid is PtdIns (Irvine, 1982). This phospholipid is first hydrolyzed by PtdIns phospholipase C and subsequently by diacyl- and monoacylglycerol lipases to release arachidonic acid from the glycerol moiety. It has been well accepted that various hormones and neurotransmitters induce the rapid turnover of PtdIns in various tissues and cells (Berridge & Irvine, 1984; Majerus *et al.*, 1988). Therefore, it is easily assumed that this pathway may be another major source of arachidonic acid. Nevertheless, PtdIns turnover is often dissociated from arachidonic acid release. For instance, arachidonic acid release was inhibited in platelets and C_6 astrocytoma by the treatment with TCLK and glucocorticoids, respectively (Walenga *et al.*, 1980; DeGeorge *et al.*, 1987), but PtdIns turnover was not blocked. These observations suggest that the activation of protein kinase C after the turnover of polyphosphoinositides by PtdIns phospholipase C results in the activation of phospholipase A_2, probably through the phosphorylation of phospholipase inhibitory proteins. This is because glucocorticoids are now known to induce the synthesis of lipomodulin/lipocortin, phospholipase A_2 inhibitory protein(s) as described below. These facts led us to study the biological role of phospholipase inhibitory proteins and their phosphorylation by various protein kinases.

Phosphorylation of phospholipase inhibitory proteins

Available evidence supports that during the perinatal period, catecholamines may perform regulatory functions in a number of important processes, including the control of placental blood flow (Bleasdale & Johnston, 1984). Norepinephrine, epinephrine, dopamine and their metabolites are found in amniotic fluid. Recently, $beta_2$ subtypes of adrenergic receptors were detected in amnion tissues. When disks of amnion tissues were incubated in pseudoamniotic fluids, isoproterenol, a beta-agonist, caused a transient increase in the formation of cyclic AMP, accompanied by a sustained stimulation of the release of arachidonic acid and prostaglandin E_2 from the disks (Bleasdale & Johnston, 1984). Since cyclic AMP was also able to stimulate prostaglandin E_2 production, this phenomenon was presumed to involve protein phosphorylation. It might be attributable to phosphorylation of either phospholipase itself or its inhibitory protein (Hirata *et al.*, 1984b).

   To examine the mechanism, we developed an in-vitro system in which porcine pancreas phospholipase A_2 and rabbit neutrophil phospholipase A_2 inhibitory protein (lipomodulin/lipocortin) were independently incubated with cyclic AMP-kinase purified from bovine heart. Cyclic AMP-dependent kinase did not activate nor inhibit the phospholipase activity. On the other hand, the antiphospholipase activity of lipomodulin/lipocortin was diminished after treatment with the protein kinase (Hirata, 1981). The incorporation of phosphate into lipomodulin/lipocortin paralleled the loss of antiphospholipase activity. Removal of phosphate by treatment with alkaline or other phosphatases resulted in the recovery of the antiphospholipase activity (Fig. 2). These observations clearly demonstrated that cyclic AMP-dependent kinase can phosphorylate lipomodulin/lipocortin. Phosphorylated lipomodulin is inactive with regard to inhibitory action against phospholipase A_2, allowing phospholipase A_2 maximal activity. This reaction is reversible; thus, the phosphorylation–dephosphorylation reaction of lipomodulin/lipocortin can regulate the cellular phospholipase A_2 activity bidirectionally. Essentially similar effects of cyclic AMP kinase on the phospholipase A_2 activity have been reported with macrophage homogenates and brain synaptosomes (Moskowitz et al., 1982; Wightman et al., 1982). These observations suggest that in the unstimulated conditions, phospholipases remain inactive by making a complex with protein inhibitors and that phosphorylation of these inhibitors is necessary for the activation of phospholipases. However, cyclic AMP caused no enhancement of arachidonic acid release from intact macrophages and/or neutrophils. They rather exhibited inhibitory effects on the fMetLeuPhe-elicited arachidonate release. The difference between results with the cell-free system and intact cells may come from the location of the substrate protein and/or protein kinase in different intracellular compartments.

Regulation of tyrosine kinase activity by protein kinase C and A

Phorbol esters, activators of protein kinase C, are mitogens of lymphocytes, while cyclic AMP is inhibitory on lymphocyte proliferation. All mitogens, phorbol esters, concanavalin A and Ca^{2+}-ionophore, increased the release of arachidonic acid with the simultaneous phosphorylation of intracellular proteins (Hirata et al., 1984a). Cyclic AMP also enhanced protein phosphorylation, but not the release of arachidonic acid. The phosphorylation of lipomodulin/lipocortin, as measured by immunoprecipitation with a monospecific antibody, paralleled the amount of arachidonic acid released (Table 3). Furthermore, cyclic AMP apparently reduced the protein phosphorylation stimulated by these mitogens. Since all mitogens employed in this study increased Ca^{2+} uptake, they seemed to stimulate Ca^{2+}-dependent kinases, at least calmodulin protein kinase and/or protein kinase C. These results suggest that cyclic AMP-dependent kinase (protein kinase A) and protein kinase C are antagonistic in certain types of cell functions rather than synergic or additive.

Since lipomodulin/lipocortin in the lymphocytes was solely phosphorylated at a tyrosine residue, it was suggested that protein kinase A and protein kinase C differentially regulate tyrosine kinase activity, which is ultimately associated

Table 3. *Arachidonic acid release and protein phosphorylation*

Treatment	Total protein (cpm × 10^{-3})	Lipomodulin (cpm)	[^{14}C]Arachidonate released (cpm per 10^6 cells)
None	48.6 ± 0.9	240 ± 50	316 ± 20
Con A	108.5 ± 1.1	1800 ± 126	920 ± 85
PMA	96.9 ± 1.0	1090 ± 108	820 ± 60
A23187	80.8 ± 0.7	660 ± 65	1360 ± 110
Cyclic AMP	98.1 ± 0.6	240 ± 50	320 ± 50
Cyclic AMP plus Con A	75.5 ± 0.8	480 ± 35	560 ± 32
Cyclic AMP plus PMA	51.9 ± 0.6	330 ± 50	480 ± 40
Cyclic AMP plus A23187	52.4 ± 0.9	540 ± 50	740 ± 62

with the proliferative activity of lymphocytes (Fig. 3). Indeed, the addition of tyrosine kinase substrates such as Src- and MT-peptides (peptides which have the same sequences of the tyrosine phosphorylation sites as Src kinase and middle T antigen, respectively) could block mitogenesis with simultaneous phosphorylation of the peptides. These results confirmed the presence and involvement of tyrosine kinase in the phosphorylation of lipomodulin in lymphocytes. Similar results were obtained with neutrophils (Hirata *et al.*, 1984b). Recently, Chackalaparampil and Shalloway reported essentially identical results using NIH 3T3-derived c-src overexpressed cells (Chackalaparampil & Shalloway, 1988). They concluded that phosphorylation at novel threonine and, possibly, serine sites within the amino 16 kd region of c-src is associated with fibroblast mitosis. At the same time, serine 17, a site which cyclic AMP generally phosphorylates, seems to be dephosphorylated. These interpretations also support the hypothesis that the proliferative action of serotonin on fibroblasts is closely associated with the decrease in cyclic AMP level (Seuwen *et al.*, 1988), since phosphorylation by protein kinase A of some key proteins involved in proliferation is apparently inhibitory against mitogenesis.

Mechanisms of action of steroids

Progesterone and glucocorticoids inhibit prostaglandin formation in the uterus, while estrogens enhance it. These steroids first bind to cytosolic receptors and the receptor–steroid complex is then transferred into nuclei to stimulate gene transcription, resulting in the synthesis of new proteins. At least, receptors for estrogen, progesterone and glucocorticoids belong to the same family of genes. These receptor proteins have different domains: a steroid-binding site located at the C terminal side, and a DNA-binding site in the middle part of the peptide. These two binding sites for DNA and steroids

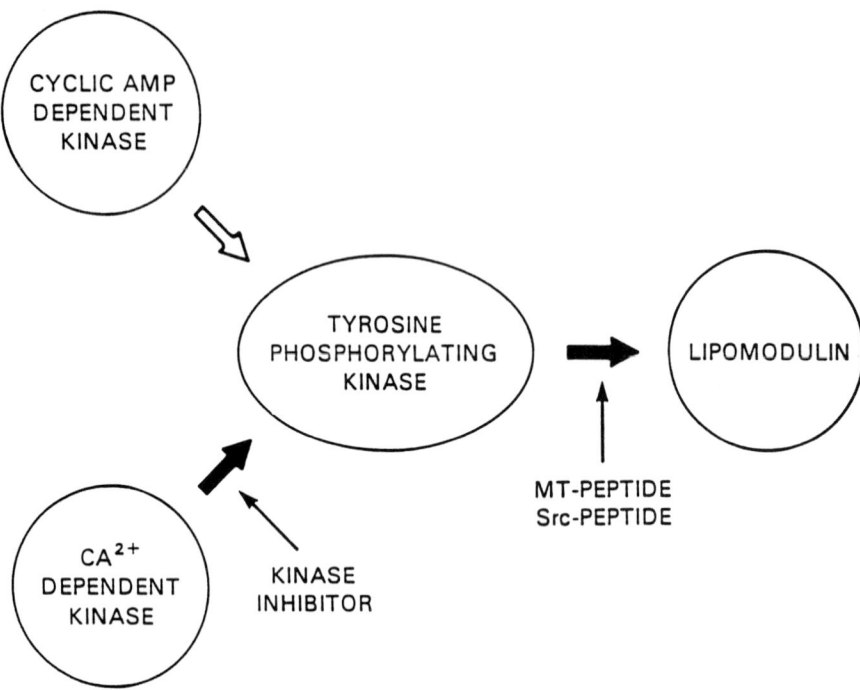

Fig. 3 Regulation of tyrosine kinase activity by protein kinase A and C.

have homology common to all steroid receptors, suggesting that steroid receptors in some tissues can cross-react with other steroids.

In the uterus, progesterone and glucocorticoids induce the synthesis of several common proteins including uteroglobulin (Mukku & Stancel, 1985). Since prostaglandin $F_{2\alpha}$ is the uterine luteolytic hormone in several species of mammals, the regulation of prostaglandin synthesis by steroid hormones is important to uterine functions. The signal for the 'switch on' of prostaglandin $F_{2\alpha}$ is assumed to be estradiol, a steroid which is released from the ovary (Thaler-Dao et al., 1983). Since the capacity to synthesize prostaglandin $F_{2\alpha}$ can always be detected in broken cells from the uterus, it is obvious that the enhanced production is due to the availability of arachidonic acid from the tissues. Although estradiol is important in the 'switching on' process, prostaglandin $F_{2\alpha}$ release from the guinea-pig uterus does not occur without progesterone priming (Thalar-Dao et al., 1983). Progesterone is now thought to regulate the release of arachidonic acid at two steps, probably cellular phospholipase and sensitivity of receptors for stimulatory ligands.

Glucocorticoids have similar effects on various tissues and organs. Especially, the anti-inflammatory action of glucocorticoids at either physiological or pharmacological doses is now proposed to be associated with the induction of the synthesis of lipomodulin/lipocortin, a phospholipase A_2 inhibitory protein (Hirata, 1988). This is based upon the findings: (a) that the anti-inflammatory action of glucocorticoids can be blocked by actinomycin D and puromycin, inhibitors of mRNA and protein synthesis, respectively; (b) that the anti-inflammatory action of glucocorticoids parallels the suppression of arachidonic acid release, ultimately formation of prostaglandins and leukotrienes, inflammatory compounds; and (c) that the synthesis of lipomodulin/lipocortin induced by glucocorticoids is inversely related to the amounts of arachidonic acid released (Hirata, 1984). As described above, we have recently identified several subtypes of phospholipase inhibitory proteins. We are not certain at the present time that the synthesis of all these phospholipase inhibitory proteins is induced by glucocorticoids.

When the molecular mechanism of phospholipase A_2 activation was studied with respect to lipomodulin/lipocortin, we found that cellular phospholipase can be activated either (a) by digestion of lipomodulin/lipocortin, or (b) by dissociation of lipocortin from phospholipase A_2 due to high Ca^{2+} concentration, phosphorylation by various kinases, or interaction with Gp protein(s) (Hirata, 1988). Therefore, it is reasonable to hypothesize that progesterone induces the synthesis of lipomodulin/lipocortin in uterine tissues, while estrogens promote the synthesis of proteases that cleave lipomodulin/lipocortin or growth factors whose receptors contain a protein kinase, typically tyrosine kinase. In fact, estrogen-mediated growth of the uterus has been shown to involve epidermal growth factor (EGF), a growth factor which stimulates cell proliferation (Mukku & Stancel, 1985). It is interesting to note that epithelial, stromal and myometrial cells contain EGF receptors.

To determine whether progesterone can induce the synthesis of lipomodulin/lipocortin in uterine tissues, we have compared the levels of prostaglandin $F_{2\alpha}$ and lipomodulin/lipocortin after treatment with progesterone and glucocorticoids. We found that glucocorticoids enhanced the synthesis of lipomodulin/lipocortin, whereas progesterone inhibited, at least, the output of this protein (Gurpide *et al.*, 1986). Since both steroids reduced the formation of prostaglandins, their mechanisms of action might be different with regard to induction of the synthesis of lipomodulin/lipocortin. An alternative explanation is that progesterone and estrogens have opposite effects on the cellular levels of Gp or other G proteins. Gp protein(s), which is coupled to various receptors, is proposed to be responsible for the activation of cellular phospholipases (Litosch & Fain, 1986). When neutrophil plasma membranes were stimulated in the presence of GTP[gamma-^{32}P] or GTP[gamma-^{35}S] with fMetLeuPhe, a synthetic chemoattractant, the activity of phospholipase A_2, as measured by the hydrolysis of exogenous 1-palmityl-2-[1-^{14}C]arachidonyl-phosphatidylcholine as substrate, was enhanced. Simultaneously, antilipocortin antibody could immunoprecipitate the radioactivity of GTP and its analogue, although purified lipocortin had no capacity to bind GTP *in vitro*

Table 4. *Interaction between G proteins and lipomodulins/lipocortins*

	Radioactivity (cpm)			
	Control	GTP[γ-^{32}P] antilipomodulin	Control	GTP[γ-^{35}S] antilipomodulin
None	512 ± 41	469 ± 32	188 ± 24	134 ± 34
ƒ MetLeuPhe (0.1 μmol/l)	554 ± 62	1852 ± 86	134 ± 26	883 ± 62

(Table 4). Although the same specific activities of GTP analogues were used for this study, GTP[gamma-^{32}P] was incorporated more into the immunoprecipitates (Hirata *et al.*, 1987). These results left a possibility that lipomodulin/lipocortin might be phosphorylated by Gp protein(s) with GTP as substrate. Ha-ras protein, which has a high homology to G proteins, is demonstrated to autophosphorylate itself with GTP but not with ATP (Shih *et al.*, 1980).

Recently, ras-**onc** gene products (which can exhibit GTP activity like G proteins) have been demonstrated persistently to activate cellular phospholipase A_2, when they were injected into intact fibroblasts. On the other hand, these products have also been proposed to be coupled to PtdIns turnover like Gp protein(s). PtdIns turnover appears to be involved in many cases of proliferating cells. In fact, homogenates of cells which were transformed by various **onc** genes have different patterns of protein phosphorylation as measured with GTP[gamma-^{32}P] or ATP[gamma-^{32}P]. Therefore, the possibility of the existence of a GTP protein kinase cannot be completely ruled out. Nevertheless, we failed to demonstrate the phosphorylation of lipomodulin/lipocortin in plasma membrane fractions with GTP[gamma-^{32}P], although we found that 20-kd and 22-kd proteins in plasma membranes were preferentially phosphorylated. Therefore, the existence of a GTP-dependent kinase associated with alteration of cellular function is an attractive hypothesis, the possibility of which is being tested in our laboratory.

Acknowledgement

This research is supported in part by NIH grants ES-04802, NS-24628, NS-23048 and ES-03505.

References

Berridge, M.J. & Irvine, R.F. (1984). Inositol triphosphate, a novel second messenger in cellular signal transduction. *Nature*, **312**:315–321.

Bleasdale, J.E. & Johnston, J.M. (1984). Prostaglandins and human parturition: regulation of arachidonic acid mobilization. *Reviews in Perinatal Medicine*, **5**:151–191.

Chackalaparampil, I. & Shalloway, D. (1988). Altered phosphorylation and activation of pp60^{c-src} during fibroblast mitosis. *Cell*, **52**:801–810.

Davidson, F.F., Dennis, E.A., Powell, M. & Glenney, J.R. (1987). Inhibition of phospholipase A$_2$ by lipocortins and calpactins. An effect of binding to substrate phospholipids. *Journal of Biological Chemistry*, **262**:1698–1705.

DeGeorge, J.J., Ousley, A.H., McCarthy, K.D., Morell, P. & Lapetina, E.G. (1987). Glucocorticoids inhibit the liberation of arachidonate but not the rapid production of phospholipase C-dependent metabolites in acetylcholine-stimulated C62B glioma cells. *Journal of Biological Chemistry*, **262**:9979–9983.

Edelman, A.M., Blumenthal, D.K. & Krebs, E.G. (1987). Protein serine/threonine kinases. *Annual Review of Biochemistry*, **56**:567–613.

Gurpide, E., Markiewicz, L., Schatz, F. & Hirata, F. (1986). Lipocortin output by human endometrium *in vitro*. *Journal of Clinical Endocrinology and Metabolism*, **63**:162–166.

Hirata, F. (1981). The regulation of lipomodulin, a phospholipase inhibitory protein, in rabbit neutrophils by phosphorylation. *Journal of Biological Chemistry*, **256**:7730–7733.

Hirata, F. (1984). Role of lipomodulin, a phospholipase inhibitory protein in immunoregulation. *Advances in Inflammation Research*, **7**:71–78.

Hirata, F. (1988). Molecular mechanism of regulation of cellular phospholipases. (In) *Cellular and Molecular Aspects of Inflammation* (Poste, G. & Crooke, S.T., eds.), pp.427–442. New York, Plenum Press.

Hirata, F., Matsuda, K., Notsu, Y., Hattori, T. & Del Carmine, R. (1984a). Phosphorylation at a tyrosine residue of lipomodulin in mitogen-stimulated murine thymocytes. *Proceedings of the National Academy of Sciences USA*, **81**:4717–4721.

Hirata, F., Notsu, Y., Matsuda, K., Vasanthakumar, G., Schiffmann, E., Wong, T.-W. & Goldberg, A.R. (1984b). Inhibition of leucocyte chemotaxis by Glu-Glu-Glu-Glu-Tyr-Pro-Met-Glu and Leu-Ile-Glu-Asp-Asn-Glu-Tyr-Thr-Ala-Arg-Gln-Gly. *Biochemical and Biophysical Research Communications*, **118**:682–690.

Hirata, F., Stracke, M.L. & Shiffmann, E. (1987). Regulation of prostaglandin formation by glucocorticoids and their second messenger, lipocortins. *Journal of Steroid Biochemistry*, **27**:1053–1056.

Huang, K.S., Wallner, B.P., Mattaliano, R.J., Tizard, R., Burne, C., Frey, A., Hession, C., McGray, P., Sinclair, L.K., Chow, E.P., Browning, J.L., Ramachandran, K.L., Tang, J., Smart, J.E. & Pepinsky, R.B. (1986). Two human 35KD inhibitors of phospholipase A$_2$ are related to substrates of pp60^{v-src} and of the epidermal growth factor receptor/kinase. *Cell*, **46**:191–199.

Hunter, T. (1987). A thousand and one protein kinases. *Cell*, **50**:823–829.

Irvine, R.F. (1982). How is the level of free arachidonic acid controlled in mammalian cells? *Biochemical Journal*, **204**:3–16.

Kretsinger, R.H. & Creutz, C.E. (1986). Cell biology – consensus in exocytosis. *Nature*, **320**:573.

Litosch, I. & Fain, J.N. (1986). Regulation of phosphoinositide breakdown by guanine nucleotides. *Life Sciences*, **39**:187–194.

Majerus, P.W., Connolly, T.M., Bansal, V.S., Inhorn, R.C. & Deckmyn, H. (1988). The mechanism of inositol phosphates. (In) *Cellular and Molecular Aspects of Inflammation* (Poste, G. & Crooke, S.T., eds.), pp.443–458. New York, Plenum Press.

Moskowitz, N., Schook, W. & Puszkin, S. (1982). Interaction of brain synaptic vesicles induced by endogenous Ca^{2+}-dependent phospholipase A_2. *Science*, **216**:305–307.

Mukku, V.R. & Stancel, G.M. (1985). Regulation of epidermal growth factor receptor by estrogen. *Journal of Biological Chemistry*, **260**:9820–9824.

Pearson, R.B., Wettenhall, R.E.H., Means, A.R., Hartshorne, D.J. & Kemp, B.E. (1988). Autoregulation of enzymes by pseudosubstrate prototypes: myosin light chain kinase. *Science*, **241**:970–973.

Seuwen, K., Magnaldo, I. & Pouysségur, J. (1988). Serotonin stimulates DNA synthesis in fibroblasts acting through $5\text{-}HT_{1B}$ receptors coupled to Gi-protein. *Nature*, **335**:254–256.

Shenolikar, S. (1988). Protein phosphorylation: hormones, drugs and bioregulation. *FASEB Journal*, **2**:2753–2764.

Shih, T.Y., Papageorge, A.G., Stokes, P.E., Weeks, M.O. & Scolnick, E.M. (1980). Guanine nucleotide-binding and autophosphorylating activities associated with the $p21^{src}$ protein of Harvey murine sarcoma virus. *Nature*, **287**:686–691.

Sugiura, T., Nakajima, M., Sekiguchi, N., Nakagawa, Y. & Waku, K. (1983). Different fatty chain compositions of alkenylacyl, alkylacyl and diacyl phospholipids in rabbit alveolar macrophages: high amounts of arachidonic acid in ether phospholipids. *Lipids*, **18**:125–129.

Taylor, S.S., Bubis, J., Toner-Webb, J., Saraswat, L.D., First, E.A., Buechler, J.A., Knighton, D.R. & Sowadski, J. (1988). cAMP-dependent protein kinase: prototype for a family of enzymes. *FASEB Journal*, **2**:2677–2685.

Thaler-Dao, H., Ramonatxo, M., Saintot, M. & Crastes de Paulet, A. (1983). Regulation by estradiol of the *in vitro* prostaglandin production by the rat and guinea pig uterus. *Advances in Prostaglandin, Thromboxane and Leukotriene Research*, **12**:429–436.

Walenga, R., Vanderhoek, J.Y. & Feinstein, M.B. (1980). Serine esterase inhibitors block stimulus-induced mobilization of arachidonic acid and phosphatidylinositide-specific phospholipase-C activity in platelets. *Journal of Biological Chemistry*, **255**:6024–6027.

Wallner, B.P., Mattaliano, R.J., Hession, C., Cate, R.L., Tizard, R., Sinclair, L.K., Foeller, C., Chow, E.P., Browning, J.L., Ramachandran, K.L. & Pepinsky, R.B. (1986). Cloning and expression of human lipocortin: a phospholipase-A_2 inhibitor with potential anti-inflammatory activity. *Nature*, **320**:77–81.

Wightman, P.D., Dahlgren, M.E. & Bonney, R.J. (1982). Protein kinase activation of phospholipase A_2 in sonicates of mouse peritoneal macrophages. *Journal of Biological Chemistry*, **257**:6650–6652.

Discussion

Casey. Dr Hirata, do you believe that lipocortin as well as uteroglobin act to inhibit phospholipase A_2 by direct interaction with the enzyme, whereas the calpactins act to inhibit the apparent phospholipase A_2 activity by binding the phospholipid?

Hirata. Yes, that is correct.

Casey. Also that glucocorticoid steroids stimulate the production of lipocortin but not calpactin?

Hirata. I do not know about calpactins. We incubated the cells *in vitro* with the glucocorticoid and failed to show an increase in the transcription of calpactins. When we treated animals with dexamethasone *in vivo* and took some tissue, we could see an increase in transcription. Therefore, the induction of calpactin might require a couple more steps.

King. From what you know about the mechanisms for the release of arachidonic acid, can you see any practical ways forward for possible developments to inhibit arachidonic acid release in the sort of system that we have been discussing here?

Hirata. One could probably give lipomodulin/lipocortin to the tissue to see whether or not prostaglandin formation is inhibited, but I have never conducted a proper experiment. Were you suggesting this as a treatment?

King. Obviously, there are situations where it might be desirable, in relation to the bleeding, to prevent arachidonic acid release. I am just trying to formulate a few ideas as to how one might proceed to investigate this.

Hirata. Not all the phospholipase inhibitor proteins can be induced by glucocorticoids, as we described in previous work. For instance, the phospholipase C inhibitory protein is not induced by glucocorticoids, and regular phospholipase C inhibitory protein seems to be induced by aspirin and non-steroidal anti-inflammatory agents. We do not know at present which drugs induce this kind of inhibitory protein.

Gurpide. How general, do you think, is the regulation of phospholipases by the lipocortin? Is it a very ubiquitous regulator? Do you think it is one essential mechanism for the regulation of phospholipase?

Hirata. I like to think that it is the essential mechanism, but I am not quite sure about that.

Gurpide. Could you say that you have a good chance to find this lipocortin in any tissue that will produce prostaglandin or arachidonic acid?

Hirata. So far, we have tested various cell lines and we can detect the protein more or less. That is all I can say.

Clark. To follow up Dr King's question, I wonder if it might be feasible to have a lipomodulin-impregnated IUD or do you think that the lipomodulin might block the contraceptive affect of the IUD?

Hirata. This would need investigation.

Findlay. According to the hypothesis of Dr Baird and Dr Smith, normal menstruation is associated with progesterone withdrawal which is leading to an increase in prostaglandin production, presumably through extra availability of arachidonic acid. Would you like to speculate on just what it is about progesterone withdrawal, and how that might in fact be facilitating the increase in availability of arachidonic acid?

Hirata. If I am allowed to speculate, probably progesterone increases the protein content and enhances the sensitivity of the various receptors for the various ligands or hormones. Therefore, I believe that progesterone is priming the cell for another stimulation. Withdrawal of progesterone should be considered at a balance with estrogen because of the enhancement of the growth factor or other factors such as the receptors. But progesterone also enhances the release, so small stimulations are starting to make more prostaglandins.

Gurpide. Different phospholipases are regulated in different ways, so I would like to understand whether the relation of lipocortins to prostaglandin production is obligatory or not. Do you visualize that the cyclo-oxygenase regulation may be determining the prostaglandins in the absence of regulation of the phospholipase?

Hirata. That is also possible. Three factors – arachidonic acid availability, the enzymes involved in synthesis and those involved in degradation – may all play a part. Whether or not phospholipase A_2 directly regulates its own special phospholipase A_2 in the cells is not known. Currently one of my students is cloning phospholipase A_2 from various cells to obtain this answer.

Macrophages and other migratory cells in endometrium: relevance to endometrial bleeding

DAVID A. CLARK* AND SALIM DAYA**

*Departments of Medicine/Obstetrics and Gynecology, Molecular Virology and Immunology Program, **Department of Obstetrics and Gynecology, McMaster University, Hamilton, Ontario, Canada.

Abstract

Macrophages and other migratory lymphomyeloid cells are present in the endometrial stroma, and a novel type of granulated lymphocyte may also be present in the epithelium. Immunohistologic studies of various lymphomyeloid cell subpopulations suggest that certain cell subtypes, and in particular granulated T lineage lymphocytes, are regulated by ovarian hormones during the menstrual cycle. Some cell subsets appear primarily related to events of implantation and early pregnancy. Other cell types appear more likely to participate in endometrial shedding and control of bleeding. This inference derives from the ability of cells such as macrophages to produce enzymes, cytokines and other mediators that affect inflammation, tissue necrosis and repair. Areas of potential future productive research are identified.

Introduction

Attempts to understand the pathophysiology of uterine bleeding have focused primarily on fibrinolytic hemostatic mechanisms and regulation of vascular tone by prostaglandins (Rybo, 1966; Hahn, 1980; Hagenfeldt, 1987). Evidence for the relevance of prostaglandins and fibrinolytic enzymes has been provided by a demonstrated reduction in spontaneous and IUD-associated menorrhagia by the antifibrinolysin ϵ-aminocaproic acid (Nilsson & Rybo, 1965; Kasonde & Bonnar, 1975) and by inhibitors of prostaglandin (PG) synthesis (Roy & Shaw, 1981; Ylikorkala & Pekonen, 1986; Hall et al., 1987, Toppozada, 1987). Increased synthesis of vasodilatory PGE_2 (Tsang et al., 1987) and PGI_2 (as contrasted with vasoconstrictive $PGF_{2\alpha}$), regulation of PG synthesis in endometrial gland epithelium by estradiol (to stimulate $PGF_{2\alpha}$ synthesis) and progesterone (that inhibits PGE_2 synthesis as well as $PGF_{2\alpha}$), (Lumsden et al., 1984; Cameron et al., 1984; Skinner et al., 1984; Moonen et al., 1985; Schatz et al., 1987; Smith & Kelly, 1988) and increased plasminogen activator activity in endometrium related to premenstrual decline in estrogen and progesterone (Bonnar & Sheppard, 1980; Paton et al., 1980; Schatz et al., 1987) provide a simple scheme of steroid-dependent regulation of uterine bleeding. Suboptimal hormone levels or subnormal progesterone-receptor levels (Gorodeski et al., 1986) associated with anovulation or oral contraceptive (OC) use could lead to a relative excess of vasodilatory PGE_2; stimulation of PGE_2 synthesis by IUDs could also produce bleeding by a shift in the balance towards vasodilatation by PGE_2 and fibrinolysis by plasmin would also play a role.

There are some problems with this simple model of endometrial bleeding. For example, substantial amounts of PGs are synthesized in stroma, and vasodilatory PGI_2, which also inhibits platelet aggregation, may be largely myometrial in origin (Smith *et al.*, 1981; Cameron *et al.*, 1984; Lumsden *et al.*, 1984). Estradiol may stimulate fibroblastic cells of stroma to produce $PGF_{2\alpha}$ and progesterone may synergize while concomitantly inhibiting production of PGE_2 and PGI_2 (Neulen *et al.*, 1988). The possible role of other cells in stroma has not been evaluated. Phospholipase A_2, a key enzyme in the generation of PGs and platelet-activating factor (PAF), is abundant in stroma and is supplemented by a contribution from gland epithelium during the secretory phase of the cycle (Bonney *et al.*, 1987). The origin of many of the lysosomal proteolytic enzymes involved in tissue destruction (Hahn, 1980; Fraser & Diczfalusy, 1980) and regeneration may be stromal as well as epithelial (Wilson, 1980). The role that cells within the stroma might play in intermediary steps that mediate the final process of tissue breakdown and bleeding has not been fully assessed.

The objective of this chapter is to review current information concerning cell populations in endometrial stroma, with particular emphasis on lymphomyeloid cells that are migratory and originate from bone marrow. Study of these cells requires an approach that differs from the usual biochemical methods employing whole-tissue homogenates. Since stroma is composed of a variety of cell types, it follows that studies of whole tissue homogenates will provide little information about the role of specific classes of cells. Methods for identification of cell subtypes in stroma include immunohistochemical methods employing sectioned material and studies of cell suspensions obtained from disaggregated tissue. Table 1 lists major cell types which have been defined by surface markers.

Types of lymphomyeloid cells in stroma and possible functions

Macrophages are bone marrow-derived cells that are common in endometrium, both proliferative and secretory, and comprise 50% of CD45-positive cells (Bulmer *et al.*, 1987a, 1987b, 1988; Kamat & Isaacson, 1987). Macrophages in endometrium occur both scattered in the stratum functionale and in aggregates adjacent to endometrial gland epithelium in the basal zone. There is one report of a 20–30% increase in macrophages in the secretory phase just prior to menses (Kamat & Isaacson, 1987).

The function of macrophages in the endometrium is unclear. Studies of uterine macrophage *function* have relied entirely on examining cells isolated from pregnancy decidua. Macrophages may have a number of functions including phagocytosis, antigen processing, release of cytotoxic mediators

Table 1. *Some lymphomyeloid populations CD45+*
(Leu 1) in human ndometrium

	Markers	
Cell Type	Present	Absent
Macrophages	HLA-DR/DP/DQ	
	CD4* (OKT-4)	CD11b (OKM-1)
	CD14 (Leu-M3)	CD15 (Leu-M1)
Langerhans cells	CD1 (Leu-6)	OKM-1
		CD11b
T lymphocytes:		
Helper/DTH	CD2/3/4*/5	CD8
Suppressor/cytotoxic	CD2/3/5/8	CD4
		CD25 (IL-2R)
Granulated lymphocytes:		
(dGL) Type I	CD2	CD3/4/5
	CD7 (Dako T2)	CD5
	Leu 19 (NKH-1)	Leu-7
		CD16 (Leu 11)
		CD25
(LGL) Type II	CD2	CD3/4/5/8
	CD7 (Dako T2)	
	Leu 7 (HNK-1)	
	Leu 19 (NKH-1)	
	CD16 (Leu-11)	
	CD11b (OKM-1)	

* Note presence on both macrophages and T cells.
Data from Bulmer & Sunderland, 1983; Bulmer *et al.*, 1987a,b,c,
1988; Morris *et al.*, 1985; Lanier & Phillips, 1986; Kamat &
Isaacson, 1987. CD2 is the receptor for binding sheep erythrocytes
(ERFC). IL-2R (CD25) is the receptor for interleukin-2. Markers
for B lymphocytes and polymorphonuclear leukocytes are not
listed.

such as H_2O_2, release of mediators including interleukin-1 (IL-1), tumour
necrosis factor α (TNF-α), PGE_2, PAF, and release of growth factors such as
TNF-α, transforming growth factor β (TGF-β), platelet-derived growth
factor-A chain (PDGF-A chain) and insulin-like growth factor (IGF)
(Rappolee *et al.*, 1988). When removed from their milieu and prepared in the
form of a single cell suspension, first trimester decidua-associated macrophages can present antigen to T cells (Oksenberg *et al.*, 1987, 1988). Possibly
this function is actually mediated by dendritic Langerhans cells as the only
phenotypic separation of the cells was based on adherence and Langerhans
cells are highly efficient at antigen presentation. Macrophages isolated from
decidua may also suppress lymphocyte responses by release of PGE_2 (Tawfik
et al., 1986a, 1986b; Lala *et al* 1986; Matthews & Searle, 1987), and possibly
might do so when present in the areas of predecidual change of late secretory

phase endometrium. Whether antigen presentation or suppression by PGE_2 synthesis is a real in-situ function of this class of cells in human endometrium is not known. In the rat, Class II MHC-positive (equivalent to HLA-D) cells were abundant in relation to gland epithelium, particularly at the time of ovulation (Head & Gaede, 1986). Intrauterine challenge with antigen was able to sensitize rats for a secondary response (Lande, 1986), but it is unclear if the sensitization took place locally or rather occurred in uterine draining lymph nodes and spleen. Lande did not note any stimulatory effect of ovarian function on immune responses that has been related to periods of estradiol production, perhaps due in part to prolonged antigen absorption from the uterus that distributed antigen over a series of hormonal (estrus) cycles (Hulka et al., 1965; Kenny et al., 1976; Krzych et al., 1978).

We have conducted some studies of suppressor function of cells isolated from human endometrium. The assay used has been the proliferation of human peripheral blood leukocytes driven by the mitogen, concanavalin A (Daya et al., 1985) – an assay of T cell proliferation. Proliferative phase endometrial cells stimulated proliferation, whereas following ovulation, the cells became progressively more inhibitory. This inhibition was not associated with a detectable soluble factor such as PGE_2, perhaps because we disaggregated our cells by a mechanical technique that appears to select against macrophages (Wood et al., 1988).

Murine pre-implantation endometrium also contains suppressor cells that, when mechanically isolated, do not release soluble factors and do not depend upon PGE_2 synthesis for their suppressive activity (Brierley & Clark, 1987). In both mouse and human, the suppressive activity is associated with large-sized cells that sediment at unit gravity at >4 mm/hour (modal velocity of 6–8 mm/hour), consistent with macrophages or large lymphoblasts. The surface phenotype of the cell in the human endometrium has not been determined, but in the mouse, the suppressor lacks the CD11b (MAC-1 complement receptor) and expresses the equivalent of CD5 and CD8, which are markers for T cells (Brierley & Clark, 1987). The activity of this cell population is hormone dependent – either due to a need for tissue recruitment or activation (Daya et al., 1985; Brierley & Clark, 1987). Interestingly, there is some evidence that CD8[+] but not CD4 cells may be induced to express progesterone receptors that then regulate cytokine activity (Szekeres-Bartho, personal communication; Szekeres-Bartho et al., 1985). These suppressor cells would appear, on the basis of surface markers, to belong to the classical T cell lineage and such cells occur in both proliferative and secretory phases of the human endometrium, with some diminution after day 20 of the cycle (Bulmer et al., 1988). At least 75% of the CD2,3-positive T cells in endometrium are CD8 (25% being CD4) and there is an apparent increase in this percentage as the menstrual cycle evolves from proliferative to secretory (Bulmer et al., 1987a, 1987b, 1988).

A third class of cells in endometrium is of particular interest. These are morphologically lymphocytic cells with cytoplasmic granules, as demonstrated by a Wright's stain or by phloxine–tartrazine. The granulated lymphocyte population can be divided into at least two classes. The first lack classical T cell markers such as CD3, 4, 5, 8, and also lack some of the markers found on natural killer (NK) cells (i.e. Leu 7 or HNK-1 and OKM-1) that belong to the granulated lymphocyte family. CD7 (Dako T2) and Leu 19 (NKH-1) (Lanier & Phillips, 1986) are present and serve to define a distinct cell population which increases in number during the secretory phase of the cycle, particularly in areas of pseudodecidualization, and dominate in early pregnancy decidua. These cells are often located with aggregates of macrophages about blood vessels and near endometrial gland epithelium (Bulmer *et al.*, 1987a, 1987b, 1988). They have been called 'endometrial granulocytes' but are in fact bone marrow-derived granulated lymphocytes (Bulmer & Sunderland, 1983; Watanabe *et al.*, 1986; Bulmer *et al.*, 1987c); 'granulocyte' is understood by many to represent a polymorphonuclear leukocyte and therefore the term 'endometrial granulocyte' is potentially misleading and should not be used. The Leu 19 + (NKH-1) subset isolated from human decidua appears to possess some degree of NK activity that would potentially include it among the intraepithelial T lineage NK-like cells described at other mucosal surfaces such as the gut (Tagliabue *et al.*, 1982) and referred to as IEL (intraepithelial lymphocytes) or gGL (gut granulated lymphocytes). The latter form of terminology would seem less confusing because the IEL-type cells may also be present in the stroma, and accordingly, it is proposed that one use neutral terminology such as 'eGL' and 'dGL' (endometrial granulated lymphocyte and decidual granulated lymphocyte). The Leu 19 + (NKH-1) subset in blood can be activated by interleukin-2 (IL-2) to become a potent killer cell (Lanier & Phillips, 1986; McMannis *et al.*, 1988). In endometrium, IL-2 receptors are not present, perhaps due to a down-regulatory effect of locally produced PGE_2 (Lala *et al.*, 1986).

The type 1 subset of eGL/dGL listed in Table 1 represents the novel T lineage cells discussed above. These cells accumulate with decidua formation (Bulmer *et al.*, 1987c, 1988), and when isolated from first trimester pregnancy decidua may exert suppressor activity distinct from that associated with macrophages (Bulmer & Ritson, 1988). There is evidence that such cells may have their suppressor activity activated by signals from trophoblast, as suggested by a close association with interstitial trophoblast (Bulmer & Sunderland, 1983), with gland epithelium that has acquired new surface phenotype-like trophoblast (Bulmer & Johnson, 1985), and by direct studies wherein trophoblast or their membranes have directly increased granulated cell number and have stimulated the appearance of small-sized suppressor cells at the murine intrauterine implantation site (Slapsys *et al.*, 1988; Daya *et al.*, 1989). Trophoblast membrane vesicles interact *in vitro* with small cells (<4 mm/hour) isolated from human luteal phase endometrium, leading to release of 44-kd and 22-kd suppressor factors that block IL-2 responses (Daya *et al.*,

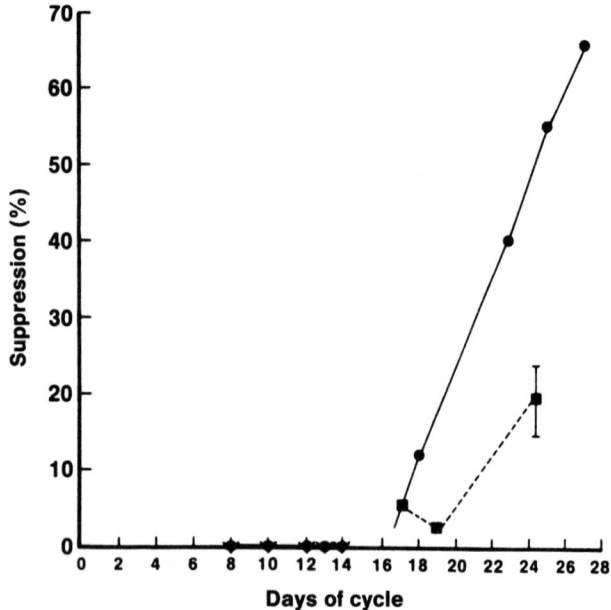

	M	Proliferative	Secretory	Late Secretory (predecidual)
Macrophages	?	+ +	+ +	+ +/+ + +
T cells	?	+	+ +	+
eGL	?	+	+	+ + +
B cells	?	±	±/+	?
Polys	+ +	–	–	?

Fig. 1 Cell types in human endometrium as a function of day of menstrual cycle. Top panel shows percent suppression of proliferation of peripheral blood lymphocytes stimulated by concanavalin A by direct addition of test cells from specimens of human endometrium (circles; adapted from Daya *et al.*, 1985). The ability of endometrial cells to generate supernatants with suppressive activity in response to 1 μg/ml human trophoblast membrane is also shown (squares; adapted from Daya *et al.*, 1989). The lower portion of the figure tabulates information on relative frequency of different subpopulations of lymphomyeloid cells. (M represents menses; ? indicates insufficient data; eGL is defined in Table 1 and related text.)

1986, 1989). Figure 1 summarizes the development of 'large' suppressor cell activity during the menstrual cycle and appearance of small cells that can interact as the trophoblast. The development of suppressor function is not likely to be related to subsequent menstrual bleeding and probably has as its purpose the preparation of the endometrium for implantation.

Type 2 granulated cells represent granulated cells with LGL morphology that possess classical NK markers such as Leu 7 (HNK-1 as contrasted with NKH-1) and Leu-11 (CD 16, a marker for one type of Fc receptor for IgG). These cells are infrequent in normal endometrium.

B lymphocytes that mediate antibody production may also be present in small numbers, scattered in the interstitium and associated with follicular collections of macrophages and T cells in the stratum basale (Morris *et al.*, 1985; Kamat & Isaacson, 1987). The B cells (bone marrow-derived lymphocytes) accumulating at mucosal surfaces tend to produce IgA which is then transported across the epithelium in association with secretory piece. Accumulation of such B cells in genital tissue is promoted by hormones and transport is enhanced during the secretory phase of the cycle, postovulation (Sullivan *et al.*, 1984). Similar data have been obtained in the mouse (McDermott *et al.*, 1980; Parr & Parr, 1985).

Polymorphonuclear leukocytes appear to enter uterine tissues only at the onset of menstruation (Hahn, 1980; Kamat & Isaacson, 1987; Bulmer *et al.*, 1988). They also rapidly enter decidua if hormonal support (i.e. progesterone) is withdrawn (Staples *et al.*, 1983).

Functional significance of lymphomyeloid cell populations in bleeding

Granulated cells

A premenstrual accumulation of granulated lymphoid cells (eGL) and their strategic location near to endometrial blood vessels in the basal zone have suggested a possible relationship to bleeding and tissue necrosis. Indeed, Dallenbach-Hellweg (1980) proposed that eGL produced bleeding via release of granules thought to contain relaxin. eGL are related to bone marrow-derived metrial gland cells that accumulate at the implantation site in rodent pregnancy (Peel *et al.*, 1983; Peel & Stewart, 1986). They do not contain relaxin (Larkin, 1974) but do contain osteopontin, an important matrix protein (Nomura *et al.*, 1988). The granules of a variety of cytotoxic lymphocytic cells (including lymphokine-activated killer cells (LAKs) and NK cells) contain perforins that mediate target cell lysis (Tschopp & Conzelmann, 1986) and there is evidence that metrial gland cells, when removed from their local environment, can lyse trophoblast cells of the conceptus (Stewart & Mukhtar, 1988). It is not clear, however, if eGL ever mediate such toxicity against blood vessels locally in response to low levels of estrogen or to progesterone withdrawal.

T cells

CD8$^+$ is associated with Class I MHC antigen recognition and cytotoxic/suppressor function. It is not known if the CD8$^+$ cells in endometrium or early pregnancy decidua possess any cytotoxic function. Some recent data suggest CD8$^+$ cells together with PGE$_2$ may inhibit development of bone marrow precursors into granulocytes and macrophages (Pelus *et al.*, 1988), but whether this is relevant to macrophage development in the endometrium is unclear.

Macrophages

Some of the possible functions of macrophages in general have already been discussed. Macrophages can be cytotoxic to tissue by release of H$_2$O$_2$, TNF-α, and various lysosomal enzymes (Ruddle, 1987; Hamilton & Adams, 1987). A variety of mediators are also released that induce function in other cells and these mediators include IL-1, TNF-α, PAF (Mencia-Huerta & Benveniste, 1979; Braquet & Rola-Pleszczynski, 1987) and growth factors (Rappolee *et al.*, 1988). One target is vascular endothelial cells that may in response produce additional PAF and IL-1 (Camussi *et al.*, 1983; Nawroth *et al.*, 1986; Bussolino *et al.*, 1988). However, there are other consequences of even greater importance. Endothelial cells may:

1. Promote clotting by secretion of tissue factor and inhibition of expression of a surface anticoagulant (thrombomodulin), thereby shifting the balance to promote clotting (Nawroth & Stern, 1986).
2. Produce inhibitors of fibrinolysis (plasminogen activator inhibitor, PAI) so that the clot plugging necrosed blood vessels is not rapidly dissolved by activation of plasminogen to plasmin (Nachman *et al.*, 1986). Plasmin is also a potent protease that may participate in tissue breakdown in general (Laiho *et al.*, 1987), so that PAI may arrest tissue digestion.
3. Promote vasodilatation via release of PGE$_2$ and PGI$_2$ and endothelium-derived relaxing factors (EDRFs) that locally relax arteriolar smooth muscle (Vanhoutte, 1988). Note: EDRFs include effects of prostacyclin, ammonia, nitrites, adenosine and possibly other, as yet undefined, factors.
4. Become sticky to polymorphonuclear leukocytes (PML) and promote tissue infiltration as part of the inflammatory process, perhaps by release of activators of PML such as leukotriene B$_4$ (LTB$_4$), PAF and IL-1 (Palmblad *et al.*, 1981; Shaw *et al.*, 1981; Camussi *et al.*, 1983; Bevilacqua *et al.*, 1985; Sayers *et al.*, 1988).
5. Become, in response to TNF-α, susceptible to killing by neutrophils (Varani *et al.*, 1988).

Polymorphonuclear leukocytes are a potent augmentor of local inflammation and in the presence of TNF-α, C5a fragments ('a' fragment of complement component number 5), or PAF, produce edema (Fernandez *et al.*, 1978; Wedmore & Williams, 1981; Shaw *et al.*, 1981). PAF plays a key role in polymorphonuclear leukocyte activation (Shaw *et al.*, 1981) and PAF blockers inhibit IL-1-induced inflammation (Rubin & Rosenbaum, 1988); blood platelet counts also drop transiently with menstruation, typical of a PAF effect (Paton *et al.*, 1980). While these events may explain how endometrial shedding occurs, they do not explain why bleeding may be excessive. In this regard, there is increasing appreciation of the potential importance of macrophages. Macrophages may also produce PAI (Chapman & Stone, 1985) and growth and differentiation factors. Macrophages in a 'wound' (of which shedding endometrium may be an example), may produce TGF-β, a potent immunosuppressive that inhibits a variety of cytotoxic cells including macrophage toxicity (Clark *et al.*, 1988; Tsunawaki *et al.*, 1988). TGF-β also stimulates production of PAI, capillary growth and fibroblast migration (Laiho *et al.*, 1987; Lund *et al.*, 1987; Postlethwaite *et al.*, 1987; Madri *et al.*, 1988) as part of the healing process. TGF-β can promote formation of adhesion proteins similar to osteopontin/osteonectin (Heine *et al.*, 1987) in some tissues and possibly could act similarly on eGL. Indeed, it has been proposed that TGF-β might prevent excessive macrophage activation and shift the balance from tissue destruction to tissue repair (Tsunawaki *et al.*, 1988).

In promotion of endometrial necrosis and bleeding, there are clearly several mediators acting in concert and, of course, antagonists that modulate and terminate the process. Investigation of macrophage mediators and their possible regulation by steroid hormones could represent a profitable focus for future research. Figure 2 illustrates some of the potentially relevant cytokine actions.

Conclusions

There are lymphomyeloid cells in human endometrium that can be defined by immunohistologic methods. These are laborious techniques that suffer from the drawback that only one marker at a time can be studied. To study several markers requires serial sections and there is always a risk of sampling error. None of the techniques currently in use defines function, and quantitation is a problem. Disaggregated cells, while easier to study, may be altered and not representative of the tissue composition (Bulmer *et al.*, 1987b). Possible ways to overcome these problems include:

(a) the use of in-situ function markers, i.e. hybridize using probes for mediator mRNA (Rappolee *et al.*, 1988);

(b) carrying out in-vivo cell depletion studies in a suitable subhuman primate that has a menstrual cycle (Fraser & Diczfalusy, 1980).

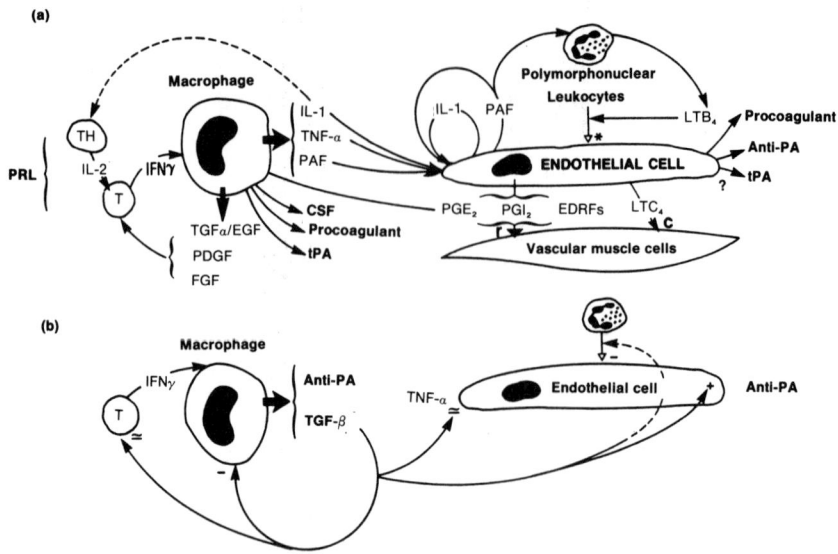

Fig. 2 Cytokine mediators and macrophage function.

(a) Agonistic circuits. Macrophages produce IL-1, TNF-α, and PAF which activate endothelial cells to produce additional IL-1 and PAF. PAF activates polymorphonuclear leukocytes which produce leukotriene B_4 (LTB$_4$) that enhances adherence and promotes killing. Viable endothelial cells can produce procoagulant, anti-PA (PAI) and leukotriene C_4 (LTC$_4$) which enhance clotting and vasoconstriction (c). Tissue plasminogen activator (tPA) enhances fibrinolysis and PGE$_2$, PGI$_2$, and EDRFs relax vascular smooth muscle. Operating in sequence, vasoconstriction and clotting would promote endometrial necrosis and subsequent bleeding would ensure wash-out of dead tissue from the uterine cavity. Note also that the macrophage can produce procoagulant and tPA as well as growth factors such as TGF-alpha (epithelial growth factor (EGF) activity), PDGF, and fibroblast growth factor (FGF) that play a role in healing and re-epithelialization and angiogenesis. T lymphocytes in endometrium may also be part of an amplification loop where IL-1 indirectly or the growth factors directly activate T cells to secrete gamma interferon (IFNγ) to activate macrophage expression of HLA-Dr and to express function (Johnson *et al.*, 1988). Note also that secretion of lymphokines by T cells appears to be dependent upon prolactin (PRL) (Bernton *et al.*, 1988).

(b) Antagonist pathways. Factors inhibiting fibrinolytic mechanisms are shown as well as TGF-β, that has the ability to inhibit T cell function, to inhibit the respiratory burst and production of toxic oxygen metabolized by macrophages, to antagonize TNF-α effects (although these data are not derived from study of endothelial cells), to inhibit killing by polymorphonuclear cells, and to promote anti-PA (PAI) synthesis (shown for several cell types). Also, it should be noted that IL-1 may inhibit the action of TNF-α so that the ratios of individual cytokines produced in (a) may also determine what happens to the endothelial cell (Cavender & Edelbaum, 1988). Recent data indicate TGF-β1 may inhibit endothelial cell growth, whereas TGF-β2 spares endothelium (Jennings *et al.*, 1988). Therefore the type of TGF-β produced in endometrium may have an important impact on healing and cessation of bleeding.

There are few published data on lymphomyeloid cell number or their function in the endometrium of women with bleeding problems. We assume they are present for a purpose. Lymphomyeloid cells may be both the source of mediators leading to excess menstrual bleeding and the source of the antagonists of these mediators that promote hemostasis and healing (i.e. TGF-β and plasminogen activator inhibitor). Since mediators of inflammation and necrosis are regulated by powerful antagonists, an *imbalance* could lead to excessive bleeding. In view of the multiplicity of potential interactions, it will be difficult to define pathophysiology by correlative and whole-tissue studies alone. It is quite possible that many of the lymphomyeloid cell types in endometrium have nothing to do with bleeding, but rather are involved in implantation and early placentation. Whoever sorts out this issue will make a major contribution to our understanding of female menstrual disorders.

Acknowledgements

Thanks are due to MRC Canada for grant support and to Mary Lynn Currington for typing the manuscript.

References

Bernton, E.W., Meltzer, M.S. & Holaday, J.W. (1988). Suppression of macrophage activation and T-lymphocyte function in hypoprolactinemic mice. *Science*, **239**:401–404.

Bevilacqua, M.P., Pober, J.S., Wheeler, M.E., Cotran, R.S. & Gimbrone, M.A. Jr (1985). Interleukin 1 acts on cultured human vascular endothelium to increase the adhesion of polymorphonuclear leukocytes, monocytes, and related leukocyte cell lines. *Journal of Clinical Investigation*, **76**:2003–2011.

Bonnar, J. & Sheppard, B.L. (1980). Endometrial changes in women using hormone-releasing intrauterine devices. (In) *Endometrial Bleeding and Steroidal Contraception* (Diczfalusy, E., Fraser, I.S. & Webb, F.T.G., eds.), pp.347–359. Bath, England, Pitman Press.

Bonney, R.C., Qizilbash, S.T. & Franks, S. (1987). Endometrial phospholipase A2 enzymes and their regulation by steroid hormones. *Journal of Steroid Biochemistry*, **27**:1057–1064.

Braquet, P. & Rola-Pleszczynski, M. (1987). Platelet activating factor and cellular immune responses. *Immunology Today*, **8**:345–352.

Brierley, J. & Clark, D.A. (1987). Characterization of hormone-dependent suppressor cells in the uterus of pregnant and pseudopregnant mice. *Journal of Reproductive Immunology*, **10**:201–217.

Bulmer, J.N., Hollings, D. & Ritson, A. (1987c). Immunocytochemical evidence that endometrial stromal granulocytes are granulated lymphocytes. *Journal of Pathology*, **153**:281–288.

Bulmer, J.N. & Johnson, P.M. (1985). Immunohistological characterization of the decidual leukocytic infiltrate related to endometrial gland epithelium in early human pregnancy. *Immunology*, **55**:35–44.

Bulmer, J.N., Johnson, P.M. & Bulmer, D. (1987b). Leukocyte populations in human decidua and endometrium. (In) *Immunoregulation and Fetal Survival* (Gill, T.J. III & Wegmann, T.G., eds.), pp.111–134. New York, Oxford University Press.

Bulmer, J.N., Lunny, D.P. & Hagin, S.V. (1988). Immunohistochemical characterization of stromal leucocytes in non-pregnant human endometrium. *American Journal of Reproductive Immunology and Microbiology*, **17**:83–90.

Bulmer, J.N. & Ritson, A. (1988). The decidua in early pregnancy. (In) *Early Pregnancy Loss: Mechanisms and Treatment* (Beard, R.W. & Sharp, F., eds.), pp.171–180. Ashton-under-Lyne, England, Peacock Press.

Bulmer, J.N., Ritson, A., Earl, U. & Hollings, D. (1987a). Immunocompetent cells in human decidua. (In) *Reproductive Immunology: Materno–Fetal Relationship*, Vol. 154 (Chaouat, G., ed.), pp.89–100. Paris, France, Colloque INSERM.

Bulmer, J.N. & Sunderland, C.A. (1983). Bone-marrow origin of endometrial granulocytes in early human placental bed. *Journal of Reproductive Immunology*, **5**:383–387.

Bussolino, F., Camussi, G. & Baglioni, C. (1988). Synthesis and release of platelet-activating factor by human vascular endothelial cells treated with tumor necrosis factor or interleukin 1α. *Journal of Biological Chemistry*, **263**:11856–11861.

Cameron, I.T., Kelly, R.W. & Baird, D.T. (1984). Prostaglandins in the human uterus: an interaction between endometrium and myometrium. *Prostaglandins and Leukotrienes in Medicine*, **17**:329–335.

Camussi, G., Aglietta, M., Malavasi, F., Tetta, C., Piacibello, W., Sanavio, F. & Bussolino, F. (1983). The release of platelet-activating factor from human endothelial cells in culture. *Journal of Immunology*, **131**:2397–2403.

Cavender, D.E. & Edelbaum, D. (1988). Inhibition by IL-1 of endothelial cell activation induced by tumor necrosis factor or lymphotoxin. *Journal of Immunology*, **141**:3111–3116.

Chapman, H.A. & Stone, O.L. (1985). Characterization of a macrophage-derived plasminogen-activator inhibitor. Similarities with placental urokinase inhibitor. *Biochemical Journal*, **230**:109–116.

Clark, D.A., Falbo, M., Rowley, R.B., Banwatt, D. & Stedronska-Clark, J. (1988). Active suppression of host-versus-graft reaction in pregnant mice. IX. Soluble suppressor activity obtained from allopregnant mouse decidua that blocks the cytolytic effector response to IL-2 is related to transforming growth factor-beta. *Journal of Immunology*, **141**:3833–3840.

Dallenbach-Hellweg, G. (1980). Discussion. (In) *Endometrial Bleeding and Steroidal Contraception* (Diczfalusy, E., Fraser, I.S. & Webb, F.T.G., eds.), pp.218–219; 359–360. Bath, England, Pitman Press.

Daya, S., Clark, D.A., Devlin, C. & Jarrell, J. (1985). Preliminary characterization of two types of suppressor cells in the human uterus. *Fertility and Sterility*, **44**:778–785.

Daya, S., Johnson, P.M. & Clark, D.A. (1986). Mechanism of activation of suppressor cells in the endometrium of the human uterus. *Journal of Reproductive Immunology*, Supplement **1**:164.

Daya, S., Johnson, P.M. & Clark, D.A. (1989). Trophoblast induction of suppressor type cell activity in human endometrial tissue. *American Journal of Reproductive Immunology*, **19**(3):65–72.

Fernandez, H.N., Henson, P.M., Otani, A. & Hugli, T.E. (1978). Chemotactic response to human C3a & C5a anaphylatoxins. Evaluation of C3a and C5a leukotaxis *in vitro* and under stimulated *in vivo* conditions. *Journal of Immunology*, **120**:109–115.

Fraser, I.S. & Diczfalusy, E. (1980). A perspective of steroidal contraception and abnormal bleeding: what are the prospects for improvement? (In) *Endometrial Bleeding and Steroidal Contraception* (Diczfalusy, E., Fraser, I.S. & Webb, F.T.G., eds.), pp.384–409. Bath, England, Pitman Press.

Gorodeski, I.G., Geier, A., Siegal, A., Beery, R., Lunenfeld, B., Langzam, J. & Bahari, C.M. (1986). Decreased ratio of total progesterone to total estradiol receptor levels in endometria of women with adult dysfunctional uterine bleeding. *Gynecologic and Obstetric Investigation*, **22**:22–28.

Hagenfeldt, K. (1987). The role of prostaglandins and allied substances in uterine haemostasis. *Contraception*, **36**:23–35.

Hahn, L. (1980). Composition of menstrual blood. (In) *Endometrial Bleeding and Steroidal Contraception* (Diczfalusy, E., Fraser, I.S. & Webb, F.T.G., eds.), pp.107–131. Bath, England, Pitman Press.

Hall, P., MacLachlan, N., Thorn, N., Nudd, M.W., Taylor, C.G. & Garrioch, D.B. (1987). Control of menorrhagia by the cyclo-oxygenase inhibitors naproxen sodium and mefenamic acid. *British Journal of Obstetrics and Gynaecology*, **94**:554–558.

Hamilton, T.A. & Adams, D.O. (1987). Molecular mechanisms of signal transduction in macrophages. *Immunology Today*, **8**:151–158.

Head, J.R. & Gaede, S.D. (1986). Ia antigen expression in the rat uterus. *Journal of Reproductive Immunology*, **9**:137–153.

Heine, U., Munoz, E.F., Flanders, K.C., Ellingsworth, L.R., Lam, H.-Y., Thompson, N.L., Roberts, A.B. & Sporn, M.B. (1987). Role of transforming growth factor-beta in the development of the mouse embryo. *Journal of Cell Biology*, **105**:2861–2876.

Hulka, J.F., Mohr, K. & Lieberman, M.W. (1965). Effect of synthetic progestational agents on allograft rejection and circulating antibody production. *Endocrinology*, **77**:897–901.

Jennings, J.C., Mohan, S., Linkhart, T.A., Widstrom, R. & Baylink, D.J. (1988). Comparison of the biological actions of TGF beta-1 and TGF beta-2: differential activity in endothelial cells. *Journal of Cellular Physiology*, **137**:167–172.

Johnson, H.M., Russel, J.K. & Torres, B.A. (1988). Structural basis for arachidonic acid second messenger signal in gamma-interferon induction. *Annals of the New York Academy of Sciences*, **524**:208–217.

Kamat, B.R. & Isaacson, P.G. (1987). The immunocytochemical distribution of leukocytic subpopulations in human endometrium. *American Journal of Pathology*, **127**:66–73.

Kasonde, J.M. & Bonnar, J. (1975). Aminocaproic acid and menstrual loss in women using intrauterine devices. *British Medical Journal*, **4**:17–19.

Kenny, J.F., Pangburn, P.C. & Trail, G. (1976). Effect of estradiol on immune competence: *in vivo* and *in vitro* studies. *Infection and Immunity*, **13**:448–456.

Krzych, U., Strausser, H.R., Bressler, J.P. & Goldstein, A.L. (1978). Quantitative differences in immune responses during the various stages of the estrous cycle in female BALB/$_c$ mice. *Journal of Immunology*, **121**:1603–1605.

Laiho, M., Saksela, O. & Keski-Oja, J. (1987). Transforming growth factor-beta induction of type-1 plasminogen activator inhibitor. Pericellular deposition and sensitivity to exogenous urokinase. *Journal of Biological Chemistry*, **262**:17467–17474.

Lala, P.K., Parhar, R.S., Kearns, M., Johnson, S. & Scodras, J. (1986). Immunologic aspects of the decidual response. (In) *Reproductive Immunology* (Clark, D.A. & Croy, B.A., eds.), pp.190–198. Amsterdam, Elsevier.

Lande, I.J. (1986). Systemic immunity developing from intrauterine antigen exposure in the non-pregnant rat. *Journal of Reproductive Immunology*, 9:57–66.

Lanier, L.L. & Phillips, J.H. (1986). Evidence for three types of human cytotoxic lymphocytes. *Immunology Today*, 7:132–134.

Larkin, L.H. (1974). Bioassay of rat metrial gland extracts for relaxin using the mouse interpubic ligament technique. *Endocrinology*, 94:567–570.

Lumsden, M.A., Brown, A. & Baird, D.T. (1984). Prostaglandin production from homogenates of separated glandular epithelium and stroma from human endometrium. *Prostaglandins*, 28:485–496.

Lund, L.R., Riccio, A., Aanreasen, P.A., Nielsen, L.S., Kristensen, P., Laiho, M., Saksela, O., Blasi, F. & Dano, K. (1987). Transforming growth factor-beta is a strong and fast acting positive regulator of the level of type-1 plasminogen activator inhibitor mRNA in WI-38 human lung fibroblasts. *EMBO Journal*, 6:1281–1286.

Madri, J.A., Pratt, B.M. & Tucker, A.M. (1988). Phenotypic modulation of endothelial cells by transforming growth factor-beta depends upon the composition and organization of the extracellular matrix. *Journal of Cell Biology*, 106:1375–1384.

Matthews, C.J. & Searle, R.F. (1987). The role of prostaglandins in the immunosuppressive effects of supernatants from adherent cells of murine decidual tissue. *Journal of Reproductive Immunology*, 12:109–124.

McDermott, M.R., Clark, D.A. & Bienenstock, J.B. (1980). Evidence for a common mucosal immunologic system. II. Influence of the estrous cycle on B immunoblast migration into genital and intestinal tissues. *Journal of Immunology*, 24:2536–2539.

McMannis, J.D., Fisher, R.I., Creekmore, S.P., Braun, D.P., Harris, J.E. & Ellis, T.M. (1988). *In vivo* effect of recombinant IL-2. I. Isolation of circulating Leu-19+ lymphokine activated killer effector cells from cancer patients receiving recombinant IL-2. *Journal of Immunology*, 140:1335–1340.

Mencia-Huerta, J.M. & Benveniste, J. (1979). Platelet-activating factor and macrophages. I. Evidence for the release from rat and mouse peritoneal macrophages and not from mastocytes. *European Journal of Immunology*, 9:409–415.

Moonen, P., Klok, G. & Keirse, M.J. (1985). Immunohistochemical localization of prostaglandin endoperoxide synthase and prostacyclin synthase in pregnant human myometrium. *European Journal of Obstetrics and Reproductive Biology*, 19:151–158.

Morris, H., Edwards, J., Tiltman, A. & Emms, M. (1985). Endometrial lymphoid tissue: an immunohistological study. *Journal of Clinical Pathology*, 38:644–652.

Nachman, R.L., Hajjar, K.A., Silverstein, R.L. & Dinarello, C.A. (1986). Interleukin 1 induces endothelial cell synthesis of plasminogen activator inhibitor. *Journal of Experimental Medicine*, 163:1595–1600.

Nawroth, P.P., Bank, I., Handley, D., Cassimeris, J., Chess, L. & Stern, D. (1986). Tumor necrosis factor/cachectin interacts with endothelial cell receptors to induce release of interleukin 1. *Journal of Experimental Medicine*, 163:1363–1375.

Nawroth, P.P. & Stern, D.M. (1986). Modulation of endothelial cell hemostatic properties by tumor necrosis factor. *Journal of Experimental Medicine*, 163:740–745.

Neulen, J., Zahradnik, H.P., Flecken, U. & Breckwoldt, M. (1988). Effects of estradiol-17-beta and progesterone on the synthesis of prostaglandin F2-alpha, prostaglandin E2 and prostaglandin I2 by fibroblasts from human endometrium *in vitro*. *Prostaglandins*, 36:17–30.

Nilsson, L. & Rybo, G. (1965). Treatment of menorrhagia with epsilon aminocaproic acid. A double blind investigation. *Acta Obstetricia et Gynecologica Scandinavica*, **44**:467–473.

Nomura, S., Wills, A.J., Edwards, D.R., Heath, J.K. & Hogan, B.L. (1988). Developmental expression of 2ar (osteopontin) and SPARC (osteonectin) RNA as revealed by *in situ* hybridization. *Journal of Cellular Biology*, **106**:441–450.

Oksenberg, J.R., Mor-Yosef, S., Ezra, Y. & Brauthbar, C. (1987). Antigen presenting cells in human decidual tissue. II. Accessory cells for the development of anti-trinitrophenyl cytotoxic T lymphocytes. *Journal of Reproductive Immunology*, **10**:309–318.

Oksenberg, J.R., Mor-Yosef, S., Ezra, Y. & Brautbar, C. (1988). Antigen presenting cells in human decidual tissue: III. Role of accessory cells in the activation of suppressor cells. *American Journal of Reproductive Immunology and Microbiology*, **16**:151–158.

Palmblad, J., Malmsten, C.L., Udén, A.M., Rådmark, O., Engstedt, L. & Samuelsson, B. (1981). Leukotriene B4 is a potent and stereospecific stimulator of neutrophil chemotaxis and adherence. *Blood*, **58**:658–661.

Parr, M.B. & Parr, E.L. (1985). Immunohistochemical localization of immunoglobulins A, G, and M in the mouse female genital tract. *Journal of Reproduction and Fertility*, **74**:361–370.

Paton, R.C., Tindall, H., Zuzel, M. & McNicol, G.P. (1980). Haemostatic mechanisms in the normal endometrium and endometrium exposed to contraceptive steroids. (In) *Endometrial Bleeding and Steroidal Contraception* (Diczfalusy, E., Fraser, I.S. & Webb, F.T.G., eds.), pp.325–341. Bath, England, Pitman Press.

Peel, S. & Stewart, I. (1986). Oestrogen and the differentiation of granulated metrial gland cells in chimeric mice. *Journal of Anatomy*, **144**:181–187.

Peel, S., Stewart, I.J. & Bulmer, D. (1983). Experimental evidence for the bone marrow origin of granulated metrial gland cells of the mouse uterus. *Cell and Tissue Research*, **233**:647–656.

Pelus, L.M., Levi, E. & Welte, K. (1988). The response of human marrow colony-forming units – granulocyte and macrophage – to inhibition by prostaglandin E and acidic isoferritins is associated with expression of MHC Class II antigens and requires the participation of CD8 + T lymphokine. *Journal of Immunology*, **141**:1658–1664.

Postlethwaite, A.E., Keski-Oja, J., Moses, H.L. & Kang, A.H. (1987). Stimulation of the chemotactic migration of human fibroblasts by transforming growth factor-beta. *Journal of Experimental Medicine*, **165**:251–256.

Rappolee, D.A., Mark, D., Banda, M.J. & Werb, Z. (1988). Wound macrophages express TGF-α and other growth factors *in vivo*: analysis by mRNA phenotyping. *Science*, **241**:708–712.

Roy, S. & Shaw, S.T. Jr (1981). Role of prostaglandins in IUD-associated uterine bleeding – effect of a prostaglandin synthetase inhibitor (ibuprofen). *Obstetrics and Gynecology*, **58**:101–106.

Rubin, R.M. & Rosenbaum, J.T. (1988). A platelet-activating factor antagonist inhibits interleukin 1-induced inflammation. *Biochemical and Biophysical Research Communications*, **154**:429–436.

Ruddle, N.H. (1987). Tumor necrosis factors and related cytotoxins. *Immunology Today*, **8**:129–130.

Rybo, G. (1966). Plasminogen activators in the endometrium. II Clinical aspects.

Variation in the concentration of plasminogen activators during the menstrual cycle and its relation to menstrual blood loss. *Acta Obstetricia et Gynecologica Scandinavica*, **45**:429–450.

Sayers, T.J., Wiltrout, T.A., Bull, C.A., Denn, A.C., Pilaro, A.M. & Lokesh, B. (1988). Effects of cytokines on polymorphonuclear neutrophil infiltration in the mouse. Prostaglandin- and leukotriene-independent induction of infiltration by IL-1 and tumor necrosis factor. *Journal of Immunology*, **141**:1670–1677.

Schatz, F., Markiewicz, L. & Gurpide, E. (1987). Estradiol enhances prostaglandin synthetase activity in epithelial but not in stromal cells of human endometrium. *Journal of Steroid Biochemistry*, **27**:1065–1071.

Shaw, J.O., Pinckard, R.N., Ferrigni, K.S., McManus, L.M. & Hanahan, D.J. (1981). Activation of human neutrophils with 1-0-hexadecyl/octadecyl-2-acetyl-**sn**-glycerol-3-phosphorylcholine (platelet-activating factor). *Journal of Immunology*, **127**:1250–1255.

Skinner, S.J., Liggins, G.-C., Wilson, T. & Neale, G. (1984). Synthesis of prostaglandin F by cultured human endometrial cells. *Prostaglandins*, **27**:821–838.

Slapsys, R.M., Younglai, E.G. & Clark, D.A. (1988). Active suppression of host-versus-graft reaction in pregnant mice. X. A novel suppressor cell is recruited to decidua by fetal trophoblast cells. *Regional Immunology*, **1**:182–189.

Smith, S.K., Abel, M.H., Kelly, R.W. & Baird, D.T. (1981). A role for prostacyclin (PGI_2) in excessive menstrual bleeding. *Lancet*, **i**:522–524.

Smith, S.K. & Kelly, R.W. (1988). The release of $PGF_{2\alpha}$ and PGE_2 from separated cells of human endometrium and decidua. *Prostaglandins, Leukotrienes and Essential Fatty Acids*, **33**:91–96.

Staples, L.D., Heap, R.B., Wooding, F.B. & King, G.J. (1983). Migration of leukocytes into the uterus after acute removal of ovarian progesterone during early pregnancy in the sheep. *Placenta*, **4**:339–349.

Stewart, I. & Mukhtar, D.D.Y. (1988). The killing of mouse trophoblast cells by granulated metrial gland cells *in vitro*. *Placenta*, **9**:417–425.

Sullivan, D.A., Richardson, G.S., MacLaughlin, D.T. & Wira, C.R. (1984). Variations in the levels of secretory component in human uterine fluid during the menstrual cycle. *Journal of Steroid Biochemistry*, **20**:509–513.

Szekeres-Bartho, J., Kilar, F., Falkay, G., Csernus, V., Torok, A. & Pacsa, A.S. (1985). The mechanism of the inhibitory effect of progesterone on lymphocyte cytotoxicity: 1. Progesterone-treated lymphocytes release a substance inhibiting cytotoxicity and prostaglandin synthesis. *American Journal of Reproductive Immunology and Microbiology*, **9**:15–18.

Tagliabue, A., Befus, A.D., Clark, D.A. & Bienenstock, J. (1982). Characteristics of natural killer cells in the murine intestinal epithelium and lamina propria. *Journal of Experimental Medicine*, **155**:1785–1796.

Tawfik, O.W., Hunt, J.S. & Wood, G.W. (1986a). Implication of prostaglandin E2 in soluble factor-mediated immune suppression by murine decidual cells. *American Journal of Reproductive Immunology and Microbiology*, **12**:111–117.

Tawfik, O.W., Hunt, J.S. & Wood, G.W. (1986b). Partial characterization of uterine cells responsible for suppression of murine maternal anti-fetal immune responses. *Journal of Reproductive Immunology*, **9**:213–224.

Toppozada, M. (1987). Treatment of increased menstrual blood loss in IUD users. *Contraception*, **36**:145–157.

Tsang, B.K., Domingo, M.T., Spence, J.E., Garner, P.R., Dudley, D.K. & Oxorn, H. (1987). Endometrial prostaglandins and menorrhagia: influence of a prostaglandin synthetase inhibitor *in vivo*. *Canadian Journal of Physiology and Pharmacology*, **65**:2081–2084.

Tschopp, J. & Conzelmann, A. (1986). Proteoglycans in secretory granules of NK cells. *Immunology Today*, **7**:135–136.

Tsunawaki, S., Sporn, M., Ding, A. & Nathan, C. (1988). Deactivation of macrophages by transforming growth factor-beta. *Nature*, **334**:260–262.

Vanhoutte, P.M. (1988). The endothelium – modulator of vascular smooth muscle tone. *New England Journal of Medicine*, **319**:512–513.

Varani, J., Bendelow, M.J., Sealey, D.E., Kunkel, S.L., Gannon, D.E., Ryan, U.S. & Ward, P.A. (1988). Tumor necrosis factor enhances susceptibility of vascular endothelial cells to neutrophil-mediated killing. *Laboratory Investigation*, **59**:292–295.

Watanabe, S., Honma, S., Kanazawa, K. & Takeuchi, S. (1986). Characterization of bone marrow derived cells in human decidua. *Journal of Reproductive Immunology*, Supplement **1**:124.

Wedmore, C.V. & Williams, T.J. (1981). Control of vascular permeability by polymorphonuclear leukocytes in inflammation. *Nature*, **289**:646–650.

Wilson, E.W. (1980). Lysosome function in normal endometrium and endometrium exposed to contraceptive steroids. (In) *Endometrial Bleeding and Steroidal Contraception* (Diczfalusy, E., Fraser, I.S. & Webb, F.T.G., eds.), pp.201–218. Bath, England, Pitman Press.

Wood, G.W., Kamel, S. & Smith, K. (1988). Immunoregulation and prostaglandin production by mechanically-derived and enzyme-derived murine decidual cells. *Journal of Reproductive Immunology*, **13**:235–248.

Ylikorkala, O. & Pekonen, F. (1986). Naproxen reduces idiopathic but not fibromyoma-induced menorrhagia. *Obstetrics and Gynecology*, **68**:10–12.

Discussion

Findlay. Can you be more specific about the method that you used to isolate those cells; it is not simply disintegrating the tissue and so freeing the lymphocytes. Do you use some sort of tissue separation or differential culturing to obtain pure cell lines?

Clark. When we are studying endometrial and decidual tissue, normally we snip it into fine pieces, press these through a 60-mesh screen, and then, to remove debris, centrifuge on isopaque Ficoll of an appropriate density. As well, we separate the cells in terms of size by velocity sedimentation which cleans up the preparation and gives physically distinct cell populations. It is also possible to do FACS (fluorescent-activated cell sorter) analysis, separating cell populations labelled with fluorescent-tagged antibodies to specific cell surface markers, and we have done that as well. Dr Bulmer has also done some studies of cell populations in human decidua using this method (Bulmer *et al.*, 1987).

Baird. I would like to ask how many of the functions of these cells which you have described are known to be influenced directly by the steroid hormones, estradiol and progesterone, which appear to play a key role in the initiation of menstruation and also in breakthrough bleeding. It is the administration of steroid hormones with either progestogenic or estrogenic activity which has an effect on the endometrium to cause it to bleed abnormally.

Clark. These lymphomyeloid cells accumulate if the tissue grows and will presumably disappear to some extent if the tissue becomes quiescent. Peel and Stewart (1986) have shown using rodents that gestational hormones stimulate accumulation of endometrial granulated lymphocytes (eGL), but that may be due to an indirect mechanism (Stewart, 1987).

Dr Casey mentioned that long-term progestogens increase the level of interleukin-1β (IL-1β) in the endometrium and there is an increase in IL-1β in the luteal phase. That would imply that progestational agents affect either the number or the function of these cells, but even if they did not, it would not be a point against involvement of lymphomyeloid cells in the process of shedding and repair because, with the initial necrosis of tissue, that necrosis will activate macrophages to then carry out their programme.

Sheppard. In your hypothesis you stressed the stimulation of the production of antiplasminogen activator from endothelial cells via macrophages. Yet it is well known from studies, particularly in IUD-induced bleeding, that macrophages produce very large amounts of plasminogen activator. How does that fit into your story?

Clark. Both macrophages and endothelial cells are producing molecules which are antagonistic in their ultimate effect, i.e. plasminogen activator and plasminogen activator inhibitor. I think we have to ask ourselves what determines which will be the dominant molecule at one particular point and what will cause a shift to the other at a different time point. We really do not understand what happens, and that could be quite relevant to problems of macrophage dysfunction if it occurs in women who have heavy bleeding or intermenstrual bleeding.

Cravioto. In hyperprolactinemic women, an inhibitory effect of the suppressor activity of peripheral T lymphocytes has been demonstrated, although we do not know the consequences of that action. Is it possible to find some similar relationship between endometrial prolactin and these immunosuppressive cells?

Clark. Yes, it is possible that prolactin may be acting on a number of cell types to alter their function, but we do not have any data as yet.

Cravioto. It seems that synthetic progestogens such as medroxyprogesterone acetate have an immunosuppressive activity. Is there any information available on this action on these cells?

Clark. Progesterone in fairly high doses can locally inhibit processes producing cell damage and graft rejection. However, pharmacological concentrations are required and these are concentrations which are not normally found, even at the choriodecidual junction where there is evidence of suppression of rejection-type responses. This information has been obtained from studies of rodents where there is not much progesterone produced by the placenta. In humans, the situation may be different. There may be effects of progestational agents on immune functions, and there may be other implications with respect to effects on systemic immunity, in contrast to my previous comments which were entirely about local mechanisms.

Bischof. If, instead of studying the mechanism of menstruation we were studying, for example, lung cancer, would your talk have been different? In other words, how specific are all these cell mechanisms to the uterus, or is it in fact what you would find in other tissues?

Clark. In the lung, which is a mucosal organ, there are granulated lymphocytes, T cells, macrophages, etc. However, there is not the hormonal regulation of the tissues, and the number of endometrial granulated lymphocytes, LEU 19-positive cells which are described in the uterus, is considerably greater than I have seen mentioned for any other site that has been looked at. I would think that there is probably a general economy in the body, whereby Mother Nature employs similar mechanisms in different organs, but each has its own unique individuality.

Naftolin. In fact the inside of the uterus uses some of the same mechanisms as in the lung. We also have to understand that the lung is a very potent steroid metabolizing organ, just as the uterus is. Some investigators have thought they found estrogen receptors in populations of macrophages; estrogen induces fems, which is colony-stimulating factor receptor; macrophages make colony-stimulating factor. This is one system that works quite happily through estrogen.

Clark. An important question is: what dose of estradiol is needed to get the effects? I found evidence for estradiol affecting macrophage function but the paper describing this was using pharmacological levels (Pfeifer & Patterson, 1985). If it occurs at physiological levels, then I think it is probably important.

Naftolin. Again, it depends on whether we talk about cells or we talk about body fluids. Since the uterus can make estrogen, there is no reason to suspect that there is not a lot of estrogen in the area of those cells. Dr Gurpide mentioned prolactin and I think it is important to point out that prolactin affects aromatase enzyme systems.

Casey. In the kidney, it is known that prolactin will enhance 1α-hydroxylation and thereby increase the production of 1,25-dihydroxy-vitamin D_3 which, as you know, will activate macrophages. This might be of some potential importance.

References

Bulmer, J.N., Ritson, A., Earl, U. & Hollings, D. (1987). Immunocompetent cells in human decidua. (In) *Reproductive Immunology: Materno–Fetal Relationship*, Vol. 154 (Chaouat, G., ed.), pp.89–100. Paris, France, Colloque INSERM.

Peel, S. & Stewart, I. (1986). Oestrogen and the differentiation of granulated metrial gland cells in chimeric mice. *Journal of Anatomy*, **144**:181–187.

Pfeifer, R.W. & Patterson, R.M. (1985). Modulation of lymphokine-induced macrophage activation by estrogen metabolites. *Journal of Immunopharmacology*, **7**:247–263.

Stewart, I. (1987). Granulated metrial gland cells in the non-traumatized regions of the uterus of ovariectomized mice with deciduomata maintained on progesterone. *Journal of Endocrinology*, **116**:11–15.

A biochemical study of lysosomal enzymes in control and levonorgestrel-treated human endometria: analysis of total activity and evidence for secretion

F.J. CORNILLIE*, I.A. BROSENS*, E. MARBAIX**, TH. VAEL**, P. BAUDHUIN** AND P.J. COURTOY**

*University Hospital Gasthuisberg, Laboratory of Gynaecological Physiopathology, K.U. Leuven, Belgium.
**International Institute of Cellular and Molecular Pathology, Louvain University Medical School, Brussels, Belgium.

Abstract

Lysosomes could be important at three stages of menstruation.

1. At the *initiation*, the active secretion of lysosomal enzymes over the last days of the cycle could trigger a substantial degradation of the extracellular matrix of the endometrium; this would result in tissue shrinkage, excessive coiling and eventually collapse of spiral arteries, and ischemia.
2. At the *onset*, the extended period of ischemia followed by reperfusion could cause irreversible damage of the lysosomal membrane resulting into autolysis (and secondarily heterolysis) of endothelial and perivascular cells, and hemorrhage.
3. At the *remodelling stage*, auto- and heterolysis could be necessary for the partial lysis required for tissue shedding and proper subsequent repair.

We measured, in 30 paired endometrial biopsies of control and levonorgestrel-treated volunteers, the total activity per unit weight (content) of four lysosomal enzymes: acid phosphatase, α-D-mannosidase, N-acetyl-β-glucosaminidase, and α-L-fucosidase. The activities were further related to the content of reference constituents – protein, DNA, lactate dehydrogenase (LDH) – and compared either to the histological dating during the control cycles, or to the bleeding pattern after treatment.

In opposition to the generally accepted view, the total activity per unit weight of the four enzymes studied decreased significantly from the early to the mid–late secretory phase of the control cycle, while reference constituents did not appreciably change. After levonorgestrel treatment, total activity N-acetyl-β-hexosaminidase was significantly increased compared to the normal mid–late secretory phase, but protein and especially LDH were markedly decreased. Thus, upon levonorgestrel treatment, lysosomal enzymes appear to be relatively spared from a general process of cytoplasmic atrophy.

We also developed a new interface organ culture system and quantified the activity of lysosomal enzymes released in the medium. To distinguish release from secretion, values were compared to the release of LDH, a crude index of cell suffering. Depending on the enzymes, the cumulative release after 24 hours of culture corresponded to 12–69% of the activity initially introduced with the control mid–late explants, and 10–

151% of that of treated explants. In both conditions, the release of hexosaminidase was significantly higher than that of LDH. It was further increased by a procedure preventing recapture of lysosomal enzymes by living cells.

Taken together, data show that control and levonorgestrel-treated endometria contain large amounts of lysosomal enzymes of which one was demonstrated to be actively secreted and partially recaptured by the living cells. However, no evidence was obtained to correlate total activities with increased likelihood of normal menstrual bleeding (the content values decreased towards menses) or abnormal endometrial bleeding (no difference between bleeders and non-bleeders).

Introduction: possible roles of lysosomes in endometrial bleeding

Lysosomes comprise an heterogeneous family of intracellular organelles, whose comprehensive equipment of hydrolytic enzymes is able to destroy virtually every biological macromolecule at the appropriate acidic pH (de Duve, 1963). Fortunately, this destructive potential is normally restricted to the interior of lysosomes by a limiting membrane which resists degradation. Hence, the other intracellular compartments, the extracellular matrix and solutes as well as the neighbouring cells, are in principle protected from the harmful lysosomal enzymes, unless they are: (1) sequestered within an autophagic or heterophagic vacuole; (2) discharged into lysosomes by membrane fusion; and (3) exposed to lysosomal enzymes at the appropriate pH. It is, however. conceivable that, under certain pathological conditions, rupture of the lysosomal membrane could allow lysosomal enzymes to escape into the whole cell, so as to be the primary cause of cell death.

Albeit this 'suicide bag' hypothesis (de Duve, 1963) has neither been formally demonstrated nor discounted, it remains relevant to the *autolysis* induced by ischemia–reperfusion, including the endothelial damage leading to secondary tissue infarction, and possibly endometrial bleeding. An experimental model is provided by the transient ligation of a rat liver lobe. In this model, reperfusion following a 2-hour ischemia leads to a secondary, irreversible increase of the non-sedimentable fraction of lysosomal enzymes of the liver homogenate (which might correspond to an in-vivo intracellular release), without obvious ultrastructural alterations (Wattiaux & Wattiaux-Deconinck, 1981). To account for enzyme release, damage of the lysosomal membrane by free radicals has been invoked.

Hence, the involvement of lysosomes in the initiation of menstruation as a consequence of extended ischemia is an attractive hypothesis (Henzl *et al.*, 1972; critically evaluated by Wilson, 1980). The direct observation of endometrial tissue implanted in the anterior chamber of the eye of the rhesus monkey showed that a prolonged spasm of spiral arteries invariably precedes menstruation (Markee, 1948). In addition, the non-sedimentable fraction of lysosomal enzymes from endometrial homogenates has been reported to increase from about 25% at the proliferative phase to about 50% at the late secretory phase, a finding interpreted as labilization of the lysosomal membranes (Rosado *et al.*, 1977). However, this increase preceded menstruation by several days, and could as well be attributed either to the secretion of lysosomal enzymes into the extracellular space, or to a structural alteration of the size or shape of lysosomes (e.g. from small, round dense bodies to large, irregular, autophagic bodies), making them more susceptible to damage by the shearing forces applied for tissue homogenization (Cohn & Hirsch, 1960). Both the explanations of secretion and enhanced autophagy are supported by cytochemical ultrastructural studies of the mid–late secretory human endometria (Henzl *et al.*, 1972). Although steroid hormones may directly labilize the membrane of isolated lysosomes (de Duve *et al.*, 1962), this is unlikely to account *per se* for autolysis and menstruation, because labilization requires pharmacological concentrations of the steroids, and is caused by the addition, not the withdrawal, of the hormones.

The *secretion* of hydrolytic (lysosomal) enzymes into the extracellular space is another mechanism that could initiate endometrial bleeding, either directly by dissociation or destruction of endothelial cells or the perivascular tissue, or indirectly by degradation of the extracellular matrix. In most cells, newly synthesized lysosomal enzymes are restricted to the interior of the cell by a direct, receptor-mediated intracellular targeting from the Golgi complex to lysosomes (for a review, see von Figura & Hasilik, 1986). In addition, lysosomal enzymes released by accident are efficiently recaptured by receptor-mediated endocytosis (Hickman & Neufeld, 1972). Both processes involve the same receptors, which recognize mannose-6-phosphate signals on the lysosomal enzymes.

However, during bone resorption, lysosomal enzymes are actively secreted into the extracellular bone resorbing lacunae, where the organic matrix can be degraded (Vaes, 1968; Baron *et al.*, 1988). Macrophages also secrete lysosomal enzymes in the inflammatory area (see, for example, Imort *et al.*, 1983) and can induce extensive tissue degradation, either directly, or indirectly via the activation of procollagenase into collagenase, the only enzyme that cleaves fibrillar collagen at neutral pH (Eeckhout, 1990). Rat liver lysosomes have proved effective in degrading extracellular matrix glycosaminoglycans, even at neutral pH (Fell & Dingle, 1963). Depolymerization of extracellular matrix constituents, especially hyaluronic acid, may also cause a considerable tissue shrinkage (Solursh *et al.*, 1979).

The rapid regression of endometrial thickness has actually been reported to be the first event which precedes menstruation in Macacus rhesus (Markee, 1948). Regression is believed to cause a disproportion between the length of the spiral arteries and the thickness of the endometrium. This would result in increased coiling and collapse of the spiral arteries, a phenomenon compromising blood supply to the functional zone of the endometrium. Morphological studies do suggest that lysosomal enzymes can indeed be secreted into the extracellular space at the mid–late secretory phase (Henzl *et al.*, 1972). The contribution of lysosomal enzymes to the remodelling of the endometrial matrix may thus be a major physiological process (albeit completely ignored), and this possible role in the initiation of menstruation should be explored.

Thirdly, it is most likely that lysosomal enzymes contribute to the partial lysis of endometrial tissue that is required for its *shedding*. However, this 'housekeeping' function may be independent from the two other mechanisms described above, and may not be relevant to endometrial bleeding.

Because we felt that possible alterations of the integrity of the lysosomal membrane in the human endometrium *in vivo* cannot be tested unambiguously by the non-sedimentable fraction of endometrial homogenates (see the effect of 1-hour ischemia in Wattiaux & Wattiaux-Deconinck, 1981), we restricted our analysis to the determination of the content of four lysosomal enzymes in biopsies of control and levonorgestrel-treated volunteers. We selected four acid hydrolases for which sensitive fluorescent assays are available: two reference enzymes, acid phosphatase (the 'traditional' lysosomal marker) and hexosaminidase (the 'current' marker), as well as two other exoglycosidases which are good candidates to act upon the extracellular matrix, a-L-fucosidase and a-D-mannosidase. We also developed a new interface culture system of endometrial tissue explants, and obtained strong evidence for the secretion of one lysosomal enzyme.

This study was part of a multicentre clinical trial on the effect of levonorgestrel on endometrial function. Other parts, following the same clinical protocol, investigated the effect of levonorgestrel on endometrial hemostasis, prostaglandin metabolism and protein synthesis; the preliminary reports of these studies are published in this volume (respectively, Hourihan *et al.*, 1990; Elder *et al.*, 1990; White *et al.*, 1990).

Materials and methods

Clinical sampling

Of the volunteers recruited among paramedical employees at the University Hospital Gasthuisberg (Leuven), 39 women with regular cycles and without any gynecological disorder or hormonal therapy were carefully selected. All women (mean: 34 years; range: 29–42 years) were first investigated during a control cycle. On the second day of the next menstrual period, a vaginal ring, designed to release 20 μg levonorgestrel/day, was inserted and left for 90 days. Women were requested to fill in bleeding charts. During the control cycle from day 10 onwards, blood was drawn three times weekly, for measurements of estradiol and progesterone. During the third treatment month, from day 60 onwards, blood was drawn three times weekly for estradiol and progesterone and once a week for levonorgestrel and sex hormone-binding globulin (SHBG) assays. Two endometrial biopsies were scheduled, at day 24–26 of the control cycle and at day 84–87 of the study period. Biopsies were performed with a Masterson aspiration curette and yielded about 50–100 mg wet weight in control cycles and 20–50 mg in study cycles. Part of the tissue was either immediately immersed in Bouin's fixative, processed for histology and dated by Dr Johannisson according to criteria reported elsewhere (Johannisson *et al.*, 1987), or processed for electron microscopy. Another sample was homogenized for the biochemical assays (described below and in Hourihan *et al.*, 1990). Finally, small pieces were transferred to Millicell™ chambers for organ cultures. For the treatment period, volunteers were grouped into normal or abnormal bleeders, the latter having at least four bleeding episodes and/or more than 20 bleeding days during treatment.

Biochemical assays

About 5–20 mg of fresh endometrial tissue were briefly blotted on gauze, washed in cold phosphate-buffered saline, solubilised in 1 ml of 1 mmol/l bicarbonate buffer, pH 7.6, containing 1 mmol/l EDTA and 0.01% Triton X-100, using a 3 ml conical glass tissue grind tube equipped with a pestle (Kontes, nominal clearance 127 μm). The extract was further sonicated for 20 seconds at 30 watts (Branson sonifier B12) and immediately assayed or frozen in aliquots at $-80°C$. When the fresh extract was sedimented at 3×10^6 $g \times$ minute, more than 85% of all lysosomal enzymes was recovered in the supernatant.

The protein content was measured by the colorimetric assay of Lowry *et al.* (1951), using bovine serum albumin as standard; a 1 mg/ml stock solution gave an absorbance at 280 nm of 0.640. DNA was measured by the fluorescent assay based on the intercalation of 4′-6-diamino-6-phenylindole (DAPI), as described by Kapuscinski and Skoczylas (1977). For standard, we used high molecular weight DNA purified from P 815 mastocytoma cells; a 20 μg/ml solution gave an absorbance at 260 nm of 0.389. Lactate dehydrogenase activity (E.C. 1.1.1.27) was determined by the rate of oxidation of 0.1 mmol/l NADH, in the presence of 3.3 mmol/l pyruvate and 100 mmol/l glycyl-glycine buffer, pH 7.4, as measured by the decrease of the optical density at 340 nm for 5 minutes at 25°C (Bergmeyer & Bernt, 1974).

feryl(4 MU)-glycosides in the conditions described in Table 1, where final concentrations are indicated. Practically, 50–80 μl of buffered substrate were mixed with 20 μl of tissue extract (diluted about 1:10) and incubated at 37°C for 2 hours. The enzymatic hydrolysis was arrested by adding 3 ml of 0.5 mol/l bicarbonate buffer, pH 10.7. Fluorescence was read in a Perkin-Elmer 1000 spectrophotometer set at 360 nm for excitation and 460 nm for emission, and compared to 0.2 μg/ml methylumbelliferone (final concentration) as standard. For blanks, the tissue extract was added after the reaction was arrested by bicarbonate. All assays were in the linear range and were performed in duplicate with less than 5% variation. The activity of acid phosphatase, N-acetyl-β-glucosaminidase and α-L-fucosidase was not appreciably affected by

Table 1. *Incubation conditions for lysosomal enzyme assays*

Enzyme		Substrate	Buffer (sodium salt)
acid phosphatase	(3.1.3.2)	12.5 mmol/l 4-MU-phosphate	125 mmol/l acetate pH 5.5
α-D-mannosidase	(3.2.1.24)	6.0 mmol/l 4-MU-α-D-manno-pyranoside	63 mmol/l citrate pH 4.5
N-acetyl-β-hexosaminidase	(3.2.1.30)	1.9 mmol/l 4-MU-2-acetamido β-D-glucopyranoside	63 mmol/l citrate pH 4.7
α-L-fucosidase	(3.2.1.38)	0.6 mmol/l 4-MU-α-L-fuco-pyranoside	63 mmol/l citrate pH 5.5

extended storage at $-80°C$, nor by freezing and thawing. In contrast, we realized that α-D-mannosidase was markedly affected by storage and/or freezing–thawing. Accordingly, only activities determined on fresh biopsies are included in this report.

Assays were performed at the optimal pH defined for human liver (Van Hoof, 1972) and were expressed according to the international units of biochemistry, i.e. 1 mU converting 1 nmol substrate/minute in the assay conditions. The pH-dependence of hydrolytic enzymes was subsequently determined for the human endometrium (Fig. 1). Data point to at least two isoenzymes for α-D-mannosidase and probably for acid phosphatase (4 MU-phosphatase, respectively). The contribution of the isoenzymes acting at more neutral pH (possibly the Golgi marker mannosidase and the endoplasmic marker glucose-6-phosphatase) was neglected. Interestingly, the isoenzyme of α-D-mannosidase acting at very acidic pH was much more sensitive to freezing–thawing and extended storage than the isoenzyme acting at more neutral pH. It should be noted that pH-dependence of activity of acid hydrolases from human endometrium markedly differs from those reported for the rabbit endometrium (Munakata *et al.*, 1986) and for rat bone (Vaes & Jacques, 1965).

Organ cultures

Ten small endometrial tissue explants not exceeding 1 mm³ were quickly layered on the membrane support of 12-mm Millicell HA culture plate inserts (Millipore), the latter fitting into four-well culture dishes (Nunc). The endometrial explants were cultured at the interphase between the gas phase (above the membrane; 5% CO_2 and 95% air) and the liquid medium phase (below the membrane). The culture medium was based on Ham's F10 (Ham, 1963) and supplemented with 5% (v/v) charcoal-treated calf serum (Gibco, lot 10 Q 9552), 5% (w/v) BSA, 235 mU/ml insulin, 100 U/ml penicillin, 1000 μg/ml streptomycin and 2.5 μg/ml fungizone (Gibco). By radioimmunoassay, the

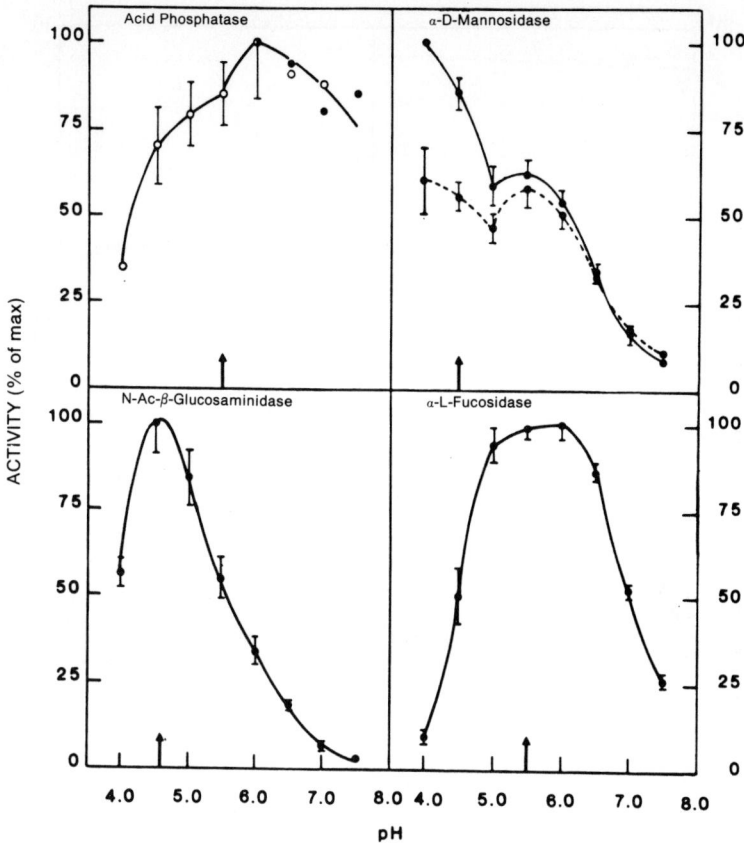

Fig. 1 pH-dependence of hydrolytic activities. Enzyme activities were measured as described under 'Materials and methods', except that pH was varied from 4.0 to 7.5 using acetate (open circles) or citrate buffer (closed circles). For mannosidase, extracts were assayed either after overnight storage at -80°C (continuous line) or after repeated freezing–thawing and prolonged storage (broken line). Values are means ± S.D. of three assays, except for acid phosphatase at pH above 6.0, and are expressed as percentage of peak values. The arrows indicate pH of routine assays of human tissue.

final concentration of steroid hormones in the medium was 0.15 pg/ml of 17-β-estradiol and 0.02 ng/ml of progesterone. The concentration of phenol red was 1.2 μg/ml (3 μmol/l) and thus one order of magnitude below that mimicking estrogen response in cultured human breast cancer cells (Kd: 20 μmol/l; Berthois *et al.*, 1986).

The culture conditions were designed as follows to optimize the detection of released enzymes. (1) We verified by autoradiography that small molecular weight solutes can diffuse by capillarity into the entire explants and we assume

390   *F.J. Cornillie* et al.

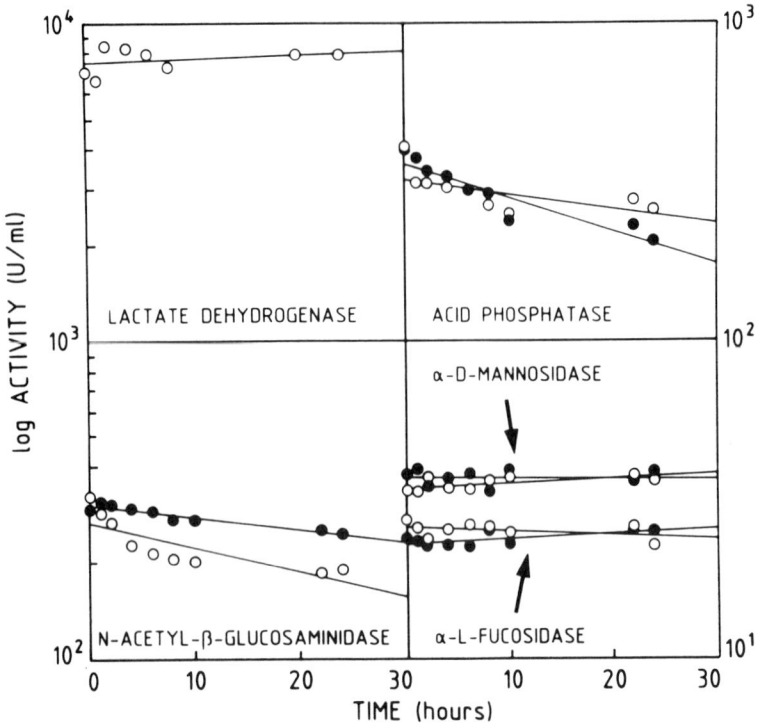

Fig. 2 Stability of enzyme activities in the culture media. An endometrial extract was diluted 1:10 in the tissue culture medium containing 5% calf serum and supplemented (closed circles) or not (open circles) with 5% BSA, and aliquots were incubated for up to 24 hours at 37°C in the tissue incubator.

that released enzymes similarly diffuse out into the medium. (2) To minimize dilution of released enzymes, the volume of the medium was brought down to 300 μl. (3) To minimize the activity of acid hydrolases normally occurring in serum, only 5% charcoal-treated calf serum was introduced. (4) To prevent enzyme adsorption and/or inactivation, 5% BSA was added as a carrier. We also verified that after a 24-hour incubation at 37°C of an endometrial extract diluted in the medium supplemented by 5% BSA, lactate dehydrogenase (LDH), α-L-fucosidase and α-D-mannosidase activities were not altered. Under those conditions, N-acetyl-β-glucosaminidase showed a minor inactivation and acid phosphatase showed a twofold inactivation after 24 hours (Fig. 2). Data were not corrected for inactivation. After culture, the explants were fixed by 1.25% glutaraldehyde in 0.1 mol/l phosphate buffer (pH 7.2), weighed and processed for histological and ultrastructural evaluation.

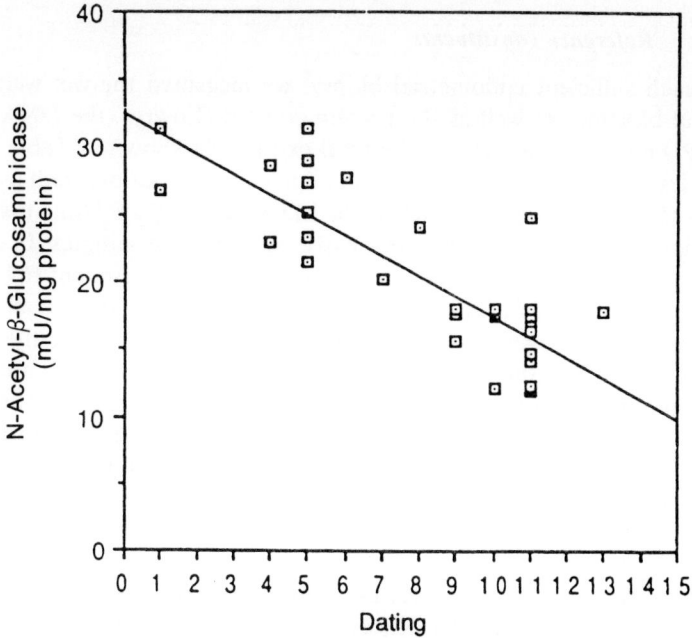

Fig. 3 Variation of specific activity of hexosaminidase in the secretory phase of the control cycle. The specific activity of N-acetyl-β-glucosaminidase in control cycles is compared to histological dating, indicated as LH+ days. r = 0.815; p $\langle$ 0.001.

Results and discussion

Accuracy of sampling

Of the 39 volunteers who entered the study, adequate biopsies were obtained from 32 women during the control cycle, and from 32 women in the treatment period, providing 30 paired samples. Retrospective histological dating (determined by Dr E. Johannisson) allowed identification of 11 samples of control cycles that clearly showed early secretory patterns, the remainder being mid or late secretory. Because we obtained good indication that the activity of acid hydrolases is significantly affected during the control cycle (Fig. 3), we felt justified in further dividing the control samples into those two groups. All treated samples showed suppressed proliferative or irregular secretory aspects. During treatment, 15 women experienced normal bleeding; irregular bleeding patterns were observed in 17.

Reference constituents

For each sufficient endometrial biopsy, we measured the wet weight after careful blotting, as well as the protein content (Lowry), the DNA content (DAPI) and LDH activity in the total extract. As shown in Table 2, in the biopsies of control cycles, the content of protein (82.7 μg/mg fresh tissue) and DNA (5.0 μg/mg tissue), as well as the LDH activity (72.0 U/mg tissue) were not significantly different between early and mid–late samples. In contrast, levonorgestrel treatment caused a decrease in protein content (69.2 μg/mg tissue) and especially LDH activity (26.3 U/mg tissue) but did not affect DNA content. Taken together, these data indicate that the water, the nuclear, cytosolic (LDH) and total protein contents do not change appreciably throughout the control cycle, as already reported by Stuermer and Stein (1951) and Stein and Stuermer (1951), with the exception of the early proliferative phase. In our study, there also appears to be no compelling reason to prefer any reference constituent for the normalization of data, since none led to a significantly lower internal variation of the other parameters (see Table 2). Data on protein content after levonorgestrel treatment indicate tissue atrophy. The marked decrease of LDH after this treatment points either to the preferential atrophy of the cell cytoplasm compared to the extracellular matrix, or to a considerable reduction of the number of erythrocytes retained in the biopsies of treated women. Histological observations favour the first explanation.

Comparison of those results with the literature is instructive. The values of protein content reported here in control endometria are very close to those reported for extracts of prepubertal pig (78 $\pm$ 9.6 μg/mg wet weight; Adamski *et al.*, 1987) or ovariectomized ewe (85–93 μg/mg wet weight; Murdoch & White, 1968). They are also comparable to the content reported by Rosado *et al.* (1977), also using the Lowry assay, on homogenates of the proliferative human endometrium (103 $\pm$ 15 μg/mg wet weight), but are about two times lower than the value reported in the same study for secretory endometria (168 $\pm$ 21 μg/mg wet weight). This difference could partially be attributed to a more extensive tissue drying in the study of Rosado *et al.*, because the DNA content was also higher than in the present report (24.2 $\pm$ 2.7 μg/mg wet weight). This is, however, unlikely to be the only explanation, since the protein:DNA ratio in the mid–late secretory phase is 15.3 in this report, 24 in the study by Rosado *et al.*, and between 5.2 and 15.6 in the control mid–late secretory volunteers studied by Hagenfeldt and co-workers (1977). Here again, our ratio in mid–late secretory phase is comparable to that reported in the proliferative phase by Rosado *et al.* (1977: 14.5). The specific activity of LDH we measured in biopsies of control secretory endometria (823 U/mg protein) is about twice as high as that found in the ovariectomized ewe endometrium (Murdoch & White, 1968: 398 U/mg protein) but about fourfold lower than reported in human endometria by Hagenfeldt *et al.* (1977). We have no

Table 2. *Reference constituents in control and treated endometria. Comparisons were done by Wilcoxon's signed rank test*

		Control			Treatment	
		Early secretory (A)	Mid–late secretory (B)		Levonorgestrel (C)	Significance (B/C; p value)
protein content (µg/mg tissue)	All	80.3 ± 14.1 (11)	83.4 ± 11.3 (21)		66.4 ± 16.8 (31)	<0.01
	Pairs		82.7 ± 11.6 (18)		69.2 ± 16.7 (18)	
DNA content (µg/mg tissue)	All	5.8 ± 1.2 (10)	4.9 ± 1.2 (20)		5.5 ± 1.9 (29)	N.S.
	Pairs		5.0 ± 1.2 (17)		5.4 ± 2.1 (17)	
protein/DNA ratio (mg/mg)	All	14.1 ± 2.9 (10)	18.0 ± 5.6 (20)		13.0 ± 5.5 (30)	<0.01
	Pairs		17.5 ± 5.1 (17)		13.6 ± 6.2 (17)	
LDH activity (U/mg tissue)	All	65.0 ± 14.6 (4)	68.5 ± 15.9 (16)		26.3 ± 19.2 (13)	<0.01
	Pairs		72.0 ± 13.1 (9)		31.6 ± 21.2 (9)	
specific activity of LDH (U/mg tissue)	All	741.5 ± 145.7 (4)	800.8 ± 165.1 (16)		418.6 ± 296.4 (13)	<0.05
	Pairs		823.4 ± 165.5 (9)		493.0 ± 331.0 (9)	
specific activity of LDH (U/µg DNA)	All	12.0 ± 2.8 (4)	15.5 ± 5.0 (16)		6.4 ± 6.8 (13)	<0.05
	Pairs		17.1 ± 5.0 (9)		7.7 ± 8.3 (9)	

Table 3. *Acid hydrolase activities in control and treated endometria. Comparisons were done by Wilcoxon's rank sum and signed rank test*

		Control			Treatment	
		Early secretory (A)	Mid-late secretory (B)	Significance (A/B; p value)	Levonorgestrel (C)	Significance (B/C; p value)
acid phosphatase						
(mU/mg tissue)	All	2.9±1.2 (11)	2.0±0.7 (21)	<0.05	1.9±0.7 (31)	N.S.
	Pairs		2.1±0.7 (18)		2.1±0.8 (18)	N.S.
(mU/mg protein)	All	38.2±16.9 (11)	23.9±8.4 (21)	<0.05	30.5±13.2 (32)	N.S.
	Pairs		25.1±8.5 (18)		30.3±11.0 (18)	N.S.
(mU/µg DNA)	All	0.52±0.21 (10)	0.39±0.12 (20)	N.S.	0.37±0.14 (31)	N.S.
	Pairs		0.38±0.10 (18)		0.39±0.15 (18)	N.S.
n-acetyl-β-glucosaminidase						
(mU/mg tissue)	All	2.1±0.2 (11)	1.4±0.3 (21)	<0.001	1.4±0.6 (31)	N.S.
	Pairs		1.3±0.3 (18)		1.4±0.5 (18)	N.S.
(mU/mg protein)	All	26.8±3.3 (11)	16.5±3.6 (21)	<0.001	22.7±8.9 (32)	<0.05
	Pairs		16.3±3.1 (18)		20.8±8.2 (18)	
(mU/µg DNA)	All	0.38±0.06 (10)	0.29±0.08 (20)	<0.01	0.28±0.11 (31)	N.S.
	Pairs		0.28±0.08 (18)		0.27±0.12 (18)	
α-L-fucosidase						
(mU/mg tissue)	All	0.28±0.05 (11)	0.21±0.07 (21)	<0.01	0.17±0.08 (31)	N.S.
	Pairs		0.20±0.06 (18)		0.17±0.09 (18)	
(mU/mg protein)	All	3.5±0.9 (11)	2.6±0.9 (21)	<0.01	2.7±1.2 (32)	N.S.
	Pairs		2.5±0.8 (18)		2.6±1.4 (18)	
(mU/mg DNA)	All	50.1±9.9 (10)	44.1±17.0 (20)	N.S.	31.0±12.3 (31)	<0.05
	Pairs		43.2±16.3 (18)		30.7±14.5 (18)	
α-D-mannosidase						
(mU/mg tissue)	All	0.10±0.06 (11)	0.05±0.04 (21)	<0.05	0.03±0.03 (33)	<0.001
	Pairs		0.06±0.04 (18)		0.03±0.03 (18)	
(mU/mg protein)	All	1.3±0.7 (11)	0.7±0.4 (21)	<0.05	0.5±0.4 (33)	<0.05
	Pairs		0.7±0.5 (18)		0.5±0.5 (18)	
(mU/mg DNA)	All	16.7±9.3 (10)	10.5±6.5 (20)	N.S.	6.3±6.4 (30)	<0.05
	Pairs		10.5±6.6 (17)		5.8±6.7 (17)	

explanation for those discrepancies. The latter authors reported, as we do, that the LDH activity in human endometrium is decreased 3 months after the implantation of a progesterone-releasing device.

Content of lysosomal enzymes

The activity of the four acid hydrolases we selected is reported in Table 3. Irrespective of the origin of the sample, the activities of acid phosphatase and of N-acetyl-β-glucosaminidase were about one order of magnitude higher than those of α-L-fucosidase and of α-D-mannosidase. In the control cycle, whereas the total and the specific activity increased during the proliferative phase (Wood *et al.*, 1969; Hagenfeldt *et al.*, 1977; our own unpublished results), they decreased during the secretory phase. This is most obvious when contents are related to histological dating (see Fig. 3). There was no good correlation between enzyme contents in the control extracts and the plasma levels of 17 β-estradiol and/or progesterone at the day of biopsy. A good correlation was found between the individual specific activities of N-acetyl-β-glucosamini-dase, acid phosphatase and α-L-fucosidase, both in control and treated samples (Fig. 4). This is compatible with the occurrence of an homogeneous population of lysosomes in the whole endometrium, irrespective of the cell type, and may indicate that the three lysosomal enzymes show a coordinate response to changes in steroid hormones. The content of N-acetyl-β-hexosaminidase was increased after levonorgestrel treatment.

Although all authors use slightly different assay conditions, we felt it would be useful to compare our results with those reported elsewhere for human tissue (Table 4) or for endometrium from animals (Table 5). Our results on the specific activity of lysosomal enzymes are in excellent agreement with those obtained by Van Hoof (1972) in human liver biopsy, under identical assay conditions, as well as those reported for acid phosphatase (paranitrophenyl-phosphatase) by Hagenfeldt *et al.* (1977). They are, however, two- to fourfold lower than those calculated from the data reported by Wood *et al.* (1969), for paranitrophenyl-phosphatase. We do not understand why the specific activities calculated from the data reported by Rosado *et al.* (1977) translate into 200-fold lower values. There are major differences in the specific activity of acid hydrolases between species and, within species, they vary considerably in activity, N-acetyl-β-glucosaminidase being one of the most active. Finally, the same hormone can elicit opposite effects on different acid hydrolases in the ovariectomized rabbit, indicating that the various lysosomal enzymes do not necessarily respond unanimously.

Secretion of lysosomal enzymes in vitro

To obtain direct evidence of secretion of lysosomal enzymes, we developed an interface culture system of endometrial explants. Our system reasonably mimicks the polarized in-situ orientation: the rapidly re-epithelialized surface

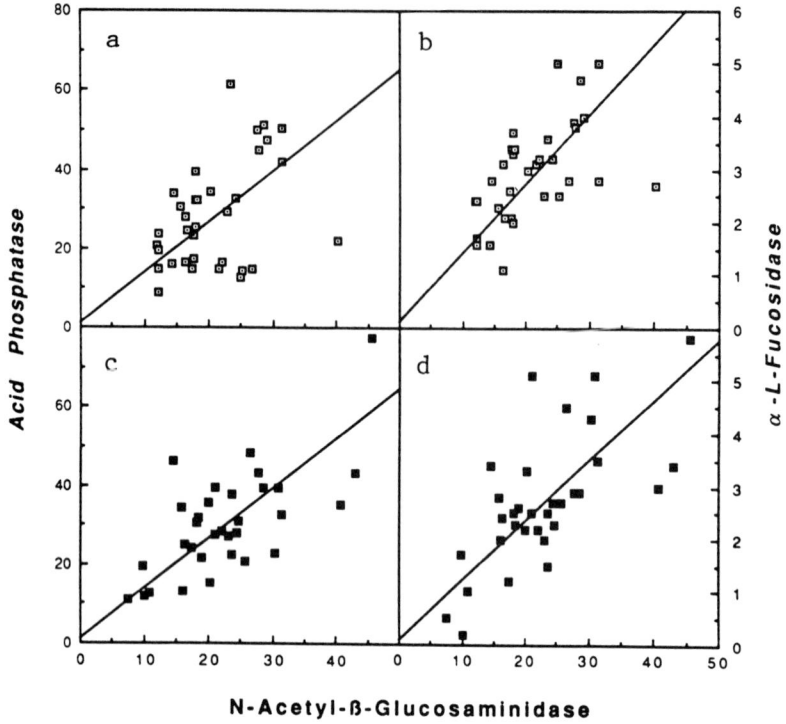

Fig. 4 Correlations between enzyme activities in endometrial extracts. The specific activity (mU/mg protein) of N-acetyl-β-glucosaminidase is compared to that of either acid phosphatase or α-L-fucosidase for each of the control (open symbols) and treated endometrial extracts (closed symbols). a: r = 0.86; b: r = 0.93; c: r = 0.92; d: r = 0.92; p < 0.001 for a–d.

faces a gas phase (20% O_2, 5% CO_2) similar to the partial tissue pressure expected for the endometrial lumen, and solutes can be exchanged through the base of the explants on the filter with a well-defined medium, also equilibrated with 20% O_2 and 5% CO_2. As shown in Fig. 5, the histological appearance showed excellent preservation up to several days.

The daily release of lysosomal enzymes and of LDH was calculated as the activity recovered in the conditioned medium collected after 24 hours from duplicate wells with explants, minus the activity in the medium of wells without explants. The fractional release index was estimated by dividing the ratio of activity released over the weight of fixed explants, by the ratio of activity over the wet weight in the fresh biopsies. The unity would indicate that the cumulative release is equal to the total activity initially placed in culture. A

Table 4. Specific activity[a] of lysosomal enzymes in humans

Enzyme	Enzyme Commission classification	Endometrium				Liver[b]
		Proliferation	Early secretory	Late secretory	3-month progestogen	
acid phosphatase	(3.1.3.2)	58.3*	71.5*; 38.2	100*; 23.0†; 23.9	27.0†; 30.5	25.2
α-D-mannosidase	(3.2.1.24)	—	1.3	0.7	0.5	0.6
N-acetyl-β-D-glucosaminidase	(3.2.1.30)	—	26.8	16.5	22.7	17.4
β-D-glucuronidase	(3.2.1.31)	6.7*	9.6*	7.3*; 0.3†	0.25†	1.8
α-L-fucosidase	(3.2.1.51)	—	3.5	2.6	2.7	1.1
cathepsin D	(3.4.23.5)	14.4*	26.0*	19.4*	—	31.2

Notes:
[a] = Expressed as mU/mg protein of the tissue extract.
[b] = Derived from Van Hoof (1972) on the basis of 220 mg protein/g wet liver.
* = Derived from Wood et al., (1969) on the basis of 80 mg protein/g wet endometrium.
† = Derived from Hagenfeldt et al., (1977).

Table 5. Specific activity[a] of lysosomal enzymes in various animals

Enzyme	Enzyme Commission classification	Pig[b] (prepubertal)	Rabbit[c] (ovariectomized)	Cow[d] (control)	Ewe[e] (ovariectomized)
acid phosphatase	(3.1.3.2)	11.0	34.6 (E↓, P↓)	7.2–11.6	1.6
acid ribonuclease	(3.1.4.22)	230.0	—	—	—
arylsulphatase	(3.1.6.1)	18.9	20.0 (E↓, P↓)	—	—
α-D-glucosidase	(3.2.1.20)	1.4	—	—	—
β-D-glucosidase	(3.2.1.21)	1.3	—	—	—
β-D-galactosidase	(3.2.1.23)	9.6	15.4 (E↓, P↑)	—	—
β-N-acetyl-D-glucosaminidase	(3.2.1.30)	195.0	76.9 (E↓, P↓)	4.0	—
β-D-glucuronidase	(3.2.1.31)	0.9	6.2 (E↓, P↓)	1.3	—
α-L-fucosidase	(3.2.1.51)	—	5.4 (E↓, P↑)	—	—
cathepsin D	(3.4.23.5)	9.1	—	1.8	—

Notes:
[a] = mU/mg protein of the tissue extract, reported as such or derived from the protein content.
Variations in the recovery of the extract and the assay conditions have been neglected.
[b] = From Adamski et al., (1987); a few values are from Sierralta et al., (1978) and Sierralta & Szendro (1983).
[c] = From Rahi & Srivastava (1983); arrows indicate increase (↑) or decrease (↓) upon estrogen (E) or progesterone (P) treatment.
[d] = From figures of Linford & Iosson (1975).
[e] = From Murdoch & White (1968).

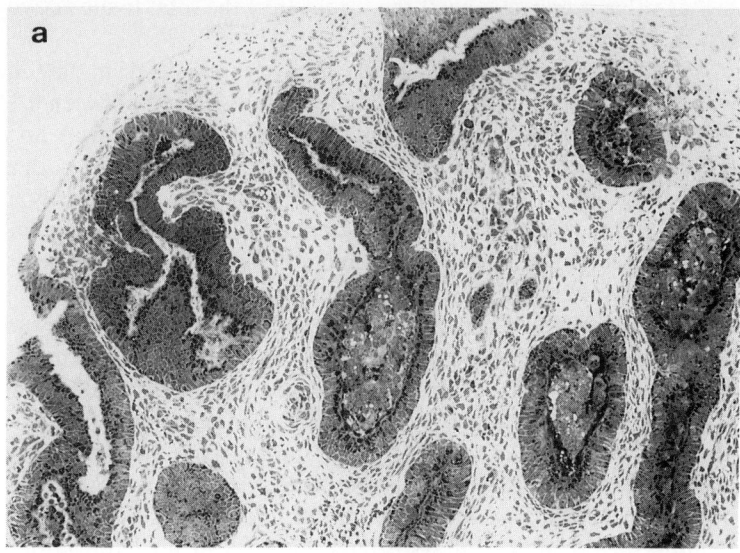

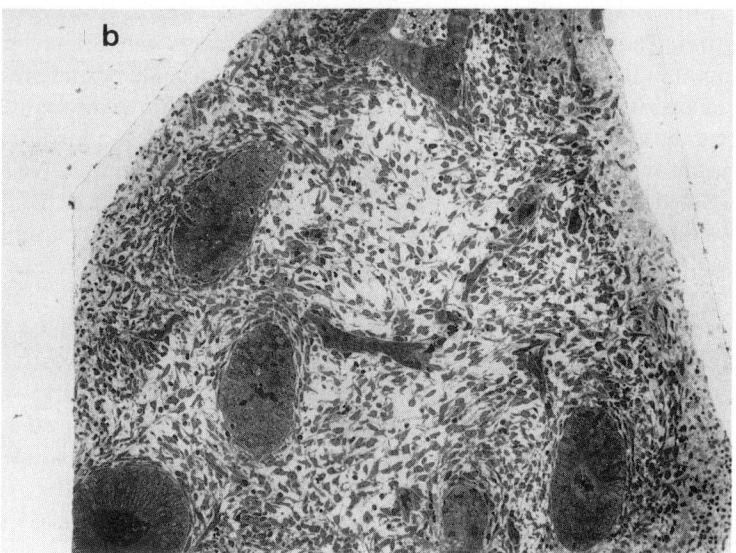

Fig. 5 Histology of interface organ cultures from a control (a) and a treated endometrium (b) after 30 hours of culture. In control explants, note the secretory differentiation of the prominent glands. There is no detectable tissue necrosis in the whole explant. After treatment, the glands are small and lack obvious secretory transformation. Semithin plastic sections, stained with toluidine-blue and PAS, × 110.

higher value is conceivable if the turnover of the total tissue activity requires less than 1 day.

As shown in Fig. 6, the mean fractional release of LDH in the control cycles was about 0.2 and that of lysosomal enzymes ranged between 0.15 and 0.5. With the possible exception of acid phosphatase, there was no detectable difference between early and mid–late secretory samples. At both phases, the fractional release of N-acetyl-β-hexosaminidase was significantly higher than that of LDH. After levonorgestrel treatment, the mean fractional release of LDH, N-acetyl-β-hexosaminidase and α-L-fucosidase were all increased, so as to sometimes exceed the unity, and that of hexosaminidase was again significantly higher than that of LDH. Interestingly, in a few preliminary experiments, the addition of 10 mmol/l mannose-6-phosphate to selectively block recapture of lysosomal enzymes by living cells, did not appreciably affect LDH release, but the fractional release of hexosaminidase was increased about 1.6-fold. Taken together, these data provide strong evidence that N-acetyl-β-hexosaminidase is actively secreted by endometrial explants.

We believe that the fractional release index is probably the best way of quantitating secretion of lysosomal enzymes in absolute terms, and that comparison with the fractional release index of LDH is the only way of distinguishing active secretion from release by dead cells. However, we are well aware that this index is open to biases and leaves some uncertainties. The amount of acid hydrolases released in the medium could be underestimated by adsorption to the tissue, recapture (as documented for hexosaminidase by the mannose-6-phosphate experiment) or inactivation in the medium (only for hexosaminidase and acid phosphatase). Secondly, the cumulative release was related to the weight of fixed tissue, because of the technical difficulty of weighing the tiny fresh explants. We do not know to what extent the weight of endometrium is affected by glutaraldehyde fixation, but this uncertainty does not invalidate the comparison of acid hydrolases and LDH. Future experiments should include the assay of DNA in explant extracts. Thirdly, we feel that the high release of LDH, especially after levonorgestrel, does not match the excellent tissue preservation demonstrated by optical and electron microscopy, and might partially reflect hemolysis. However, we were unable to replace LDH by another cytosolic enzyme which is absent from erythrocytes, such as phosphoglucomutase, because the latter enzyme was quickly inactivated upon incubation in the culture medium at 37°C.

In at least three animal species, progesterone (and to a lower extent progesterone combined with estrogen) strongly stimulated the release of acid hydrolases into the uterine lumen (Hansen *et al.*, 1985). Interestingly, large variations among the enzymes were reported: acid phosphatase, N-acetyl-β-glucosaminidase and β-glucosidase showed a 900-fold, 300-fold and 10-fold increase respectively. Animal endometrial explants were also shown to synthesize and secrete N-acetyl-β-glucosaminidase. The hydrolase released could not be distinguished from the two authentic lysosomal isoenzymes

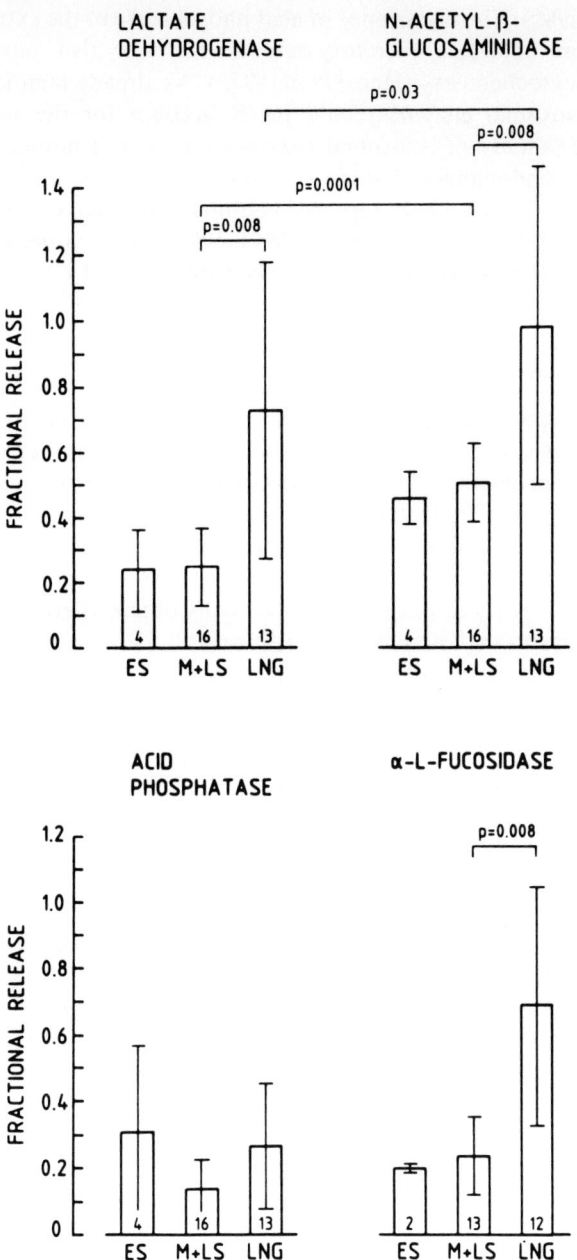

Fig. 6 Fractional release of LDH and acid hydrolases by organ cultures from control early secretory (ES), control mid–late secretory (M + LS) and levonorgestrel-treated endometria (LNG). Statistical comparison was done by the Wilcoxon signed rank test.

(Hansen *et al.*, 1985). The occurrence of acid phosphatase in the extracellular space of human mid–late secretory endometria was also reported by ultrastructural cytochemistry (Henzl *et al.*, 1972). As already mentioned, the secretion of lysosomal enzymes could partly account for the substantial increase of free activity of lysosomal enzymes reported in homogenates of secretory human endometria (Rosado *et al.*, 1977). The preferential secretion of hexosaminidase has also been reported in human fibroblasts (Halley *et al.*, 1978), and upon the induction of phagocytosis in human macrophages (Imort *et al.*, 1983). In the latter case, secretion reached 70% of total activity within a few hours.

Conclusions and perspectives

Our results provide some arguments both in favour of and against the involvement of lysosomal enzymes in endometrial bleeding, but certainly they do not solve the problem at this stage. In favour of the lysosomal concept, there is a high content of hydrolytic (lysosomal) enzymes both in secretory and levonorgestrel-treated endometria. We also obtained good evidence that at least one lysosomal enzyme (hexosaminidase) is actively secreted and that secretion is enhanced by levonorgestrel. We finally obtained evidence for the persistence of lysosomal activity towards neutral pH for another (a-L-fucosidase). Against the lysosomal concept, the content of lysosomal enzymes was significantly decreased from the early to mid–late secretory control cycle, and unaffected (acid phosphatase and a-L-fucosidase), decreased (a-D-mannosidase) or increased (hexosaminidase) upon treatment with levonorgestrel. Furthermore, there was no significant difference in the content of enzymes between normal and abnormal bleeders after levonorgestrel treatment.

We should, thus, pay more attention to the non-lysosomal enzymes and address the following questions.

1. Are endometrial hydrolytic enzymes all of lysosomal origin? This could be tested by selective inhibition (Vaes & Jacques, 1965; Garcia-Bunuel & Brandes, 1966), activation (Vaes & Jacques, 1965), or inactivation (Beaufay & de Duve, 1954). Isoenzymes could be resolved by chromatofocusing (Munakata *et al.*, 1986) or immunoprecipitation (Hansen *et al.*, 1985). We could improve subcellular fractionation by placing emphasis on optimal initial latency (e.g. by controlling shearing forces: Adamsky *et al.*, 1987). Finally, lysosomal enzymes can now be demonstrated by light and ultrastructural immunocytochemistry on fixed sections and several antibodies are already available.

2. Are all hydrolytic enzymes equally secreted? Can secretion be quantified? Is it regulated by hormones? These questions could be addressed in the organ culture system, with the improvements indicated under 'Results and discussion'. This culture system allows close control of the hormonal environment in the medium.

3. Do secreted enzymes act upon the extracellular matrix at neutral pH? The hydrolytic activity of conditioned media from organ cultures could be assessed on radiolabelled artificial matrices (Peeters-Joris *et al.*, 1981) or, perhaps more relevant, on endometrial explants which have been metabolically labelled and heat inactivated (see below).

4. What is the turnover of the endometrial extracellular matrix? The organ culture system may also be ideal to address this essential question. Primary experiments performed in our laboratory show that endometrial explants efficiently and linearly incorporate radiolabelled precursors over more than 24 hours, with negligible incorporation in heat-inactivated samples. The system is now amenable to the analysis of the chemistry and the distribution of labelled species, to kinetic pulse chase and steady-state analysis, and to the study of hormonal effects.

Acknowledgements

This work was supported by grants from the WHO Special Programme of Research and Research Training in Human Reproduction (project No. 85904), and partly by the Belgian State – Prime Minister's Office – Science Policy Programming (concerted actions, Grant 82/87-39, a framework of interuniversity attraction poles, Grant 7). P.J. Courtoy is Research Associate at the Belgian Fonds National de la Recherche Scientifique.

The dedicated technical help of Michèle Leruth-Deridder, Nicole Delflasse, Francesca N'Kuli-Pyrrhou and Lieve Verbist, and the typing assistance of Michèle Geist are gratefully acknowledged.

References

Adamski, J., Sierralta, W.D. & Jungblut, P.W. (1987). Harvesting and separation of two populations of lysosomes from porcine endometrium. *European Journal of Cell Biology*, **45**:238–245.

Baron, R., Neff, L., Brown, W., Courtoy, P.J., Louvard, D. & Farquhar, M.G. (1988). Polarized secretion of lysosomal enzymes: co-distribution of cation-independent mannose-6-phosphate receptors and lysosomal enzymes along the osteoclast exocytic pathway. *Journal of Cell Biology*, **106**:1863–1872.

Beaufay, H. & de Duve, C. (1954). Le système hexose-phosphatasique. IV. Spécificité de la glucose-6-phosphatase. *Bulletin de la Société de Chimie Biologique*, **26**:1525–1537.

Bergmeyer, H.V. & Bernt, E. (1974). Lactate dehydrogenase. (In) *Methods of Enzymatic Analysis*, Vol. 2 (Bergmeyer, H.V., ed.), p.574. New York, Academic Press.

Berthois, Y., Katzenellenbogen, J.A. & Katzenellenbogen, B.S. (1986). Phenol red in tissue culture media is a weak estrogen: implications concerning the study of estrogen-responsive cells in culture. *Proceedings of the National Academy of Sciences USA*, **83**:2496–2500.

Cohn, Z.A. & Hirsch, J.G. (1960). The influence of phagocytosis on the intracellular distribution of granule-associated components of polymorphonuclear leucocytes. *Journal of Experimental Medicine*, 112:1015–1022.

de Duve, C. (1963). General properties of lysosomes: the lysosome concept. (In) *Ciba Foundation Symposium on Lysosomes* (De Reuck, A.V.S. & Cameron, M.P., eds.), pp.1–31. London, Churchill.

de Duve, C., Wattiaux, R. & Wibo, M. (1962). Effect of fat-soluble compounds on lysosomes *in vitro. Biochemical Pharmacology*, 9:97–116.

Eeckhout, Y. (1990). Tissue breakdown. (In) *Contraception and Mechanisms of Endometrial Bleeding* (d'Arcangues, C., Fraser, I.S., Newton, J.R. & Odlind, V., eds.), pp.431–438. Cambridge, England, Cambridge University Press.

Elder, M.G., Patel, L. & White, J.O. (1990). Effects of contraceptive progestogens on prostaglandins. (In) *Contraception and Mechanisms of Endometrial Bleeding* (d'Arcangues, C., Fraser, I.S., Newton, J.R. & Odlind, V., eds.), pp.279–286. Cambridge, England, Cambridge University Press.

Fell, H.B. & Dingle, J.T. (1963). Studies on the mode of action of excess of vitamin A. 6. Lysosomal protease and the degradation of cartilage matrix. *Biochemical Journal*, 87:403–408.

Garcia-Bunuel, R. & Brandes, D. (1966). Lysosomal enzymes in human endometrium. A histochemical study of acid phosphatase, nonspecific esterase, and E-600 resistant esterase. *American Journal of Obstetrics and Gynecology*, 94:1045–1055.

Hagenfeldt, K., Landgren, B.M., Edstrom, K. & Johannisson, E. (1977). Biochemical and morphological changes in the human endometrium induced by the Progestasert device. *Contraception*, 16:183–197.

Halley, D.J.J., De Wit-Verbeek, H.A., Reuser, A.J.J. & Galjaard, H. (1978). The distribution of hydrolytic enzyme activities in human fibroblast cultures and their intercellular transfer. *Biochemical and Biophysical Research Communications*, 82:1176–1182.

Ham, R.G. (1963). An improved nutrient solution for diploid Chinese hamster and human cell lines. *Experimental Cell Research*, 29:515–526.

Hansen, P.J., Bazer, F.W. & Roberts, R.M. (1985). Appearance of β-hexosaminidase and other lysosomal-like enzymes in the uterine lumen of gilts, ewes and mares in response to progesterone and estrogens. *Journal of Reproduction and Fertility*, 73:411–424.

Henzl, M.R., Smith, R.E., Boost, G. & Tyler, E.T. (1972). Lysosomal concept of menstrual bleeding in humans. *Journal of Clinical Endocrinology and Metabolism*, 34:860–875.

Hickman, S. & Neufeld, E.F. (1972). A hypothesis for I-cell disease: defective hydrolases that do not enter lysosomes. *Biochemical and Biophysical Research Communications*, 49:992–999.

Hourihan, H.M., Sheppard, B.L. & Brosens, I.A. (1990). Endometrial hemostasis. (In) *Contraception and Mechanisms of Endometrial Bleeding* (d'Arcangues, C., Fraser, I.S., Newton, J.R. & Odlind, V., eds.), pp.95–114. Cambridge, England, Cambridge University Press.

Imort, M., Zuehlsdorf, M., Feige, U., Hasilik, A. & Von Figura, K. (1983). Biosynthesis and transport of lysosomal enzymes in human monocytes and macrophages. Effects of ammonium chloride, zymosan and tunicamycin. *Biochemical Journal*, 214:671–678.

Johannisson, E., Landgren, B.-M., Rohr, H.P. & Diczfalusy, E. (1987). Endometrial morphology and peripheral hormone levels in women with regular menstrual cycles. *Fertility and Sterility*, **48**:401–408.

Kapuscinski, J. & Skoczylas, B. (1977). Simple and rapid fluorimetric method for DNA microassay. *Analytical Biochemistry*, **83**:252–257.

Linford, E. & Iosson, J.M. (1975). A quantitative study of some lysosomal enzymes in the bovine endometrium during early pregnancy. *Journal of Reproduction and Fertility*, **44**:249–260.

Lowry, O.H., Rosebrough, N.J., Farr, A.L. & Randall, R.J. (1951). Protein measurement with the Folin phenol reagent. *Journal of Biological Chemistry*, **193**:265–275.

Markee, J.E. (1948). Morphological basis for menstrual bleeding: relation of regression to initiation of bleeding. *Bulletin of the New York Academy of Medicine*, **24**:253–268.

Munakata, H., Isemura, M. & Yosizawa, Z. (1986). Hormonal effects on the activities of glycosidases in the endometrium of rabbit uterus. *Biochemical Medicine and Metabolic Biology*, **35**:179–183.

Murdoch, R.N. & White, I.G. (1968). The effect of oestradiol and progesterone on the activity of enzymes in the endometrium and caruncles of the ovariectomized ewe. *Journal of Endocrinology*, **42**:187–192.

Peeters-Joris, C., Emonds-Alt, X. & Vaes, G. (1981). A direct simultaneous plate assay of proteoglycan and collagen degradation by cells in culture and its application to synovial cells. *Biochemical Journal*, **196**:95–104.

Rahi, H. & Srivastava, P.N. (1983). Hormonal regulation of lysosomal hydrolases in the reproductive tract of the rabbits. *Journal of Reproduction and Fertility*, **67**:447–455.

Rosado, A., Mercado, E., Gallegos, A.J., De Los Angeles-Wens, M. & Aznar, R. (1977). Subcellular distribution of lysosomal enzymes in the human endometrium. I. Normal menstrual cycle. *Contraception*, **16**:287–298.

Sierralta, W.D. & Szendro, P.I. (1983). Characterization of microsomal subfractions from porcine endometrium cells. *Hoppe-Seyler's Zeitschrift für Physiologische Chemie*, **364**:1329–1335.

Sierralta, W., Truitt, A.J. & Jungblut, P.W. (1978). Studies on the involvement of lysosomes in estrogen action. I. Isolation and enzymatic properties of pig endometrial lysosomes. *Hoppe-Seyler's Zeitschrift für Physiologische Chemie*, **359**:517–528.

Solursh, M., Fisher, M., Meier, S. & Singley, C.T. (1979). The role of extracellular matrix in the formation of the sclerotome. *Journal of Embryology and Experimental Morphology*, **54**:75–98.

Stein, R.J. & Stuermer, V.M. (1951). Cytodynamic properties of the human endometrium. III. Variations in the nucleo-protein content of the endometrium during the menstrual cycle. *American Journal of Obstetrics and Gynecology*, **61**:414–417.

Stuermer, V.M. & Stein, R.J. (1951). Cytodynamic properties of the human endometrium. IV. Water content of human endometrium during the various phases of the menstrual cycle. *American Journal of Obstetrics and Gynecology*, **61**:668–669.

Vaes, A. (1968). On the mechanisms of bone resorption. The action of parathyroid hormone on the excretion and synthesis of lysosomal enzymes and on the extracellular release of acid by bone cells. *Journal of Cell Biology*, **36**:676–697.

Vaes, G. & Jacques, P. (1965). Studies on bone enzymes. The assay of acid hydrolases and other enzymes in bone tissue. *Biochemical Journal*, **97**:380–388.

Van Hoof, F. (1972). Les mucopolysaccharidoses en tant que thesaurismoses lysosomiales. Thèse d'agrégation de l'enseignement supérieur (Vander, Louvain), pp.285.

Von Figura, K. & Hasilik, A. (1986). Lysosomal enzymes and their receptors. *Annual Review of Biochemistry*, **55**:167–193.

Wattiaux, R. & Wattiaux-Deconinck, S. (1981). Effect of a transitory ischaemia on the structure-linked latency of rat liver acid phosphatase and beta-galactosidase. *Biochemical Journal*, **196**:861–866.

White, J.O., Croxtall, J.D. & Elder, M.G. (1990). Effects of contraceptive progestogens on endometrial proteins. (In) *Contraception and Mechanisms of Endometrial Bleeding* (d'Arcangues, C., Fraser, I.S., Newton, J.R. & Odlind, V., eds.), pp.233–239. Cambridge, England, Cambridge University Press.

Wilson, E.W. (1980). Lysosome function in normal endometrium and endometrium exposed to contraceptive steroids. (In) *Endometrial Bleeding and Steroidal Contraception* (Diczfalusy, E., Fraser, I.S. & Webb, F.T.G., eds.), pp.201–221. Bath, England, Pitman Press.

Wood, J.C., Williams, E.A., Barley, V.L. & Cowdell, R.H. (1969). The activity of hydrolytic enzymes in the human endometrium during the menstrual cycle. *Journal of Obstetrics and Gynaecology of the British Commonwealth*, **76**:724–728.

Discussion

Wilson. Several points: did you try to distinguish between free and membrane-bound enzyme in your homogenates of fresh tissue, because there are several authors who have described differences in the free and membrane-bound content throughout the cycle? Secondly, can you give us some idea why you did not do more histochemical studies. You clearly had the tissue available; it was good quality tissue, and it seems to me that any study on lysosomes needs the complementary information that histochemistry gives to biochemical studies. My last point is about Dr K. Hagenfeld and co-workers who looked at lysosomal as well as other enzymes in Progestasert IUD users over quite a long period of time (Hagenfeldt *et al.*, 1977), and the Mexican group (Mercado *et al.*, 1977) who also looked at endometrial biopsies from Progestasert IUD users. These did distinguish between free and bound fractions and showed, at least for acid phosphatase, that there was a major shift between the bound and free fractions in the late part of the cycle in progesterone-releasing IUD users.

Cornillie. First of all, the activities measured here are total activities measured in homogenate. We did not feel it appropriate to look at free or latent activity and Dr Courtoy will discuss this in a moment. We embarked on studies of this hypothesis with limited time available, and agreed to study biochemical aspects as a priority. However, I would fully agree that further work requires histochemical staining techniques, at light and electron-microscopic level.

Courtoy. It is very difficult to determine whether change in the ratio of free activity is reflecting something that occurred *in vivo* or is an *in vitro* artefact. Actually, it is generally agreed that changes of latency are an all-or-none phenomenon. In other words, lysosomes are tight or they are fully permeable. What struck me when I read in detail the paper of Henzl and co-workers (1972) was the change in appearance of the lysosomes in human endometrium in the proliferative and early secretory versus late secretory phases. They report a considerable increase in the number of large, autophagic structures. A possible explanation for the increase of the free activity reported by Rosado and co-workers in Mexico (Mercado *et al.*, 1977) is that the small, dense bodies are more resistant to the shearing forces of homogenization, whereas large autophagic structures are much more vulnerable. So this may not reflect a release of lysosomal enzymes in the living cells *in situ*, but is a reflection of laboratory artefact, which tells us something about the difference in size and shape of the structure but does not allow us to conclude on a release of lysosomal enzymes into the cytosol. In Namur, Wattiaux and co-workers (Wattiaux & Wattiaux-Deconinck, 1981) did a study in the rat where they ligated one liver lobe for 1 hour or 2 hours, then released the ligation and measured the free enzyme activities immediately after release and after reperfusion. With reperfusion, they observed first an increase in free activity and then a progressive recovery over 1 hour. It is difficult to envisage that during 1 hour the lysosomes can recapture selectively the lysosomal enzymes of the cytosol. So they concluded that there was a change, perhaps a swelling of the lysosomes, which caused an artificial increase of the free activity due to vulnerability to homogenization. For all of these reasons, we decided not to perform studies of latency.

Naftolin. Our primary interest is to look at steroid effects on cells. I am concerned about the interpretation of this work, mostly because such a generalized process has to be carefully scrutinized statistically. I have no evidence that there is a normal distribution of the effects that you have shown us, and I am not sure that that is a statistically significant difference. I would ask you to do non-parametric statistics and find out whether that is truly a statistically significant effect. Once you have done that, then you still have to deal with the general issue of interpretation, and the only way you can do this is to study the time-course of development of these lysosomal changes.

Cornillie. Statistics were acutally done with non-parametric tests. We agree that our results now require a more detailed study of the time-course of lysosomal changes and we also plan to do longer incubations with steroids in the organ cultures.

Smith. The hypothesis that we are trying to grapple with is that the initiation of bleeding from the endometrium follows some event, probably an increase of some agent; now your data suggesting that there is a decline of these enzymes is inconsistent with the view that they are the initiators of the onset of menstrual bleeding. Whether they respond to subsequent ischemia is a separate question. The second hypothesis, as I understand it, is that lysosomal enzyme release is associated with increase in cell death. Yet your data show not only that there is greatest release in activity in the early secretory phase of the cycle when the endometrium could not be healthier, but furthermore that you are getting release of these lysosomes in explants which you have yourself said are very healthy looking. Your findings are inconsistent with a role for lysosomes, at least in the initiation of menstrual bleeding.

Cornillie. Our study was not designed to study carefully the late secretory phase of the normal cycle and we have not yet analyzed menstrual bleeding data in the progestogen-treated women. Therefore we cannot say much about the initiation of bleeding. These cultures were short-term cultures, and we did not prolong them because we wanted to know what was happening at the time the tissue was taken. We do not fully understand the significance of the increased release of lactate dehydrogenase (LDH) into the cultures. This suggests that there was quite a lot of membrane damage to many cells without this being obvious on histology. I think there is indeed some early necrosis in the levonorgestrel-treated explants, and this is reflected by the high, up to 80% in some cases, release of LDH into cultures.

Elder. You have made suggestions on what is going on in cultures from the early secretory phase of the cycle compared with other times. Am I right in thinking you had only four samples? Do you really think you can draw valid conclusions from that small number?

Cornillie. I agree with your comment in general; however, I think that early secretory measurements can be regarded as good preliminary information.

Casey. You showed us some excellent micrographs of the endometrium in organotypic cultures, one from a normal secretory endometrium and one after treatment with progestogen. My interpretation, looking at those two briefly, was that there was a great proliferation of the glandular tissue at the edges of the explants after treatment with the progestogen. I would ask you if that is a correct interpretation, and if so, do you interpret it as being withdrawal, or recovery from the progestogen in the culture dish, and could that contribute to the findings that you have seen with the lysosomal enzymes?

Cornillie. I do not believe there was is a major difference between glandular proliferation at the edges of explants after progestogen exposure compared to controls.

King. I have conceptual problems with the whole system and with the interpretation of the data, but let me just mention two points that I think are important. We know from the literature that the time-course of effect of levonorgestrel on the induction of enzymes is much longer than the ones you have been assaying. Maximum induction occurs by between days 4 and 6 and, on a per cell basis, the activities of those enzymes then decrease. So taking the samples at the times you are doing so, I think you may be missing the major effects. The second point I would make is that when you take pieces of endometrium, then approximately half of the protein in that piece of tissue is extracellular, and again, there are many publications in the literature saying that if you assay by anything except activity per DNA, you can get erroneous results. There are at least six publications indicating that you can induce certain enzymes in endometrium with progestogens if you measure on a per cell basis. But if you measure it on a per protein basis, you will not see any effects.

Odlind. You explained at the onset of your talk that you aimed to take all the control samples on day 24; however, not all patients were sampled on that day. Is that not creating an artefact?

Cornillie. We tried to schedule all biopsies at the end of the cycle, around day 24 of the cycle, but we were not able to measure luteinizing hormone (LH) peaks. Some of the patients ovulated unexpectedly early or late. However, retrospective dating was accurate according to endocrine data and dating of biopsies. I would like to come back to the technique of organ culture of endometrium, in which very small pieces of endometrium are cultured without any blood flow at all. If these cultures are kept for several days in the absence of progesterone, they develop cellular features resembling the premenstrual changes seen *in vivo*. These cultures are done with 5% serum which is deprived or nearly deprived of steroids. To me this suggests that there is something programmed in endometrial cells. We have observed that endometrial epithelial cells from the proliferative phase put in culture without any progesterone can turn into secretory endometrial cells.

Smith. One takes your point about the preprogramming of the cells *in vitro*, which is of course a reflection of the tissue *in vivo*, but surely it is wrong to remove completely the influence of steroids when we have spent our time discussing the ability of progesterone withdrawal in estrogen-primed endometrium and the predictability of that in terms of inducing menstruation. Yet there may be some preprogramming of the cells. Could I ask you, what features of secretory change are you talking about in your cell system? How would you characterize the secretory change in this endometrium and are these the glands or the stroma, or both?

Cornillie. The changes include basal vacuolation and the accumulation and secretion of glycogen *in vitro*. The human endometrial stroma is a unique stroma because you cannot normally get decidualization just by a mechanical stimulus, although there is some evidence that it may be possible. But in rodents, as shown by Finn (1986), you need mechanical or oil-drop stimulation or the presence of a blastocyst contacting the uterine lining epithelium to get decidual reaction. Predecidual reaction occurs even in non-fertile cycles in women. This seems to be an end-point of differentiation. If there is no implantation, this tissue will die and will be shed and this would fit with the hypothesis which you presented that menstruation results from implantation failure.

References

Finn, C.A. (1986). Implantation, menstruation and inflammation. *Biological Reviews*, Cambridge Philosophical Society, 61:313–328.

Hagenfeldt, K., Landgren, B.M., Edstrom, K. & Johannisson, E. (1977). Biochemical and morphological changes in the human endometrium induced by the Progestasert device. *Contraception*, 16:183–197.

Henzl, M.R., Smith, R.E., Boost, G. & Tyler, E.T. (1972). Lysosomal concept of menstrual bleeding in humans. *Journal of Clinical Endocrinology and Metabolism*, 24:860–875.

Mercado, E., Aznar, R., Gallegos, A.J., Dominguez, R. & Rosada, A. (1977). Subcellular distribution of lysosomal enzymes in the human endometrium. II. Effect of the inert, and copper and progesterone-releasing T intrauterine devices. *Contraception*, 16:299–312.

Wattiaux, R. & Wattiaux-Deconinck, S. (1981). Effect of a transitory ischaemia on the structure-linked latency of rat liver acid phosphatase and beta-galactosidase. *Biochemical Journal*, 196:861–866.

Oxygen radicals, bleeding and tissue injury

CATHERINE RICE-EVANS AND BRIAN COOKE

Department of Biochemistry and Chemistry, Royal Free Hospital School of Medicine, London, UK.

Abstract

It is currently considered that menstruation arises from the induction of local tissue ischemia by a prolonged vasoconstriction of the end arterioles of the spiral arteries, possibly induced by specific prostaglandins secreted during the second half of the ovarian cycle. Increased production of oxygen-derived free radicals post-ischemia results from increased leukocyte infiltration, abnormal arachidonic acid metabolism and disrupted mitochondrial function. In addition, release of hydrolytic and oxidative enzymes, as well as iron decompartmentalization from hemoglobin, may initiate a sequence of events culminating in the onset of endometrial bleeding.

Introduction

Free radicals are essential for many normal biological processes: they are intermediates in enzyme-catalyzed reactions, they are involved in the eicosanoid pathways in the synthesis of prostaglandins and leukotrienes, and they are an essential intermediary in the response of tissues to invading micro-organisms. However, free radicals can be highly destructive if not tightly controlled.

It is not yet clear whether free radical reactions are a cause of tissue damage or an accompaniment to or a consequence of such injury. Nevertheless, it is clear that diseased or damaged tissues undergo radical reactions more readily than normal tissues, thus exacerbating the primary injury.

Oxygen-derived free radicals have been implicated as a general mechanism of cellular and tissue injury in oxygen toxicity, post-ischemic reperfusion damage, inflammatory disorders and many other pathological states (Slater, 1984). This is a consequence of the fact that one of the major intermediaries in damaging radical reactions is oxygen. Oxygen is toxic not because of its own reactivity, which is rather feeble, but because it has the capacity to undergo a series of one-electron reductions producing a variety of potentially damaging intermediates, such as superoxide radical, $O_2\cdot^-$, hydroperoxy radical, $HO_2\cdot$, or the peroxide anion of hydrogen peroxide. These species may be directly damaging or may interact under some conditions to form the highly reactive cytotoxic species, the hydroxyl radical, $\cdot OH$, which can attack almost every molecule in living cells – DNA, lipids, proteins, carbohydrates.

In this chapter, a description will be given of how free radicals damage cells, how the consequences of such damage amplify cellular injury and have further

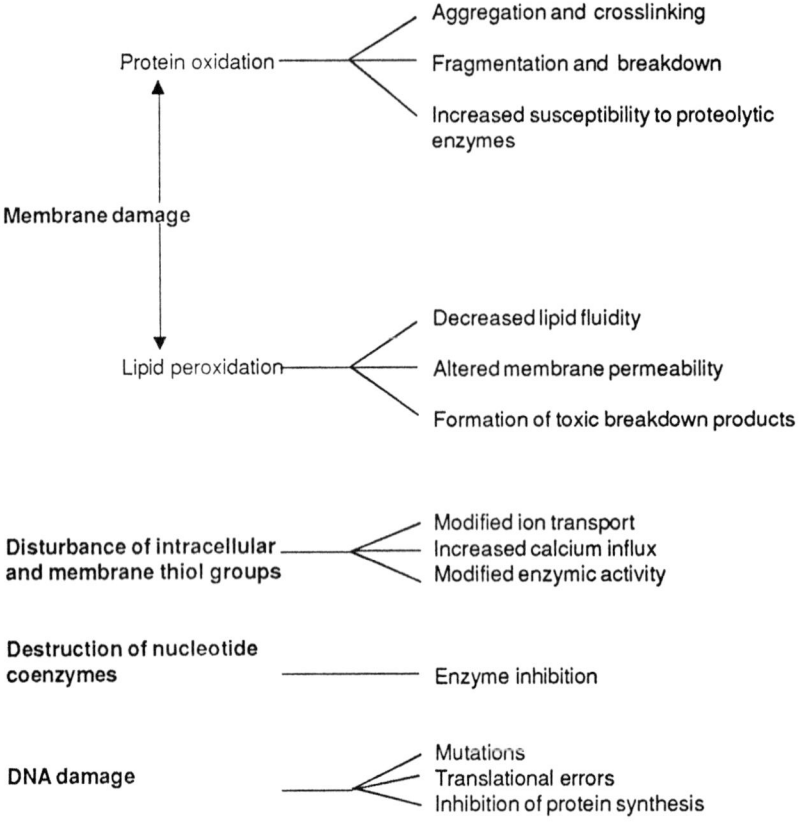

Fig. 1 How do free radicals damage cells?

deleterious effects on cellular function; how free radicals can arise in tissues, cells and membranes; and the potential roles of oxygen radicals and hemoglobin in tissue breakdown in endometrial bleeding.

Mechanisms of cellular and tissue damage mediated by oxygen-derived free radicals

The different cellular targets that are susceptible to free radical attack and the possible consequences are shown in Fig. 1.

Peroxidative damage to lipids and its consequences

One mechanism whereby the generation of free radicals within biological tissues may result in damage is due to the ability of certain species to peroxidize the polyunsaturated fatty acids of the membrane lipids. This may occur either enzymically, utilizing such substrates as arachidonic acid released from

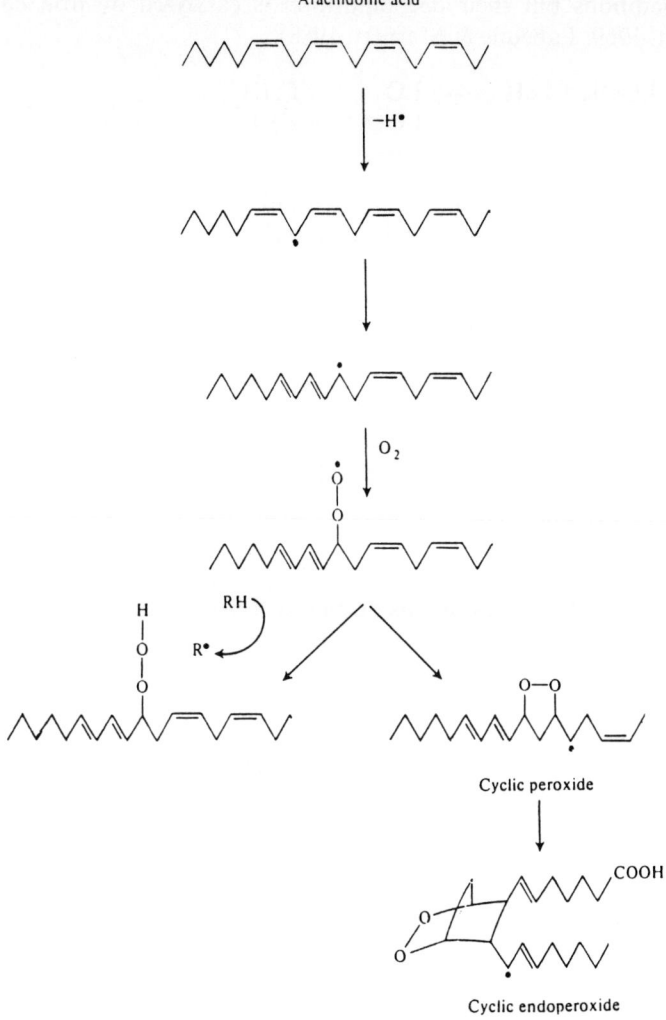

Arachidonic acid

−H•

O₂

RH
R•

Cyclic peroxide

COOH

Cyclic endoperoxide

Fig. 2 Mechanism of the peroxidative degradation of a polyunsaturated fatty acid.

phospholipid side-chains, or non-enzymically since the polyunsaturated fatty acid side-chain in the phospholipid is a highly vulnerable target to hydrogen abstraction initiated by a free radical species. As shown in Fig. 2, once the initiating species is formed, propagation of the chain may occur and the subsequent radical intermediates – peroxy radicals, fatty acyl radicals, lipid radicals – may initiate further chain reactions thereby amplifying the cellular damage. Lipid hydroperoxides are relatively stable molecules under physiological conditions but their decomposition is catalyzed by iron complexes (O'Brien, 1969; Labeque & Marnett, 1988).

$$LOOH + FeII ------\rangle LO. \qquad + FeIII$$
$$ LOO. \quad + FeII$$
$$ peroxy$$

$$LOOH + FeIII ------\rangle LO. \qquad + FeIV = O$$
$$ alkoxy \;\; ferryl$$
$$ LO- \qquad + FeV = O$$

As shown in this sequence of equations, both iron II and iron III are effective catalysts for hydroperoxide degradation, but the former more so. Such complexes include heme, hemoglobin, hemochrome, complexes of iron salts, some non-heme iron proteins. Peroxy radicals formed are more stable and selective in their reactivity than alkoxy radicals and possess half-lives that enable them to diffuse relatively far from their site of production in cells. Alkoxy radicals and metal–oxo complexes such as the ferryl species are potent oxidants that approach the hydroxyl radical in reactivity (Pryor, 1986) and thus participate in the amplification of the peroxidation process.

Cleavage of the carbon bonds during such peroxidative reactions (Fig. 3) results in the formation of a variety of secondary metabolites of the cyclic endoperoxide or fatty acyl hydroperoxide intermediates, including alkanals (Tappel, 1980), alkenals, 4-hydroxy alkenals (Esterbauer, 1985; Dianzani, 1989), alkenes, alkanes (Tappel & Dillard, 1981). Many of these compounds exert toxic effects on the cell. For example, alkanals such as malonaldehyde can bind to protein thiols, cross-link amino groups of lipids and proteins forming chromolipids and aggregated proteins; an hydroxy alkenal, such as 4-hydroxy nonenal, is very biologically active and modifies adenylate cyclase activity, acts as a substrate for glutathione transferases, stimulates chemotaxis and inhibits platelet aggregation.

Consequences of lipid peroxidation

The production of a highly reactive free radical leads to primary reactions and damage in the immediate surroundings of where the radical is produced. It will not diffuse far before it interacts within its microenvironment, which in a membrane would include the initiation of lipid peroxidation. Secondary products of peroxidative events, such as lipid peroxy radicals and lipid hydroperoxides, may diffuse in the plane of the membrane before reacting further, thereby spreading the biochemical lesion. Such processes, therefore, not only affect the structural and functional integrity of the membranes, but also the breakdown products of lipid peroxidation can further damage cellular function. For example, alkenals, alkanals and lipid hydroperoxides may undergo degradative reactions and be metabolized rapidly; some of these, e.g.

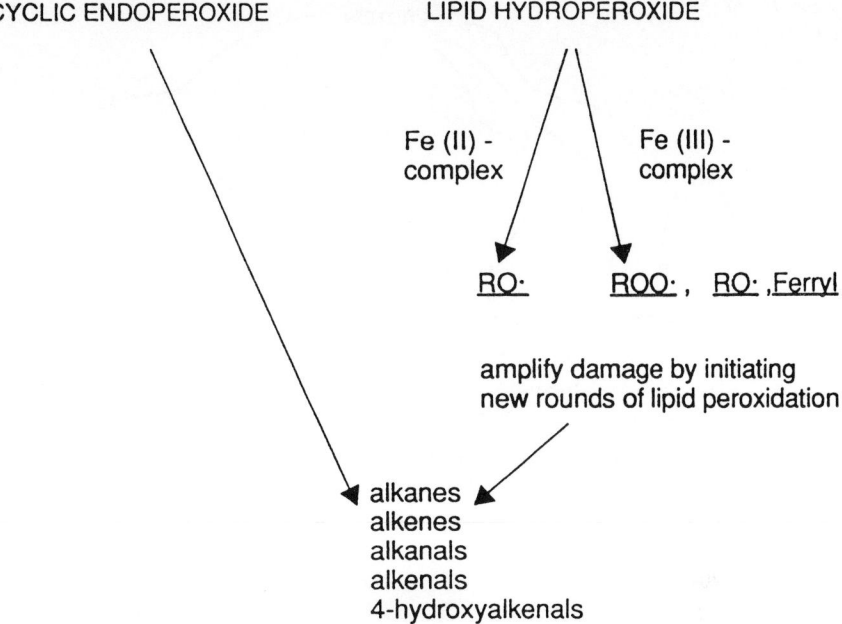

Fig. 3 Cleavage of carbon bonds during lipid peroxidation processes.

the lower molecular weight hydroperoxides, aldehydes and 4-hydroxyalke-nals, can escape from the membrane and cause disturbances at a distance. Therefore, a reaction that originally produces a radical which interacts within its microenvironment may induce a sequence of later events that direct disturbances throughout the cell, its membrane and, in some instances, into the extracellular domain.

Radical-mediated protein oxidation

Proteins are critical targets for free radical attack and, because many are catalytic, modifications may have an amplified effect. Several amino acids crucial for protein function are particularly vulnerable to radical damage (Sies, 1986), as shown in Fig. 4, with the consequence of such oxidative modification. It is generally accepted that highly reactive species such as hydroxyl radicals can react at several of these sites on a protein. However, it is becoming increasingly evident that once protein radicals are formed at a specific amino acyl site, they can be rapidly transferred to other sites within the protein infrastructure, the pathway so far proven being illustrated in Fig. 5 (Butler *et al.*, 1988). Proteins are also particularly susceptible to attack from radical intermediates of lipid peroxidation, alkoxy LO. and peroxy LOO. radicals. These may react with proteins closely associated with the peroxidi-

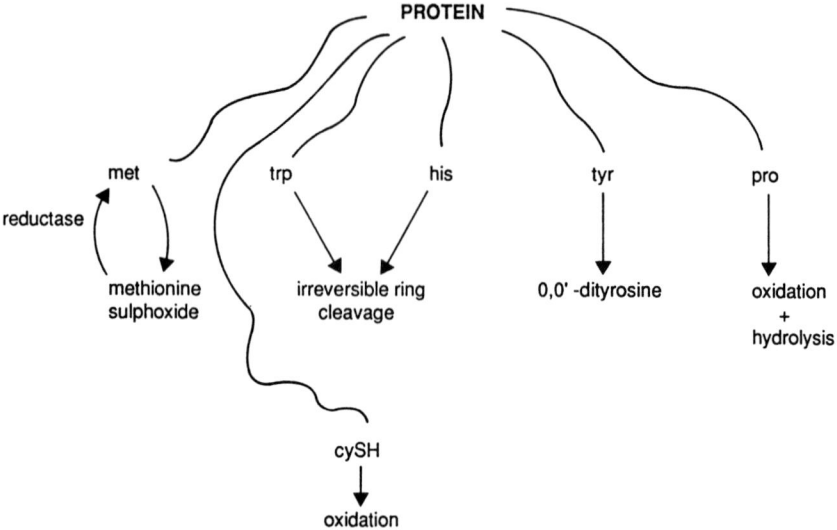

Fig. 4 Vulnerability of proteins to oxygen radical-mediated damage.

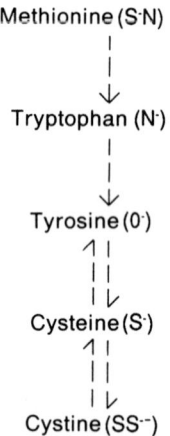

Fig. 5 Radical transfers within proteins.

zing lipids. The consequences of such damage may be aggregation and cross-linking or protein degradation and fragmentation, depending on the nature of the vulnerable protein component and the attacking radical species (Wolff *et al.*, 1986; Wolff & Dean, 1986).

The consequences of oxidative modification to proteins may be altered enzymic activity and altered membrane and cellular function resulting from degradation or cross-linking (Davies & Goldberg, 1987). Such damage to the membrane transport proteins, for example, would affect the ionic homeostasis of the cells leading to calcium accumulation. The resulting potential for activation of phospholipases, proteases and accumulation of mitochondrial calcium may lead to extensive membrane and cellular deterioration and gross exacerbation of the initial lesion.

Oxidative modification of proteins renders them more susceptible to proteolytic attack and enzymic hydrolysis (Wolff *et al.*, 1986). Hence, if generation of active oxygen species occurs significantly *in vivo*, one consequence may be accelerated hydrolysis of damaged proteins. Therefore, radical generation at inappropriate sites may lead to pathological tissue degradation.

Factors controlling the release of oxygen-derived free radicals

Increased oxidative stress may be the result of three major defects arising during tissue injury (Fig. 6) (Halliwell & Gutteridge, 1985; Rice-Evans, 1986, 1987; Cross *et al.*, 1987). Increased production of superoxide radicals may be generated by activated leukocytes and disrupted mitochondrial electron transport, and altered arachidonic acid metabolism can lead to excessive generation of active oxygen species. These sources of active oxygen species, superoxide radical, and hydrogen peroxide from its dismutation, provide direct production of cytotoxic oxidizing species. Once triggered, these processes may lead to modified antioxidant enzyme activity and to release of iron, which may all mutually interact amplifying the initial triggering event.

Modified antioxidant defences

In the normal course of events, cells have adequate antiradical defence mechanisms located intracellularly, extracellularly and bound to the membrane, as shown in Table 1 (Rice-Evans, 1988). Any pathological situation which increases the turnover of the antioxidant cycle, whether increased oxidative stress or modified antiradical defences, can lead to progressive cellular and membrane damage.

Increased leukocyte activation

Increased leukocyte infiltration may result from stimulation of chemotaxis in post-ischemic reperfusion mechanisms and in inflammatory responses. As an important part of their antibacterial defences, neutrophils possess a mem-

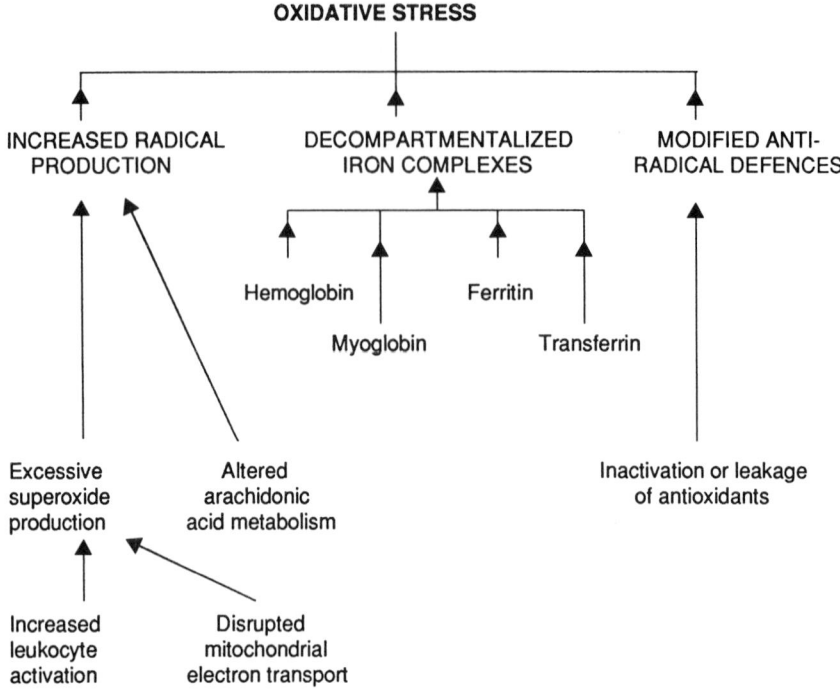

Fig. 6 Factors controlling increased oxygen radical production in cells and tissues.

brane-bound NADPH-oxidase (Babior, 1978) which produces superoxide radical when metabolically activated. The released superoxide seems to amplify the inflammatory response by activation of a latent chemoattractant present in extracellular fluids.

In vivo, ischemia and inflammation may be synergistic (McCord, 1988), leading under certain conditions to the cycle in Fig. 7. Vasoconstriction leads to ischemia which may produce an increased flux of superoxide radical production on reperfusion from the xanthine oxidase reaction or disrupted mitochondrial electron transport, for example (see below), which activates a latent chemoattractant perfusing the tissue. The presence of such chemotactic factors causes neutrophils to adhere to the endothelium and not only release hydrolytic and oxidative enzymes, thereby damaging the surrounding tissues, but also extravasate entering the interstices. The adherent neutrophils plug the capillary beds (Engler *et al.*, 1983, 1986), leading to further impairment of the circulation, exacerbating the ischemia. Increased capillary permeability creates edema and increases interstitial pressure which eventually may cause a local circulatory shutdown creating greater ischemia.

Table 1. *Protective antioxidant systems*

Non-enzymic
(i)   Alpha tocopherol
      bound to membranes and in plasma bound to lipoproteins
      chain breaking antioxidant and hydroxyl radical scavenger
(ii) Ascorbate
      water soluble antioxidant which acts synergistically with tocopherol.

Major extracellular protection mechanisms
(i)   Uric acid
       scavenges hydroxyl radical and singlet oxygen
       iron and copper chelator.
(ii)   Ceruloplasmin
       acts as an antioxidant by virtue of its ferroxidase activity.
(iii) Transferrin
       sequesters iron (III) rendering it unavailable for catalyzing the Haber-Weiss reaction,
       initiating lipid peroxidation or catalyzing the decomposition of lipid hydroperoxides.
(iv)   Albumin
       binds metals, especially copper but also iron weakly.
(v)   Beta carotene

Enzymic antioxidant defences
(i)   Superoxide dismutase
       disposes of superoxide radicals.
(ii)   Catalase
       detoxifies hydrogen peroxide.
(iii) Glutathione peroxidase
       detoxifies hydrogen peroxide and lipid peroxides in the presence of reduced glutathione.

Disrupted mitochondrial electron transport

During ischemia, the adenine nucleotide pool is partially degraded, energy limitations cause the elevation of calcium levels, and the mitochondrial electron carriers accumulate, reducing equivalents. When reperfusion occurs (McCord, 1985), electron egress through cytochrome oxidase will be diminished due to lack of adenosine diphosphate, even though oxygen is now available, hence electron leakage occurs forming superoxide radical. Concomitantly, as a result of the ischemia, the mitochondrial radical scavenging ability is rendered less able to deal with the increased radical flux, due to modified enzymic activity, glutathione responses etc. As the mitochondrial injury progresses, more disruption of normal electron flow occurs, leading to elevated fluxes of radical production.

Altered arachidonic acid metabolism

Increased production of eicosanoids has been shown to occur in a variety of pathological states, and their metabolism is accompanied by the generation and subsequent utilization of oxygen-derived free radicals. Arachidonic acid,

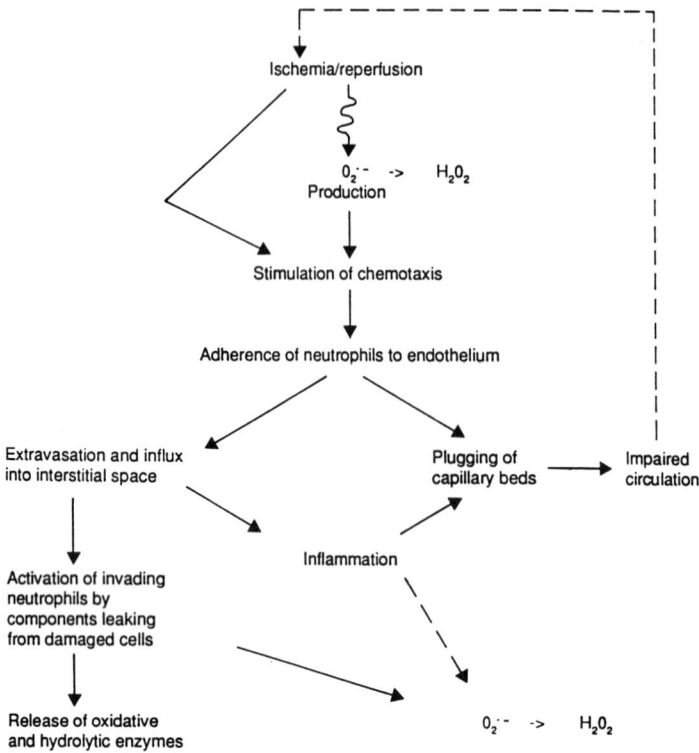

Fig. 7 Links between ischemia/reperfusion mechanisms and inflammation.

released from lipids as a result of activation of phospholipases by tissue injury or by hormones, may be metabolized by the prostaglandin (PG) or leukotriene pathways. The peroxidase-catalyzed conversion of PGG_2 to PGH_2 (Lands, 1979) (Fig. 8) and the mechanism of hydroperoxy fatty acid to the hydroxy fatty acid conversion (Fig. 8) both yield oxygen radicals (Miyamoto *et al.*, 1976; Kuehl *et al.*, 1977; Van der Ouderra *et al.*, 1977; Yamamoto *et al.*, 1980). These radicals can be detected by electron spin resonance (ESR) spectroscopy at low temperatures and can be captured by antioxidant compounds with consequent stimulation of PGG_2 to PGH_2 and subsequent prostanoids. One of the consequences of scavenging the reactive oxygen species is to prevent the irreversible degradation of the cyclo-oxygenase enzyme (Hemler & Lands, 1980; Yamamoto *et al.*, 1980). The radical species, depicted as [Ox], has many of the properties of the hydroxyl radical, although it is known not to be this species. It has been postulated that an active iron–oxygen species such as a ferryl iron–oxygen radical [FeIV = O]. is formed in the peroxidase reaction (Kuehl *et al.*, 1980). It has also been proposed that the heme iron in the cyclo-oxygenase enzyme must be reduced for maximal activity (Peterson *et al.*, 1981)

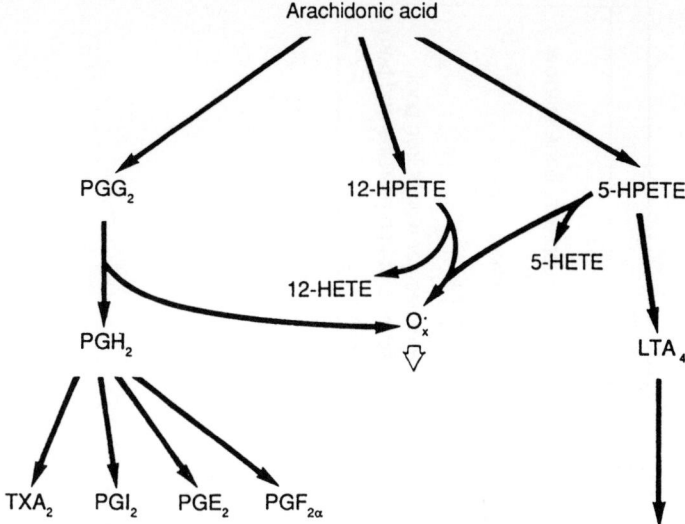

Fig. 8 Release of active oxygen species during arachidonic acid
metabolism.

and that superoxide radical, lipid hydroperoxides and hydrogen peroxide can
satisfy this criterion. Hence the stimulatory effects of hydroperoxides and
hydrogen peroxide on the activity of this enzyme.

The inhibition of these reactions may have profound effects on the overall
functions of arachidonic acid metabolism. Inhibition of prostaglandin
production at the cyclo-oxygenase part of the pathway may lead to
overproduction of leukotrienes, hydro(per)oxy fatty acids, e.g. 5- or 12-
HETE, and peroxidase-derived free radicals, all of which will have profound
pathophysiological effects (Deby & Deby-Dupont, 1980).

Decompartmentalization of iron

The iron in the human body is normally compartmented into its functional
localizations in the heme-containing and iron-binding proteins and enzymes
(Fig. 9). The majority (65%) of the iron is in the divalent state in hemoglobin
and myoglobin, the rest being distributed between storage sites, bound to
ferritin, in the low molecular weight iron pool awaiting synthesis of iron-
containing proteins, or bound to transferrin for transport and to lactoferrin.
The question therefore arises as to what forms of iron are available *in vivo*
which are capable of catalyzing the formation of damaging initiating species,
as normally the only 'free' iron available is that in the low molecular weight
iron pool which is normally sequestered from exerting toxic effects. In certain
pathological situations, iron may be released from its normal functional

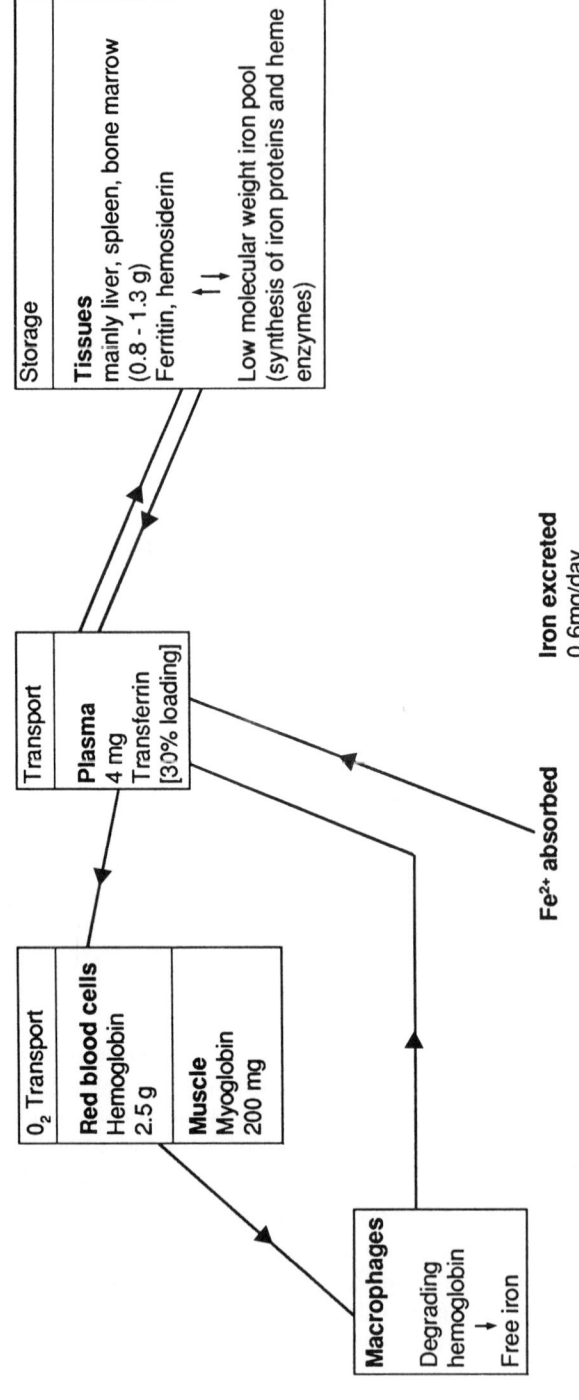

Fig. 9 Normal functional localizations of iron in the human body.

compartments: mobilization of iron from ferritin by superoxide radical, ascorbate and other reducing agents has been demonstrated (Biemond *et al.*, 1984, 1988). This might occur in endothelial cells, which contain high levels of ferritin, on generation of superoxide radicals (Shingu *et al.*, 1985) at sites of damage, or on reperfusion post-ischemia, as observed in the inflamed rheumatoid joint, for example. Evidence is accumulating that when hemoglobin is released via microbleeding processes, it becomes toxic (White *et al.*, 1986); microbleeding has been observed in the eye causing retinal damage (Doly *et al.*, 1986), in the brain, in certain tumours (Rowland & Symons, 1988) and at sites of inflammation (Yoshino *et al.*, 1985). Iron can be released from hemoglobin by hydrogen peroxide formed from superoxide radical (Gutteridge, 1986) and such released iron may catalyze the formation of the hydroxyl radical via the iron-catalyzed Haber-Weiss reaction:

$$Fe^{3+} + O_2^{\cdot-} \longrightarrow Fe^{2+} + O_2$$
$$O_2^{\cdot-} \longrightarrow H_2O_2$$
$$Fe^{2+} + H_2O_2 \longrightarrow \cdot OH + OH^- + Fe^{3+}$$

The mechanism of iron release from hemoglobin during interaction with excess hydrogen peroxide may involve the intermediary of ferryl hemoglobin (Symons, 1989), as outlined in the equations below.

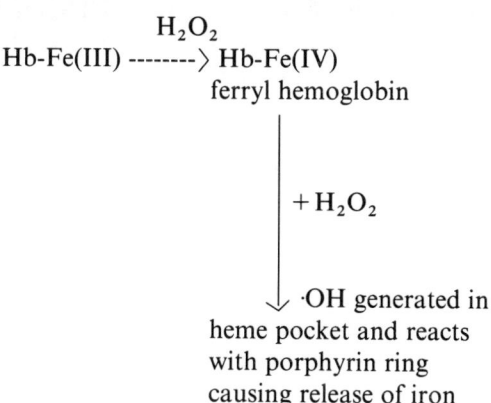

$$\overset{H_2O_2}{Hb\text{-}Fe(III) \longrightarrow Hb\text{-}Fe(IV)}$$
ferryl hemoglobin

$+ H_2O_2$

$\cdot OH$ generated in
heme pocket and reacts
with porphyrin ring
causing release of iron

The hydroxyl radical is formed in the heme pocket and hence will not generally escape but will interact in the close vicinity of its site of generation. It may require several cycles to give enough damage to the heme pocket to release the iron. However, ferryl hemoglobin itself is extremely reactive and can exert toxic oxidative effects.

Implications for the initiation and regulation of menstrual bleeding

During the normal ovarian cycle, withdrawal of steroids is the prime event leading to breakdown of the endometrium. The human endometrium has the capacity to form several different prostaglandins including PGE_2 and PGF_{2a}, thromboxane (TXA_2) and prostacyclin (PGI_2) (Green *et al.*, 1981). Levels of prostaglandins in human endometrium in normal and pathological situations are practically difficult to assess since they are subject to artefactual biosynthesis during tissue handling. It nevertheless seems that progressive increases in the concentration of PGF_{2a} and PGE_2 occur from the proliferative phase to the secretory phase, reaching peak levels during menstruation. Phospholipase A_2 activity peaks at ovulation and resumes normal basal levels at menstruation when prostaglandins are at their highest. Additionally, irregular and dysfunctional bleeding seems to be associated with overproduction of prostaglandins E and F (Bydgeman & Lundström, 1988).

Menstruation is thought to arise from the induction of local ischemia by a prolonged vasoconstriction of the end arterioles of the spiral arteries induced by prostaglandins such as PGF_{2a} and possibly leukotrienes such as the LTC_4 family, which are secreted during the second half of the ovarian cycle. This creates a scenario for increased oxygen radical generation. The release of leukotriene-type inflammatory mediators, e.g. LTB_4, results in the massive infiltration of leukocytes which occurs in the premenstrual phase. The contributions of prostaglandin and lipoxygenase products released from the white cell components of the blood remain to be established. The release of leukotrienes has high biological significance: one type (LTB_4) induces the accumulation of leukocytes by chemotaxis and subsequent adhesion to endothelium, which is known to precede passage of cells into tissues; the other type (LTC_4-E_4) causes increased vascular permeability leading to extravasation and migration to sites of damage.

Superoxide radical is released by metabolically activated neutrophils which can serve to amplify the inflammatory responses by further activation of latent chemoattractants. Such processes not only induce release of oxidative and hydrolytic enzymes but also active oxygen species are formed, thereby damaging surrounding tissue. Interaction between such active oxygen species and hemoglobin leads to the formation of highly reactive cytotoxic free radicals which may be involved in the mechanisms of the breakdown of endometrial cells.

The potential for the generation of oxygen-derived free radicals from a variety of sources post-ischemia (including stimulation of prostaglandin and lipoxygenase products from macrophages, for example) in association with decompartmentalization of iron complexes may be important factors in the initiation and control of menstrual bleeding.

References

Babior, B.M. (1978). Oxygen-dependent microbial killing by phagocytes. *New England Journal of Medicine*, **298**:659–668.

Biemond, P., Swaak, A.J.G., Van Eijk, H.G. & Koster, J.F. (1988). Superoxide dependent iron release from ferritin in inflammatory diseases. *Free Radical Biology and Medicine*, **4**:185–198.

Biemond, P., Van Eijk, H.G., Swaak, A.J.G. & Koster, J.F. (1984). Iron mobilisation from ferritin by superoxide derived from stimulated polymorphonuclear leukocytes: possible mechanisms in inflammatory diseases. *Journal of Clinical Investigation*, **73**:1576–1579.

Butler, J., Hoey, B.M. & Lea, J.S. (1988). The measurement of radicals by pulse radiolysis. (In) *Free Radicals: Methodology and Concepts* (Rice-Evans, C. & Halliwell, B., eds.), pp.457–479. London, Richelieu Press.

Bydgeman, M. & Lundström, V. (1988). Menstruation and dysmenorrhoea. (In) *Prostaglandins* (Curtis-Pryor, P.B., ed.), pp.490–495. Edinburgh, Churchill Livingstone.

Cross, C.E., Halliwell, B., Borish, E.T., Pryor, W.A., Ames, B.N., Saul, R.L., McCord, J.M. & Harman, D. (1987). Oxygen radicals and human disease. *Annals of Internal Medicine*, **107**:526–545.

Davies, K.J. & Goldberg, A.L. (1987). Oxygen radicals stimulate intracellular proteolysis and lipid peroxidation by independent mechanisms in erythrocytes. *Journal of Biological Chemistry*, **262**:8220–8226.

Deby, C. & Deby-Dupont, G. (1980). Oxygen species in prostaglandin biosynthesis *in vitro* and *in vivo*. (In) *Biological and Clinical Aspects of Superoxide and Superoxide Dismutase* (Bannister, W.H. & Bannister, J.V., eds.), pp.84–97. Amsterdam, Elsevier/North-Holland.

Dianzani, M.U. (1989). (In) *Free Radicals, Metal Ions and Biopolymers* (Beaumont, P., Deeble, D., Parsons, B. & Rice-Evans, C., eds.), in press. London, Richelieu Press.

Doly, M., Bonhomme, B. & Vennat, J.C. (1986). Experimental study of the retinal toxicity of haemoglobinic iron. *Ophthalmic Research*, **18**:21–27.

Engler, R.L., Dahlgren, M.D., Peterson, M.A., Dobbs, A. & Schmid-Schoenbein, G.W. (1986). Accumulation of polymorphonuclear leukocytes during 3h experimental myocardial ischaemia. *American Journal of Physiology*, **251**:H93–H100.

Engler, R.L., Schmid-Schoenbein, G.W. & Pavelec, R.S. (1983). Leukocyte capillary plugging in myocardial ischaemia and reperfusion in the dog. *American Journal of Pathology*, **111**:98–111.

Esterbauer, H. (1985). Lipid peroxidation products: formation, chemical properties and biological activation. (In) *Free Radicals in Liver Injury* (Poli, G., Cheeseman, K.H., Dianzani, M.U. & Slater, T.F., eds.), pp.29–47. Washington, IRL Press.

Green, K., Christensen, N.Y. & Bydgeman, M. (1981). The chemistry and pharmacology of prostaglandins with reference to human reproduction. *Journal of Reproductive Fertility*, **62**:269–281.

Gutteridge, J.M.C. (1986). Iron promoters of the Fenton reaction and lipid peroxidation can be released from haemoglobin by peroxides. *FEBS Letters*, **201**:291–295.

Halliwell, B. & Gutteridge, J.M.C. (1985). The importance of free radicals and catalytic metal ions in human diseases. *Molecular Aspects of Medicine*, **8**:89–193.

Hemler, M.E. & Lands, W.E.M. (1980). Evidence for a peroxide-initiated free radical mechanism of prostaglandin biosynthesis. *Journal of Biological Chemistry*, **255**:6253–6261.

Kuehl, F.A., Humes, J.L., Egan, R.W., Ham, E.A., Beveridge, G.C. & Van Arman, C.G. (1977). Role of prostaglandin endoperoxide PGG_2 in inflammatory processes. *Nature*, **265**:170–173.

Kuehl, F.A., Humes, J.L., Ham, E.A., Egan, R.W. & Dougherty, H.W. (1980). Inflammation: the role of peroxidase-derived products. *Advances in Prostaglandin and Thromboxane Research*, **6**:77–86.

Labeque, R. & Marnett, L.J. (1988). Reaction of hematin with allylic fatty acid hydroperoxides: identification of products and implications for pathways of hydroperoxide-dependent epoxidation of 7,8-dihydroxy-7,8-dihydrobenzo(a)pyrene. *Biochemistry*, **27**:7060–7070.

Lands, W.E.M. (1979). The biosynthesis and metabolism of prostaglandins. *Annual Review of Physiology*, **41**:633–652.

McCord, J.M. (1985). Oxygen-derived free radicals in post-ischaemic tissue injury. *New England Journal of Medicine*, **312**:159–163.

McCord, J.M. (1988). Free radicals and myocardial ischaemia: overview and outlook. *Free Radical Biology and Medicine*, **4**:9–14.

Miyamoto, T., Ogino, N., Yamamoto, S. & Hayaishi, O. (1976). Purification of prostaglandin endoperoxide synthetase from bovine vesicular gland microsomes. *Journal of Biological Chemistry*, **251**:2629–2636.

O'Brien, P.J. (1969). Intracellular mechanisms for the decomposition of a lipid hydroperoxide. I. Decomposition of a lipid peroxide by metal ions, heme compounds and nucleophiles. *Canadian Journal of Biochemistry*, **47**:485–492.

Peterson, D.A., Gerrard, J.M., Rao, G.H. & White, J.G. (1981). Reduction of heme by lipid peroxides and its potential relevance to understanding the control of cyclooxygenase activity. *Progress in Lipid Research*, **20**:299–301.

Pryor, W.A. (1986). Oxy-radicals and related species: their formation, lifetimes and reactions. *Annual Review of Physiology*, **48**:657–667.

Rice-Evans, C., ed. (1986). *Free Radicals, Cell Damage and Disease*. London, Richelieu Press.

Rice-Evans, C., ed. (1987). *Free Radicals, Oxidant Stress and Drug Action*. London, Richelieu Press.

Rice-Evans, C. (1988). Free radicals in health and disease: implications for drug delivery and drug targeting. (In) *Targeting of Drugs: Anatomical and Physiological Considerations* (Gregoriadis, G. & Poste, G., eds.), pp.53–67. New York and London, Plenum Press.

Rowland, I.J. & Symons, M.C.R. (1988). Tumours and iron: the use of electron spin resonance. (In) *Free Radicals: Methodology and Concepts* (Rice-Evans, C. & Halliwell, B., eds.), pp.169–184. London, Richelieu Press.

Shingu, M., Yoshioka, K., Nobunaga, M. & Yoshida, K. (1985). Human vascular smooth muscle cells and endothelial cells lack catalase activity and are susceptible to hydrogen peroxide. *Inflammation*, **9**:309–320.

Sies, H. (1986). Biochemistry of oxidative stress. *Angewandte Chemie*, **25**:1058–1071.

Slater, T.F. (1984). Free-radical mechanisms in tissue injury. *Biochemical Journal*, **222**:1–15.

Symons, M.C.R. (1989). Applications of radiation and ESR spectroscopy to the study of ferryl haemoglobin and myoglobin. *Journal of the Chemical Society Faraday Transactions*, in press.

Tappel, A.L. (1980). Measurement and protection from *in vivo* lipid peroxidation. (In)

Free Radicals in Biology and Medicine, Vol IV (Pryor, W.A., ed.), pp.1–45. New York, Academic Press.

Tappel, A.L. & Dillard, C.J. (1981). *In vivo* lipid peroxidation: measurement via exhaled pentane and protection by vitamin E. *Federation Proceedings*, **40**:174–178.

Van der Ouderra, F.J., Buytenhek, M., Nugteren, D.H. & Van Dorp, D.A. (1977). Purification and characterisation of prostaglandin endoperoxide synthetase from sheep vesicular glands. *Biochimica Biophysica Acta*, **487**:315–331.

White, C.T., Murray, A.J., Greene, J.R., Smith, D.J., Medina, F., Makovec, G.T., Martin, E.J. & Bolin, R.B. (1986). Toxicity of human haemoglobin solution infused into rabbits. *Journal of Laboratory and Clinical Medicine*, **108**:121–131.

Wolff, S.P. & Dean, R.T. (1986). Fragmentation of proteins by free radicals and its effect on their susceptibility to enzymic hydrolysis. *Biochemical Journal*, **234**:399–403.

Wolff, S.P., Garner, A. & Dean, R.T. (1986). Free radicals, lipids and protein degradation. *Trends in Biochemical Sciences*, **11**:27–31.

Yamamoto, S., Ohki, S., Ogino, N., Shimizu, T., Yoshomoto, T., Watanabe, K. & Hayaishi, O. (1980). Enzymes involved in the formation and further transformations of prostaglandin endoperoxides. *Advances in Prostaglandin and Thromboxane Research*, **6**:27–34.

Yoshino, S., Blake, D.R., Hewitt, S., Morris, C. & Bacon, P.A. (1985). Effect of blood on the activity and persistence of antigen-induced inflammation in the rat air pouch. *Annals of Rheumatic Diseases*, **44**:485–490.

Discussion

Naftolin. I am interested in the fact that estrogens form superoxides, they form catechols, and some of those catechols then are superoxides. Can you comment on steroid superoxides?

Rice-Evans. I can only comment in the sense that catecholamines have been implicated in mechanisms of superoxide production under ischemia/reperfusion conditions. But no clear data have yet emerged, in the presence or absence of steroids, in the systems I am discussing.

Naftolin. Superoxide dismutase also responds to steroids and so does peroxidase, which is clearly induced by estrogen which rises during this time in the uterus. What role do you see it playing in ameliorating or making these processes work?

Rice-Evans. Peroxidases are involved in all sorts of cell types in the body and may participate in the controlled production of free radicals under certain circumstances.

Naftolin. I just wanted to look at membrane fluidity because this changes during the cycle in many sex steroid-responsive tissues. Generally, this is studied by looking at changes in fluorescence. Estrogen, for example, plays a role in capping and patching the intramembranous protein particles. How rapidly can these effects occur on membranes?

Rice-Evans. Well, you have picked on one measure that occurs very early on, because as soon as a radical attacks a lipid in the membrane, a change of fluidity occurs. Once a polyunsaturated fatty acid releases an electron, there is a rearrangement of double bonds in the formation of conjugated di-enes before it has taken up the oxygen. So it is possible to see changes in membrane fluidity. Of course, you have to be very careful when you measure membrane fluidity because if you use certain types of probes, you are not sure whether they are just probing the lipid region or whether they are reaching the protein portion.

Clark. I was fascinated by the role that iron plays in this particular process and I wondered if perhaps merely allowing women who have recurrent bleeding to become iron deficient in terms of their body stores should not correct the bleeding by decreasing the availability of iron, and thereby decreasing availability of free radicals. Related to that is the fact that if you give radiotherapy for cancer, you generate free radicals, and I am puzzled as to why that does not produce acute hemorrhage. Could you comment on those two points?

Rice-Evans. I can comment on your first question. The point is that in menstrual disturbance and iron deficiency, there is a lack of iron where it ought to be, but some of it is escaping into tissue where hemoglobin is not normally found. So it is not just a question of the total body iron but deposition of iron protein in tissue. I think it would be interesting to look at endometrial tissue from various stages in the cycle, from individuals who are being treated on iron chelation therapy. Unfortunately, the only group of patients that I know of who are treated on iron chelation therapy are those who are iron deficient or anemic because they have beta-thalassemia. These women are being transfused regularly to correct their anemia and therefore suffer from iron overload. Iron chelation therapy is given to correct the iron overload, and unfortunately, one of the sites where iron deposition occurs is in the endocrine glands.

Courtoy. I would like to know if this cascade leading to the production of free radicals shows a critical temperature dependence. The reason I ask this question is in relation to the observations of Dr Wattiaux and Dr Wattiaux-Deconinck (1981). When they reperfused the rat liver, they observed marked increase in the apparent free activity at 38°C. But this is completely abrogated at 36°C. So I would like to know if there is a marked change in the Arrhenius plot of this system.

Rice-Evans. That is a very small temperature change in relation to free radical generation. My experience is with organ storage for transplantation and, as you know, when organs are removed and rendered ischemic they are usually kept at about 2–4°C. We have done some work on kidney storage for transplantation looking at various mechanisms for free radical production. We actually observed more damage in those stored at 2°C than in those stored at 37°C.

Findlay. The gene for superoxide dismutase is located on chromosome 21 in the human, and it is located in the same area as the Down's syndrome locus. Do any of the clinicians here know whether female Down's syndrome subjects have abnormal endometrial bleeding?

Rees. In Oxford, quite a few hysterectomies have been carried out on Down's syndrome patients because of abnormal endometrial bleeding, but the volume has not been quantitated. The indication is usually inability to cope with bleeding rather than true menorrhagia.

Fraser. I would like to ask whether free radical generation is more likely to be involved as an amplification process of the damage process once it has started, or do you think it really is a prime candidate for being involved in the initiation of bleeding?

Rice-Evans. I am quite convinced that it is prostaglandin $F_{2\alpha}$ that initiates the initial vasoconstriction in normal bleeding. But I am not convinced about the levels needed and what other factors need to be included; following the $F_{2\alpha}$ initial vasoconstrictive/vasodilatory event, what other effects are occurring that amplify the levels of prostaglandins and then may lead to more serious ischemia reperfusion? I believe that while free radical generation may be secondary to the prime event, it nevertheless plays an important role.

Breakthrough bleeding is very interesting because there is no vasoconstriction, so we are not starting from the same point. Some questions need to be answered. Could we look and see what sort of products are released with breakthrough bleeding compared with the various tissues in the normal cycle? We would need to look at antioxidant levels, peroxidative breakdown products and the toxic products: in the presence and absence of progestogens; in the presence and absence of antioxidants and iron chelators in women with breakthrough bleeding and normal cycles to get a feel for the different contributions of each mechanism in the two situations.

Naftolin. Could anybody comment on the role of vitamin E in potentially aborting this system and therefore changing bleeding patterns? In view of the recent interest in the dismutases, it would be appropriate to complete a small clinical trial of vitamin E and see what it does in these cases of progestogen-induced bleeding.

Rice-Evans. This would be worth exploring.

References

Wattiaux, R. & Wattiaux-Deconinck, S. (1981). Effect of a transitory ischaemia on the structure-linked latency of rat liver acid phosphatase and beta-galactosidase. *Biochemical Journal*, **196**:861–866.

Tissue breakdown

Y. EECKHOUT

Laboratoire de Chimie Physiologique, Université de Louvain, and Institute of Cellular and Molecular Pathology, Brussels, Belgium.

Abstract

The cellular and molecular mechanisms and control of endometrial bleeding are still obscure. Lack of progress might be the result of hitherto insufficient attention being paid to the extracellular matrix and to the involvement of non-lysosomal mechanisms. Therefore, an overview of different and sometimes better documented processes of physiological tissue breakdown is expected to elicit new conceptual and methodological approaches for future research in endometrial breakdown.

Relevant properties of the major proteinases implicated in mammalian tissue resorption are first surveyed: lysosomal acid proteinases (the aspartic proteinase cathepsin D, and the collagenolytic cysteine proteinases cathepsins B and L), neutral matrix metalloproteinases (collagenase and the related gelatinase and stromelysin) and serine proteinases (principally those of the plasminogen activator–plasmin cascade).

Lysis of connective tissue fibres appears to represent a critical step in many instances of tissue involution, including endometrial breakdown. Therefore, the second part of this contribution focuses on the enzymatic degradation mechanisms of interstitial collagen, which represents the major fibrillar component of the extracellular matrix. The respective roles of collagenase, collagen depolymerases and of gelatinolytic proteinases are examined in extracellular and intracellular degradation of collagen. Attention is also given to the influence of age, intermolecular cross-linking and type of collagen on its susceptibility towards proteolytic enzymes and to the mechanisms controlling the production and activity of collagenase.

Part three summarizes recent data and mechanisms of two processes of tissue involution related to mammalian reproduction: postpartum involution of the uterus, and cervical ripening and dilatation. Our present knowledge of the respective roles of collagenase, lysosomal cysteine proteinases, plasminogen activators, osteoclasts and osteoblasts in bone resorption is presented in part four.

The last part proposes some questions and research perspectives on the enzymes, cells and regulatory molecules possibly involved in endometrial degradation. It stresses the need for considering the extracellular matrix as well as non-lysosomal proteinases for a better understanding of endometrial tissue breakdown.

Introduction

Endometrial tissue breakdown represents a key process in menstruation but its precise nature, localization, timing and mechanism still remain obscure (Smith, 1990; Johannisson, 1990). Lack of progress in the understanding of endometrial degradation could result in part from hitherto insufficient attention being paid to the involvement of both the extracellular matrix and non-lysosomal mechanisms. Therefore, a survey of the salient properties of the major proteinases implicated in tissue breakdown, the mechanisms of collagen degradation and a few better documented processes of tissue resorption, is expected to suggest new approaches for future research in endometrial breakdown.

Proteinases implicated in tissue breakdown

Several proteolytic enzymes have been implicated in tissue breakdown (for reviews see Lorand, 1981; Harris *et al.*, 1984;, Jeffrey, 1986; Eeckhout *et al.*, 1988; Hart & Rehemtulla, 1988; Moscatelli & Rifkin, 1988). Salient properties of the major ones are summarized in Table 1. They belong to four different classes. The aspartic lysosomal proteinase cathepsin D is generally active at pH values lower than 4. Its involvement in tissue breakdown has been postulated since its discovery in the lysosomes, but it remains poorly documented and has been overshadowed by the more recently discovered lysosomal cysteine proteinases. The latter are active at more physiologic pH values and are now considered to play a major role in intracellular (heterophagic or autophagic) digestion and also, when secreted by specialized cells such as macrophages or osteoclasts, in slightly acidic extracellular microenvironments. Their ability to depolymerize crosslinked collagen as well as to activate procollagenase (see next sections of this chapter) points to their possible intervention in the degradation of the extracellular matrix.

Most metallo- and serine proteinases are secreted as inactive proenzymes and act outside the cell at neutral pH, either at the cell surface or in extracellular matrices or fluids. Their activity is limited in space and in time by the presence of specific proteolytic activators and of potent endogenous inhibitors. The closely related matrix metalloproteinases (collagenase, gelatinase and stromelysin) are capable of degrading most matrix proteins, including interstitial collagens, basement membrane collagen, proteoglycans, laminin and fibronectin. On the other hand, several serine proteinases are potential activators of procollagenase, and polymorphonuclear leukocyte elastase is collagenolytic (Burleigh, 1977).

Physiological mechanisms of collagen degradation

Collagen represents the major fibrous protein of the extracellular matrix. The native triple helical domain of the most abundant (type I) collagen (Fig. 1) is resistant towards all proteolytic enzymes except collagenase which cleaves it into a three-quarter N-terminal and a one-quarter C-terminal fragment. At 37°C these fragments become susceptible to the action of gelatinolytic proteinases. Type III collagen, which is more abundant in fetal and newly formed tissues (thus probably in endometrium), can in addition be fragmented by non-specific proteinases.

Table 1. *Mammalian proteinases implicated in tissue breakdown*

Class	Name	Localization	Properties	Inhibitors[a]	
				Endogenous	Exogenous
Aspartic	Cathepsin D	Lysosomal	pH optimum <4 for most substrates		Pepstatin
Cysteine	Cathepsins B and L	Lysosomal	pH optimum 5–6; collagenolytic; activation of procollagenase	Cystatins	E-64, Z-Phe-Ala-CHN$_2$ p-CMB and other SH-reagents
Metallo-	Collagenase and related gelatinase and stromelysin	Secreted as proenzymes; not stored (except in PMN leukocytes)	Degradation of collagens, proteoglycans and other matrix proteins at neutral pH	TIMP	CI-1
Serine	Plasminogen activators and plasmin	Peri- and extracellular	Neutral optimum pH; activation of procollagenase	α_1-proteinase inhibitor	DIPF, PMSF
	PMN-leukocyte elastase and cathepsin G	Azurophil granules	Collagenolytic		
	Mast cell proteinases	Mast cell granules	Activation of procollagenase		

[a] Most proteinases of the four catalytic classes are irreversibly inhibited by α_2-macroglobulin (Barrett, 1981).

Abbreviations:

CI-1: collagenase inhibitor 1 (Delaissé et al., 1985)
CMB: parachloromercuribenzoate
DIPF: diisopropylfluorophosphate
E-64: *trans*-epoxy-succinyl-L-leucylamido-(4-guanidino)-butane
PMN: polymorphonuclear leukocytes
PMSF: phenylmethanesulfonylfluoride
TIMP: tissue inhibitor of metalloproteinases
Z-Phe-Ala-CHN$_2$: benzyloxycarbonyl-phenylalanine-alanyl diazomethane

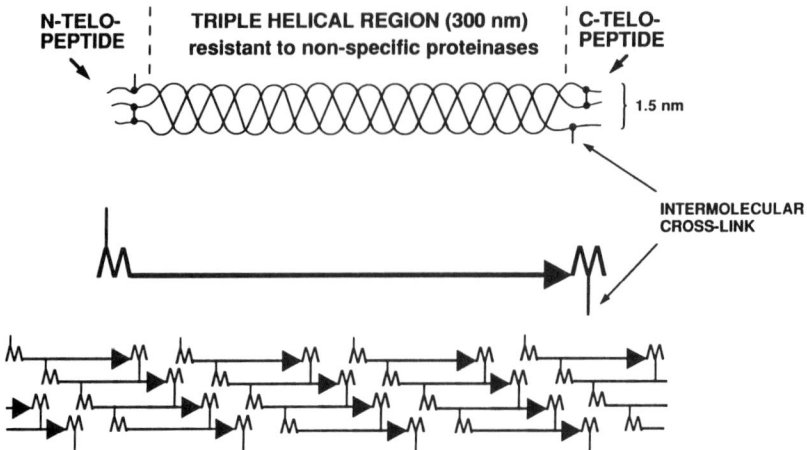

Fig. 1 Diagram to illustrate the structure and cross-linking of interstitial collagen.

At 37°C the collagen molecules organize spontaneously into fibrils. Covalent intermolecular cross-links, whose number and/or stability increase with maturation, contribute to the high tensile strength of the collagen fibrils and to their decreased susceptibility to digestion by collagenase. However, some tissue proteinases (for a review see Burleigh, 1977), e.g. the lysosomal cysteine proteinases cathepsins B and L and granulocyte elastase, are capable of cleaving the collagen telopeptides proximally to the cross-links. This results in depolymerization and solubilization of the collagen molecules which can be further digested either extracellularly by collagenase and gelatinase or, after endocytosis, in the intracellular acid lysosomal environment.

Regulation of mammalian collagenase

There is now much evidence for the involvement of collagenase in the degradation of collagen in fetal and young tissues, e.g. postpartum uterus and woven bone (see next sections of this chapter). It is therefore sound to hypothesize an intervention of collagenase in the initiation or (and) in a later step of endometrial breakdown. Many cell types are known to produce collagenase when stimulated, e.g. fibroblasts, myometrial smooth muscle cells, macrophages and endothelial cells. Several hormones, cytokines, prostaglandins and growth factors were found to regulate collagenase production by these cells (for recent reviews see Harris *et al.*, 1984; Vaes, 1985; Jeffrey, 1986).

Collagenase is secreted as an inactive proenzyme which can be activated by several tissue proteinases including plasmin (or plasminogen activator in the presence of plasminogen), kallikrein, the lysosomal cysteine proteinase cathepsin B and a mast cell serine proteinase. On the other hand, collagenase activity is restricted to focal microenvironments by the presence of potent irreversible inhibitors: the tissue inhibitor of metalloproteinases (TIMP) in the interstitial matrix and α_2-macroglobulin in the blood plasma.

Tissue involutions related to mammalian reproduction

Tissue involutions related to mammalian reproduction represent useful models for the study of endometrial breakdown. The postpartum involution of the uterus has been the most extensively studied (for reviews see Woessner, 1980, 1982; Jeffrey, 1986). Approximately 700 g wet human uterine tissue, including 24 g collagen, are resorbed in 8 days. Several observations point to the participation of both collagenase, probably produced by smooth muscle cells (Blair *et al.*, 1986; Roswit *et al.*, 1988), and lysosomal enzymes, probably contained within macrophages. Estradiol and progesterone exert striking inhibitory effects on the production of collagenase, on collagenolysis and on the accumulation of macrophages in the postpartum uterus. In the last case the abundance of type III collagen (at least 10%) and of poorly cross-linked collagen is noticeable.

Stromal tissue and collagen are predominant in the uterine cervix, whose ripening and dilatation result mainly from connective tissue remodelling (Woessner, 1982). Increased ground substance, total hexosamines and water content, and reduced cross-linking of collagen were noticed at term. Type III collagen represents one-fifth of total collagen. Prostaglandin E_2, which induces dilatation of the uterine cervix, stimulates the production of collagenase by cultured rabbit cervical fibroblasts, whereas PGI_2 does not (Goshowaki *et al.*, 1988). Interleukin-1α stimulated the production of collagenase in these cervical fibroblasts and estradiol-17β increased their sensitivity to interleukin-1 (Ito *et al.*, 1988). On the other hand, several data suggest that ripening and dilatation of the uterine cervix do not result from collagen breakdown but from slippage of collagen fibrils past one another. This slippage would originate from modifications of glycosaminoglycan ground substances or (and) from depolymerization of collagen. Increase of collagenase and collagen degradation (Rath *et al.*, 1987) would then not reflect dilatation but postpartum involution of the uterine cervix.

The data summarized above and the numerous influences of sex steroid hormones on the metabolism of extracellular matrix proteins (Cutroneo *et al.*, 1986) strongly suggest that remodelling of the extracellular matrix could represent a key process in endometrial tissue breakdown.

Bone resorption

There is now ample evidence for the involvement of both collagenase and lysosomal cysteine proteinase in bone resorption (Eeckhout *et al.*, 1988;

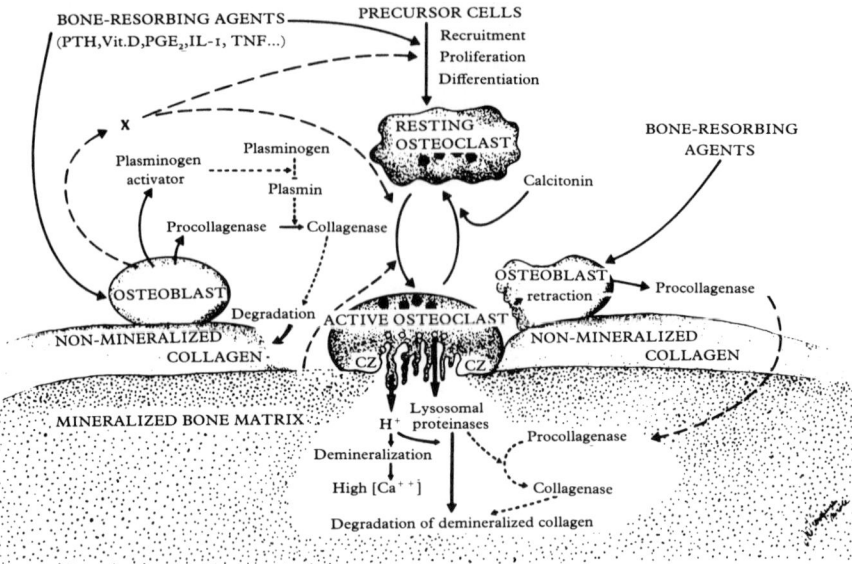

Fig. 2 Scheme illustrating the presumed roles of proteinases in bone resorption. Broken arrows represent processes which, in bone tissue, are more hypothetical. Abbreviations: CZ, clear zone; PTH, parathyroid hormone; Vit. D, 1,25 $(OH)_2$ vitamin D_3; PGE_2, prostaglandin E_2; IL1, interleukin 1; TNF, tumour necrosis factor. (From Glauert (1988), with permission.)

Eeckhout & Delaissé, 1988; Vaes, 1988). Our present view on the mechanisms of bone resorption is schematically illustrated in Fig. 2. The major bone-eroding cell is the osteoclast which, once activated, closely adheres to the mineralized matrix through a specialized annular cell structure, the sealing or clear zone. The ruffled border membrane of the adhering osteoclast secretes both acid, which dissolves bone mineral, and lysosomal enzymes, including very probably cysteine proteinases, which depolymerize and solubilize bone collagen. Osteoclasts are directly inactivated by calcitonin but they are not directly activated by bone-resorbing agents. Osteoblastic cells, but not osteoclasts, have receptors for parathyroid hormone, for 1,25-dihydroxyvita-min D_3 and probably for most other bone-resorbing agents, which induce them to produce procollagenase and plasminogen activator.

Plasmin is able to transform procollagenase into active collagenase. Collagenase would degrade the non-mineralized collagen which protects the mineralized matrix from osteoclastic attack. Moreover, other data suggest that stimulated osteoblasts release an osteoclast-activating factor (X on Fig. 2) or (and) retract themselves. Procollagenase, which has been extracted from mineralized bone matrix, could in addition participate together with lysosomal cysteine proteinases in the subosteoclastic resorption of the organic bone matrix.

Conclusions

A better understanding of the mechanisms and control of tissue breakdown in menstruation will, it is hoped, contribute to the development of new strategies to prevent abnormal endometrial bleeding. Our present knowledge of the endometrial degradation mechanisms compared to that of a few other physiological processes of tissue breakdown indicates that more attention should be given to the extracellular matrix, to the collagenolytic lysosomal cysteine proteinases and to non-lysosomal proteinases. Remodelling of stromal collagen and/or ground substance (hyaluronic acid and proteoglycans) could take part in the initiation of menstruation (Johannisson, 1990). Therefore, the participation of neutral matrix-degrading metalloproteinases and of the plasminogen activator–plasmin cascade should be investigated in endometrial breakdown. Methods exist for assaying the major matrix components and the enzymes implicated in their degradation. Reagents are now also available allowing immunoassays, immunolocalizations and in-situ mRNA hybridization of these agents in human endometrial biopsies or cultures. Such investigations, associated with studies of cytokines, prostaglandins and growth factors implicated in endometrial breakdown, should contribute to a noticeable progress in the understanding and control of endometrial bleeding.

Acknowledgements

This work was supported by the Belgian Fonds de la Recherche Scientifique Médicale. The author wishes also to thank Dr Pierre Courtoy for his friendly encouragement in the preparation of this manuscript and Mr Yves Marchand for skilled secretarial and library assistance.

References

Barrett, A.J. (1981). α_2-Macroglobulin. (In) *Proteolytic Enzymes. Methods in Enzymology*, Vol. 80 (Lorand, L., ed.), pp.737–754. New York, Academic Press.

Blair, H.C., Teitelbaum, S.L., Ehlich, L.S. & Jeffrey, J.J. (1986). Collagenase production by smooth muscle: correlation of immunoreactive with functional enzyme in the myometrium. *Journal of Cellular Physiology*, **129**:111–123.

Burleigh, M.C. (1977). Degradation of collagen by non-specific proteinases. (In) *Proteinases in Mammalian Cells and Tissues* (Barrett, A.J., ed.), pp.285–309. Amsterdam, Elsevier/North-Holland.

Cutroneo, K.R., Sterling, K.M. Jr & Shull, S. (1986). Steroid hormone regulation of extracellular matrix proteins. (In) *Regulation of Matrix Accumulation* (Mecham, R.P., ed.), pp.119–176. Orlando, Academic Press.

Delaissé, J.M., Eeckhout, Y., Sear, C., Galloway, A., McCullagh, K. & Vaes, G. (1985). A new synthetic inhibitor of mammalian tissue collagenase inhibits bone resorption in culture. *Biochemical and Biophysical Research Communications*, **133**:483–490.

Eeckhout, Y. & Delaissé, J.M. (1988). The role of collagenase in bone resorption. An overview. *Pathologie Biologie*, **36**:1139–1146.

Eeckhout, Y., Delaissé, J.M., Ledent, P. & Vaes, G. (1988). The proteinases of bone resorption. (In) *The Control of Tissue Damage* (Glauert, A.M., ed.), pp.297–313. Amsterdam, Elsevier.

Glauert, A.M. (1988). *The Control of Tissue Damage* Amsterdam, Elsevier.

Goshowaki, H., Ito, A. & Mori, Y. (1988). Effects of prostaglandins on the production of collagenase by rabbit uterine cervical fibroblasts. *Prostaglandins*, **36**:107–114.

Harris, E.D., Welgus, H.G. & Krane, S.M. (1984). Regulation of the mammalian collagenases. A review. *Collagen and Related Research*, **4**:493–512.

Hart, D.A. & Rehemtulla, A. (1988). Plasminogen activators and their inhibitors: regulators of extracellular proteolysis and cell function. *Comparative Biochemistry and Physiology*, **90B**:691–708.

Ito, A., Goshowaki, H., Sato, T., Mori, Y., Yamashita, K., Hayakawa, T. & Nagase, H. (1988). Human recombinant interleukin-1α-mediated stimulation of procollagenase production and suppression of biosynthesis of tissue inhibitor of metalloproteinases in rabbit uterine cervical fibroblasts. *FEBS Letters*, **234**:326–330.

Jeffrey, J.J. (1986). The biological regulation of collagenase activity. (In) *Regulation of Matrix Accumulation* (Mecham, R.P., ed.), pp.53–98. Orlando, Academic Press.

Johannisson, E. (1990). Endometrial morphology during the normal cycle and under the influence of contraceptive steroids. (In) *Contraception and Mechanisms of Endometrial Bleeding* (d'Arcangues, C., Fraser, I.S., Newton, J.R. & Odlind, V., eds.), pp.53–72. Cambridge, England, Cambridge University Press.

Lorand, L. (1981). Proteolytic enzymes. (In) *Methods in Enzymology*, Vol. 80, Part C (Colowick, S. & Kaplan, N., eds.), pp.1–919. New York, Academic Press.

Moscatelli, D. & Rifkin, D.B. (1988). Membrane and matrix localization of proteinases: a common theme in tumor cell invasion and angiogenesis. *Biochimica et Biophysica Acta*, **948**:67–85.

Rath, W., Adelman-Grill, B.C., Pieper, U. & Kuhn, W. (1987). Collagen degradation in the pregnant human cervix at term and after prostaglandin-induced cervical ripening. *Archives of Gynecology*, **240**:177–184.

Roswit, W.T., Rifas, L., Gast, M.J., Welgus, H.G. & Jeffrey, J.J. (1988). Purification and characterization of human myometrial smooth muscle collagenase. *Archives of Biochemistry and Biophysics*, **262**:67–75.

Smith, S.K. (1990). The physiology of menstruation. (In) *Contraception and Mechanisms of Endometrial Bleeding* (d'Arcangues, C., Fraser, I.S., Newton, J.R. & Odlind, V., eds.), pp.33–44. Cambridge, England, Cambridge University Press.

Vaes, G. (1985) Macrophage secretory products and connective tissue remodelling: role of macrophage enzymes and of 'matrix regulatory monokines'. (In) *Developments in Cell Biology. 1. Secretory Processes* (Dean, R.T. & Stahl, P., eds.), pp.99–117. London, Butterworths.

Vaes, G. (1988). Cellular biology and biochemical mechanism of bone resorption. A review of recent developments on the formation, activation, and the mode of action of osteoclasts. *Clinical Orthopaedics and Related Research*, **231**:239–271.

Woessner, J.F. (1980). Collagenase in uterine resorption. (In) *Collagenase in Normal and Pathological Connective Tissues* (Woolley, D. & Evanson, J.M., eds.), pp.223–239. Chichester, England, John Wiley & Sons.
Woessner, J.F. (1982). Uterus, cervix and ovary. (In) *Collagen in Health and Disease* (Weiss, J.B. & Jayson, M.I.V., eds.), pp.506–527. Edinburgh, Churchill Livingstone.

Discussion

Weintraub. I think there is some evidence that cytoskeletal proteins in the cytoplasm are not only involved in and attached to proteins in cell membranes, but may actually be linked with non-collagen proteins that are in the immediate cellular matrix via desmosomes or other structures.

Eeckhout. We have to consider that local, microenvironment and cytoskeletal proteins play a very important role in maintaining contact and communication between cells. For example, macrophages are able to create under themselves a microenvironment which can be very acidic and where lysosomal enzymes can be active because the pH is between 5 and 6. Cytoskeletal proteins probably also play a role in this morphological control of tissue destruction. I think it is always controlled, everywhere, very locally.

Naftolin. Although we have little information about tissue destruction in the myometrium and endometrium, we have considerable evidence about the cervix. The cervix contains primarily type I and type III collagen, and estrogen induces collagenolysis through collagenase. I think that similar actions may apply to the vessels that you are talking about. It has been our opinion that the primary event may be collagenase activation but cathepsins and other enzymes may also attack collagen. Why are they able to attack the collagen so well? It is because estrogen induces hyaluronic acid. Hyaluronic acid is a polyhydrated glycosaminoglycan which makes for a much more soluble environment in which these actions occur. I think that cervical ripening is a good model for collagenase action. Every obstetrician who has ever felt the cervix knows what happens: it ripens, it gets soft, it becomes so hydrated that sometimes it cannot be felt. Histologically, ultrastructurally, biochemically, we see these same things occurring when exogenous prostaglandin is applied. I see close parallels with the present situation and I would urge people to take the same techniques and apply them to the study of uterine and endometrial vessels.

Ludwig. Gynecologists have known for more than 20 years that menstrual blood is full of fibrin degradation products and must follow considerable activation of fibrinolysis. I would like to ask you, from which cells in the tissue are plasminogen activators released?

Eeckhout. There are two main sources for plasminogen activator. One is vascular and the other is from certain tissues. Many proteolytic enzymes are also able to activate plasminogen. But the other aspect is a deficiency of inhibitors. In general, in the blood, everything is controlled by an abundance and excess of inhibitors, and maybe in endometrial bleeding, you have a situation where there is an escape of plasminogen-activator activity from the inhibitors which are neutralized by other proteolytic enzymes.

Bischof. I wonder if there is a local regulatory mechanism. You know that the extracellular matrix is full of glycosaminoglycans and they are usually co-factors of inhibitors, for instance antithrombin III, which heparin accelerates. I wonder if the endometrial smooth muscle cells are capable of activating local enzymes so that, through estradiol or progesterone effects, you would have a regulatory mechanism?

Eeckhout. The effect of glycosaminoglycans, and especially heparin, on enzymes is non-specific. These are polyanionic molecules, and you will find, for example, that heparin has an effect on 50% of the enzymes studied, and this, I think, is non-specific.

Naftolin. The reproductive tract contains the 'renin–angiotensin' system and plasminogen activator activates renin from inactive renin. These tissues all have angiotensin receptors and if you make angiotensin, you could activate this cascade.

Sheppard. In response to Dr Ludwig's comment, we now have a reasonable amount of evidence to suggest that the tissue plasminogen activator is being produced by vascular endothelial cells in endometrium.

Casey. Endometrial stromal cells do, in fact, make tissue plasminogen activator as well as urokinase. This was demonstrated *in vitro* by an activity assay and there was no plasminogen-activator inhibitor produced in that particular cell culture.

Endometrium: tissue remodelling and regeneration

HANS LUDWIG*, HILDEGARD METZGER** AND MARTINE FRAULI*

*Dapartment of Obstetrics and Gynecology, University of Basel, Basel, Switzerland.
**Department of Obstetrics and Gynecology, University of Freiburg, Freiburg, Federal Republic of Germany.

Abstract

A series of micrographs obtained on specimens from 22 uteri is presented. The elective hysterectomy was dated according to the menstrual cycle. Cases with known endometrial pathology, gross uterine pathology or preceding irregular menstrual bleeding were excluded from the evaluation. Uterine specimens from day 1 through day 8 of the cycle were collected; small parts of the endometrium were critical-point dried, gold sputtered and prepared for scanning electron microscopy.

Twenty-four hours after the onset of menstrual bleeding, the uterine cavity shows desquamation of most parts of the lining surface epithelium but glandular stumps are well preserved. This result is in contrast with some other investigations based on biopsies from menstrual endometrium. On the first day of menstrual bleeding, opened sections of small endometrial vessel segments can be observed running parallel to the surface. Those vessel segments are devoid of clots. On the second and third day of the menstrual cycle, the remaining glandular stumps are transformed by outgrowing epithelium. The outgrowing process is directed towards the denuded endometrial stroma surrounding the glands which is then partially covered by fibrin mesh. Lysosomes and macrophages can be identified. The peak activity of those components taking part in the clearing process of the uterine slough appears to be on the third and fourth day. On the fourth day the newly formed lining surface epithelium already covers most parts of the interglandular area. Epithelial excess proliferations can then be seen resulting in transient micropolyp formation. On the fifth and sixth day of the menstrual cycle, the endometrial wound is completely re-epithelialized and it is only after that that the stromal tissue starts to grow and to remodel the internal surface of the uterine cavity. The total thickness of the endometrium increases by then. Final clearing of the uterine cavity takes place by extrusion of single cells out of the lining epithelium. The cellular surface of the lining epithelium starts to exhibit further differentiation with cilioneogenesis and the formation of microvilli.

Introduction

The endometrium is a tissue unique in that it undergoes cyclic breakdown and repair. No cicatrization takes place during the process of 'healing'. Desquamation and regeneration coexist, shedding appearing to be almost complete by 60 hours, whereas the regeneration of the surface lining epithelium of the endometrium starts as early as 36 hours after the onset of menstruation. The regeneration of the endometrium is completed by 140 hours after the initiation of the menstrual shedding (Nogales-Ortiz *et al.*, 1978) or even earlier (Ludwig & Metzger, 1976).

Materials and methods

The preparations shown have been collected during two decades from 22 dated hysterectomy specimens. The present study includes three cases which have been described in a previous publication (Ludwig & Metzger, 1976).

The *dating* was according to basal body temperature chart and history confirmed by estradiol serum level, which was checked the day before surgery. The ages of the patients were in the range of 24–50 years old. Cases with known endometrial pathology or with irregular uterine bleeding were excluded from this series. Those criteria for exclusion made the investigation time consuming and difficult. Only a few cases per year were finally eligible. The patients were surgically treated by the first author in the Departments of Obstetrics and Gynecology in either Essen (1972–83) or Basel (1983–88).

Preparation

The specimens are transferred as rapidly as possible into 0.9% saline solution. They are properly washed several times before further procedure. The following steps of the preparation procedure are performed under continuous observation with the dissecting microscope ($\times$ 6.3 to $\times$ 16). The side to be examined is placed upwards and pinned to a thin cork plate. The cork plate is put into the fixation medium, keeping the pinned samples upside down in the fluid. The fixative is 2.5% solution of glutaraldehyde. Diluent is 0.1 mol/l phosphate buffer pH 7.4 (osmolarity 300 mosmol). After a fixation time of approximately 24 hours, the tissue sample is minced in order to achieve its definitive size (4x4 mm). After repinning these small particles are fixed for another 8 hours. The second fixation medium is a renewed solution of glutaraldehyde. The specimens are then dehydrated in a graded ethanol series (30–50–70–80–90–96–100% ethanol), each specimen being twice in each concentration for 2–4 hours. The last bath is pure amylacetate. Then the probes are subjected to critical-point drying with carbon dioxide followed by sputter coating with gold in a high-vacuum evaporator. The coating thickness achieved is 10–20 nm. After coating, the specimens are stored again in a desiccator containing silica gel until examination by scanning electron microscopy (SEM). The material is observed at different tilts, usually 30° and the SEM (Cambridge Instrument Comp. S 4-10) is adjusted at an accelerating voltage of 20 keV during analysis and microphotography. Different apertures are used.

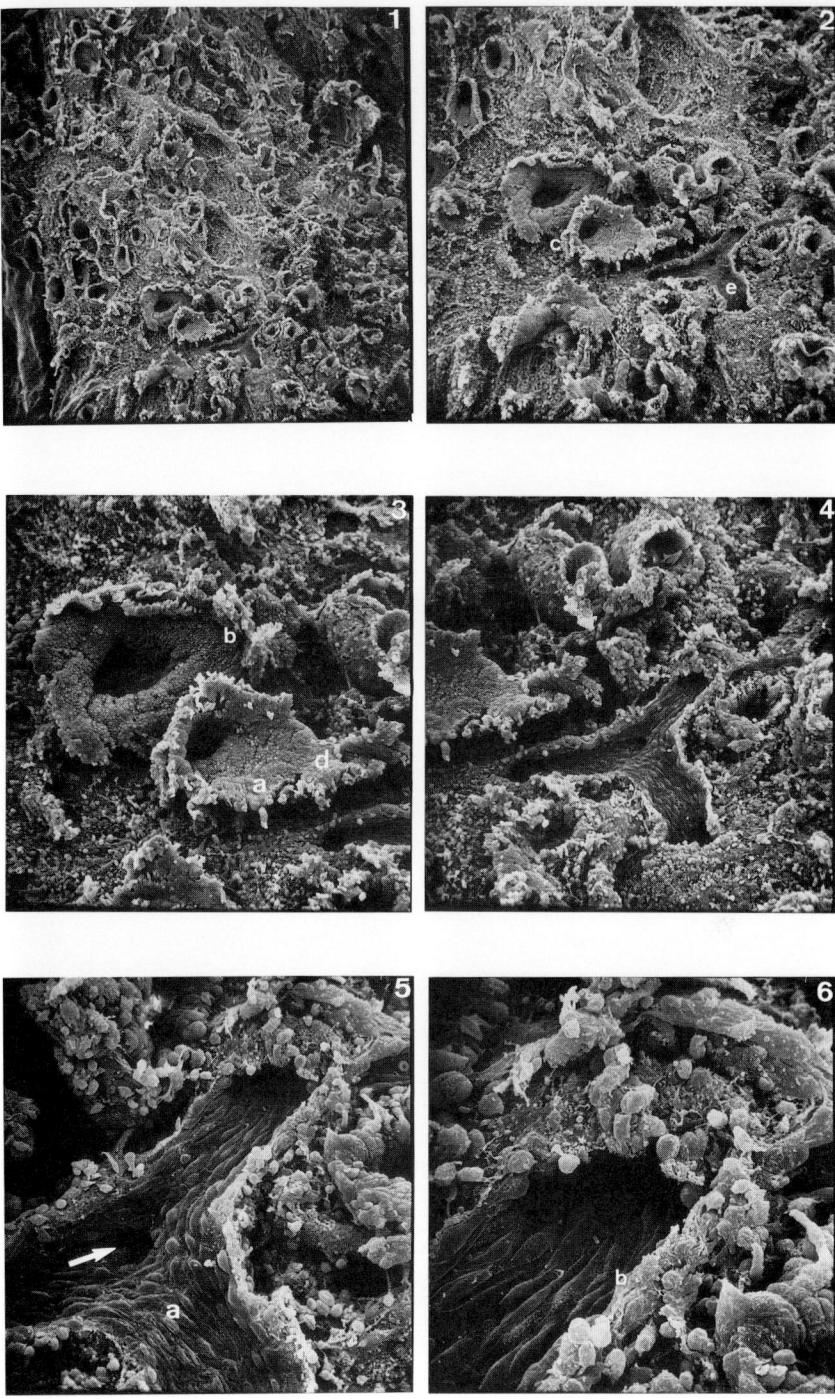

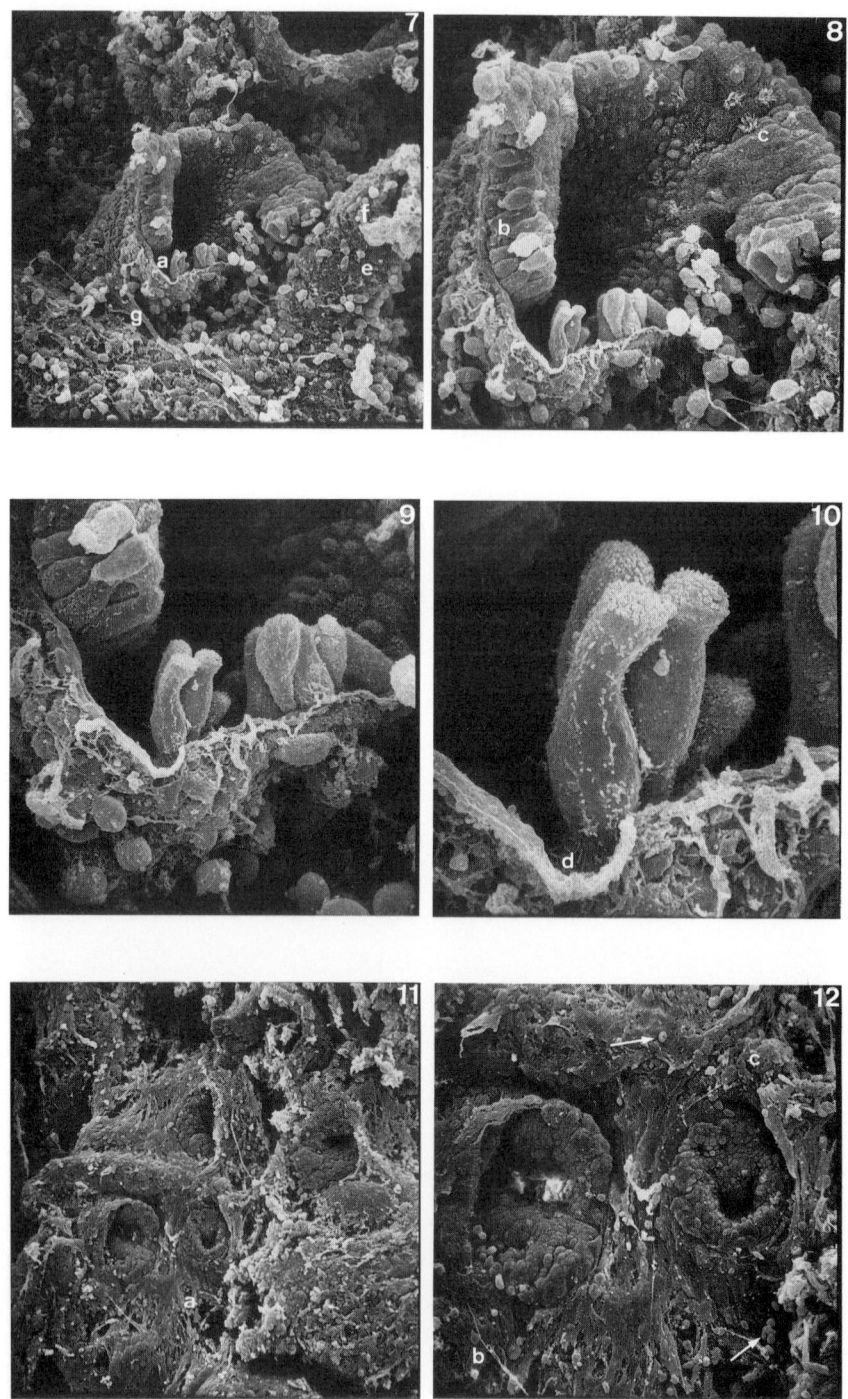

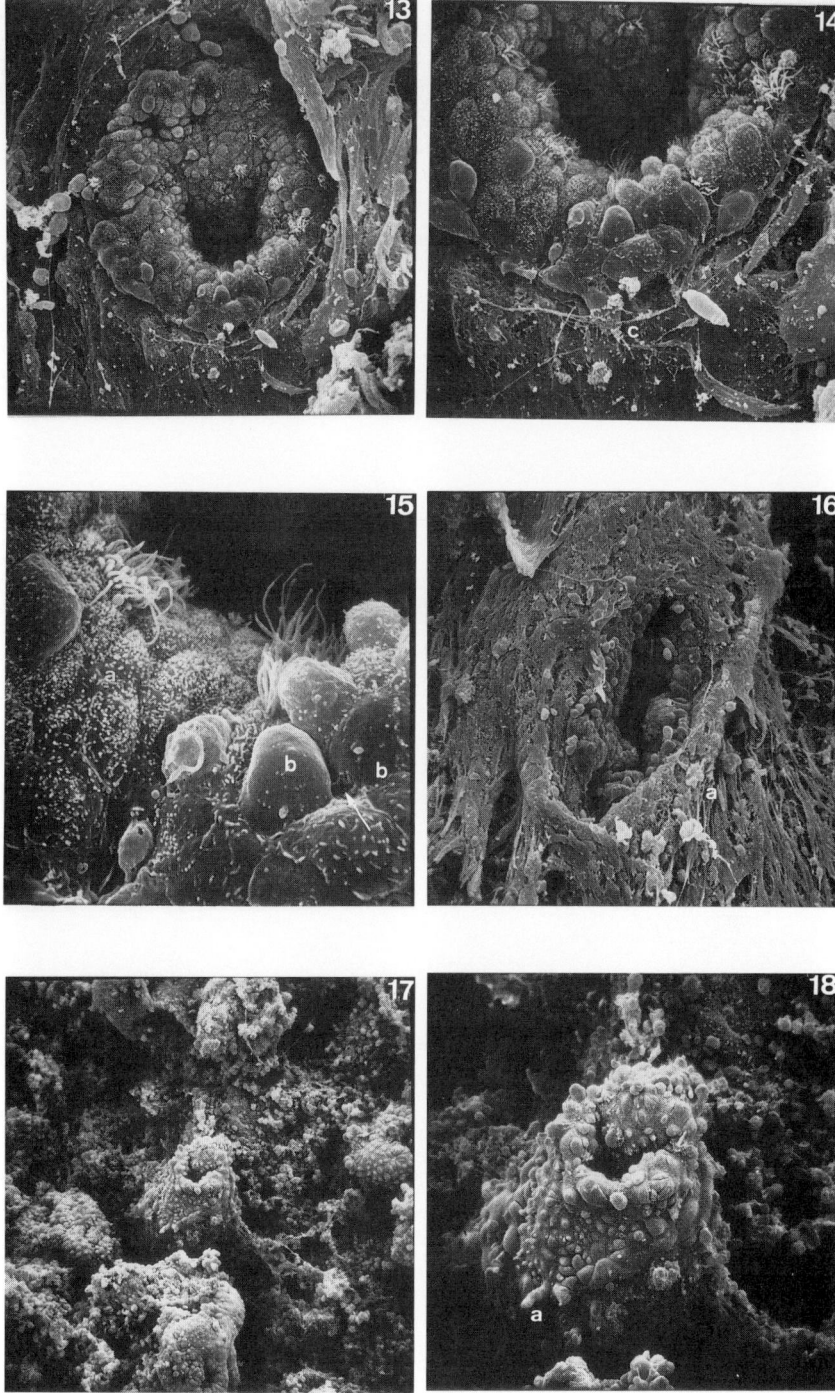

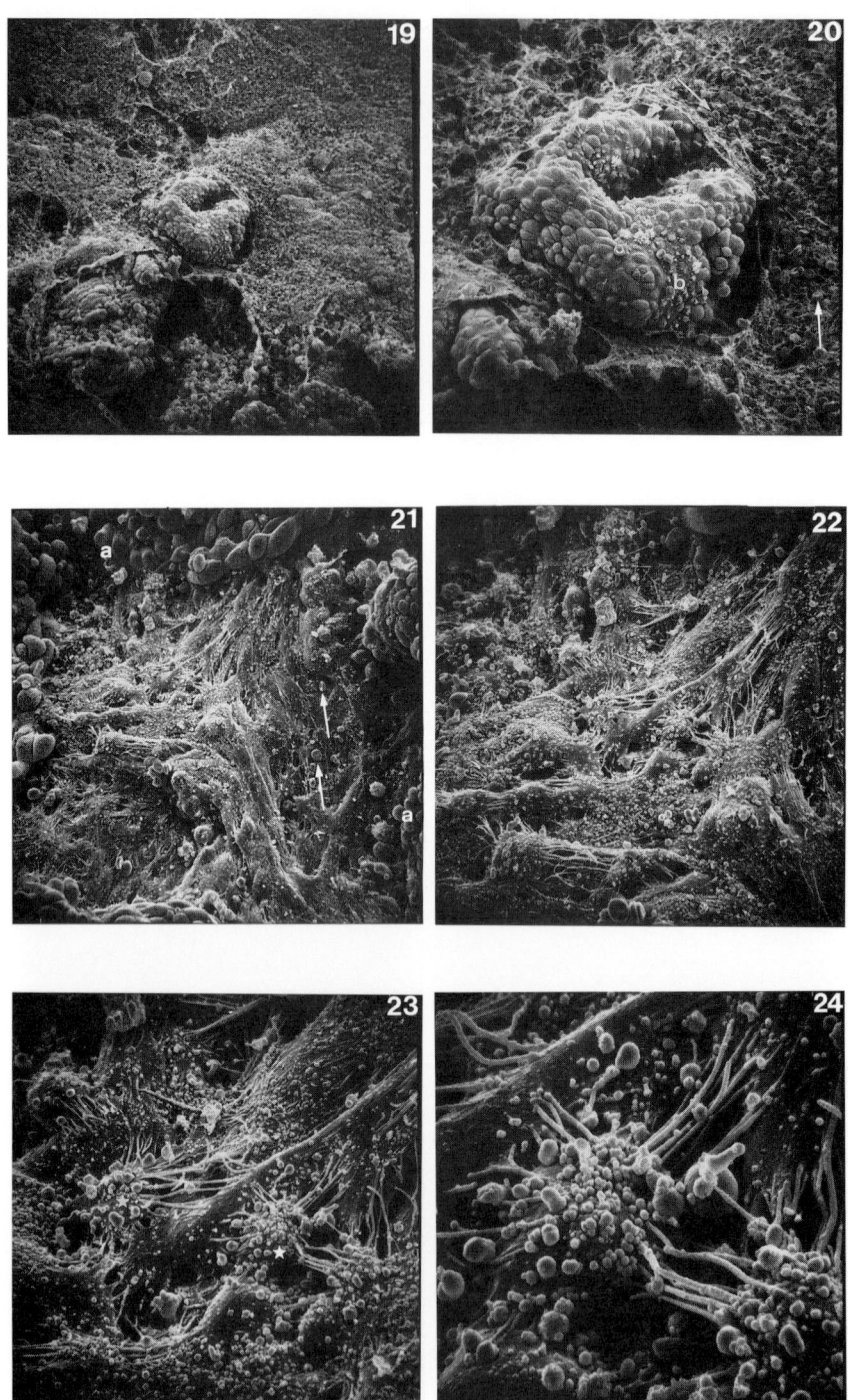

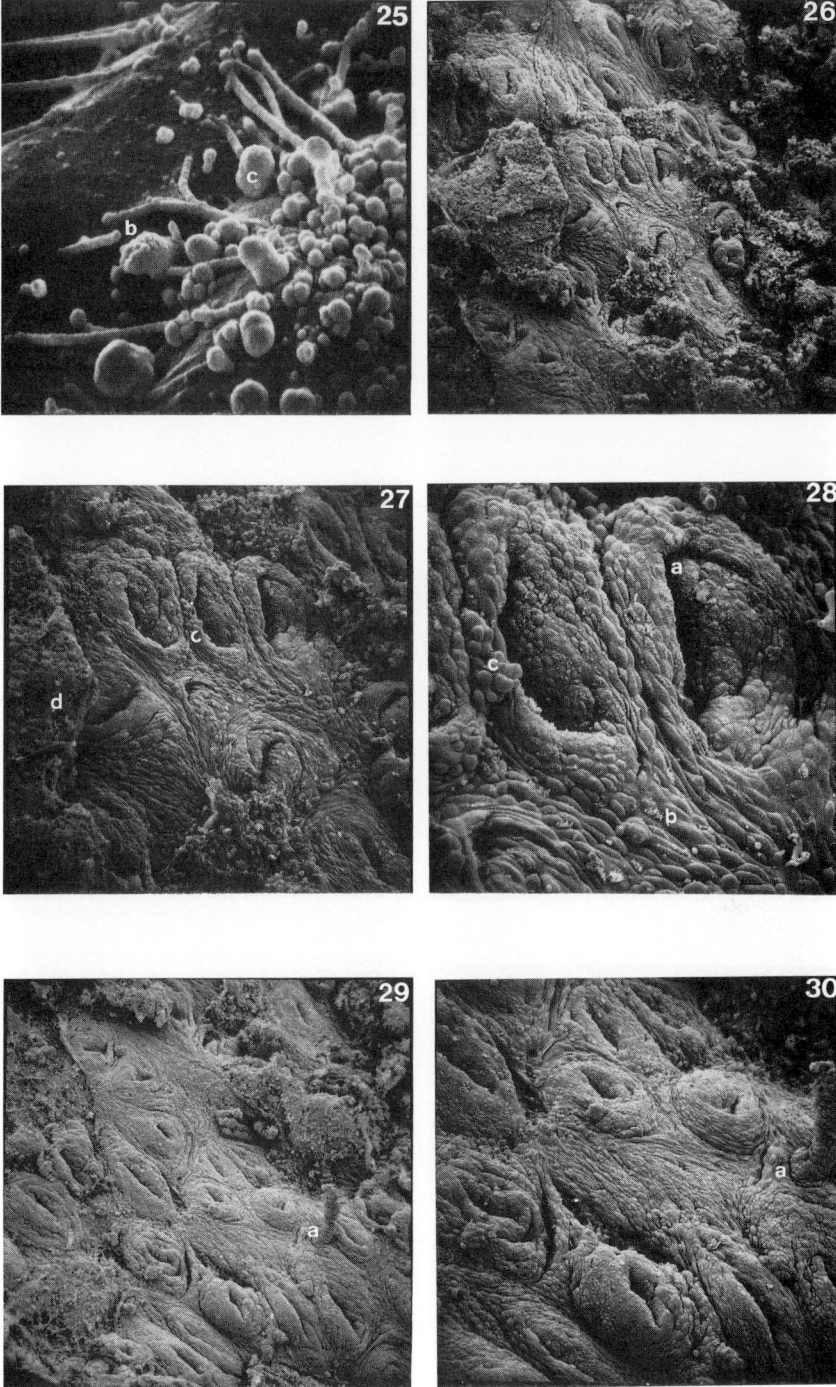

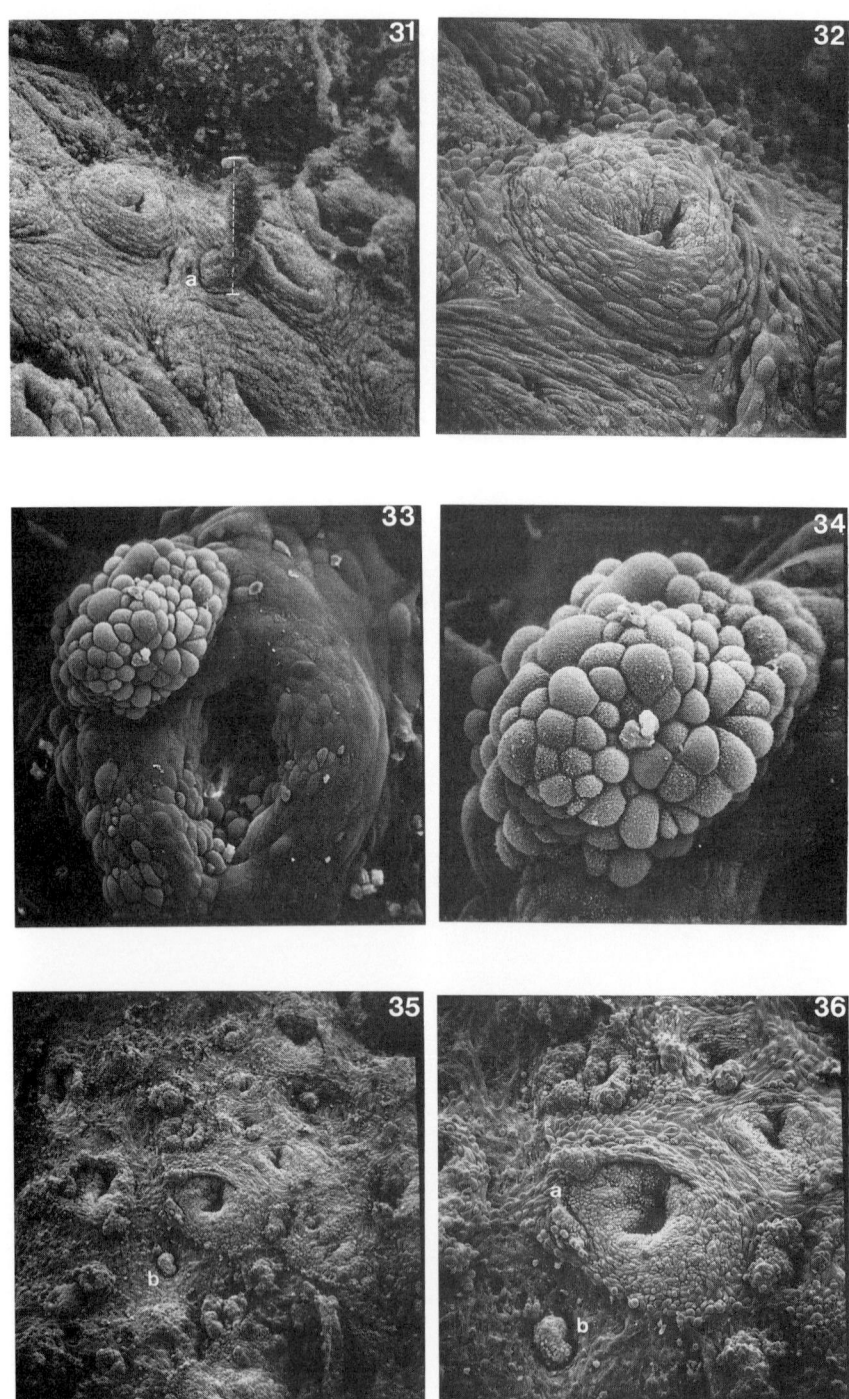

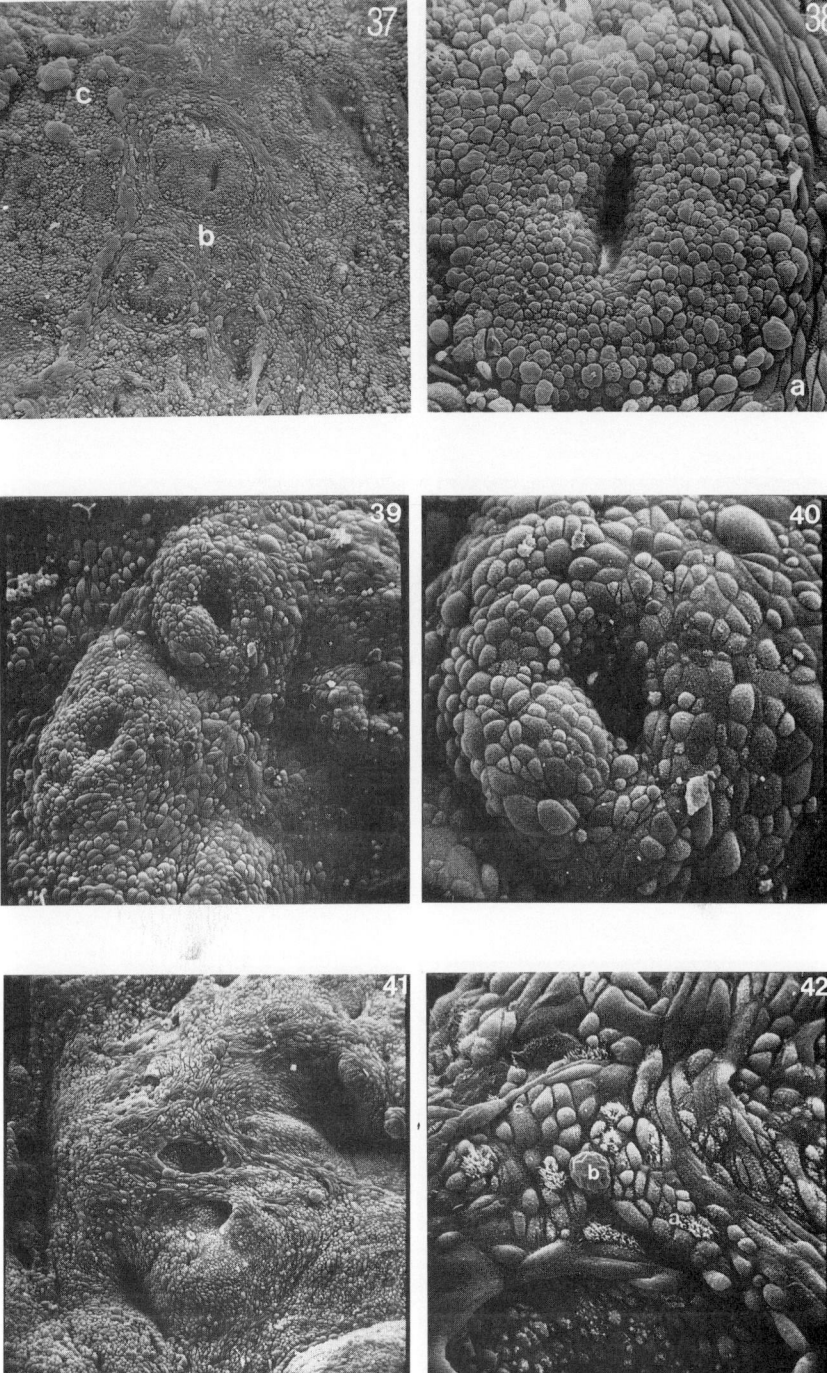

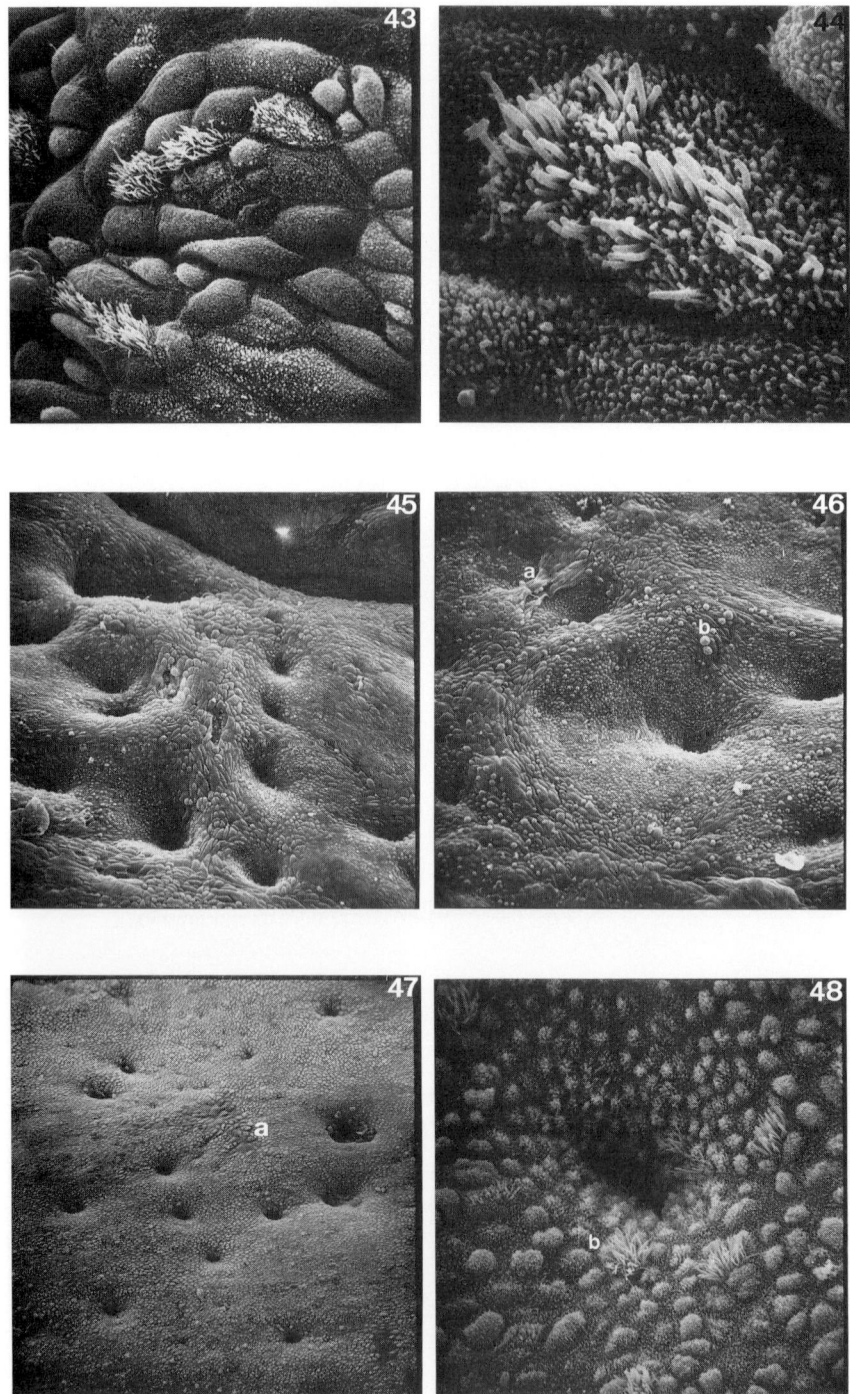

Figs. 1–48 Scanning electron microscopy photomicrographs.
Figs. 1 (× 50), **2** (× 100) and **3** (× 200) *24 hours after the onset of menstrual bleeding.*
A segment of the fundal area is shown. The striking feature is the numerous glandular openings which differ in their respective luminal width: 60–120 μm. The margins of the glandular stumps expose torn monolayer epithelium (a in Fig. 3), partially lined by epithelial debris (b in Fig. 3).

These stumps stand out from the surface level (c in Fig. 2) of the menstrual uterine wound, which is approximately 50 μm below the upper margin of the remaining glandular stump. Parts of the lining surface epithelium are preserved (d in Fig. 3), but only so when adjacent to the glandular stumps and in non-interrupted connection with them. Most of the interglandular surface is destroyed by menstrual tissue desquamation, and stromal components can be seen: connective tissue fibres and round-shaped single cells lying at the surface. During the preparation, blood components and slough which might have been loosely attached to the uterine wound structures were washed away. Near the glandular openings, some of which are still in connection with collar remnants of lining surface epithelium, a few small blood vessels (e in Fig. 2) can be identified. They are lying open; their endothelium is intact and devoid of thrombotic material. These open sections of superficial endometrial vessels represent the *original sites of menstrual bleeding.*

Figs. 4 (× 200), **5** (× 500) and **6** (× 1000) These figures demonstrate a section of Figs. 1 and 2. *24 hours after the onset of menstrual bleeding.* The micrograph section shows the branching of a small endometrial vein which was obviously torn open during the process of menstrual desquamation of the zona compacta. The layer of endothelial cells (a in Fig. 5) forms the vessel wall. From their shape and formation, they can clearly be identified as endothelial rather than epithelial (Figs. 4 and 5). The vessel wall is thin; its only layer consists of endothelial cells which are attached to a basement membrane (b in Fig. 6). Note the opening of a small joining vessel located at the area of ramification (arrow). There is no thrombotic material within the vascular lumen. Small isles of lining surface epithelium are in connection with parts of the collar of the gland openings.

Figs. 7 (× 500), **8** (× 1000), **9** (× 2000) and **10** (× 5000) *24 hours after the onset of menstrual bleeding.* The *microarchitecture* of a remaining gland opening is shown within the uterine menstrual wound. The composition of the glandular epithelium can be followed along the upper margin. Parts of the uppermost edge were obviously torn and destroyed, presumably by the process of menstrual desquamation. Across the funnel-shaped opening left over, the margin of glandular epithelium is seen bending horizontally and turning into lining surface epithelium. The latter is characterized by slightly flattened cells (a in Fig. 7). The glandular epithelium is a monolayer of cylindrical-shaped cells (b in Fig 8). A few ciliated cells (c in Fig. 8) are interspersed among the secretory cells.

Larger magnification shows the cylindrical shape of these cells. Their slight bulgings are alternatively luminal or basal. These changes of shape result in a certain veneering effect for stabilization of the epithelial monolayer. The tender anchoring of glandular cells in the basement membrane (d in Fig. l0) is demonstrated.

Adjacent to the glandular stump, a small endometrial vessel is seen sticking out from the stromal ground. The lumen of this vessel (e in Fig. 7) is narrow compared to the glandular width. The vessel bears a crown of thrombotic debris (f in Fig. 7). A collagen fibre is inserted at the flank of the glandular stump (g in Fig. 7). This fibre is presumably part of the stabilizing structures of the endometrial stroma.

Figs. 11 (× 200) and **12** (× 500) *Second day of the normal cycle.*
Several gland openings are embedded in an non-homogeneous layer of slough material which is formed by the menstrual desquamative process. This material contains coarse fibres of the endometrial stroma (a in Fig. 11), blood cells (arrows in Fig. 12), fibrin fibres (b in Fig. 12), and remnants of incompletely shed lining surface epithelium (c in Fig. 12). The gland openings are clearly visible. Their margins appear rounded or smooth due to the newly formed cells of the collar. The shape change of those cells located at the margin of the glandular collar is interpreted as a sign of glandular epithelial growth. It is the *step of the re-epithelialization* of the menstrual wound, i.e. the de-epithelialized zone between the remains of the numerous endometrial glands.

Figs. 13 (× l000), **14** (× 2000) and **15** (× 5000) These figures demonstrate a section of Figs. 11 and 12. *Second day of the normal cycle.*
The collar of a gland opening is shown in more detail. Ciliated and non-ciliated cells of the glandular epithelium can be identified. Some of them are close to the margin. The apical portions of the non-ciliated glandular cells exhibit a differentiation of fine microvilli (a in Fig. 15). More laterally, the newly formed cells of the collar have considerably fewer microvilli. Their cell body is larger, their apical portion protruding (b in Fig. 15), some intercellular gaps are wider (arrow in Fig. 15) compared to the persisting glandular epithelium. Along the flank of the glandular stump one can see fibrin fibres with platelets attached (c in Fig. 14).

Fig. 16 (× 500) *Second day of the normal cycle; stabilization of the remaining glands.*
The remaining endometrial gland is stabilized by a fibrous network originating from the endometrial stroma. The collagen fibres (a) are inserted at the basement membrane of the gland along its flank. They form a kind of *sheath* (outside connective tissue, inside epithelium) which might protect the persisting endometrial gland from collapsing during the process of epithelial growth from the gland.

Figs. 17 (× 200), **18** (× 500), **19** (× 200) and **20** (× 500) *Third day of the normal cycle.*
The endometrial glands grow. Their appearance is *cone*-shaped (Figs. 17 and 18) or *cake*-shaped (Figs. 19 and 20). The margins of the gland openings do not show the tears seen previously due to the desquamative menstrual process, but they are completely rounded because of the new formation of *polymorphic* glandular cells. Occasionally small cellular

protrusions can be seen (a in Fig. 18). These protrusions consist of very few cells and might represent the beginning of transitional micropolyps (see sixth day preparations). Groups of newly generated *ciliated* cells – all in the state of cilioneogenesis – can assemble by forming small descending streaks along the collar of outgrowing glandular epithelium (b in Fig. 20). The menstrual wound around the glands still remains to be covered by shreds of fibrin mesh which contain all forms of blood cells. Note the erythrocytes (arrows in Fig. 20) for better understanding of the size relation of the different compounds.

Figs. 21 (× 500), **22** (× 1000), **23** (× 2000), **24** (× 5000) and **25** (× 10000) *Fourth day of the normal cycle.*
The clearing of the postmenstrual slough and the re-epithelialization of the uterine cavity occur in parallel. Fig. 21 shows a still de-epithelialized centre of naked stroma surrounded by newly formed lining surface epithelium (a in Fig. 21). This central field is occupied by a triangle consisting of coarse fibres. The fibres represent part of the yet uncovered stromal ground on top of the basal endometrium which has survived menstrual desquamation. However, the structure is filled with globules of differing size (0.1–5.0 μm).

The globules are thought to be *lysosomes*. Their function is to clear the menstrual wound from cell debris and blood remnants and, by so doing, facilitate the re-epithelialization of the uterine cavity. The proliferating cells of the newly formed lining surface epithelium sprout from all directions towards the uncovered centre. Presumably the presence of lysosomes will enhance the closing of remaining epithelial defects.

With larger magnifications (Figs. 22–25), some giant cells (stars in Fig. 23) with multiple, slender *pseudopodia* can be identified beneath the layer of scattered lysosomal particles. The appearance of those cells with pseudopodia is known from *macrophages* in culture. Note the pseudopodia of the supposed macrophages protruding from the cell body and reaching out for the various fibrous structures in their immediate surroundings (b in Fig. 25) and the lysosomes of differing size (c in Fig. 25). The arrows in Fig. 21 show the erythrocytes.

Figs. 26 (× 100), **27** (× 200) and **28** (× 500) *Fourth day of the normal cycle.*
The lining surface epithelium covers almost completely the areas between the gland openings. The process of outgrowing of the epithelium from the glands temporarily produces bulgings just beneath the orifices (a in Fig. 28). The newly formed lining surface epithelium consists of fusiform cells; some prospective ciliated cells show *cilioneogenesis* (b in Fig. 28). Shape and arrangement of cells change once they have left the gland: cells are larger and the arrangement of the new lining reflects the dynamics of fast growth. The pattern of the interglandular lining epithelium resembles confluences of streaks of outgrowing epithelium convening from different directions: multiple rows of strands of cells in triangular and arched forms come into existence. A considerable variation of forms – known from epithelial tissue cultures – can be observed in those natural preparations, all modelling the process of growing.

In several parts, but always close to glands, piles of epithelial cells might heap up into *micropolyps* (c in Figs. 27 and 28). Patches of fibrin meshes can be identified where the closure of the uterine menstrual wound is not yet completed (d in Fig. 27). At this stage the endometrium is thin, the new stroma beneath the epithelial layer meagre. The distance between single and slightly prominent gland openings is small, their orifices rather large, and the areas of the interglandular lining epithelium is flat or even sunk down.

Figs. 29 (× 100), **30** (× 200), **31** (× 200), **32** (× 500), **33** (× 500) and **34** (× 1000) *Fourth day of the normal cycle.*

The formation of *micropolyps* can be observed at this stage of re-epithelialization of the postmenstrual uterine wound. Some are even piled up in cellular pillars measuring up to 35 μm in height (a in Figs. 29, 30 and 31); others are smaller but bulkier with broader diameters, proliferating from the very edge of endometrial glands. The latter exhibit a certain cake-shaped prominence (Fig. 32) and are surrounded by rows of newly formed lining surface epithelium.

Figs. 35 (× 100) and **36** (× 200) *Fourth day of the normal cycle.*

The section shows an area partly covered by newly formed lining surface epithelium and partly still uncovered (lower left corner of micrograph in Fig. 35). The irregular appearance of this part of the postmenstrual uterine cavity is due to a transitional multiple micropolyp formation in the course of re-epithelialization (a in Fig. 36). These micropolyps are obviously avascular and form as small multicellular proliferations from outgrowing epithelium. Thus they are located close to the gland orifices. Clumps of cells can also be seen in some denuded holes – preformed spaces in the stroma for glands not yet developed or destroyed by the menstrual desquamative process? (b in Fig. 35). The epithelium which is growing out of the glands leaves the glandular structure by forming parallel strands of fusiform cells. The direction of growth of these strands describes a spiral form (Fig. 36). At the extreme end of the epithelial spiral, a multicellular polyp is ultimately formed, probably as the result of a certain degree of overgrowth. The rounded cake-shaped architecture of the gland, where the re-epithelialization has started from, obviously influences the alignment of the rows of newly formed cells which become the lining surface epithelium.

Figs. 37 (× 100) and **38** (× 500) (Posterior wall of the uterine fundus.)
Figs. 39 (× 200) and **40** (× 500) (Side wall of the uterine fundus.) *Fifth day of the normal cycle.*

Endometrial gland openings are encased in an uninterrupted layer of lining surface epithelium. The postmenstrual endometrial wound is closed. The appearance of the lining surface epithelium is determined by slightly polymorphic cells without detectable apical differentiation (absence of microvilli). Adjacent to the gland orifice, the lining cells are preferentially fusiform (a in Fig. 38); further away from the glands they assume the aspect of a more cobblestone-like pattern (b in Fig. 37). Scattered fields of some larger polygonal cells can be observed. They appear to be lifted from the ground level by their size and composition. These formations are interpreted as micropolyps in the state of levelling off (c in Fig. 37). Other gland orifices, preferentially those from the sides of the fundal endometrium, are still prominent and open out from a small cone of cells, but again the general appearance of their cellular composition is that of a slightly polymorphic layer of densely packed polygonal epithelial cells (Figs. 39 and 40).

Figs. 41 (× 200), **42** (× 1000), **43** (× 2000) and **44** (× 10000) *Seventh day of the normal cycle.*

The lining surface epithelium is completely restored. *Cilioneogenesis* starts simultaneously with the faster growth of the endometrial stromal tissue. The consequence is the increase of the interglandular endometrial stroma which leads to the formation of cushion-like bulgings of the endometrial surface. Consequently, the gland openings sink down below surface level.

Ciliated cells are clearly visible, but sprouting *cilia* are not yet fully developed at this stage (a in Fig. 42). Detail magnifications show ciliated cells in various phases of cilioneogenesis (Figs. 43 and 44). The cilia in most of these cells have reached only half of their final length. Whereas *microvilli* of the ciliated cells are normally developed at this time, most of the non-ciliated cells just start to produce this type of apical differentiation (Fig. 43). Few single standing cells within the compound of the lining surface epithelium exhibit wrinkles in their apical membranes and, although large, seem to be deflated (b in Fig. 42). They also seem to be involved in a process of detachment through a loosening of their intercellular connections. This phenomenon is interpreted as a further sign of *clearing* of the endometrial surface. Some other cells which keep their fusiform shapes and their tightness form small bridges above the epithelial surface layer (c in Fig. 42).

Figs. 45 (× 200) and **46** (× 200) *Eighth day of the normal cycle.*

The endometrial surface has become homogeneous and smooth. However, the orifices of the endometrial glands are still seen to be sunk deeply below surface level. This is due to an increase of the stroma between the ascending parts of the glands together with a slight but remarkable decrease of the proliferation of the endometrial glands to full length. The endometrial stroma forms 'cushions' which bulge in the interglandular areas of the endometrial surface (Figs. 45 and 46). Cells lying adjacent to the orifices of the glands are considerably smaller and more homogeneous than the cells of the newly formed lining surface epithelium located far away from the glands. Obviously the lining surface epithelial cells – once outgrown from the endometrial glands – proliferate independently from the glandular epithelial cells. The encircling of gland openings by rows of lining surface epithelium occasionally produces cell bridges (a in Fig. 46). Globular protrusions of single cells (b in Fig. 46) could not be studied in further detail.

Figs. 47 (× 200) and **48** (× 2000) *Midcycle endometrial surface.*

For comparison with the previous micrographs, which demonstrate the remodelling of the endometrium stepwise after menstrual desquamation, the appearance of the normal midcycle endometrium is shown in order to illustrate the end-point of the *microtopographic* restoration of the endometrium during the first half of the normal cycle. The surface represents an almost homogeneous epithelial layer, only interrupted by glands. The gland openings are situated at greater distances from each other than before. The underlying stroma has produced greater distance as well as quite an even surface level free of the bulgings which have characterized the endometrium of the 7th/8th day of the cycle. Besides one small field of some larger polygonal lining surface epithelial cells (a in Fig. 47), the epithelium is composed of small polygonal cells, all bearing a dense turf of microvilli as their apical differentiation. At larger magnifications, fully developed ciliated cells (b in Fig. 48) and non-ciliated cells can be identified by their typical surface criteria. The transition from lining surface epithelium to periglandular and intraglandular epithelium – previously clearly visible – is now steplessly smooth.

Results

The results of the study are illustrated in a series of micrographs (see Figs. 1–48). Selected micrographs illustrate the sequence of events during the process of endometrial remodelling after menstrual desquamation. In preparations taken during the first 24 hours after the onset of menstruation, the stumps of endometrial glands are preserved. They stick out from the preserved basal layer of the endometrium. Examining whole-uterus specimens after hysterectomy (timed according to cycle dates), it can be stated that the functional endometrium of the uterine cavity is desquamated completely or at least to a great extent (more than 80%). Menstrual bleeding originates from open endometrial vessels which can be identified next to the openings of the preserved gland stumps. The wall of those vessels consists of an endothelial layer and a basement membrane. They have no media structure and might be classified as capillaries.

Since no thrombotic material could be detected in the lumina of those vessels, platelet aggregates and fibrin depositions as usually found in or around a bleeding vessel could not have been formed with any stability during the first 24 hours of menstruation, or may have been washed away by the menstrual blood flow. In other preparations which are rinsed and washed cautiously before further preparation, we do see remnants of blood clotting at the edges of a torn vessel. At the beginning of menstruation the blood loss must be regulated or limited by other means than by forming hemostatic plugs in the torn vessels. Extravascular debris and intravascular thrombotic material might easily be washed away by the menstrual bleeding at the first day of menstruation. This would not have been the case if hemostatic plugs had established the usual close contact between the injured vessel wall and platelet aggregates which soon become stabilized by fibrin. All those events fail to be seen in preparations from the bleeding menstrual wound.

Preparations of the second and third days of the cycle – menstrual bleeding still present – reveal considerable activities of the glandular epithelium. These activities result in outgrowing of strands of fusiform cells to form the lining surface epithelium. There are at this time wide areas left where the stromal tissue is still naked. At the bare stromal fibres, macrophage and lysosomal action for clearing the postmenstrual uterine cavity can be observed. Around the third day, maximum macrophage activity – as seen by surface ultramicroscopy – is reached and an abundant liberation of lysosomal globules (solid globes of different sizes) takes place along stromal fibres.

The proliferating process within the lining surface epithelium gives rise to certain epithelial growths which can be seen in preparations from the fourth to the sixth day of the normal cycle. Whether or not these epithelial growths occur in cycles other than normal is unknown. Under normal conditions the micropolyps appear and then fade away after the sixth day of the cycle, most probably by being discharged with the menstrual afterflow. A few of them might be levelled off or resorbed at the restoring endometrial surface. Although the micropolyps appear to be solid cellular compositions and hence avascular, their tearing off from the lining surface epithelium might nevertheless injure small vessels immediately beneath the epithelial surface, and the discharge of solid micropolyps can produce spotting at this particular time of the cycle.

Under regular conditions the postmenstrual uterine wound is covered *de novo* on the fifth or sixth day of the cycle. The interglandular stroma then starts to mould the endometrial cushion, which is at first bulky and uneven until the eighth day and then becomes smooth and even until midcycle, in parallel with the increase in thickness of the whole endometrial layer. Cilioneogenesis is seen at the lining surface epithelium from the fifth day on. Various forms of incomplete ciliation, i.e. cilia of unequal length and reduced in number, are observed. Ciliated cells will develop rapidly. Some days later, most of the ciliated cells bear 80–90 kinocilia, each of them 4–5 μm long. The microvillous brush of the ciliated cells develops earlier than the microvilli at the apical membrane of the non-ciliated cells. Since the lining surface epithelium of the endometrium originates from glandular epithelium, the ciliated cells of the lining surface are glandular derivatives. The information to create cilia must be carried with the outgrowing epithelial cell, and cilia do not start to sprout before the matrix cell has reached its definitive position within the epithelial compound. We were not able to show morphologic differences between the two types of ciliated cells, those with de-novo synthesis and others surviving the menstrual desquamation as part of the intraglandular epithelium.

After complete remodelling of the endometrial surface, some clearing process is still continuing: single cells are seen in a state of extrusion from the epithelial layer; others form bridges adjacent to the gland openings. These bridges from fusiform epithelial cells are also transitional signs of remodelling of the endometrial surface. The cells devoid of function are mostly more prominent than others, but their apical dome-shaped portion is wrinkled, a sign that evokes the impression of cell deflation.

Table 1. *Remodelling of the endometrium after menstrual desquamation:*
sequence of events by morphologic (SEM) observation of the uterine cavity

24 hours after onset of menstrual bleeding	Menstrual desquamation under *preservation of stumps* of endometrial glands
	Bleeding from opened endometrial vessels
	Washing away of menstrual debris
2nd/3rd day	Forming of endometrial gland stumps into *cones*
	Outgrowing of epithelium from endometrial glands
	Fibrin mesh formed
	Start of re-epithelialization
	Activity of *lysosomes* and *macrophages* for the clearing of debris
4th day	Forming of new lining surface epithelium
	Fibrin replaced by epithelium
	Epithelial excess proliferation and forming of *micropolyps*
5th/6th day	*Closure of the postmenstrual endometrial wound* by re-epithelialization
	Levelling off of micropolyps and *clearing* of epithelial excess proliferations
	Start of stromal growth
7th/8th day	Final clearing of the uterine cavity by extrusion of single cells
	Cilioneogenesis in ciliated cells of the lining surface epithelium
	Enhanced stroma formation (interglandular stroma growing fast, formation of 'cushions', gland openings sink down)
	Apical differentiation of cells of the lining surface epithelium (appearance of microvilli)

The sequence of main events during the remodelling process as seen by SEM in whole uterus preparations is summarized in Table 1.

Comments

Much of the present understanding of the phenomena of vascular breakdown and endometrial shedding is derived from experimentation with menstruating primates (Markee, 1940, 1950; Hartmann, 1962), in particular by autotransplanting the endometrium to the anterior chamber of the eye of the rhesus monkey. These early investigations stress the importance of marked spasms of the spiral arteries immediately preceding the onset of menstruation. This vascular reaction is followed by a rapid decrease in the thickness of the endometrial layer.

There is still controversy about the extent of the tissue shedding at menstruation. It was stated from examinations of human biopsy material that: 'at no time during menstruation was there extensive denudation of surface epithelium. In fact, the largest breaks were not more than 2 mm in diameter and most were less than 100 μm' (Flowers & Wilborn, 1978). The endometrial regions of the lower uterine pole and of the peritubal ostia (cornual area) seem to be more resistant to menstrual desquamation than the fundal endometrium (Ferenczy, 1976a, 1976b; Ferenczy *et al.*, 1979). The extensive investigation of hysterectomy specimens with SEM through the entire phase of menstruation starting 24 hours after the onset of menstrual bleeding revealed, however, that most parts of surface lining epithelium are shed, with only the epithelium at the glandular stumps left and, adjacent to it, naked endometrial stroma forming the surface. Isles of non-shed endometrium may be preserved within the fundal cavity (Bartelmez, 1957; Davie *et al.*, 1977; Nogalez-Ortiz *et al.*, 1978) preferably at the side walls (own observations) or at the cornua and at the isthmus. Flowers and Wilborn (Flowers & Wilborn, 1978; Wilborn & Flowers, 1984), using transmission electron microscopy, describe autophagia, hetero-phagia, extrusion of secretory products and elimination of fluids through intercellular spaces during the breakdown phase. Vessel wall lesions as characterized by holes in the endothelial layer, and interruptions of the basement membrane were found (Christiaens *et al.*, 1980). Our technique did not allow the investigation of deeper sections of the endometrial vasculature. The endothelium of the most superficial capillaries was intact as far as the open segments of the torn vessels could be followed.

Cell debris, macrophages and lymphocytes are seen at the large intercellular spaces immediately before breakdown (Davie *et al.*, 1977; Cornillie *et al.*, 1985). Macrophages were identified in the spaces of the stroma where they take part in the postmenstrual clearing process. It seems reasonable to assume that the accumulation of macrophages starts in the stroma in the last days of the cycle and remains present until the postmenstrual clearing of the endometrial surface is completed. On the third day of the normal cycle, if not before, fibres of the stromal network of the endometrium are surrounded by extracellular lysosomes which might have escaped from disintegrating stromal cells, from glandular or lining epithelial cells and from extravascular leukocytes. By rupturing, these lysosomes liberate enzymes, the principal being acid phosphatase, and digest many of the fibres exposed at the surface of the endometrial wound during the first days of menstruation. Phagocytosis of collagenous fibres by predecidual stromal cells has been reported by Cornillie *et al.* (1985).

The desquamative process probably follows a topographic sequence and the process might not have reached the same stage in each segment of the uterine cavity. Whether or not relaxin plays a role in the dissolution of reticulum fibres (Hoffmeister & Schulz, 1961) is not clear. Relaxin has been reported to stimulate dilatation and congestion of thin-walled capillaries located just beneath the surface (Dallenbach & Dallenbach-Hellweg, 1964; Bitensky & Cohen, 1965). The premenstrual congestion of the vasculature obviously facilitates the occurrence of tears and lesions in the vessel wall, so that torn vessels are present at the onset of menstrual bleeding. The overt bleeding is preceded by diapedesis, but at the onset of true menstrual bleeding ('first day of the cycle'), real vascular defects must be present. They were demonstrated here, as examination of the endothelium of the vessel was possible.

The activity of plasminogen activators rises just before menstruation and reaches a second peak on the first day of menstrual bleeding (Rybo, 1966;

Casslén & Åstedt, 1981). These fibrinolytic enzymes are possibly acting locally and they are confined to the intima of small arterioles, capillaries and venules, as well as to the stromal cells (Jirásek & Dyková, 1964) around the glands of the functional superficial layer of the endometrium (Weiss & Beller, 1969) and to the granulocytes (Henzl *et al.*, 1972). Progesterone intensifies the estrogen-primed accumulation of acid phosphatase in lysosomes (Godfrey *et al.*, 1981). Alkaline phosphatase increases cell membrane permeability, leading to the liberation of acid phosphatase (Sawaragi & Wynn, 1969). The preparation of their breakdown process and the clearing of the postmenstrual endometrial wound are parts of the same perimenstrual event. By means of morphology, some end-points of enzymatic processes can be visualized; their functional background must be elucidated by interpreting the results of investigation with different models and experimental conditions.

The predominant proliferative activity during endometrial regeneration is confined to the formation of a new surface epithelium, to the growth of surviving endometrial glands from stumps and – after the completion of the surface lining – the increase of the interglandular endometrial stroma. It is noteworthy that the stroma of the endometrium remains relatively inactive until the epithelial surface is restored. The first signs of epithelial regeneration are observed 24 hours after the onset of menstruation and complete surface re-epithelialization occurs at cycle day 5. The major part of the surface epithelium is regenerated from the glandular epithelium preserved in the glandular stumps, but the possibility cannot be excluded that, to a lesser degree, there is proliferation within the newly formed lining surface epithelium (see also Ferenczy, 1976b; Ferenczy *et al.*, 1979). The glandular edges form collars of new epithelium which extend toward the adjacent denuded surface. The direction of growth describes spiral paths around the cone-shaped or cake-shaped gland stumps (Ferenczy, 1976a, 1976b; Ludwig & Metzger, 1976). Epithelial bridges may arise close to the orifices (Ferenczy, 1976a). The glandular trunks are stabilized by connective tissue fibres (Ludwig & Metzger, 1976), which can act as strings guiding the epithelial rows. During the first 48 hours of the regenerative period, spreading and migration appear to be the principal means for rapid re-epithelization, whereas DNA synthesis, cell division and migration continue simultaneously thereafter until complete regeneration of the lining surface epithelium by the fifth or sixth day (Ferenczy *et al.*, 1979). Most of the denuded areas are covered with newly formed epithelium by day 4 of the normal cycle, coinciding with the decreased or eventually ceased menstrual blood flow.

We observed excess formation of epithelial sprouts resulting occasionally in micropolyps. Discharging those polyps might again create oozing or spotting after the menstrual blood flow has ceased. Once the epithelial cells of the lining surface entirely cover the uterine cavity, the layer looks like a cobblestone pavement. At this time the stroma is flat and underdeveloped; then it starts to form interglandular bulgings. Later on, towards midcycle, the surface gets gradually smoother and evenly formed, the gland openings still sunk down a little in between the surrounding tissue.

The proliferating process involves the capillaries as well. Endothelial cells start to show mitotic activity around day 4/5 of the normal cycle concurrently with the start of the growth of stromal tissue (Ferenczy, 1976b; present observations).

Conclusion

To our knowledge, the only recent study related to the mechanism of endometrial desquamation or regeneration is that of Wilborn and Flowers (1984). Questions concerning both desquamation and repair still remain open. It has been shown that the process of endometrial repair is initiated only when and where the zona basalis is denuded from the overlying spongiosa (Ferenczy, 1976a). The factors triggering the repair process are unknown. It remains to be determined, as suggested by Ferenczy *et al.* (1979), if it is a diffusible substance or the loss of an inhibitory substance that is responsible for the initiation of repair. However, a serial investigation of the morphology of the endometrial surface has shown that there exists an interrelationship between: (1) epithelial outgrowth from remaining glandular stumps, (2) formation of a new uninterrupted lining, and (3) initiation of the growth of the stromal tissue.

Acknowledgements

The work described in this chaper was supported by Schweizerischer Nationfonds zur Förderung der wissenschaftlichen Forschung, 3.082-0.87.

References

Bartelmez, G.W. (1957). The phases of the menstrual cycle and their interpretation in terms of the pregnancy cycle. *American Journal of Obstetrics and Gynecology*, **74**:931–955.

Bitensky, L. & Cohen, S. (1965). The variation of endometrial acid phosphatase activity with the menstrual cycle. *Journal of Obstetrics and Gynaecology of the British Commonwealth*, **72**:769–774.

Casslén, B. & Åstedt, B. (1981). Fibrinolytic activity of human uterine fluid. *Acta Obstetricia et Gynecologica Scandinavica*, **60**:55–58.

Christiaens, G.C.M.L., Sixma, J.J. & Haspels, A.A. (1980). Morphology of haemostasis in menstrual endometrium. *British Journal of Obstetrics and Gynaecology*, **87**:425–439.

Cornillie, F.J., Lauweryns, J.M. & Brosens, I.A. (1985). Normal human endometrium. An ultrastructural survey. *Gynecologic and Obstetric Investigation*, **20**:113–129.

Dallenbach, F.D. & Dallenbach-Hellweg, G. (1964). Immunohistologische Untersuchungen zur Lokalisation des Relaxins in menschlicher Placenta und Decidua.

Virchows Archiv für Pathologische Anatomie und Physiologie und für Klinische Medizin, **337**:301–316.

Davie, R., Hopwood, D. & Levison, D.A. (1977). Intercellular spaces and cell junctions in endometrial glands: their possible role in menstruation. *British Journal of Obstetrics and Gynaecology*, **84**:467–476.

Ferenczy, A. (1976a). Studies on the cytodynamics of human endometrial regeneration. I. Scanning electron microscopy. *American Journal of Obstetrics and Gynecology*, **124**:64–74.

Ferenczy, A. (1976b). Studies on the cytodynamics of human endometrial regeneration. II. Transmission electron microscopy and histochemistry. *American Journal of Obstetrics and Gynecology*, **124**:582–595.

Ferenczy, A., Bertrand, G. & Gelfand, M.M. (1979). Studies on the cytodynamics of human endometrial regeneration. III. *In vitro* short-term incubation historadioautography. *American Journal of Obstetrics and Gynecology*, **134**:297–304.

Flowers, C.E. Jr & Wilborn, W.H. (1978). New observations on the physiology of menstruation. *Obstetrics and Gynecology*, **51**:16–24.

Godfrey, K.A., Aspillaga, M.O., Taylor, A. & Lind, T. (1981). The relation of circulating progesterone and oestradiol concentrations to the onset of menstruation. *British Journal of Obstetrics and Gynaecology*, **88**:899–903.

Hartman, C.G. (1962). *Science and the Safe Period*. Baltimore, Williams and Wilkins.

Henzl, M.R., Smith, R.E., Boost, G. & Tyler, E.T. (1972). Lysosomal concept of menstrual bleeding in humans. *Journal of Clinical Endocrinology and Metabolism*, **34**:860–875.

Hoffmeister, H. & Schulz, H. (1961). Lichtoptische und elektronenoptische Befunde am Endometrium der geschlechtsreifen Frau während der Proliferations- und Sekretionsphase unter besonderer Berücksichtigung der Faserstrukturen. *Beiträge zur Pathologischen Anatomie und zur Allgemeinen Pathologie*, **124**:415–446.

Jirásek, J.E. & Dyková, H. (1964). Esterasepositive endometriale Stromazellen. *Gynaecologia (Basel)*, **157**:3–8.

Ludwig, H. & Metzger, H. (1976). The re-epithelization of endometrium after menstrual desquamation. *Archives of Gynaecology*, **221**:51–60.

Markee, J.E. (1940). Menstruation in intraocular endometrial transplants in the rhesus monkey. *Contributions to Embryology*. Carnegie Institution of Washington Publication No. 518, **28**(No. 177):219–308.

Markee, J.E. (1950). The relation of blood flow to endometrial growth and the inception of menstruation. (In) *Menstruation and its Disorders* (Engle, E.T., ed.), pp.165–185. Springfield, Illinois, Charles C Thomas.

Nogalez-Ortiz, F., Puerta, J. & Nogalez, F.F. Jr (1978). The normal menstrual cycle. Chronology and mechanism of endometrial desquamation. *Obstetrics and Gynecology*, **51**:259–264.

Rybo, G. (1966). Plasminogen activators in the endometrium. II. Clinical aspects. Variation in the concentration of plasminogen activators during the menstrual cycle and its relation to menstrual blood loss. *Acta Obstetricia et Gynecologica Scandinavica*, **45**:429–450.

Sawaragi, I. & Wynn, R.M. (1969). Ultrastructural localization of metabolic enzymes during the human endometrial cycle. *Obstetrics and Gynecology*, **34**:50–61.

Weiss, G. & Beller, F.K. (1969). Tissue activator of the fibrinolytic enzyme in the female reproductive system. *Obstetrics and Gynecology*, **34**:809–819.

Wilborn, W.H. & Flowers, C.E. Jr (1984). Cellular mechanisms for endometrial conservation during menstrual bleeding. *Seminars in Reproductive Endocrinology*, 2:307–341.

Discussion

Baird. Thank you, Dr Ludwig, for showing us an amazing collection of information about the process of normal menstruation. I think we should remember in the discussion that we are investigating whether we can identify a cause for abnormal bleeding and whether these appearances are also seen in women who have anovulatory bleeding, or bleeding with progestogens.

Ludwig. We have four uteri from progestogen-treated patients examined in the same way, and you see alterations of the endometrial picture. There is a lack of differentiation of the lining epithelium and there is a complete change in the number of ciliated cells. We have also found defective ciliated cells, and disrupted intercellular connections. But this is only a descriptive impression; we should now carefully examine it histochemically.

Brosens. How do you explain the fact that you see so few open vessels? Could it be that you get retraction of the spiral arteries?

Ludwig. The purpose of our study was to have information about the dynamics of restoration of the epithelium, so perhaps we did not pay too much attention to the vessel walls. I am sure that if I go through our specimens again we may see more open vessels. I do not think there is any vessel contraction because this occurs in the capillary network within the spongiosa of the shed endometrium or just on the border between basal endometrium and the shedding endometrium.

Baird. If I remember Markee's (1940) original description, the bleeding was focal – not all parts of the endometrium bled at the same time. Indeed, if one does calculations, if every single capillary in the endometrium was patent and bleeding, it would take the woman about half-an-hour to die. In fact the remarkable thing is that she only loses 30 ml over 5 days, so at any one time, there must be very few vessels bleeding. Now, is this due to the fact that there are only relatively few vessels damaged at a time or is it because the blood supply to a tree of vessels is obstructed or constricted intermittently?

Ludwig. I think the latter is true. We cannot see vasoconstriction by our method. What we see is hemostatic plug formation, fibrin formation, but during the preparation of the specimen, we wash away those clots which are mobile. In the hemostasis of endometrium, there are three factors playing a role. First, vasoconstriction; second, a hemostasis which is a balance between coagulation and fibrinolysis; and third, the rapid growth of epithelium which *de novo* covers open vessels. To find those naturally open vessels one needs chance or to know exactly where to look for them.

Courtoy. You have described in detail granules which are apparently resting on flattened epithelial cells. Have you performed transmission electron microscopy to see if those are blebs or granules and what is their content?

Ludwig. Yes, we did: they are not blebs, they are granules. I cannot tell you exactly what the content is, but it is a non-structural content which is electron dense. We can re-examine our preparations to get more information.

Johannisson. I have a question with regard to the breakthrough bleeding. Some years ago, Wilborn and co-workers did a study in which they administered to baboons various types of progestogens and they studied the endometrium with scanning electron-microscopy (unpublished observations). They found denudation and breaks in the lining epithelium and came up with the hypothesis that this could be responsible for the breakthrough bleeding. I wonder if you have seen anything like that in the human endometrium in these patients who have been treated with long-term progestogens?

Ludwig. Unfortunately, the picture in our progestogen users was not similar to that in the baboon.

Sheppard. I wish to ask two questions related to intermenstrual bleeding. First, am I correct in understanding that there was no loss of surface epithelium in breakthrough bleeding? The second question refers to the study that Dr Johannisson mentioned by Wilborn and co-workers. They also found an increase in the number of these micropolyps which you alluded to in the normal cycle and we have also found an increase in micropolyps in the endocervix in patients on low-dose oral progestogens. Do you know whether these micropolyps are vascularized or are they are just epithelial cells?

Ludwig. In answer to the first question, I do not think that intermenstrual bleeding is always linked with an intact surface layer. There are defects in the surface layer which means the loss of single cells or groups of cells, allowing visualization of the basement membrane of the underlying tissue. So breakthrough bleeding, to my knowledge and from our preparations, is at least partially linked with the loss of lining endothelium. With regard to your second question: yes, we have observed some tiny capillaries in cross-sections of micropolyps.

Naftolin. I am interested in what the glycocalyx of these cells is like because it is certainly responsive to sex steroids. Do you know if anybody has tried to find out whether the recognition molecules that are represented in the glycocalyx are different at different times of the cycle?

Ludwig. I am not aware of anybody having studied this topographically.

Åkerlund. In the late 1970s, we looked at the blood flow in the non-pregnant uterus and used beta-adrenoreceptor stimulants such as terbutaline, and relaxed the contractile activity (Åkerlund *et al.*, 1976). Then we got a very marked increase in blood flow. So we must not forget the contractile activity of the uterus, which can be extremely high at menstruation, with pressures far above systolic blood pressure.

Baird. I am glad you brought that up, Dr Åkerlund. The blood vessels that supply the endometrium have to get through the myometrium and I suspect that the myometrium can have a crucial influence on blood flow.

Findlay. In subjects who are on long-term progestogen therapy, is there any evidence of increased levels of white blood cells, macrophages, etc., which could provide the initial stimulus for breakthrough bleeding?

Ludwig. I have no evidence of that. As far as I know from the literature, there are no quantitative studies in this respect.

Sheppard. I would like to back that up. There is absolutely nothing in the literature to suggest that there is an increase in leukocyte infiltration in patients taking oral progestogens for a long time. The only time that has been quoted is obviously in relation to the hormone-releasing IUDs. But that is a foreign-body response. In our own studies, where we have looked at patients on low-dose oral progestogens, there have definitely been no differences in the number of leukocytes in the endometrium in the patients that were on this therapy.

Fraser. I do not believe that the morphologists have looked adequately for an influx of white cells in the endometrium of women exposed to progestogens who are bleeding. White cells have not been obvious to morphologists who have been scanning the sections, or perhaps there are relatively small numbers of these cells which are highly active and produce substances that could be locally toxic to cells.

References

Åkerlund, M., Andersson, K.-E. & Ingermarsson, I. (1976). Effects of terbutaline on myometrial activity, uterine blood flow and lower abdominal pain in women with primary dysmenorrhoea. *British Journal of Obstetrics and Gynaecology*, **83**:673–678.

Markee, J.E. (1940). Menstruation in intraocular endometrial transplants in the rhesus monkey. *Contributions to Embryology*. Carnegie Institution of Washington Publication No. 518, **28**(No. 177):219–308.

Angiogenic factors

PETER BÖHLEN

American Cyanamid Company, Medical Research Division, Pearl River, USA.

Abstract

Angiogenesis, the formation of new capillaries from existing blood vessels, occurs in normal tissue development and growth, inflammation, tissue repair and in a variety of pathological conditions, most notably tumour growth. It is characterized by several specific endothelial cell functions, including (a) local degradation of basement membranes surrounding existing blood vessels, (b) migration, (c) proliferation, (d) structural reorganization (lumen formation), and (e) functional maturation. Recently, a number of proteins, all potent inducers of blood vessel formation, have been chemically and biologically characterized. They include basic and acidic fibroblast growth factors (bFGF, aFGF), transforming growth factors-α and β (TGF-α and TGF-β), tumour necrosis factor-α (TNF-α) and angiogenin. Although very little is still known about the molecular mechanisms underlying angiogenesis, the biological study of angiogenic factors is beginning to provide insight into this complex process.

The FGFs may be considered prototype angiogenic factors because they stimulate all of the above-listed functions associated with new blood vessel formation. FGFs are widely distributed in vascularized tissues. The growth factors are largely stored in extracellular matrices of tissues, bound to heparan sulfate proteoglycans, and their activity may be regulated by cellular signals which liberate bound (and presumably inactive) mitogen by degrading extracellular matrix components. Such growth factor-activation mechanisms may be important in neovascularization associated with tissue development and repair, and in tumour metastasis and growth.

The angiogenic activity of TGF-β is based on an entirely different mechanism of action. TGF-β does not possess the aforementioned properties; in fact, it is inhibitory to some of them (migration, proliferation, extracellular matrix degradation). TGF-β is a potent chemoattractant for macrophages which are known to produce angiogenesis factors such as bFGF, TGF-α, and TNF. It is possible that TGF-β exerts angiogenic activity indirectly by attracting macrophages which in turn release angiogenic substances. Like FGF, TGF-β is distributed widely in tissues and therefore placed strategically to be involved in tissue development and repair.

TNF, like TGF-β, is a potent inhibitor of endothelial cell proliferation *in vitro*. Some evidence suggests that TNF may be a principal angiogenic activity of macrophages which may mediate neovascularization in inflammatory processes and wound healing.

Less is known about the mechanisms of action of the other angiogenic factors. TGF-α is mitogenic for endothelial cells *in vitro*. Angiogenin is not known to affect endothelial cells *in vitro*, but possesses some ribonuclease activity. The physiological involvement of TGF-α and angiogenin in neovascularization remains unclear.

The phenomenon of angiogenesis

Angiogenesis, or neovascularization, the formation of new capillaries from existing blood vessels, is a highly complex and still poorly understood process. The vascular endothelial cell, the principal cell type making up a capillary blood vessel, is intimately involved in this specialized form of organogenesis. Detailed observation of the angiogenic process, mainly at the morphological level, has provided evidence for the involvement of the endothelial cell in a number of cellular events. They include: (a) the local degradation of the extracellular basement membrane surrounding an existing blood vessel; (b) sprout formation, i.e. the coordinated migration of endothelial cells from an existing vessel outwards into the space created by the previous destruction of the extracellular matrix; (c) the proliferation of endothelial cells which, together with further outwards migration of the cells, contributes to sprout elongation; (d) the formation of a lumen by the endothelial cells making up the new sprout; (e) the joining of two vascular sprouts to form a functional capillary loop; and (f) the maturation of vascular cells for assumption of specific functions, e.g. the development of the blood–brain barrier (Folkman, 1984a; Folkman, 1986; Folkman & Klagsbrun, 1987; D'Amore & Thompson, 1987; Joseph-Silverstein & Rifkin, 1987; Zetter, 1988). It is currently thought that many, if not all, of those events are triggered and regulated by soluble factors that are released locally by vascular cells or by other cells that are located in close proximity to blood vessels. This concept originated from observations that tumours secrete diffusible factors which are capable of stimulating the growth of new blood capillaries in animals (Greenblatt & Shubi, 1968; Folkman et al., 1971). Although no tumour-specific angiogenesis factor has so far been discovered, the concept has been validated by the molecular characterization of angiogenic substances and endothelial cell growth factors common to normal tissues and tumours (Folkman, 1984b; Baird et al., 1986; Gospodarowicz et al., 1986).

Angiogenesis is a tightly regulated process. Under normal circumstances, endothelial cell turnover in blood vessels is very slow (in the order of years). However, vascular endothelial cells have the capacity to proliferate rapidly under the influence of appropriate stimuli. For example, in an adult healthy man neovascularization is practically absent, but it is induced dramatically by the occurrence of a wound. Regulation of neovascularization is even more evident in women where angiogenesis occurs cyclically during the menstrual cycle (maturation of follicles, formation of endometrium) and in pregnancy (placenta formation). Finally, unregulated neovascularization is a characteristic of many pathological states that include such diseases as chronic inflammatory states (arthritis, psoriasis), retinopathies and, most notably, solid tumours.

Angiogenesis occurs in almost all tissues under certain circumstances (organ growth or repair). Endogenous substances that can induce neovascularization have been found in many tissues and it is thought that such agents are present in most if not all tissues. Despite this, angiogenesis does not occur spontaneously, which points to the existence of distinct regulatory mechanisms. Furthermore, all evidence suggests that various angiogenic events may be regulated by quite different mechanisms. For example, angiogenesis associated with the female menstrual cycle is most likely to be regulated in some manner by sex steroid action which is almost certainly different from the regulation of wound healing or tumour-associated angiogenesis. Nevertheless, virtually nothing is presently known about the mechanisms that regulate various aspects of neovascularization and the action of angiogenic factors.

This is also true with respect to endometrial angiogenesis. While angiogenic activity has been found in endometrial tissue (Fuchs *et al.*, 1985), and some evidence suggests that many aspects of new blood vessel formation in the endometrium (Findlay, 1986) may be common to those occurring in other tissues under entirely different physiological or pathological situations, the physiological significance of this activity and its mode of action remain to be elucidated. Considering the very limited knowledge that is available on the subject of endometrial neovascularization, it will be most useful, at least for the time being, to review this topic in rather general terms. This chapter will therefore focus on angiogenic factors known today and their potential roles in neovascularization without regard for tissue-specific aspects that may exist.

Angiogenic factors

Fibroblast growth factor

Fibroblast growth factor (FGF) is by far the best understood angiogenic activity known. Two molecular forms of FGF exist: they are referred to as basic FGF (bFGF) and acidic FGF (aFGF). They were isolated, structurally characterized and their genes cloned in 1984–1986 (Thomas *et al.*, 1984; Böhlen *et al.*, 1984, 1985; Gimenez-Gallego *et al.*, 1985; Esch *et al.*, 1985; Abraham *et al.*, 1986a, 1986b; Jaye *et al.*, 1986). Both mitogens are proteins with molecular weights of 15–18 kd. A larger form of immunoreactive bFGF (25 kd) has also been detected (Moscatelli *et al.*, 1987). This, and other evidence (Abraham *et al.*, 1986a; Sommer *et al.*, 1987), suggests that bFGF, but not aFGF (Jaye *et al.*, 1986), may be synthesized from a larger protein precursor. Acidic and basic FGF are structurally related (55% sequence homology), suggesting evolution of the two mitogens from a common ancestral gene. Furthermore, bFGFs from different species (and to a lesser degree also aFGFs) are extremely conserved, indicating possibly strong evolutionary pressure to conserve an important biological function. Both types of FGF bind to the same cellular receptor and display similar biological activities; however, in most biological systems, bFGF is 10–100-fold more potent. For the purpose of this review, both FGFs are therefore referred to as FGF, except when specifically indicated.

Basic FGF has been isolated from many normal and tumour tissues; it is synthesized by many different normal and tumour cell types (Böhlen, 1989) and probably occurs in most if not all tissues. Acidic FGF, originally thought to be restricted to nervous tissues, was more recently also found in a number of other tissues and cell types. However, the distributions of aFGF and bFGF are not identical. For example, the vascular endothelial cell, an ubiquitous bFGF-producing cell (Schweigerer *et al.*, 1987), does not synthesize aFGF mRNA (Winkles *et al.*, 1987). FGFs have also been found in some body fluids, particularly in those of patients with diseases that have an important angiogenic element [urine of bladder carcinoma patients (Chodak *et al.*, 1988), ocular fluid of retinopathy patients (Baird *et al.*, 1985b), synovial fluid of patients with chronic inflammatory joint diseases (Hamerman *et al.*, 1987)]. Interestingly, however, FGFs have not been detected in blood (Thomas, 1987; Böhlen, 1989).

Many different cell types respond to FGF. For most of these, FGF is mitogenic, but in a variety of cells, FGF also induces non-mitogenic activities, e.g. the stimulation or suppression of the synthesis of particular cellular proteins, the induction or suppression of cellular differentiation, and the induction of cellular motility and migration. Basic FGF is a very potent agent: in most in-vitro test systems it is active at low picomolar concentrations and nanogram quantities elicit local in-vivo responses. The large variety of biological activities of FGF can now be understood in the context of potential physiological functions proposed for it. These include the promotion of angiogenesis, tissue repair and regeneration, a potential role in embryogenesis and cellular differentiation, the maintenance of certain neural functions, and modulation of some endocrine systems. In broader terms, FGF may constitute an important tissue hormone involved in the formation, maintenance and repair of tissues (reviewed by Baird *et al.*, 1986; Gospodarowicz *et al.*, 1986; Thomas, 1987; Böhlen, 1989).

The in-vivo angiogenic activity of the FGFs was established by a number of investigators (Gospodarowicz & Thakral, 1978; Gospodarowicz *et al.*, 1979; Esch *et al.*, 1985; Lobb *et al.*, 1985; ; Shing *et al.*, 1985; Thomas *et al.*, 1985; Moscatelli *et al.*, 1986). The angiogenic effects of FGFs were mainly studied in such animal models as the rabbit corneal implant assay (Gimbrone *et al.*, 1974), or the chick chorioallantoic membrane assay (Ausprunk *et al.*, 1975), which permit the observation of a developing capillary vasculature in areas of low-density vascularity. The mechanism of action of FGF in neovascularization is still unknown. However, as one might expect from an angiogenic factor, FGF acts on vascular endothelial cells in a number of ways thought to be relevant to angiogenesis. For example, FGF stimulates the proliferation of cultured vascular endothelial cells *in vitro* (Gospodarowicz *et al.*, 1976; Maciag *et al.*, 1982; Böhlen *et al.*, 1984, 1985) and *in vivo* (Buntrock *et al.*, 1984). It also promotes the migration of these cells (Terranova *et al.*, 1985; Presta *et al.*, 1986) and the release from them of the matrix-degrading proteases collagenase and plasminogen activator (Presta *et al.*, 1986; Moscatelli, 1987). Moreover, FGF induces a variety of additional in-vitro effects in endothelial cells, the potential role of which is not well understood but which might also support the process of neovascularization. These include (a) the maintenance of a properly differentiated state in cultured endothelial cells, expression of a non-thrombogenic apical surface (Vlodavsky *et al.*, 1979), preferential synthesis of certain types of collagen (Tseng *et al.*, 1982), delayed cell senescence (Gospodarowicz *et al.*, 1986), attachment to the substratum (Schubert *et al.*, 1987); and (b) the shaping of endothelial cells into tubular structures resembling blood capillaries (angiogenesis *in vitro*) (Jaye *et al.*, 1985; Montesano *et al.*, 1986). Furthermore, FGF induces the proliferation of smooth muscle cells (Gospodarowicz *et al.*, 1985a) and of pericytes (Buntrock *et al.*, 1984), both of which are associated with new blood vessels.

The question as to whether FGF is involved in the physiological or pathophysiological regulation of new blood vessel growth is obviously of great interest. Although there is no definite answer available at this time, the above mentioned activities of FGF on endothelial cells and the following additional evidence strongly support this notion. First, bFGF is present in relatively high quantity in probably all vascularized tissues, including tumour tissues. It would thus be strategically located to induce angiogenesis almost anywhere. Second, it is now known that during embryonic development of the kidney and brain, bFGF is expressed in these tissues at the time when vascularization of them begins (Risau, 1986; Risau & Ekblom, 1986; Risau *et al.*, 1988). Similarly, a role of FGF in tissue vascularization has also been suggested in the development and maturation of the ovarian corpus luteum in which a vascular network develops around the follicle and invades the previously avascular granulosa cell layer, presumably to facilitate luteinization and for nourishment of the developing corpus luteum. To this end, angiogenesis factors and endothelial cell mitogens have been found in the corpus luteum, follicles and follicular fluid (Jakob *et al.*, 1977; Gospodarowicz & Thakral, 1978; Koos & Lemaire, 1983; Frederick *et al.*, 1984) and at least some of these factors are now identified as bFGF (Gospodarowicz *et al.*, 1985b). More recently, it was shown that the granulosa cells, the target of this neovascularization, synthesize bFGF (Neufeld *et al.*, 1987) and thus may be responsible for capillary blood vessel attraction.

Another important issue pertains to the question as to how the action of FGF is regulated. It is interesting that FGF occurs rather ubiquitously in most tissues in significant quantities yet under normal circumstances the endogenous FGF does not seem to induce any obvious proliferative, angiogenic or other biological effects. It has been speculated that FGF is stored intracellularly and may be released from cells by some unknown mechanism or upon cell death. In support of this hypothesis, it was shown that bFGF is not secreted from cultured cells in appreciable quantities into the culture medium (Vlodavsky *et al.*, 1987a), presumably because FGFs are not synthesized as precursors containing a signal peptide sequence typical of secreted proteins (Jaye *et al.*, 1986; Abraham *et al.*, 1986a, 1986b). On the other hand, endothelial cells seem capable of secreting bFGF by an unknown mechanism through the apical side of the cell into the extracellular matrix (Vlodavsky *et al.*, 1987b). This, and the findings that bFGF is present in extracellular matrices in large quantities (Baird & Ling, 1987; Folkman *et al.*, 1988), binds with high affinity to the sulfated glycosaminoglycan heparin and the related heparan sulfate proteoglycans present in extracellular matrix (Gospodarowicz *et al.*, 1984; Shing *et al.*, 1984), and can be released from the extracellular matrix by treatment with matrix component-degrading enzymes such as heparinases (Baird & Ling, 1987), have given rise to another hypothesis concerning the regulation of FGF. Accordingly, FGF may be constitutively secreted at a slow rate from cells into the surrounding extracellular matrix where it accumulates in a bound, inactive form as a consequence of its high affinity for heparin-like sulfated glycosaminoglycans. FGFs bound in this manner may be biologically inactive. Glycosaminoglycan-degrading enzymes may be responsible for activating the FGFs by liberating them from their bound state. Thus, the controlled secretion of such enzymes from cells may provide a mechanism to regulate the proliferative and angiogenic activities of FGFs. Such a mechanism would reconcile the seemingly contradictory facts of abundant but apparently inactive FGF in tissues. Furthermore, the hypothesis could explain how such obviously different phenomena as angiogenesis in wound healing, tumour growth, and organogenesis might be regulated via a common mechanism.

Transforming growth factor-beta

Transforming growth factor-beta (TGF-β) was originally identified as a growth factor from virus-transformed cells which possesses the ability to convey a transformed phenotype to normal cells (Roberts *et al.*, 1981). On the basis of this activity, it was later purified to homogeneity from kidney, placenta, and platelets (Sporn *et al.*, 1987), and its chemical structure was determined by cDNA cloning (Derynck *et al.*, 1985). TGF-β is a homodimeric protein (mol. wt 25 kd) consisting of two identical disulfide-linked polypeptide chains of 112 residues. The protein is synthesized in cells as a larger precursor protein (Derynck *et al.*, 1985) and is secreted in a latent, biologically inactive form of a high molecular weight complex (Pircher *et al.*, 1986; Miyazono *et al.*, 1988). Presumably, latent TGF-β is activated outside the cell, probably involving a protease activity liberating the 25-kd TGF-β which could serve as a regulatory device. The amino acid sequences of TGF-β from a number of species are extremely highly conserved, indicating strong evolutionary pressure to maintain important biological function.

Like FGF, TGF-β is found in most tissues and is synthesized by many varied cell types (Derynck *et al.*, 1985). TGF-β also acts on many different cells. It is mitogenic for some cells but functions as a highly potent growth inhibitor for many others and has diverse cellular effects not related to proliferation (Sporn *et al.*, 1987). The biological activities of TGF-β strongly suggest that this cytokine may have physiological functions in such diverse processes as embryogenesis; tissue growth, differentiation and repair; inflammation; and modulation of immune response (Sporn *et al.*, 1986, 1987).

TGF-β stimulates blood vessel formation when injected subcutaneously into newborn mice (Roberts *et al.*, 1986), or implanted into the rabbit cornea (Folkman & Klagsbrun, 1987). Little is known about how TGF-β stimulates neovascularization. Interestingly, TGF-β seems to antagonize several events thought to be of importance in angiogenesis: it is a potent in-vitro inhibitor of endothelial cell proliferation (Frater-Schroeder *et al.*, 1986; Baird & Durkin, 1986; Heimark *et al.*, 1986), of endothelial cell migration (Heimark *et al.*, 1986) and of morphogenic properties of endothelial cells sometimes referred to as angiogenesis *in vitro* (Müller *et al.*, 1987). One observation could explain how TGF-β might be angiogenic despite its inhibitory effects on endothelial cells: TGF-β is exquisitely potent as a chemotaxis stimulator for monocytes (Wahl *et al.*, 1987). Furthermore, TGF-β implanted in the rabbit cornea was shown to induce the influx of leukocytes into the cornea which precedes angiogenesis (Folkman and Klagsbrun, 1987). Hence, TGF-β might exert its angiogenic activity by attracting such cells as monocytes/macrophages which are now known to contain and/or secrete several angiogenic proteins including bFGF (Baird *et al.*, 1985a), TGF-β (Assoian *et al.*, 1987), TGF-α (Madtes *et al.*, 1988) and tumour necrosis factor-α (Austgulen *et al.*, 1987; see also below). A further, albeit speculative possibility is that TGF-β may stimulate the production of prostaglandins E in tissues, as is known to be the case with bone tissue (Tashjian *et al.*, 1985). Prostaglandins E are known to have angiogenic activity (Ben Ezra, 1978; Ziche *et al.*, 1982; Form & Auerbach, 1983).

Tumour necrosis factor-alpha

Tumour necrosis factor-alpha (TNF-α), also known as cachectin, is a major macrophage secretory protein, the structure of which was determined by cDNA cloning (Pennica *et al.*, 1984; Beutler *et al.*, 1985). TNF-α is a cytokine affecting many cell types. It is characterized by mitogenic, growth inhibitory, and cytotoxic activities, as well as many not related to cell growth (Oettgen & Old, 1987). TNF-α is thought to have a physiological function in many aspects of macrophage-mediated regulation of metabolism and inflammatory responses (Beutler & Cerami, 1988).

TNF-α has been shown to induce capillary blood vessel growth in the rabbit cornea and the chicken chorioallantoic membrane assays (Frater-Schroeder *et al.*, 1987; Leibovich *et al.*, 1987). The mechanism of action of TNF-α in angiogenesis is unclear. In many respects, TNF-α-induced activities in endothelial cells resemble those caused by TGF-β. Like TGF-β, TNF-α is a potent inhibitor of endothelial cell proliferation *in vitro* (Stolpen *et al.*, 1986; Sato *et al.*, 1986; Frater-Schroeder *et al.*, 1987). Angiogenesis induced by TNF-α is also characterized by infiltration of white cells into the site of TNF-α application (Frater-Schroeder *et al.*, 1987; Leibovich *et al.*, 1987), suggesting that TNF-α-mediated angiogenesis is secondary to leukocyte action. Furthermore, TNF-α seems to inhibit the migration of endothelial cells (Mano-Hirano *et al.*, 1987); however, this activity is controversial since migration-stimulatory activity has also been observed (Leibovich *et al.*, 1987). Finally, TNF-α is able to stimulate prostaglandin E production, at least in certain cell types (Dayer *et al.*, 1985; Bachwich *et al.*, 1986). Therefore, a mechanism involving prostaglandin E-mediated neovascularization should not be ruled out. In contrast to the effects of TGF-β, TNF-α has been reported to stimulate the formation of capillary-like tube structures from endothelial cells cultured in collagen gels (angiogenesis *in vitro*) (Leibovich *et al.*, 1987). Finally, TNF-α, like FGF, seems to promote extracellular matrix degradation in some systems (Dayer *et al.*, 1985; Saklatvala, 1986; Nakagawa *et al.*, 1987).

Secretory substances from macrophages are well known to induce neovascularization (Polverini *et al.*, 1977). Although macrophages produce several of the known angiogenesis factors (bFGF, TGF-β, TNF-α, TGF-α), TNF-α appears to be the most important one because anti-TNF-α antibodies largely inhibit macrophage-dependent blood vessel formation (Leibovich *et al.*, 1987). This suggests that TNF-α may be a physiologic angiogenic agent in macrophages, and may be involved in neovascularization associated with macrophage-mediated processes such as inflammation and wound healing.

Transforming growth factor-alpha

Like TGF-β, transforming growth factor-alpha (TGF-α) was first identified as a tumour cell product having cell-transforming properties (DeLarco & Todaro, 1978). TGF-α is a 50-residue polypeptide which possesses considerable sequence homology to epidermal growth factor (EGF) (Marquardt *et al.*, 1984). The biosynthetic precursor of TGF-α has been cloned (Derynck *et al.*, 1984). TGF-α and EGF bind to the same cellular receptor and share many, but not all, biological activities. In contrast, TGF-α and TGF-β are structurally unrelated, bind to different receptors and share few biological activities. TGF-α is synthesized by a variety of normal and tumour cells (Lee *et al.*, 1985; Derynck *et al.*, 1987) but occurs in tissues in relatively small quantities.

Like most other growth factors, TGF-α acts on many cell types (Derynck, 1986) to cause mitogenic and various non-mitogenic effects. These include the stimulation of bone resorption and the inhibition of bone formation (Derynck, 1986), the acceleration of wound healing (Schultz *et al.*, 1987), the stimulation of angiogenesis (Schreiber *et al.*, 1986), and developmental effects (Derynck, 1986). The possible physiological significance(s) of the known activities of TGF-α is unclear. Because TGF-α is synthesized in early fetal development and in many cancer cells, it is thought potentially to play a role in embryonic tissue formation and in neoplastic pathogenesis.

The angiogenic activity of TGF-α has so far only been studied in the hamster cheek pouch assay. This animal model is not commonly used by other investigators who study angiogenesis factors and it is therefore difficult to compare the angiogenic effects of TGF-α to those of other factors. Nothing is known about the possible mechanism of action of TGF-α other than that it stimulates the proliferation of endothelial cells *in vitro* (Schreiber *et al.*, 1986). It is interesting to note that the structurally and biologically related EGF possesses much weaker angiogenic activity than TGF-α, whereas it is equally potent as an endothelial cell mitogen (Derynck, 1986). EGF is therefore not commonly considered an angiogenic factor.

Angiogenin

Angiogenin is a 14-kd protein of known sequence (Strydom *et al.*, 1985) which was first isolated from a carcinoma cell line (Fett *et al.*, 1985). The angiogenin sequence is 35% homologous to ribonucleases (Strydom *et al.*, 1985) and possesses ribonuclease activity for large RNA (Shapiro *et al.*, 1986). The protein is found in plasma (Shapiro *et al.*, 1987). Furthermore, angiogenin mRNA is abundant in liver (Weiner *et al.*, 1987) and was also found to a lesser degree in many other normal and tumour tissues (Rybak *et al.*, 1987). Angiogenin stimulates neovascularization in the chick chorioallantoic membrane and rabbit cornea assays (Fett *et al.*, 1985). Its mechanism of action is not understood. Endothelial cells seem to have receptors for angiogenin (Bicknell & Vallee, 1988), but angiogenin does not affect proliferation of this cell (Folkman & Klagsbrun, 1987). Furthermore, relatively high levels of angiogenin are circulating without the apparent stimulation of angiogenesis, and the expression of the angiogenin gene does not seem to be temporally related to the development of the vascular system of the rat (Weiner *et al.*, 1987). In the absence of more data, the physiological relevance of angiogenin in capillary vessel growth is therefore difficult to evaluate.

Other cytokines

Most recently, investigators using DNA probes and other molecular tools derived from existing angiogenic cytokines have uncovered the existence of a number of additional genes coding for proteins which are highly homologous to several of the above-mentioned angiogenesis factors. Thus, int-2 (Dickson & Peters, 1987), hst/KS3 (Delli Bovi *et al.*, 1987; Yoshida *et al.*, 1987), and FGF-5 (Zhan *et al.*, 1988) are new oncogene members of the FGF gene family. TGF-β2 (DeMartin *et al.*, 1987; Hanks *et al.*, 1988; Madisen *et al.*, 1988), TGF-β3 (Ten Dijke *et al.*, 1988; Derynck *et al.*, 1988), and heterodimeric TGF-β1/2 (Cheifetz *et al.*, 1988) belong to the TGF-β family (TGF-β as described above is now referred to as TGF-β1). Lymphotoxin or TNF-β (Gray et al., 1984) is another known member of the TNF gene family. Finally, vaccinia growth factor (VGF) is related to EGF/TGF-α (Stroobant et al., 1985; Brown et al., 1985). In general, the members of these cytokine families share biological activities, although activity and distribution differences between family members exist. It is presently not known whether any of these cytokines possesses angiogenic activity. However, based on biological and structural similarities to FGF, TGF-β, TGF-α, or TNF, it is reasonable to speculate that most of them would have such activity and potentially may be physiological angiogenic factors.

In addition to these potentially angiogenic factors, a number of angiogenic activities have been described (Folkman & Klagsbrun, 1987) which are still largely uncharacterized and therefore difficult to evaluate.

Modulators of angiogenesis

There is ample evidence that a number of well-defined endogenous substances can either interfere with or augment neovascularization without having a direct angiogenic or antiangiogenic activity. It is generally thought that these substances modulate in some largely unknown ways, the activity of angiogenic factors. The best known of these modulators is heparin, which interacts with endothelial cells in a number of ways (effects on proliferation and migration) and also binds strongly to FGF. Heparin can augment growth factor-induced angiogenesis or inhibit it when certain steroids are present (Folkman & Klagsbrun, 1987; Joseph-Silverstein & Rifkin, 1987).

Copper ions are another potential physiological modulator of neovascularization. Several copper-binding naturally occurring substances such as heparin, the serum tripeptide Gly-His-Lys, and ceruloplasmin, are angiogenic in the copper-bound state but not when free of copper (Folkman & Klagsbrun, 1987). In the absence of more data, it is difficult to evaluate the potential function of copper in angiogenesis.

Conclusions

Table 1 lists in summary form the properties of the known angiogenic cytokines which are thought to be potentially relevant in angiogenesis. It is rather obvious that these factors must act by multiple distinct mechanisms. Perhaps it is useful to distinguish between 'direct' and 'indirect' angiogenesis factors. The former would be those which act directly on capillary endothelial cells, while the indirectly acting factors could be characterized as those factors which do not stimulate the endothelial cell directly but in some way recruit other direct-acting factors. Recruitment of angiogenic factors might be achieved in a number of different ways which at this time are largely

Table 1. *Properties of angiogenic factors potentially relevant to their mechanisms of action*

Factor	Proliferation of EC	Migration of EC	ECM degradation	Angiogenesis *in vitro*	Leukocyte/ monocyte chemotaxis
FGF	+	+	+	+	
TGF-β	-	-	-	-	+
TNF-α	-	+-	+	+	+
TGF-α	+				
Angiogenin	No effect				

Notes:
EC, endothelial cell; ECM, extracellular matrix; +, stimulatory effect; -, inhibitory effect; blank space, effect not known.
Appropriate references are cited in the text.

speculative in nature: indirect angiogenesis factors might act by (a) attracting cells which contain 'direct' angiogenesis factors (e.g. macrophages), (b) stimulating the release of extracellular matrix-degrading enzymes from cells, thus liberating matrix-bound growth factors, or (c) stimulating the release of direct-acting angiogenesis factors from cells.

FGF is likely to be a direct-acting angiogenic factor because of its multiple stimulatory effects on endothelial cells. In contrast, TGF-β might be best described as an 'indirect' angiogenesis factor. In this manner, the apparently contradictory facts that TGF-β is both angiogenic (which presumably requires endothelial cell proliferation) and inhibitory for endothelial cell growth, could be reconciled. The finding that TGF-β potently attracts monocytes which are known to contain several angiogenic factors would support this classification. However, not enough is known about the possible mechanisms of action of FGF or TGF-β for this classification to be firmly established. The situation is even less clear with the other angiogenic cytokines, for which not enough relevant data exist to make even a tentative assignment.

It is presently unclear whether all of the known angiogenic factors are physiologically involved in the control of neovascularization. It has been suggested (Zetter, 1988) that the apparent redundancy of angiogenic substances may be a consequence of the vital importance of the angiogenic process. Angiogenesis is essential for the growth, maintenance and repair of most tissues and an adequate angiogenic response can be best provided by the availability of multiple factors as part of independent regulatory systems. Furthermore, angiogenic demands of the organism are quite diverse (e.g. spontaneous injury-induced angiogenesis versus hormonally regulated angiogenesis in ovarian follicle development) and it seems reasonable that they be met by the evolution of distinct control mechanisms.

References

Abraham, J.A., Mergia, A., Whang, J.L., Tumolo, A., Friedman, J., Hjerrild, K.A., Gospodarowicz, D. & Fiddes, J.C. (1986a). Nucleotide sequence of a bovine clone encoding the angiogenic protein, basic fibroblast growth factor. *Science*, **233**:545–548.

Abraham, J.A., Whang, J.L., Tumolo, A., Mergia, A. & Fiddes, J.C. (1986b). Human basic fibroblast growth factor: nucleotide sequence, genomic organization, and expression in mammalian cells. *Cold Spring Harbor Symposia on Quantitative Biology*, **51**:657–668.

Assoian, R.K., Fleurdelys, B.E., Stevenson, H.C., Miller, P.J., Madtes, D.K., Raines, E.W., Ross, R. & Sporn, M.B. (1987). Expression and secretion of type β transforming growth factor by activated human macrophages. *Proceedings of the National Academy of Sciences USA*, **84**:6020–6024.

Ausprunk, D.H., Knighton, D.R. & Folkman, J. (1975). Vascularization of normal and neoplastic tissues grafted to the chick chorioallantois. Role of host and pre-existing graft blood vessels. *American Journal of Pathology*, **79**:597–628.

Austgulen, R., Espevik, T. & Nissen-Meyer, J. (1987). Fibroblast growth-stimulatory activity released from human monocytes. The contribution of tumour necrosis factor. *Scandinavian Journal of Immunology*, **26**:621–629.

Bachwich, P.R., Chensue, S.W., Larrick, J.W. & Kunkel, S.L. (1986). Tumor necrosis factor stimulates interleukin-1 and prostaglandin E2 production in resting macrophages. *Biochemical and Biophysical Research Communications*, **136**:94–101.

Baird, A., Culler, F., Jones, K.L. & Guillemin, R. (1985b). Angiogenic factor in human ocular fluid. *Lancet*, **ii**:563.

Baird, A. & Durkin, T. (1986). Inhibition of endothelial cell proliferation by type beta-transforming growth factor: interactions with acidic and basic fibroblast growth factors. *Biochemical and Biophysical Research Communications*, **138**:476–482.

Baird, A., Esch, F., Mormede, P., Ueno, N., Ling, N., Böhlen, P., Ying, S.Y., Wehrenberg, W.B. & Guillemin, R. (1986). Molecular characterization of fibroblast growth factor: distribution and biological activities in various tissues. *Recent Progress in Hormone Research*, **42**:143–205.

Baird, A. & Ling, N. (1987). Fibroblast growth factors are present in the extracellular matrix produced by endothelial cells *in vitro*: implications for a role of heparinase-like enzymes in the neovascular response. *Biochemical and Biophysical Research Communications*, **142**:428–435.

Baird, A., Mormede, P. & Böhlen, P. (1985a). Immunoreactive fibroblast growth factor in cells of peritoneal exudate suggests its identity with macrophage-derived growth factor. *Biochemical and Biophysical Research Communications*, **126**:358–364.

Ben Ezra, D. (1978). Neovasculogenic ability of prostaglandins, growth factors and synthetic chemoattractants. *American Journal of Ophthalmology*, **86**:455–461.

Beutler, B. & Cerami, A. (1988). Cachectin (tumor necrosis factor): a macrophage hormone governing cellular metabolism and inflammatory response. *Endocrine Reviews*, **9**:57–66.

Beutler, B., Greenwald, D., Hulmes, J.D., Chang, M., Pan, Y.-C.E., Mathison, J., Ulevitch, R. & Cerami, A. (1985). Identity of tumor necrosis factor and the macrophage-secreted factor cachectin. *Nature*, **316**:552–554.

Derynck, R., Jarrett, J.A., Chen, E.Y., Eaton, D.H., Bell, J.R., Assoian, R.K., Bicknell, R. & Vallee, B.L. (1988). Angiogenin activates endothelial cell phospholipase C. *Proceedings of the National Academy of Sciences USA*, **85**:5961–5965.

Böhlen, P. (1989). Fibroblast growth factor. (In) *Macrophage-Derived Cell Regulatory Factors. Cytokines*, Vol. 1 (Sorg, C., ed.), pp.204–228. Basel, Switzerland, Karger.

Böhlen, P., Baird, A., Esch, F., Ling, N. & Gospodarowicz, D.(1984). Isolation and partial molecular characterization of pituitary fibroblast growth factor. *Proceedings of the National Academy of Sciences USA*, **81**:5364–5368.

Böhlen, P., Esch, F., Baird, A. & Gospodarowicz, D. (1985). Acidic fibroblast growth factor (FGF) from bovine brain: amino-terminal sequence and comparison with basic FGF. *EMBO Journal*, **4**:1951–1956.

Brown, J.P., Twardzik, D.R., Marquardt, H. & Todaro, G.J. (1985). Vaccinia virus encodes a polypeptide homologous to epidermal growth factor and transforming growth factor. *Nature*, **313**:491–492.

Buntrock, P., Buntrock, M., Marx, I., Kranz, D., Jentzsch, K.D. & Heder, G. (1984). Stimulation of wound healing, using brain extract with fibroblast growth factor (FGF) activity. III. Electron microscopy, autoradiography, ultrastructural autoradiography of granulation tissue. *Experimental Pathology*, **26**:247–254.

Cheifetz, S., Bassols, A., Stanley, K., Ohta, M., Greenberger, J. & Massague, J. (1988). Heterodimeric transforming growth factor-β. Biological properties and interaction with three types of cell surface receptors. *Journal of Biological Chemistry*, **263**:10783–10789.

Chodak, G.W., Hospelhorn, V., Judge, S.M., Mayforth, R., Koeppen, H. & Sasse, J. (1988). Increased levels of fibroblast growth factor-like activity in urine from patients with bladder or kidney cancer. *Cancer Research*, **48**:2083–2088.

D'Amore, P.A. & Thompson, R.W. (1987). Mechanisms of angiogenesis. *Annual Review of Physiology*, **49**:453–464.

Dayer, J.M., Beutler, B. & Cerami, A. (1985). Cachectin/tumor necrosis factor stimulates collagenase and prostaglandin E2 production by human synovial cells and dermal fibroblasts. *Journal of Experimental Medicine*, **162**:2163–2168.

DeLarco, J.E. & Todaro, G.J. (1978). Growth factors from murine sarcoma virus-transformed cells. *Proceedings of the National Academy of Sciences USA*, **75**:4001–4005.

Delli Bovi, P., Curatola, A.M., Kern, F.G., Greco, A., Ittmann, M. & Basilico, C. (1987). An oncogene isolated by transfection of Kaposi's sarcoma DNA encodes a growth factor that is a member of the FGF family. *Cell*, **50**:729–737.

DeMartin, R., Haendler, B., Hofer-Warbinek, R., Gaugitsch, H., Wrann, M., Schlüsener, H., Seifert, J.M., Bodmer, S., Fontana, A. & Hofer, E. (1987). Complementary DNA for human glioblastoma-derived T cell suppressor factor, a novel member of the transforming growth factor-β gene family. *EMBO Journal*, **6**:3673–3677.

Derynck, R. (1986). Transforming growth factor-α: structure and biological activities. *Journal of Cellular Biochemistry*, **32**:293–304.

Derynck, R., Goeddel, D.V., Ullrich, A., Gutterman, J.U., Williams, R.D., Bringman, T.S. & Berger, W.H. (1987). Synthesis of messenger RNAs for transforming growth factors α and β and the epidermal growth factor receptor by human tumors. *Cancer Research*, **47**:707–712.

Roberts, A.B., Sporn, M.B. & Goeddel, D.V. (1985). Human transforming growth factor-β complementary DNA sequence and expression in normal and transformed cells. *Nature*, **316**:701–705.

Derynck, R., Lindquist, P.B., Lee, A., Wen, D., Tamm, J., Graycar, J.L., Rhee, E.L., Mason, A.J., Miller, D.A., Coffey, R.J., Moses, H.L. & Chen, E.Y. (1988). A new type of transforming growth factor-β, TGF-β3. *EMBO Journal*, **7**:3737–3743.

Derynck, R., Roberts, A.B., Winkler, M.E., Chen, E.Y. & Goeddel, D.V. (1984). Human transforming growth factor-α: precursor structure and expression in E. coli. *Cell*, **38**:287–297.

Dickson, C. & Peters, G. (1987). Potential oncogene product related to growth factors. *Nature*, **326**:833.

Esch, F., Baird, A., Ling, N., Ueno, N., Hill, F., Denoroy, L., Klepper, R., Gospodarowicz, D., Böhlen, P. & Guillemin, R. (1985). Primary structure of bovine pituitary basic fibroblast growth factor (FGF) and comparison with the amino-terminal sequence of bovine brain acidic FGF. *Proceedings of the National Academy of Sciences USA*, **82**:6507–6511.

Fett, J.W., Strydom, D.J., Lobb, R.R., Alderman, E.M., Bethune, J.L., Riordan, J.F. & Vallee, B.L. (1985). Isolation and characterization of angiogenin, an angiogenic protein from human carcinoma cells. *Biochemistry*, **24**:5480–5486.

Findlay, J.K. (1986). Angiogenesis in reproductive tissues. *Journal of Endocrinology*, **111**:357–366.

Folkman, J. (1984a). What is the role of endothelial cells in angiogenesis? *Laboratory Investigation*, **51**:601–604.

Folkman, J. (1984b). Angiogenesis. (In) *Biology of Endothelial Cells* (Jaffe, E., ed.), pp.412–428. Boston, USA, Martimus Nijhoff.

Folkman, J. (1986). How is blood vessel growth regulated in normal and neoplastic tissue? G.H.A. Clowes memorial Award lecture. *Cancer Research*, **46**:467–473.

Folkman, J. & Klagsbrun, M. (1987). Angiogenic factors. *Science*, **235**:442–447.

Folkman, J., Klagsbrun, M., Sasse, J., Wadzinski, M., Ingber, D. & Vlodavsky, I. (1988). A heparin-binding angiogenic protein – basic fibroblast growth factor – is stored within basement membrane. *American Journal of Pathology*, **130**:393–400.

Folkman, J., Merler, E., Abernathy, C. & Williams, G.J. (1971). Isolation of a tumor factor responsible for angiogenesis. *Journal of Experimental Medicine*, **133**:275–283.

Form, D.M. & Auerbach, R. (1983). PGE2 and angiogenesis. *Proceedings of the Society for Experimental Biology and Medicine*, **172**:214–218.

Frater-Schroeder, M., Müller, G., Birchmeier, W. & Böhlen, P. (1986). Transforming growth factor-β inhibits endothelial cell proliferation. *Biochemical and Biophysical Research Communications*, **137**:295–302.

Frater-Schroeder, M., Risau, W., Hallmann, R., Gautschi, P. & Böhlen, P. (1987). Tumor necrosis factor type α, a potent inhibitor of endothelial cell growth *in vitro*, is angiogenic *in vivo*. *Proceedings of the National Academy of Sciences USA*, **84**:5277–5281.

Frederick, J.L., Shimanuki, T. & Di Zerega, G.S. (1984). Initiation of angiogenesis by human follicular fluid. *Science*, **224**:389–390.

Fuchs, A., Lindenbaum, E. & Marcoudas, N.G. (1985). Location of the angiogenic activity in the pregnant human uterus. *Acta Anatomica, Basel*, **124**:241–244.

Gimbrone, M.A., Cotran, R.S., Leapman, S.B. & Folkman, J. (1974). Tumor growth and neovascularization: an experimental model using the rabbit cornea. *Journal of the National Cancer Institute*, **52**:413–427.

Gimenez-Gallego, G., Rodkey, K., Bennett, C., Rios-Candelore, M., Di Salvo, J. & Thomas, K. (1985). Brain-derived acidic fibroblast growth factor: complete amino acid sequence and homologies. *Science*, **230**:1385–1388.

Gospodarowicz, D., Bialecki, H. & Thakral, K.K. (1979). The angiogenic activity of the fibroblast and epidermal growth factor. *Experimental Eye Research*, **28**:501–514.

Gospodarowicz, D., Cheng, J., Lui, G.M., Baird, A. & Böhlen, P. (1984). Isolation of brain fibroblast growth factor by heparin-sepharose affinity chromatography: Identity with pituitary fibroblast growth factor. *Proceedings of the National Academy of Sciences USA*, **81**:6963–6967.

Gospodarowicz, D., Cheng, J., Lui, G.M., Baird, A., Esch, F. & Böhlen, P. (1985b). Corpus luteum angiogenic factor is related to fibroblast growth factor. *Endocrinology*, **117**:2383–2391.

Gospodarowicz, D., Massoglia, S., Cheng, J., Lui, G.M. & Böhlen, P. (1985a). Isolation of pituitary fibroblast growth factor by fast protein liquid chromatography (FPLC): partial chemical and biological characterization. *Journal of Cellular Physiology*, **122**:323–332.

Gospodarowicz, D., Moran, J., Braun, D. & Birdwell, C. (1976). Clonal growth of bovine vascular endothelial cells: fibroblast growth factor as a survival agent. *Proceedings of the National Academy of Sciences USA*, **73**:4120–4124.

Gospodarowicz, D., Neufeld, G. & Schweigerer, L. (1986). Fibroblast growth factor. *Molecular Cell Endocrinology*, **46**:187–204.

Gospodarowicz, D. & Thakral, K.K. (1978). Production of a corpus luteum angiogenic factor responsible for proliferation of capillaries and neovascularization of the corpus luteum. *Proceedings of the National Academy of Sciences USA*, **75**:847–851.

Gray, P.W., Aggarwal, B.B., Benton, C.L., Bringman, T.S., Henzel, W.J., Jarrett, J.A., Leung, D.W., Moffat, B., Ng, P., Svedersky, L.P., Palladino, M.A. & Nedwin, G.E. (1984). Cloning and expression of cDNA for human lymphotoxin, a lymphokine with tumor necrosis activity. *Nature*, **312**:721–724.

Greenblatt, M. & Shubi, P. (1968). Tumor angiogenesis: transfilter diffusion studies in the hamster by the transparent chamber study. *Journal of the National Cancer Institute*, **41**:111–124.

Hamerman, D., Taylor, S., Kirschenbaum, I., Klagsbrun, M., Raines, E.W., Ross, R. & Thomas, K.A. (1987). Growth factors with heparin binding affinity in human synovial fluid. *Proceedings of the Society for Experimental Biology and Medicine*, **186**:384–389.

Hanks, S.K., Armour, R., Baldwin, J.H., Maldonado, F., Spiess, J. & Holley, R.W. (1988). Amino acid sequence of BSC-1 cell growth inhibitor (polyergin) deduced from the nucleotide sequence of the cDNA. *Proceedings of the National Academy of Sciences USA*, **85**:79–82.

Heimark, R.L., Twardzik, D.R. & Schwartz, S.M. (1986). Inhibition of endothelial regeneration by type beta-transforming growth factor from platelets. *Science*, **233**:1078–1080.

Jakob, W., Jentzsch, K.D., Mauersberger, B. & Oehme, P. (1977). Demonstration of angiogenesis-activity in the corpus luteum of cattle. *Experimental Pathology*, **13**:231–236.

Jaye, M., Howk, R., Burgess, W., Ricca, G.A., Chiu, I.M., Ravera, M.W., O'Brien, S.J., Modi, W.S., Maciag, T. & Drohan, W.N. (1986). Human endothelial cell growth factor: cloning, nucleotide sequence, and chromosome localization. *Science*, **233**:541–545.

Jaye, M., McConathy, E., Drohan, W., Tong, B., Deuel, T. & Maciag, T. (1985). Modulation of the sis gene transcript during endothelial cell differentiation *in vitro*. *Science*, **228**:882–885.

Joseph-Silverstein, J. & Rifkin, D.B. (1987). Endothelial cell growth factors and the vessel wall. *Seminars in Thrombosis and Hemostasis*, **13**:504–513.

Koos, R.D. & Lemaire, W.J. (1983). Evidence for an angiogenic factor from rat follicles. (In) *Factors Regulating Ovarian Function* (Greenwald, G.S. & Terranova, P.F., eds.), pp.191–195. New York, Raven Press.

Lee, D.C., Rochford, R.M., Todaro, G.J. & Villareal, L.P. (1985). Developmental expression of rat transforming growth factor-α mRNA. *Molecular and Cellular Biology*, **5**:3644–3646.

Leibovich, S.J., Polverini, P.J., Shepard, H.M., Wiseman, D.M., Shively, V. & Nuseir, N. (1987). Macrophage-induced angiogenesis is mediated by tumour necrosis factor-α. *Nature*, **329**:630–632.

Lobb, R.R., Alderman, E.M. & Fett, J.W. (1985). Induction of angiogenesis by bovine brain-derived class 1 heparin-binding growth factor. *Biochemistry*, **24**:4969–4973.

Maciag, T., Hoover, G.A. & Weinstein, R. (1982). High and low molecular weight forms of endothelial cell growth factor. *Journal of Biological Chemistry*, **257**:5333–5336.

Madisen, L., Webb, N.R., Rose, T.M., Marquardt, H., Ikeda, T., Twardzik, D., Seyedin, S. & Purchio, A.F. (1988). Transforming growth factor-β2: cDNA cloning and sequence analysis. *DNA*, **7**:1–8.

Madtes, D.K., Raines, E.W., Sakariassen, K.S., Assoian, R.K., Sporn, M.B., Bell, G.I. & Ross, R. (1988). Induction of transforming growth factor α in activated alveolar macrophages. *Cell*, **53**:285–293.

Mano-Hirano, Y., Sato, N., Sawasaki, Y., Haranaka, K., Satomi, N., Nariuchi, H. & Goto, T. (1987). Inhibition of tumor-induced migration of bovine capillary endothelial cells by mouse and rabbit tumor necrosis factor. *Journal of the National Cancer Institute*, **78**:115–120.

Marquardt, H., Hunkapiller, M.W., Hood, L.E. & Todaro, G.J. (1984). Rat transforming growth factor type I: structure and relation to epidermal growth factor. *Science*, **223**:1079–1082.

Miyazono, K., Hellmann, U., Wernstedt, C. & Heldin, C.H. (1988). Latent high molecular weight complex of transforming growth factor-β. 1. Purification from human platelets and structural characterization. *Journal of Biological Chemistry*, **263**:6407–6415.

Montesano, R., Vasalli, J.D., Baird, A., Guillemin, R. & Orci, L. (1986). Basic fibroblast growth factor induces angiogenesis *in vitro*. *Proceedings of the National Academy of Sciences USA*, **83**:7297–7301.

Moscatelli, D. (1987). High and low affinity binding sites for basic fibroblast growth factor on cultured cells: absence of a role for low affinity binding in the stimulation of plasminogen activator production by bovine capillary endothelial cells. *Journal of Cellular Physiology*, **131**:123–130.

Moscatelli, D., Joseph-Silverstein, J., Manejias, R. & Rifkin, D.B. (1987). Mr 25,000 heparin-binding protein from guinea pig brain is a high molecular weight form of basic fibroblast growth factor. *Proceedings of the National Academy of Sciences USA*, **84**:5778–5782.

Moscatelli, D.A., Presta, M., Mignatti, P., Mullins, D., Crowe, R.M. & Rifkin, D.B. (1986). Purification and biological activities of an angiogenesis factor from human placenta. *Anticancer Research*, **6**:861–863.

Müller, G., Behrens, J., Nussbaumer, U., Böhlen, P. & Birchmeier, W. (1987). Inhibitory action of transforming growth factor-β on endothelial cells. *Proceedings of the National Academy of Sciences USA*, **84**:5600–5604.

Nakagawa, H., Kitagawa, H. & Aikawa, Y. (1987). Tumor necrosis factor stimulates gelatinase and collagenase production by granulation tissue in culture. *Biochemical and Biophysical Research Communications*, **142**:791–797.

Neufeld, G., Ferrara, N., Schweigerer, L., Mitchell, R. & Gospodarowicz, D. (1987). Bovine granulosa cells produce basic fibroblast growth factor. *Endocrinology*, **121**:597–603.

Oettgen, H.F. & Old, L.J. (1987). Tumor necrosis factor. *Important Advances in Oncology 1987*, pp.105–130.

Pennica, D., Nedwin, G.E., Hayflick, J.S., Seeburg, P.H., Derynck, R., Palladino, M.A., Kohr, W.J., Aggarwal, B.B. & Goeddel, D.V. (1984). Human tumor necrosis factor: precursor structure, expression and homology to lymphotoxin. *Nature*, **312**:724–729.

Pircher, R., Jullien, P. & Lawrence, D.A. (1986). β Transforming growth factor is stored in human blood platelets as a latent high molecular weight complex. *Biochemical and Biophysical Research Communications*, **136**:30–37.

Polverini, P.J., Cotran, R.S., Gimbrone, M.A. & Unanue, E.R. (1977). Activated macrophages induce vascular proliferation. *Nature*, **269**:804–806.

Presta, M., Moscatelli, D., Joseph-Silverstein, J. & Rifkin, D.B. (1986). Purification from a human hepatoma cell line of a basic fibroblast growth factor-like molecule that stimulates capillary endothelial cell plasminogen activator production, DNA synthesis, migration. *Molecular and Cellular Biology*, **6**:4060–4066.

Risau, W. (1986). Developing brain produces an angiogenesis factor. *Proceedings of the National Academy of Sciences USA*, **83**:3855–3859.

Risau, W. & Ekblom, P. (1986). Production of a heparin-binding angiogenesis factor by the embryonic kidney. *Journal of Cell Biology*, **103**:1101–1107.

Risau, W., Gautschi-Sova, P. & Böhlen, P. (1988). Endothelial cell growth factors in embryonic and adult chick brain are related to human acidic fibroblast growth factor. *EMBO Journal*, **7**:959–962.

Roberts, A.B., Anzano, M.A., Lamb, L.C., Smith, J.M. & Sporn, M.B. (1981). New class of transforming growth factors potentiated by epidermal growth factor: isolation from non-neoplastic tissues. *Proceedings of the National Academy of Sciences USA*, **78**:5339–5343.

Roberts, A.B., Sporn, M.B., Assoian, R.K., Smith, J.M., Roche, N.S., Wakefield, L.M., Heine, U.I., Liotta, L.A., Falanga, V., Kehrl, J.H. & Fauci, A.S. (1986). Transforming growth factor type β: rapid induction of fibrosis and angiogenesis *in vivo* and stimulation of collagen formation *in vitro*. *Proceedings of the National Academy of Sciences USA*, **83**:4167–4171.

Rybak, S.M., Fett, J.W., Yao, Q.Z. & Vallee, B.L. (1987). Angiogenin mRNA in human tumor and normal cells. *Biochemical and Biophysical Research Communications*, **146**:1240–1248.

Saklatvala, J. (1986). Tumor necrosis factor alpha stimulates resorption and inhibits synthesis of proteoglycan in cartilage. *Nature*, **322**:547–549.

Sato, N., Goto, T., Haranaka, K., Satomi, N., Nariuchi, H., Mano-Hirano, Y. & Sawasaki, Y. (1986). Actions of tumor necrosis factor on cultured vascular endothelial cells: morphologic modulation, growth inhibition, and cytotoxicity. *Journal of the National Cancer Institute*, **76**:1113–1121.

Schreiber, A.B., Winkler, M.E. & Derynck, R. (1986). Transforming growth factor-α: a more potent angiogenic mediator than epidermal growth factor. *Science*, **232**:1250–1253.

Schubert, D., Ling, N. & Baird, A. (1987). Multiple influences of a heparin-binding growth factor on neuronal development. *Journal of Cell Biology*, **104**:635–643.

Schultz, G.S., White, M., Mitchell, R., Brown, G., Lynch, J., Twardzik, D.R. & Todaro, G.J. (1987). Epithelial wound healing enhanced by transforming growth factor-α and vaccinia growth factor. *Science*, **235**:350–352.

Schweigerer, L., Neufeld, G., Friedman, J., Abraham, J.A., Fiddes, J.C. & Gospodarowicz, D. (1987). Capillary endothelial cells express basic fibroblast growth factor, a mitogen that promotes their own growth. *Nature*, **325**:257–259.

Shapiro, R., Riordan, J.F. & Vallee, B.L. (1986). Characteristic ribonucleolytic activity of human angiogenin. *Biochemistry*, **25**:3527–3532. (And published erratum in *Biochemistry* (1986), **25**:6730.)

Shapiro, R., Strydom, D.J., Olson, K.A. & Vallee, B.L. (1987). Isolation of angiogenin from normal human plasma. *Biochemistry*, **26**:5141–5146.

Shing, Y., Folkman, J., Haudenschild, C., Lund, D., Crum, R. & Klagsbrun, M. (1985). Angiogenesis is stimulated by a tumor-derived endothelial cell growth factor. *Journal of Cellular Biochemistry*, **29**:275–287.

Shing, Y., Folkman, J., Sullivan, R., Butterfield, C., Murray, J. & Klagsbrun, M. (1984). Heparin affinity: purification of a tumor-derived capillary endothelial cell growth factor. *Science*, **223**:1296–1299.

Sommer, A., Brewer, M.T., Thompson, R.C., Moscatelli, D., Presta, M. & Rifkin, D.B. (1987). A form of human basic fibroblast growth factor with an extended amino terminus. *Biochemical and Biophysical Research Communications*, **144**:543–550.

Sporn, M.B., Roberts, A.B., Wakefield, L.M. & Assoian, R.K. (1986). Transforming growth factor-β: biological function and chemical structure. *Science*, **233**:532–534.

Sporn, M.B., Roberts, A.B., Wakefield, L.M. & Decrombrugghe, B. (1987). Some recent advances in the chemistry and biology of transforming growth factor-β. *Journal of Cell Biology*, **105**:1039–1045.

Stolpen, A.H., Guinan, E.C., Fiers, W. & Pober, J.S. (1986). Recombinant tumor necrosis factor and immune interferon act singly and in combination to reorganize human vascular endothelial cell monolayers. *American Journal of Pathology*, **123**:16–24.

Stroobant, P., Rice, A.P., Gullick, W.J., Cheng, D.J., Kerr, I.M. & Waterfield, M.D. (1985). Purification and characterization of vaccinia virus growth factor. *Cell*, **42**:383–393.

Strydom, D.J., Fett, J.W., Lobb, R.R., Alderman, E.M., Bethune, J.L., Riordan, J.F.

& Vallee, B.L. (1985). Amino acid sequence of human tumor-derived angiogenin. *Biochemistry*, **24**:5486–5494.

Tashjian, A.H., Voelkel, E.F., Lazzaro, M., Singer, F.R., Roberts, A.B., Derynck, R., Winkler, M.E. & Levine, L. (1985). α and β human transforming growth factors stimulate prostaglandin production and bone resorption in cultured mouse calvaria. *Proceedings of the National Academy of Sciences USA*, **82**:4535–4538.

Ten Dijke, P., Hansen, P., Iwata, K.K., Pieler, C. & Foulkes, J.G. (1988). Identification of another member of the transforming growth factor type β gene family. *Proceedings of the National Academy of Sciences USA*, **85**:4715–4719.

Terranova, V.P., Diflorio, R., Lyall, R.M., Hic, S., Friesel, R. & Maciag, T. (1985). Human endothelial cells are chemotactic to endothelial cell growth factor and heparin. *Journal of Cell Biology*, **101**:2330–2334.

Thomas, K.A. (1987). Fibroblast growth factors. *FASEB Journal*, **1**:434–440.

Thomas, K.A., Rios-Candelore, M. & Fitzpatrick, S. (1984). Purification and characterization of acidic fibroblast growth factor from bovine brain. *Proceedings of the National Academy of Sciences USA*, **81**:357–361.

Thomas, K.A., Rios-Candelore, M., Gimenez-Gallego, G., Di Salvo, J., Bennett, C., Rodkey, J. & Fitzpatrick, S. (1985). Pure brain-derived acidic fibroblast growth factor is a potent angiogenic vascular endothelial cell mitogen with sequence homology to interleukin-1. *Proceedings of the National Academy of Sciences USA*, **82**:6409–6413.

Tseng, S.C., Savion, N., Stern, R. & Gospodarowicz, D. (1982). Fibroblast growth factor modulates synthesis of collagen in cultured vascular endothelial cells. *European Journal of Biochemistry*, **122**:355–360.

Vlodavsky, I., Folkman, J., Sullivan, R., Fridman, R., Ishai-Michaeli, R., Sasse, J. & Klagsbrun, M. (1987b). Endothelial cell-derived basic fibroblast growth factor: synthesis and deposition into subendothelial extracellular matrix. *Proceedings of the National Academy of Sciences USA*, **84**:2292–2296.

Vlodavsky, I., Fridman, R., Sullivan, R., Sasse, J. & Klagsbrun, M. (1987a). Aortic endothelial cells synthesize basic fibroblast growth factor which remains cell associated and platelet-derived growth factor-like protein which is secreted. *Journal of Cellular Physiology*, **131**:402–408.

Vlodavsky, I., Johnson, L.K., Greenburg, G. & Gospodarowicz, D. (1979). Vascular endothelial cells maintained in the absence of fibroblast growth factor undergo structural and functional alterations that are incompatible with their *in vivo* differentiated properties. *Journal of Cell Biology*, **83**:468–486.

Wahl, S.M., Hunt, D.A., Wakefield, L.M., McCartney-Francis, N., Wahl, L.M., Roberts, A.B. & Sporn, M.B. (1987). Transforming growth factor type β induces monocyte chemotaxis and growth factor production. *Proceedings of the National Academy of Sciences USA*, **84**:5788–5792.

Weiner, H.L., Weiner, L.H. & Swain, J.L. (1987). Tissue distribution and developmental expression of the messenger RNA encoding angiogenin. *Science*, **237**:280–282.

Winkles, J.A., Friesel, R., Burgess, W.H., Howk, R., Mehlman, T., Weinstein, R. & Maciag, T. (1987). Human vascular smooth muscle cells both express and respond to heparin-binding growth factor I (endothelial cell growth factor). *Proceedings of the National Academy of Sciences USA*, **84**:7124–7128.

Yoshida, T., Miyagawa, K., Odagiri, H., Sakamoto, H., Little, P.F., Terada, M. &

Sugimura, T. (1987). Genomic sequence of hst, a transforming gene encoding a protein homologous to fibroblast growth factors and the int-2-encoded protein. *Proceedings of the National Academy of Sciences USA*, **84**:7305–7309.

Zetter, B. (1988). Angiogenesis, state of the art. *Chest*, **93**(Supplement 3):159S–166S.

Zhan, X., Bates, B., Hu, X. & Goldfarb, M. (1988). The human FGF-5 oncogene encodes a novel protein related to fibroblast growth factors. *Molecular and Cellular Biology*, **8**:3487–3495.

Ziche, M., Jones, J. & Gullino, P.M. (1982). Role of prostaglandin E1 and copper in angiogenesis. *Journal of the National Cancer Institute*, **69**:475–482.

Discussion

Archer. In the rabbit cornea model, when you remove the FGF stimulus, do these new vessels regress or remain and how long does it take before they begin to regress?

Böhlen. They regress, but I do not know after what time.

Courtoy. You mentioned that TGF-β is abundant, as abundant as TNF. Is the morphology of the vessel induced by TNF similar to or different from that induced by TGF-β in the in-vivo system?

Böhlen. TGF-β is abundant. It is produced by almost all cells, so that it is strategically located to start angiogenesis wherever that would begin. TNF is carried by macrophages which can also go to all the strategic locations, but it is definitely not as abundant as TGF-β or αFGF. As far as the morphology of the vessels go, I have not done experiments with TGF-β myself, and therefore I cannot comment on whether they are different to TNF.

Findlay. Just for the record, there have been two reports of FGF in endometrium: one from Brigstock *et al.* (1989) who purified it from porcine endometrium, the other from Fujii and Lee (1987) in California with evidence for FGF in bovine endometrium. I wanted to ask a question about the potential origin of angiogenic factors in the endometrium. It is my understanding that there has to be some chemotactic effect in order to get the budding from a capillary. So, presumably, in the case of the endometrium, it has to be in cells distal from the vessels, perhaps epithelial cells.

Böhlen. I would like to entertain the hypothesis that it is not important which cell really makes FGF, but what is important is the fact that FGF is deposited in the extracellular matrix in a kind of diluted or unorganized fashion. Then activation comes from specific endothelial cells.

Findlay. If you take that line of thinking, every cell may have FGF in its extracellular matrix and it is whatever can cause the release of that FGF that is going to be important for stimulating angiogenesis.

Böhlen. Not every cell has FGF because we know cells which do not make FGF. It is true that the signals that come from perhaps a very small number of cells to activate the pool of FGF in the extracellular matrix may be very important molecules.

Clark. I would like to raise a point and ask for your comment. It has to do with the observation that there are several members of the TGF-β family; there are at least three and probably more members and there are at least three receptors for TGF-β. In comparing TGF-β1 and TGF-β2, it is clear that different cells will show different responses to the two members of the family based on the types of receptors that they express. Now, you have shown us that there may be five members of the FGF family. Are there also different receptors for FGF and might there be different responses depending on which of the family is about?

Böhlen. As far as we know, there is only one FGF receptor which occurs in two molecular forms. Probably the difference is the glycosylation and all cells seem to have this kind of receptor, so the diversity probably does not come from there. With respect to TGF-β family, it is now known (data from Andrew Baird, Salk Institute; personal communication) that TGF-β2 is a far less potent endothelial cell inhibitor than TGF-β1.

Baird. We have heard that the events in the uterus are primarily stimulated in an endocrine fashion, for example by the interaction of estradiol with its steroid receptor. How many of these potential angiogenic factors are influenced by particular steroid hormones?

Böhlen. I have no knowledge as to how any of these angiogenic factors would be affected by steroid treatment.

Baird. Angiogenesis continues long after the tissue has repaired, the endometrium has totally re-epithelialized by day 5 and there is massive new growth of capillaries occurring through the next 10 days.

Bischof. We know that decidual cells produce heparin sulfate very quickly; endometrial cells can also produce heparin sulfate in the matrix. So when damage occurs, angiogenesis would not continue, because if your hypothesis is correct, then FGF would just be trapped in the extracellular matrix.

Clark. I wish to bring up a point relating to available evidence that production of these growth factors may be stimulated by endocrine mechanisms. I do not think we know what happens in the endometrium. But in the ovary, the development of the follicle is stimulated by TGF-α, and either TGF-β or a factor related to Müllerian inhibitory substance. The production of these factors is believed to be triggered by the pituitary hormones that turn on the process in the ovary. So it would not be surprising to find other cells in the reproductive tract that could respond to endocrine signals to increase the production of growth factors.

Ludwig. Are there any factors known which govern the direction in which the vessels grow? It is one thing to start angioneogenesis, and another to continue growth within the fully developed endometrium. In the rabbit anterior chamber experiments, we have seen vessels growing in parallel. What orientates this growth?

Böhlen. I cannot explain why they grow parallel in the cornea experiment, but I have one possible explanation, and that is that we are dealing with an unnatural gradient. We have a large amount of FGF, localized in the cornea, and all the vessels grow towards that stimulus, and that is in fact in keeping with the hypothesis on tumour angiogenic factors whereby vessels grow into tumour tissue because of the presence of a gradient of the growth factors.

Naftolin. I want to point out how difficult the rabbit corneal assay is. It is very susceptible to any form of inflammation. This requires histological proof of absence of an inflammatory response. Moreover, the chorioamniotic membrane assay has exactly the same problems, so that if one is to assess these issues, it is probably not too useful to use the rabbit cornea. We should use something else like the ovary or the uterus. For example, angiotensin clearly is angiogenic in the cornea, but it does it by bringing in leukocytes. It does not do it in the ovary itself if we use a specific blocker, saralasin, to show that this is a specific effect.

Böhlen. It is an important point and I agree that it is essential to include controls and to look for absence of white cells.

Casey. Tumour necrosis factor-α is known to be a growth factor in almost every normal cell type except that it is cytolytic in tumour cells. In your model, you indicated that prior to the growth effect that was required for angiogenesis, you need something to disrupt the extracellular matrix. I wonder if you could comment on the state of the endometrial extracellular matrix at the time angiogenesis would be taking place?

Böhlen. I cannot comment on the last part of your question. However, I would like to oppose your notion that TNF-α is a growth factor for most cells. I would say it is an inhibitor for most normal cells. It is a growth factor for some cells, under certain conditions, for instance for fibroblasts, but not under all in-vitro conditions.

Casey. Can you be more specific? I have tested about 25 different cell lines and endometrial cells and a host of other investigators also have tested a variety of cells and it is only cytolytic in tumour cells.

Böhlen. TNF-α is an inhibitor of the smooth muscle cell and of the epithelial lens cell, at least.

References

Brigstock, D.R., Heap, R.B. & Brown, K.D. (1989). Polypeptide growth factors in uterine tissues and secretions. *Journal of Reproduction and Fertility*, **85** (2):747–758.
Fujii, D.K. & Lee, E. (1987). Growth and hormonal responsiveness of cultured bovine uterine epithelium. *Proceedings of the US Endocrinology Society*, **69**:127.

Towards a better understanding of the effects of progestogens on the mechanisms of endometrial bleeding: recommendations for research

IAN S. FRASER

Department of Obstetrics and Gynaecology, University of Sydney, Sydney, Australia.

Abstract

Long-acting progestogen-only contraceptives lead to a troublesome incidence of amenorrhea and irregular, frequent or prolonged endometrial bleeding. The causes of these bleeding disturbances are not understood, and simple and reliable treatment regimens have not yet been adequately investigated. An improved knowledge of the underlying endometrial events and biochemical mechanisms could be expected to lead to improved long-acting methods with reduced bleeding disturbances and to improved means of treatment of the disturbances.

There are still considerable gaps in our knowledge of the sequence of events and endometrial mechanisms of normal menstruation, but it seems likely that substantial differences exist in the mechanisms of breakthrough bleeding with progestogens. It seems probable that a major part of the bleeding during normal menstruation comes from the spiral arterioles and is actively limited in volume by vasoconstriction. On the other hand, breakthrough bleeding is probably of capillary origin, limited to particular areas of the endometrial surface at any one time, and repair of vessels and epithelium may be limited by a deficiency of estrogen receptors. Beyond these hypotheses, relatively little is understood about breakthrough bleeding and the way in which mechanisms could vary with different types of progestogen exposure.

In this chapter, a number of clinical questions have been outlined and a range of research needs suggested in relation to the clinical problem of contraceptive-related bleeding disturbances and to normal menstruation. There is an urgent need for collaborative research between clinicians and basic scientists with access to newer laboratory technologies in order to start unravelling what is undoubtedly a complex but fascinating biological problem.

Introduction

In 1979 the Task Force on Long-Acting Methods for Fertility Regulation of the Special Programme of Research, Development and Research Training in Human Reproduction of the World Health Organization convened an invited symposium to review what was known about endometrial bleeding and bleeding disturbances in relation to the use of different types of hormonal contraception, in particular, those using progestogens alone. The proceedings from that symposium still provide an important background to our present basis of knowledge (Diczfalusy *et al.*, 1980) and most of that background has not been repeated or included in this symposium. Interested readers should also consult the Serono Symposium on 'Mechanisms of menstrual bleeding' (Baird & Michie, 1985).

The 1979 symposium culminated with a comprehensive summary of the state of knowledge of endometrial bleeding and hormonal contraception, and systematic recommendations for a range of approaches to future research: 'A perspective of steroidal contraception and abnormal bleeding: what are the prospects for improvement?' (Fraser & Diczfalusy, 1980). Nine years later we are in a much better position to focus more clearly and ask better questions. In addition, we now have access to a wealth of information on molecular interactions which regulate cell and tissue processes which may have a bearing on endometrial breakdown and bleeding. New technologies are continuing to be developed at an ever-increasing rate and may be of great value if the right questions are asked. On the other hand, there are very considerable difficulties in studying this problem systematically, not just because of the difficulty of defining the problem in simple terms, but also in the collection of defined and relevant human endometrial tissues for study.

This chapter is intended to provide a framework for productive future discussion of research priorities.

Clinical background

Important clinical patterns of abnormal bleeding

It is worth emphasizing those disturbances of bleeding which women most frequently report as being disturbing, and which are often cited as reasons for method discontinuation (Odlind & Fraser, 1990). It is likely that the endometrial mechanisms underlying these clinical problems may differ quantitatively, if not qualitatively.

1. Frequent and unpredictable.
2. Prolonged.
3. Heavy (uncommon with hormonal methods).
4. Amenorrhea.

Endocrine background

Types of spontaneous endometrial bleeding

The endocrine background preceding individual episodes of endometrial bleeding may vary considerably, and this highlights the possibility that different local mechanisms may be involved in the tissue breakdown.

1. Estrogen and progesterone withdrawal following unopposed estrogen with subsequent estrogen and progesterone/progestogen exposure.

(a) True menstruation: in this situation most of the bleeding is thought to come from the spiral arterioles (Markee, 1940).

(b) Combined pill withdrawal bleed: bleeding here is thought to come from defectively developed spiral arterioles.

2. Estrogen withdrawal from endometrium exposed to estrogen alone.

(a) Anovulatory bleeding: this may occur from proliferative or hyperplastic endometrium.

3. Continuous progestogen exposure – breakthrough bleed.

(a) Low-dose progestogen with fluctuating follicular estradiol secretion (sometimes with endogenous progesterone secretion also): this type of bleeding is thought to arise mainly from capillaries, and is seen with low-dose continuous-release subdermal implants and vaginal rings (Odlind & Fraser, 1990).

(b) Medium- to high-dose progestogen exposure with low estradiol secretion: this bleeding is also of capillary origin. This pattern of exposure is seen in users of depo-medroxyprogesterone acetate, norethisterone enantate and sometimes in the first year of use of subcutaneous implants such as Norplant[R].

(c) Very high-dose progestogen exposure with cyclical ovarian function: this type of exposure is seen with levonorgestrel-releasing intrauterine devices, and bleeding is usually scanty.

4. Amenorrhea. Although this is not a type of spontaneous bleeding, it is a disturbance of the menstrual pattern which may hold some useful clues to the understanding of bleeding disturbances with different hormonal contraceptives. It would be helpful to know why women do not bleed under these circumstances.

(a) Low estrogen and low progestogen exposure: this is seen in the physiological conditions of postmenopause and lactation.

(b) Low estrogen and high progestogen exposure: this is typically seen in users of depo-medroxyprogesterone acetate, but may also occur in other hormonal contraceptive users under circumstances where other women may be bleeding erratically.

(c) High estrogen and high progestogen exposure: this is a situation seen in pregnancy.

An integrated picture of normal menstruation

At this point it is appropriate to review what we do know and what we do not know about this physiological process. A schematic overview of the possible mechanisms and sequence of events is summarized in Fig. 1.

It is clear that complex interrelationships exist between the many families of regulatory molecules during tissue breakdown and repair. A simplistic attempt to highlight some of these interactions is illustrated in Fig. 2, orientated around a possible central role for migratory white cells.

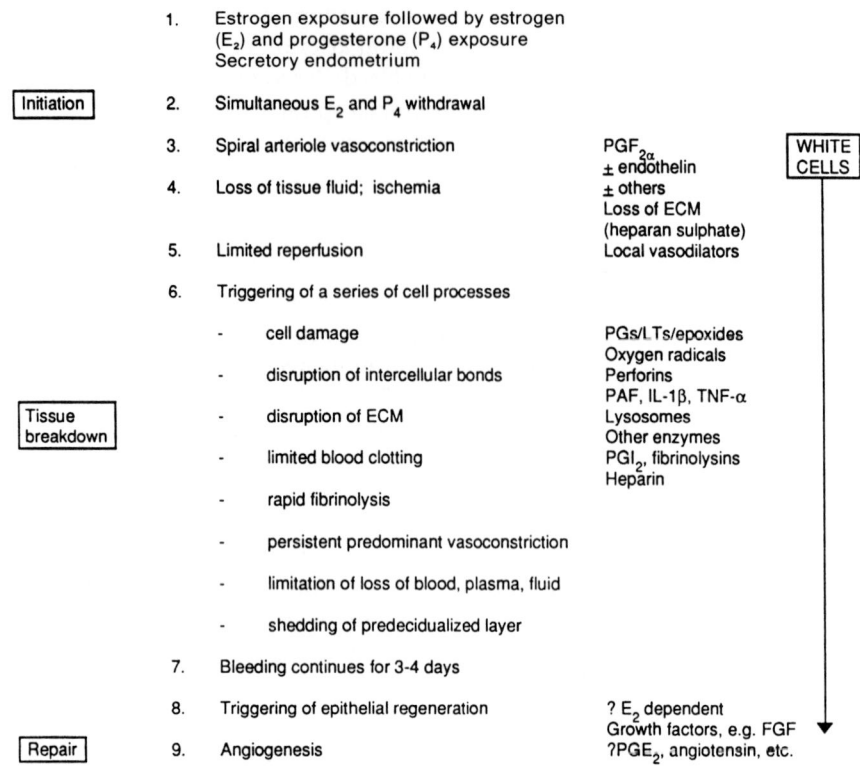

Fig. 1 Normal menstruation. What are the current views on mechanisms?
Key: E_2 = estradiol; P_4 = progesterone; PG = prostaglandin;
ECM = extracellular matrix; LTs = leukotrienes; PAF = platelet-activating
factor; Il-1β = interleukin-1β; TNF-α = tumour necrosis factor α;
FGF = fibroblast growth factor.

An integrated picture of breakthrough bleeding

A schematic view of possible mechanisms is illustrated in Fig. 3. Most of the
steps illustrated are hypotheses, but it is suggested that each of them can be
tested.

A research strategy

It is clear from the preceding discussion that a huge number of questions can
already be asked, yet few of them can currently be answered satisfactorily.
Hence, it is worthwhile looking at different priorities for investment of
resources. In this context, it is appropriate to review the most important
clinical questions and then to determine possible research needs.

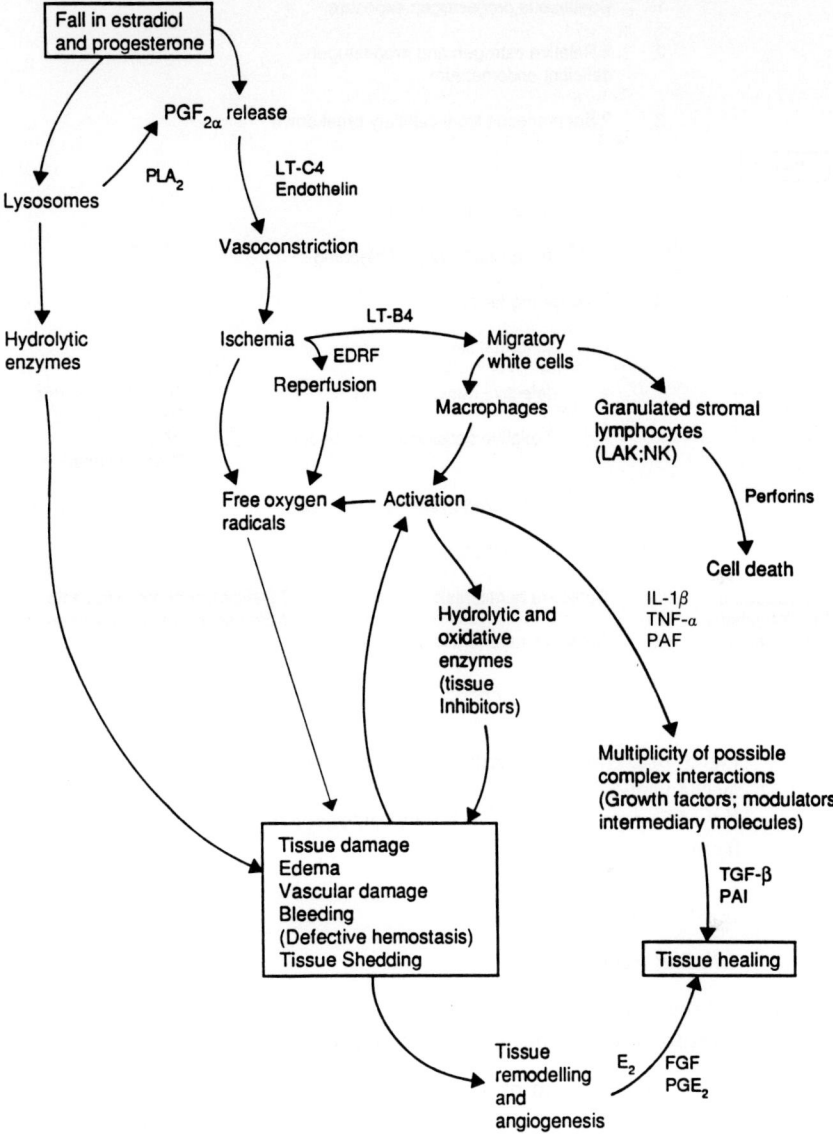

Fig. 2 A possible scheme of interactions between regulatory molecules in the endometrium during menstruation. No attempt has been made to distinguish stromal from glandular actions.

Key: PG = prostaglandin; LAK = lymphokine-activated killer cells; NK = natural killer cells; PLA_2 = phospholipase A_2; LT-B4 = leukotriene B4; LT-C4 = leukotriene C4; PAI = plasminogen activator inhibitor; EDRF = endothelium-derived relaxing factor; PAF = platelet-activating factor; FGF = fibroblast growth factor; IL-1β = interleukin 1β; TNF-α = tumour necrosis factor α; TGF-β = transforming growth factor β.

1. Continuous progestogen exposure

2. ? Relative estrogen and progestogen-deficient endometrium

3. ? Spontaneous focal capillary breakdown

Initiation
- subepithelial

- microbleeds/spotting

- recognizable vaginal bleeding

4. ? Triggering factors

- abnormal capillary morphology

- defective decidualization   PGs/LTs/epoxides
    Oxygen radicals
- ? relative deficiency of white cells   PAF
    Other intermediary
    molecules
- ? localized ischemia/reperfusion   Hydrolase enzymes

- ? activation of other mechanisms

Prolongation of bleeding

5. Defective hemostasis   ? Deficiency of procoagulants
    ? Excess activity of anticoagulants

6. Defective regeneration

    ? Estrogen deficiency
7. Defective angiogenesis   ? Growth factor deficiency
    ? Excess inhibitor activity

Fig. 3 Breakthrough bleeding. What are the current views on mechanisms?
Key: PG = prostaglandin; LT = leukotriene; PAF = platelet-activating factor.

Clinical questions

In users of long-acting progestogen-only contraceptives there are a number of priority questions which merit an early attempt at finding answers.

1. What variations in morphology occur in the endometrial arterioles, capillaries and venules in long-term progestogen users?
2. What is the endometrial and vascular histology during bleeding episodes? Does this vary in women with breakthrough bleeding compared with those who do not show breakthrough bleeding? Do these changes only occur in localized areas of the endometrium?
3. What is the appearance of the endometrial surface during bleeding episodes? Are the changes localized?
4. What are the extent and uniformity of decidualization of the endometrium following different durations of exposure to progestogens?

5. What is the extent of white cell infiltration of the endometrium in progestogen users? Does this change during episodes of bleeding? Can the cells involved in localized changes be identified?
6. Is the endometrium of progestogen users relatively deficient in estrogen and progestogen receptors? Can these receptor concentrations be measured? Are there localized variations in receptor concentration?
7. What volumes of blood and tissue fluid are lost during episodes of breakthrough bleeding?
8. Can different treatment regimens reliably stop episodes of breakthrough bleeding? What is the efficacy of different low dose estrogen regimens? Do agents such as antiprostaglandins, antihistamines, antifibrinolytic agents or vitamin E have any influence on different types of breakthrough bleeding? Are there other agents currently worth testing to see if they influence breakthrough bleeding?
9. Do estrogen and progestogen receptors reappear in the endometrium during successful treatment?

Clinical research needs

The clinical questions mentioned above can be translated into a number of research priorities and some suggestions are made under four headings below.

1. To define thoroughly the morphological appearances and some functions of progestogen-exposed endometrium (with and without bleeding).
1.1 Users should have been on treatment for a period of more than 3 months and should be using a specified progestogen delivered by a method providing constant release.
1.2 Specimens should only be obtained from timed hysterectomies.
1.3 There should be a defined endocrine background requiring repeated hormone sampling preoperatively.
1.4 There should be a study of the full depth of endometrial vasculature, looking specifically for dilated capillaries, endothelial proliferation, spiral arterioles, venules, lymphatics, subepithelial bleeding and scanning electron microscopy of the surface endometrium (especially if bleeding sites can be identified).
1.5 The extent of decidualization should be studied.
1.6 Migratory white cells should be sought and, if possible, identified by immunocytochemical typing.
1.7 Estrogen and progestogen receptors should be identified by immunocytochemistry in glands, stroma and vessels.
2. To define the endometrial surface appearances during breakthrough bleeding.
2.1 Subjects should have been on treatment for more than 3 months and the methods of use should be carefully defined.

2.2 The endometrial surface should be explored using contact hystero-scopy. By preference, one of the new narrow-diameter, flexible hysteroscopes with biopsy capability should be used.

2.3 Areas of endometrium showing subepithelial hemorrhage and specific bleeding points should be compared with non-bleeding areas. The appearances should be recorded by video and still-photography and directed biopsies should be carried out.

3. To explore simple therapies for treatment of prolonged or frequent bleeding.

3.1 Appropriate models include first-year users of Norplant[R] or progestogen-releasing vaginal rings.

3.2 Women experiencing an episode of bleeding greater than 8 days, or several episodes of bleeding where the bleeding-free interval is less than 10 days, could be considered for treatment.

3.3 Prospective menstrual diary cards should be kept.

3.4 Treatment groups should be randomized and treatment should be given in a double-blind manner. Possible treatment groups include the following.

3.4.1 Placebo.

3.4.2 Estradiol skin patches for 21 days (varying dosages).

3.4.3 Combined oral contraceptives for 21 days (consider varying regimens). Combined oral contraceptive pills have been included since these are widely and cheaply available in the developing world and are extensively and anecdotally used for treatment of bleeding disturbances with long-acting progestogens.

3.4.4 Vitamin E (varying doses).

3.5 The reversal of various endometrial markers during treatment should be studied in endometrial biopsies.

3.6 Intrauterine instillation of other possible therapies should be considered in exploratory studies.

4. To explore steroid mediation of breakthrough bleeding in more detail.

4.1 Users of progestogen-only methods, not experiencing breakthrough bleeding, should be studied. Markers of progestogen and estrogen status in timed biopsies should be studied using immunohistochemistry and biochemical techniques. The following markers should be considered: estradiol dehydrogenase; isocitric dehydrogenase; estrogen receptors; progestogen receptors; prolactin and PP 14.

4.2 Users of progestogen-only methods experiencing breakthrough bleeding should be studied. Markers of progestogen and estrogen status in timed endometrial biopsies should be studied in the same manner as 4.1.

4.3 The antiprogesterone agent RU486 could be used as a model to simulate progestogen withdrawal in users of long-acting progestogen-only methods. The ability of RU486 administration to produce a withdrawal bleed should be explored. Endometrial events in timed endometrial biopsies could be directly related to the timing of RU486 administration (see subsequent sections for endometrial events which require study).

Normal menstruation

Do we understand normal menstruation sufficiently well, or do we need to explore mechanisms in more detail as a matter of priority? It seems to me that there is an urgent need to explore the role of various factors in the initiation and maintenance of normal menstrual bleeding. I believe that this process is still relatively poorly understood.

1. Only women experiencing regular (25–35 day) cycles should be studied.
2. Detailed endocrinology of each study cycle should be obtained with at least three times weekly blood sampling.
3. Timed endometrial biopsies should be collected in relation to the onset of menstruation. Ideally these sections should be collected by timed hysterectomy since this allows much more accurate and detailed assessment of the full depth of endometrium as well as underlying myometrium.
4. Migratory white cells should be identified and quantified.
5. Tissue iron should be studied by electron spin resonance and tissue antioxidants should be assessed.
6. Lysosomal enzymes should be studied in more detail.
7. Non-lysosomal enzymes require detailed study.
8. The complex interactions of intermediary regulators require a series of co-ordinated studies.
9. Endothelin and endothelium-derived relaxing factors in endometrium require evaluation.
10. The direct and indirect influences of myometrium also require exploration.

Breakthrough bleeding

What events occur within the endometrium of progestogen-only users immediately before and during an episode of breakthrough bleeding; and what factors prolong a particular episode of bleeding? Practical priority studies need to be designed and careful attention needs to be paid to the types of experiment which can be done with endometrial biopsy specimens alone compared with the much better defined specimens which can be obtained from hysterectomy material.

A possible scheme of investigations is outlined in Fig. 4. This is mainly based

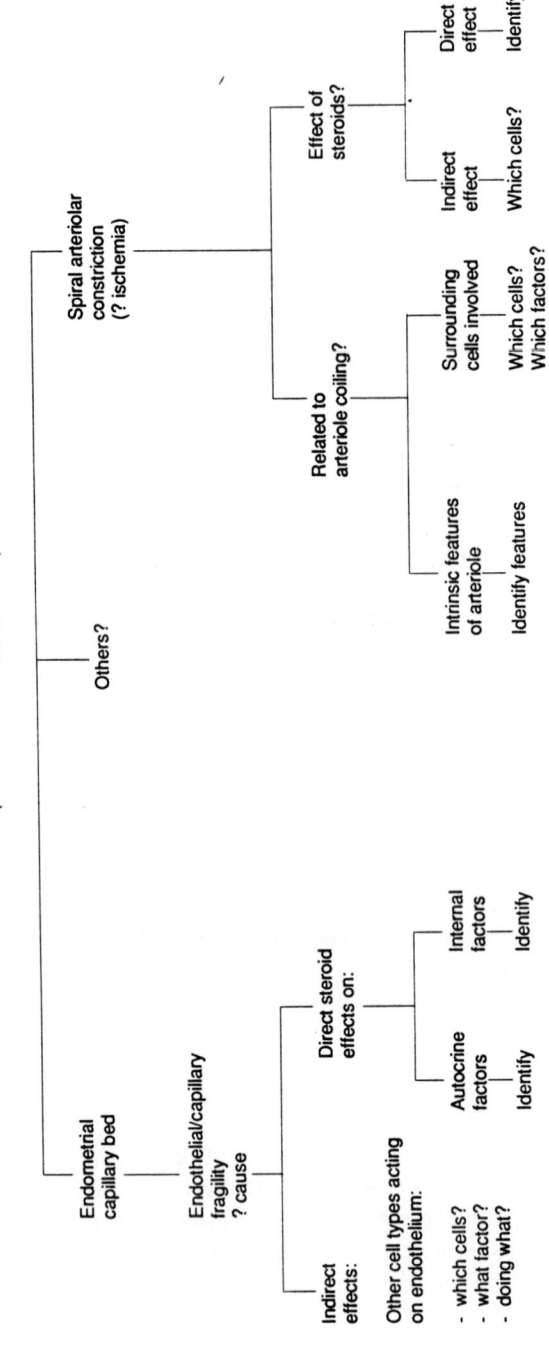

Possible factors involved: Arachidonic acid metabolism, prostaglandins, epoxides, lipocortins, PAF, paracrine effects, interleukin-1β, tumour necrosis factor-α, migratory white cells, free oxygen radicals, lysosomes, other enzymes, cytoskeleton.

Fig. 4 Flow chart suggesting possible routes for investigation of endometrial mechanisms involved in breakthrough bleeding (based on suggestions from Dr R.J.B. King).

on a plan suggested by Dr Roger J. B. King. In considering this model, it may be worthwhile bearing in mind the question of whether there is a final common metabolic pathway within the endometrium compared with the tissue breakdown and bleeding which occurs with normal menstruation.

In women experiencing prolonged episodes of bleeding, it is worth considering what direct and indirect effects occur within the endometrium in relation to hemostasis, tissue and cytoskeleton regeneration and angiogenesis.

Amenorrhea should not be forgotten since women experiencing this condition could serve as a form of control for comparisons with women experiencing breakthrough bleeding.

Animal models

Animal models need to be considered although we should carefully define what questions might be asked which cannot be answered by study of women themselves.

Subhuman primates have been considered, although anecdotally it appears that it is difficult to produce breakthrough bleeding in these animals. The primate which has been studied in most detail in relation to progestogen usage is the baboon (Fotherby & Goldzieher, 1980). It appears that this animal has an endometrium which is similar to, although not identical in response to, the human endometrium. Other models which may be considered further include mice treated so that the endometrium is decidualized (Finn & Pope, 1984) and human endometrial explants in hamster cheek pouch (Abel *et al.*, 1982). The advantages of these models are likely to lie in the direction of the assessment of in-vivo vascular changes under the influence of different factors. On the other hand, if an animal model of breakthrough bleeding could be identified, this would provide considerable opportunities for research study.

Menstruation in primates and the opportunities for research have been reviewed previously (Kraemer, 1980).

Conclusions

The opportunity now exists for the application of modern technologies to the elucidation of the complex interaction of different biochemical processes within the endometrium in relation to normal menstruation, breakthrough bleeding and amenorrhea. Many questions can be asked, but in the absence of unlimited research funding there is an urgent need to establish research priorities. A number of suggestions have been put forward in this chapter, and these should be read in relation to the highly detailed suggestions provided in a series of research papers read at this symposium. A further distillation of ideas is summarized in the Subgroup Reports which form the final chapter of this publication.

References

Abel, M.H., Zhu, C. & Baird, D.T. (1982). An animal model to study menstrual bleeding. *Research and Clinical Forums*, **4**(4):25–34.
Baird, D.T. & Michie, E.A., eds. (1985). *Mechanism of Menstrual Bleeding*. Serono Symposia Publications, Vol. 25. New York, Raven Press.
Diczfalusy, E., Fraser, I.S. & Webb, F.T.G., eds. (1980). *Endometrial Bleeding and Steroidal Contraception*. Bath, England, Pitman Press.
Finn, C.A. & Pope, M. (1984). Vascular and cellular changes in the decidualized endometrium of the ovariectomized mouse following cessation of hormone treatment: a possible model for menstruation. *Journal of Endocrinology*, **100**:295–300.
Fotherby, K. & Goldzieher, J.W. (1980). Animal models for the development of long-acting injectable contraceptives. (In) *Animal Models in Human Reproduction* (Serio, M. & Martini, L., eds.), pp.461–473. New York, Raven Press.
Fraser, I.S. & Diczfalusy, E. (1980). A perspective of steroidal contraception and abnormal bleeding: what are the prospects for improvement? (In) *Endometrial Bleeding and Steroidal Contraception* (Diczfalusy, E., Fraser, I.S. & Webb, F.T.G., eds.), pp.384–413. Bath, England, Pitman Press.
Kraemer, D.C. (1980). Comparative assessment of endometrial morphology and function in nonhuman primate models. (In) *Endometrial Bleeding and Steroidal Contraception* (Diczfalusy, E., Fraser, I.S. & Webb, F.T.G., eds.), pp.366–383. Bath, England, Pitman Press.
Markee, J.E. (1940). Menstruation in intraocular endometrial transplants in the rhesus monkey. *Contributions to Embryology*. Carnegie Institution of Washington Publication No. 518, **28**(No. 177):219–308.
Odlind, V. & Fraser, I.S. (1990). Contraception and menstrual bleeding disturbances. A clinical overview. (In) *Contraception and Mechanisms of Endometrial Bleeding* (d'Arcangues, C., Fraser, I.S., Newton, J.R. & Odlind, V., eds.), pp.5–29. Cambridge, England, Cambridge University Press.

Discussion

There was extensive general discussion which focused on two main areas: (a) normal menstruation, and (b) breakthrough bleeding and abnormal bleeding.

Normal menstruation

Baird. In this general discussion I think we should try to concentrate on those elements which may be relevant to solving the problem of breakthrough bleeding. In order to do this, we have to have some understanding of the mechanism of normal menstruation, the mechanism of tissue breakdown, and the possible cellular and biochemical events which may accompany this process of tissue breakdown. The establishment of normal menstruation is clearly a very complex event which has enormous evolutionary pressures on it to make sure that it does not compromise subsequent reproductive function. As Dr Clark mentioned, it is a very unusual event, that inside the body you can lose a gram of tissue over a period of 5 days and start again from where you started last month. The lack of coagulation during menstruation is absolutely essential for preservation of reproductive function. The sequence of hormonal events which induce the changes in the endometrium can be disturbed very little without compromising the pattern of menstruation. So I think it is relevant that we discuss what is the mechanism by which the endometrium normally bleeds. Because I think there have been considerable advances over the last 9 years since the last meeting in both the means of looking at the function of the endometrium and the uterus and the way in which it is controlled hormonally. I think some of these findings are relevant to development of methods for controlling abnormal bleeding with hormonal contraceptives. So I would like to start with what we know about normal menstruation.

Menstruation normally occurs from the secretory endometrium, in response to a fall in the concentration of progesterone and estradiol, and is associated with a characteristic pattern of myometrial activity. Normal menstruation is associated with a discarding of most of the superficial layers of the endometrium and this is maybe where it differs from some of the other abnormal bleeding episodes that we see. Lastly, it is of limited duration. Now, would anybody like to add anything other than that as an essential core to the process of normal menstruation?

Ludwig. I just want to add that it is not only a discarding, it is also a process of restoration, which has an effect on the duration of menstruation.

Baird. Yes. I was going to come on to the three separate events within the process of menstruation, namely the actual initiation of normal menstruation, the maintenance of bleeding and the regeneration leading to the cessation of bleeding. What is the trigger which initiates menstruation in response to steroid withdrawal? We heard from Dr Smith (Smith, 1990), that there have been various hypotheses of the mechanism of menstruation, some of which have been reiterated at this meeting. The initial event is a vascular one, basically an ischemic one. However, I would like to point out that the vascular events described by Markee (1940) involved not only vasoconstriction, but also rather striking vasodilatation, and I think any vascular theory has to encompass not just constriction of the vessels, but also vasodilatation. We have heard mentioned several times the theory of lysosomal instability. I think we have to say that any theory for the onset of menstruation has to be sensitive to steroid hormones, because it is steroid hormones that are actually initiating events. Would anybody like to discuss this?

Clark. There is an important point which should be brought up, I think, and that is this vasoconstriction which occurs as one of the very early events. To my understanding, this does not occur in a proliferative endometrium, it requires an endometrium which is primed and in the secretory phase. It is for that reason that I put vasoconstriction further down in the list of events and put the trigger as the drop in effective levels of progesterone and what I would prefer to call the detonator, and, next in line, the production of $PGF_{2\alpha}$. Because, in the absence of a suitably prepared endometrium, there will not be necessarily a response that will produce bleeding.

Smith. I wonder if the study of the factors inhibiting menstruation in early pregnancy will also give us insight into the initiation of menstruation?

Naftolin. In relation to normal menstruation, we are not talking about the withdrawal of progesterone, but about the regression of the corpus luteum which invariably leads to withdrawal of estrogen and progesterone.

Clark. I wish to comment further on the changes that prevent bleeding in normal pregnancy, because there seem to be two chemical actions that have been discussed during this meeting. The first is suppression of prostaglandin formation by steroidal hormones, the second is the presence in the decidua of transforming growth factor β (TGFβ)-like molecules. TGFβ is known to convert macrophages from an unfriendly superoxide-producing form to one which may be more compatible with lack of tissue destruction. Therefore, there may be these two factors involved in preventing the tissue destruction that occurs during a normal menstruation.

Baird. It is not only the maintenance of progesterone levels, but it is also highly likely that the embryo or embryonic products are producing factors which are suppressing a prostaglandin release; based on the sheep model, it is likely there might be an interferon-like substance. Certainly, with those species like the sheep and the guinea-pig and the rat in which suppression of uterine prostaglandin production and release is absolutely essential for the maintenance of the corpus luteum, there is very good evidence that the embryo is producing some factors which are suppressing prostaglandin release.

Courtoy. If I remember correctly from the early studies, one of the first steps which was pointed out by Markee was not only vasoconstriction but also collapse; so I think this should not be disregarded, as perhaps one of the initiating steps.

Rees. I was going to add to the definition that the bleeding will come principally from spiral arterioles rather than capillaries and venules based on the Markee model for normal menstruation. Does one say which blood vessel the blood comes from principally in our definition?

Baird. What Markee observed was that the constriction is occurring somewhere in the area of the myometrial/endometrial junction. Now what Dr Smith and I have suggested is that that constriction is due to the release of $PGF_{2\alpha}$ from the glands under the influence of the withdrawal of progesterone.

Cornillie. I think that we did not pay enough attention to the basal endometrium. Seeing this constriction in the myometrial/endometrial junction, and having in mind that, maybe, arterioles or larger venules are bleeding in endometria under the influence of long-acting progestogens, I think that the morphological picture of the endometrium we see is much more like a basal structure than a fully differentiated, superficial endometrium. So, when studying normal menstruation, we should also study the basal endometrium.

Bouchard. It is obvious that the basal endometrium is playing a role because there are steroid receptors present. How they are regulated has not been finalized as yet. The fall of progesterone was mentioned as initiating normal menstruation, then Dr Naftolin said that it is the fall of estradiol and progesterone. I think that if we refer to what Dr Sitruk-Ware presented (Sitruk-Ware *et al.*, 1990), it is a fall of estradiol in secretory endometrium, because when you give RU486 during the luteal phase, bleeding occurs. Now if luteolysis is not achieved, menstrual bleeding occurs 5 or 6 days later, so the fall of progesterone *per se* is not initiating menstruation.

Brosens. I wonder whether the vasoconstriction may not be an artefact in the sense that the upper part of the spiral arteries is the segment which is well developed and will develop more than the basal part, so that you get a bottle-neck at the endometrium/myometrium junction, and a bottle-neck may look like a spasm. It is only by increasing the amount of steroids that the bottle-neck may be released at the end of menstruation, and in a number of cases, the fall of steroids and the bleeding may just be coincidental.

Smith. But we have other evidence to suggest that the vasoconstriction is an important feature. Markee clearly stated that every episode of bleeding was preceded by vasoconstriction. Most of it, in Bartelmez's work (1937), occurs in the basal area of the endometrium, incidentally, not in the upper areas. So the point about vasoconstriction is true in Markee's work and is also true in hysteroscopic studies showing focal areas of ischemia.

Findlay. I just wanted to comment on your perception that there may have been some difference of opinion about the role of PG initiating that vasoconstriction. I suspect that actually reflects our ignorance about the specific action of PG, whether it is a specific action directly on the smooth muscle cells, or whether it involves some other vasoconstrictors and vasodilators.

Baird. I would be prepared to accept that it may not be a direct effect, but as you say, whether it is direct or indirect it is probably due to a release of vasoactive substance, maybe the prostaglandins. In fact, Dr Åkerlund, did you not tell me that if you give a big enough dose of vasopressin, you can induce bleeding?

Åkerlund. Yes, I agree there is a vasoconstriction. What causes it, however we do not know, as yet.

Wilson. I think there is one step you are missing out. Before there is vasoconstriction, there is dehydration whereby the tissue reduces significantly in height.

Baird. So, to sum up the initiation of menstruation, there is reasonable evidence that vasoconstriction of the arteries is probably an important insult to the endometrium and that it is probably due to the release of prostaglandins. Many of the events that we have discussed since then are probably a consequence of that tissue damage, because ischemia of tissue results in a whole range of changes in cellular function which are going to result in holes in the capillaries and further bleeding.

Perhaps now we can discuss the second step, which is the maintenance of bleeding. This is probably more relevant to what causes heavy bleeding and what might be associated with breakthrough bleeding. There is evidence that the maintenance of bleeding during the 4 or 5 days of menstruation is dependent on vasodilatation, on an inhibition of platelet aggregation and on inhibition of the normal coagulation response to tissue injury. That is a point that we have not discussed very much at this symposium. We did discuss it extensively in 1979 when the data from Dr Sixma's group (Sixma *et al.*, 1980) and others on the changes of the coagulation system was new, but I do not think we should forget it.

Clark. In the case of an ischemic injury of the brain or the heart, there is not usually a 40–50 ml bleed into that necrotic area subsequently. There may be some necrosis but, in the case of the uterus, perhaps there is a special mechanism to ensure that the blood does not clot, thereby destroying its subsequent function, but at a cost of some blood loss on a regular basis. Does the uterus have this characteristic, and could this be involved in much of the bleeding that occurs whenever there is an injury to it?

Sheppard. We have carried out studies to show that it is due to a very high level of fibrinolytic activity, but the blood does actually clot, and in fact in the 1979 meeting report (Sixma *et al.*, 1980), there are two electron micrographs showing fibrin in menstrual clots. There is no doubt about this. Due to the fibrinolytic activity, the blood does clot and then lyses.

Baird. But in general, the hemostatic response, which stops you bleeding within 4 minutes when you have cut your finger, is very seriously impaired within the uterus. The platelet plugs hardly get a chance to stay there. They disappear; you do not get fibrin in among the plugs, and the whole process of tissue repair does not take place.

Ludwig. I want to add something to what Dr Clark mentioned. He addressed myocardial infarction and brain infarction and stated that there was necrosis but not necessarily bleeding. In the endometrium, when we have initiation by vasoconstriction and then maintenance by vasodilatation, it is a different picture because we have a refilling of vascular space which has been, prior to this event, undergoing vasoconstriction. So the stroma of the endometrium on the first day of bleeding, when it is not completely destroyed but still filled with blood, extravasate and so on, looks like an organ after shock being recirculated. So this is very different to other pathological events where there is an irreversible arrest of bleeding. In the endometrium, there is continuous bleeding with an impaired endometrial tissue.

Rice-Evans. You certainly do get bleeding in the brain after an ischemic episode. After a myocardial infarction, what you can get is actually a leakage of myoglobin, so it is not bleeding in the same way, but nevertheless you are getting substances moving out of cells and across the system.

Clark. You do not usually get massive hemorrhage into your heart or brain infarct; however, I did not say that you did not get clotting, but rather that the uterus seemed to be specialized towards antagonizing that clot and dissolving it. My question was, does this make what occurs in the uterus different from what happens in other organs when you have an ischemic insult?

Baird. I think we would all agree that it does.

Cooke. Dr McNicol actually demonstrated that there was heparin in the uterus that was not circulating in the general circulation. That would tie up quite well with the activation of macrophages and potential dissolution of the extracellular matrix, because there are large concentrations of sulfated mucopolysaccharides in the ground substance.

Baird. Dr Rees demonstrated in her talk (Rees, 1990) and Dr McNicol's group presented very convincing evidence that platelets, once they have been through the uterine vasculature, are totally spent and degranulated and those which return into general circulation via the uterine vein are unable to clot. So something has happened to those platelets in their passage through the uterus, yet they have not actually formed plugs.

Rees. Platelets in uterine vein are able to aggregate normally and to metabolize arachidonic acid to thromboxane B_2, so they are able to function normally. The only thing they cannot do is adhere to glass beads, but you wonder what that actually means.

Findlay. I have a specific question in relation to the time-frame involved. For example, in the Markee model, how long does it take to go from the initial vasoconstriction event until you see extravasation or diapedesis?

Baird. I can tell you from the hamster cheek pouch: from the time of progesterone withdrawal and blanching, it takes about 48 hours before you get bleeding.

Fraser. I wonder whether someone might indicate whether they think there is a contribution from prostacyclin at this particular time during menstruation.

Baird. Dr Abel and Dr Kelly made some experiments, where they, like Poyser and others, noticed that prostacyclin was the major metabolite of arachidonic acid from the myometrium in contrast to the endometrium. The production of prostacyclin could be enhanced markedly by the myometrium if you added either homogenates of endometrium or supernatant from endometrium to myometrium. Subsequently, Dr Cameron demonstrated a similar effect using explants or chunks of tissue co-incubated together. Dr Abel proposed the hypothesis that platelets were prevented from clumping by the release of prostacyclin from the intima of the radial arteries. Now, as far as I know, nobody has ever been able to confirm or provide further evidence for this theory, but it certainly would be one explanation as to why the platelets fail to adhere at the point of tissue damage.

Smith. The observation in heavy periods was that the combined production of endometrial/myometrial prostacyclin was greater when the endometrium was taken from women with heavy periods compared to women who did not have heavy periods. If I could just come back to Dr Rees' comment: I thought that the platelets in menstrual blood, once they had gone through the uterus, were not able to respond to ADP and collagen. In which case prostacyclin would seem to me the most likely reason for this changed platelet function.

Baird. Yes, but what Dr Rees said was that uterine vein platelets were normal.

Rees. Yes, they are normal; but I wanted to add another point. If you take menstrual blood and spin off the supernatant serum and then you add the serum to normal peripheral venous platelets, they aggregate. So menstrual serum has a pro-aggregatory compound in it, and this aggregation is inhibited by pre-incubating the platelets with aspirin. We had expected that menstrual serum would inhibit aggregation, whereas in fact it promoted it; we think that menstrual blood platelets do not aggregate because they are spent and degranulated and have already aggregated in the endometrium.

Harper. In connection with this discussion on platelets, I would like to remind you that when platelets are exposed to platelet-activating factor (PAF), they degranulate, but they are also desensitized and their response to PAF is reduced or ablated (Keraly & Benveniste, 1982; Tokumura *et al.*, 1985; Homma *et al.*, 1987). So I think this fits in very well with the model.

Åkerlund. There is something I missed and that is tissue expulsion. That made me think of how the uterus functions with regard to contractile activity at menstruation. One can prove, by recording intrauterine pressure at different places in the uterus, that there is a propagation of contractions which, presumably, serves for expulsion of the content. This is good for hemostasis but one could also imagine a milking effect of this contractile activity, perhaps increasing the blood loss.

Baird. Could somebody remind me when most of the tissue is actually expelled?

Ludwig. There is no expulsion of tissue on only one day. The uterus expels tissue for 3 days in the normal cycle. We have evidence from some uteri that before the tissue is expelled, it remains in the uterine cavity for hours and then gets proteolytically destroyed. So that if we look at menstrual discharge, we still find tissue, but in very small amounts and nearly not identifiable.

Rees. Collecting menstrual fluid, I noticed I collected viable tissue, and in fact you can grow endometrial cells collected in menstrual fluid and the yield of cells per unit of time is greater on the first 2 days of menstruation than on subsequent days.

Breakthrough bleeding and abnormal bleeding

Baird. I would like to move on to breakthrough bleeding. I propose that what we talk about now is any bleeding not associated with normal menstruation.

Naftolin. One question we have not addressed is whether every woman can be made to develop breakthrough bleeding when faced with a certain amount of progestogen. This might be helpful in understanding the genesis of the disturbance. I would suggest that one of the clinical protocols that might be considered is a carefully selected group exposed to stepwise changes in progestogens over varying periods of time. If we can create a group of breakthrough bleeders, then we could apply some of the specific technologies selectively.

Fraser. To my knowledge, that has never been done. We do have much information about the pharmacokinetics and pharmacodynamics of various progestogens and we do see individuals with identical blood levels of exogenous progestogen who have totally different bleeding patterns. On the other hand, I am unaware of any investigators who have set out to cause breakthrough bleeding in particular individuals by stepwise variation in their progestogen exposure.

Diaz. Actually, some women never experience bleeding problems with progestogens, but the same woman may change with time, even when exposed to the same doses of the steroid. When we replace Norplant implants in long-term users, they receive the same dose and blood levels they were exposed to during the first month, 5 years previously, when they experienced prolonged bleeding, but this does not recur when they are re-exposed to the higher daily dosage.

Naftolin. I believe that every woman, at some point, must be able to be made to have breakthrough bleeding. If that is not true, that is an important piece of information, but, intuitively, I think that if you give either enough or insufficient amounts for some period of time, every woman's endometrium will finally say 'I will not support this'.

Fraser. The concept is an interesting one. I suspect that one of the clinical problems is that some women will not show breakthrough bleeding in the first 1–3 months and will then suddenly embark upon a dreadful pattern, even with the same continuing exposure. So you might need to expose the women to each dose for several months at a time before moving to a different dose to study them again.

Diaz. The experiment is quite difficult because when women receive a given progestogen after a hormone-free period, they react in a certain way. If they receive that progestogen at the same dose after previous treatment, they may react in a different way. So I cannot imagine how we can do such an experiment, and what numbers of women should be included to make that statistically meaningful.

Toppozada. I have a small comment here about the suggested clinical trials. We know that estrogens probably work in a percentage of patients, particularly amongst those who have prolonged spotting or prolonged bleeding, but have you considered adding some studies with antiprostaglandins or with the antifibrinolytic agents?

Fraser. Yes, but I deliberately put those as a lower priority because we have preliminary evidence from Dr Diaz that a prostaglandin inhibitor given in high dose seems to be less effective than estrogen. It is something that might well benefit from further exploration, but I do not see it as one of the highest priorities. The same applies to the antifibrinolytic agents which generally require to be taken in quite high dosage, and although there is also evidence that they may reduce the duration of episodes of bleeding and spotting, they are probably not quite as good in this area as estrogen would be.

Gurpide. I wonder if another model could be useful to study the effects on capillary beds, for instance of different ratios of prostaglandins. That could be extracorporal perfusion of the human uterus, a technique well developed in Italy, at least for perfusion of isolated cotyledons in the placenta. You could really test in a reproducible manner relative effects of vasoconstrictors and dilators.

Ludwig. For macrocirculatory studies, you need very fresh material free of artefact. The most valuable information in breakthrough bleeding would be to obtain tissue just before the bleeding begins, because when bleeding starts, we see destruction in the upper layers just beneath the lining epithelium. I cannot see a way to plan collection of such tissue, except perhaps by careful history review in a high-risk group of patients.

Sheppard. As far as I can see, we cannot obtain the same sort of information that we had in the events leading up to normal menstruation in breakthrough bleeding because of its irregularity and unpredictability.

Brosens. Maybe one could try to detect microbleeders (using sensitive cervical detection) so that you are not working on material which is exposed to heavy bleeding. My second point is whether a stepwise increase in progestogens would be worth studying to see if this could stop breakthrough bleeding.

Clark. Since you are trying to study an unpredictable event, perhaps it might be possible to get some information by having hysterectomy specimens from a control group without the problem, and specimens from the group with the problem. And if you expect 50% of the women to develop breakthrough bleeding at some time, then if you find abnormalities in a certain proportion of those uteri, you could infer that they might be relevant to the problem. In order directly to implicate those changes in the process of breakthrough bleeding, you really need a manipulable model where you can reproduce that type of situation.

Fraser. You may also obtain predictive information by studying different areas of the same uterus in the patient who is bleeding from only one or two small areas. I would suggest that we also consider whether prolonged bleeding is due to one area that starts bleeding and then continues bleeding, or whether it is repetitive initiation of new bleeds from different areas. You could also take a group of women who do not appear to have much of a bleeding problem on a particular progestogen dosage, and a group who do have repeated problems, and then look at different parts of the endometrial surface.

Naftolin. I am interested in a very old model of the monkey with a uterine fistula, which has produced a lot of information in years past, to investigate estrogen and progestogen responses. As far as I know, it has not been applied to any of these recent questions. This is a model that Dean Moyer developed 20 years ago (Good & Moyer, 1966) and I think would be extremely useful for the investigation of progestogen-induced bleeding. Is there a reason why a monkey model could not be used now to test some well-defined questions?

Fraser. Ten years ago we considered Dean Moyer's uterine fistula model as a way of finding out what was happening in the endometrium. We decided not to use it for a number of reasons, although some of those reasons may now be superseded. At that time we felt that we could biopsy women under specific circumstances of treatment with progestogens and other agents and get better information from human endometrium. Also, the rhesus monkey endometrium may not be identical to the human endometrium. Secondly, we had information that it was very difficult to make monkeys have breakthrough bleeds and therefore would prefer to stay with the human model where we know there is a bleeding problem. Perhaps the only advantage in an animal model situation would be that we could take more biopsies. However, we were also concerned that by doing one biopsy we might alter what was happening in the endometrium at the time the next biopsy was taken. On the other hand, I am sure you could design useful experiments by asking questions that could be answered specifically in a monkey model.

Harper. I would like some clarification about the unsuitability of a subhuman primate model. I am not clear whether it was that you could not really induce the condition in the baboon or rhesus monkey or whether it was a question of cost. Secondly, and this is part of the same question, has any systematic attempt ever really been made to try to induce an inappropriate or abnormal endometrial bleeding in some subhuman primate by appropriate hormonal regimens?

Fraser. We did consider this, and our primate experts told us that they had never been able to find breakthrough bleeding in baboons or rhesus monkeys treated with the long-acting agents. However, they had not systematically set out to study those models with different dosages to see if they could induce breakthrough bleeding. And, of course, breakthrough bleeding in those animals might be very light and only be detectable by a cotton-tipped swab in the vagina, looking for very small amounts of bleeding, and it may not be really obvious at the entrance of the vagina. So, there may well be a place for exploring such a model further, but you need to consider what questions you can answer with that model which you cannot answer in women.

Cornillie. I think there is substantial evidence that breakthrough bleeding is only a very focal event in the whole endometrium. We cannot be sure that biopsies are giving the correct piece of tissue. I would suggest that using hysteroscopic localization, we try to take microbiopsies from bleeding and non-bleeding foci in the endometrium, so that each endometrium has its own control. This would provide us with material for morphological and biochemical studies from the same endometrium under the same hormonal conditions.

Baird. I do not think it matters too much that we try to identify exactly what happens during a bleeding episode. We know that under certain hormonal regimens, a large percentage of women will experience breakthrough bleeding at some time or another and that must indicate some fundamental change in the biochemistry of that endometrium or that uterus which makes it susceptible to abnormal bleeding. I do not think we want to be concerned that we will time the biopsy during an episode of bleeding. If there is an abnormality, it should occur in response to the steroids to make that endometrium more susceptible to it, and if we can identify the abnormality, then we can start to try to correct it.

Diaz. I also want to warn you that endometrium from these women is thin and gives rather small amounts of tissue, so that after the first few hours of bleeding you may not obtain any biopsy sample.

Weintraub. I would like to talk about a model of focal bleeding which may help us find the factors that initiate bleeding. This is a model of cerebral malaria in mice in which there are hemorrhages in the brain from capillaries; it has been shown that endothelial destruction was mediated by immune-activated cells and also by tumour necrosis factor (TNF). I think it may be possible to look in biopsies for these kinds of effects on endothelial cells without actually waiting for the start of bleeding. This is obviously a non-steroidal mediated model, and although it may seem a little distant from what we are talking about today, it at least provides a pathway for discussing how endothelia become permeable.

Fraser. I understand that malaria is a condition where there are extraordinarily high initial circulating levels of TNF, and I think that TNF is said to be responsible for a whole series of the symptoms and signs of severe malaria. It remains to be seen whether high TNF levels are released in the endometrium. Do women with acute malarial infection start bleeding from the endometrium?

Clark. If one obtained hysterectomy specimens from a population of women with a 50% risk of bleeding and you found in 50% of those uteri that there were focal areas of increased mRNA for TNF, then one might have some direct information implicating such a mechanism in bleeding.

Diaz. It happens that the majority of women who use these methods are young, fertile women who do not require a hysterectomy. Therefore protocols to look for tissue at hysterectomy specimens may need to be big, international collaborative studies.

Fraser. You need to identify those women who are already scheduled to have a hysterectomy for benign disease and then treat them with Norplant[R]. These include women with uterine prolapse, but they may still be few and far between. Dr Ludwig has collected 35 in 18 years. However, I really believe that hysterectomy specimens set up in this way are going to provide enormous advantages over biopsies.

Smith. I do not agree that these should be difficult to get. There are 20 000 hysterectomies performed a year in Britain alone for so-called menstrual problems, of whom only 60% have major symptoms.

Johannisson. I would like to say that with good biopsy material, and particularly with directed biopsies which have been taken by hysteroscopy, we have the possibility to study the vasculature in the functional layer, and perhaps also to carry out biochemical studies in the same material.

Ludwig. It is not easy to convince clinicians to arrange hysterectomies at a particular time and date, and to have an endocrine profile before operation. I think it could be one of the purposes of this group in their respective regions to encourage cooperation with surgeons and to convince them that essential information can be provided by properly dating a hysterectomy in a premenopausal woman or in a woman with some cyclic events on Norplant[R].

Naftolin. I think that, in a pragmatic sense, it would be inappropriate to start out with the idea that we are going to depend on hysterectomies. I think that the hope is to do proper, deep hysteroscopic biopsies and to try to establish a model in women using the protocol that I suggested. If that fails, then one might consider going to the much more extreme and unbelievably more complex idea of trying to get enough hysterectomies and obtain them in well-matched conditions. I do not think it is wise to make an experiment any more complex than you really need.

Wilson. As I look round this table, the majority of participants are from developed countries, and yet there is a wealth of resources, both human and material, in developing country institutions, which I would suggest are much closer to the problem than most of you. I would urge, simply, that any research programmes, such as those outlined by Dr Fraser, should have the active participation of developing country scientists at all levels.

Brosens. I agree with Dr Naftolin that you do not need a large number of hysterectomy specimens, but if you combine a proper hysteroscopy at the time of hysterectomy, you have the correlation between hysteroscopy with assessment of bleeding with tissue from a few hysterectomy specimens examined in detail.

Rees. Hysteroscopy specimens may have some value, but they only provide endometrium, and we should compare studies of endometrium with myometrium because myometrium is the greatest bulk of tissue of the uterus. Myometrium produces prostacyclin which is the principal prostaglandin produced by the uterus.

Smith. I agree with Dr Brosens that you probably need both approaches. I would suspect that the hysteroscopically directed biopsy is only going to provide enough tissue to do immunohistochemistry. You are not going to obtain more than, say, 20 mg of tissue, and if you want to study messengers and regulation of messengers, you will need at least 100, maybe 200 mg of tissue. Once the woman is taking progestogens, the amount of biopsy tissue will be very limited.

Naftolin. Again, I would just plead for simplicity and for very carefully defined goals. The idea of doing in-situ hybridization, for example, is far too complex for this stage of the investigation. What I see is that we have no histology, so let us satisfy ourselves that we are first going to get some decent histology. I think that is accomplishable.

Clark. I wonder if I might ask a provocative question. Do we not already have treatments to prevent breakthrough bleeding? If there are anovulatory cycles, we can give sequential contraceptive agents. If there is progestogen-only bleeding, can we not give ethinyl estradiol? If an IUD is causing heavy periods, we can give a non-steroidal agent, and if we cannot correct the breakthrough bleeding, can we not remove it and give something else? Why are we expending the energy to try to define the mechanisms if we already have treatment for these problems?

Diaz. I want to point out that we do not have a treatment for irregular bleeding in progestogen-only contraceptors. We have a single study in which ethinyl estradiol seems to work to control prolonged bleeding in progestogen-only contraceptive users. It is a single study; we cannot draw that conclusion from that study.

Odlind. Even if we did have a positive effect of estrogen treatment in these women, it is going to be very controversial, because one of the objectives of the long-acting contraception is the ease of administration. It has to be pointed out that you want people to continue to use this method. So the only way of making it acceptable to women is to make it very easy to use and not induce side-effects. Estrogens are also connected with side-effects and risks and are less acceptable. But even if we did have that treatment, it is very impractical.

Cooke. I just wanted to say that Dr Odlind's despair was really generated from the epidemiology and toxicology of much higher doses of estrogen from a long time ago. Now there is very good percutaneous estrogen administration of estradiol with maintenance of quite low levels, which are likely to have much less morbidity. So I think they are entirely different opportunities for looking at potential treatment and one ought to look at the mechanism and see the different treatment modalities over a longer period of time.

Fraser. Just to follow on from Dr Cooke: I think that estrogen is an option if you are going to be able to use it short-term, perhaps for one treatment course to help a woman over a period of bleeding problems. I do not think it is an option in the long term because one of the major advantages of these methods is that they are simple, they are long acting, and the women see major advantages in that approach, and it becomes much more complicated if you add something else. The estradiol patches may well be an advantage in terms of providing constant low levels of estrogen in a somewhat easier way, but they are expensive. Certainly, the WHO Programme would regard this as a considerable problem if they were providing huge numbers of patches for women in the developing world, so I think we have to bear those practical problems in mind. In answer to Dr Clark: stopping treatment is an inferior option when these methods do involve considerable advantages, and I think it is important to have those clinical perspectives rather than just saying, 'we will opt out' or 'we will use other treatments'.

Bischof. Instead of giving the estrogen with skin patches, why not include the estradiol directly into the implant, and study a mixed implant?

Diaz. Because we are looking for an estrogen-free method.

Smith. We have tried progestogens alone, and in 50% of the women there is abnormal bleeding. Many women are going to need some additional medication and it is more than likely going to be some sort of estrogen preparation on an intermittent basis.

Clark. We have heard that the simple solution of adding estrogen is not going to be widely acceptable, notwithstanding the suggestion that patches be tried as one remedy. Therefore, it would seem that the hope is that by applying modern scientific techniques and some of the newer technologies, we might be lucky and discover mechanisms producing the bleeding where we could intervene with some alternative measure which would be acceptable with progestogen-only contraceptive users.

Casey. Dr Baird, the comments you made earlier about the reluctance of acceptance of the hypothesis that you and Dr Smith put forward are somewhat confusing to me, for there are many investigators in this room who have spent many years of work to evaluate that in some detail and, in fact, I think it is quite well accepted. In addition to that, Dr Diaz has undertaken a study in which she has treated women on progestogens with the inhibitor of prostaglandin synthesis and was fairly successful in showing that there was a reduction in bleeding. Albeit she has suggested that it is only one study, it was in fact one that leads you to think there might be some further studies to be done based on that fact. So I think we should all keep that in mind.

Baird. It is possible that only an endometrium which has undergone predecidual or decidual change, having been exposed to estrogen and then followed by progesterone, can respond to vasoconstriction or insult by tissue necrosis and sloughing. One hypothesis is that breakthrough bleeding which occurs in women who are exposed continuously to progestogens is due to the fact that the endometrium is never allowed to go through a period of unopposed estrogen, and hence never gets the opportunity to develop an adequate number of either estradiol or progesterone receptors and therefore is in a functional state of progesterone deficiency. Now, I think that hypothesis is amenable to testing. It should be tested before we embark on very tedious and expensive trials or to repeat the sort of work that Dr Diaz has done. If it did confirm that there is a deficiency of progesterone receptors and that one could correct this deficiency by the administration of estrogen, then I think there is every hope that you should try to develop an appropriate system for delivering estrogen to cope with breakthrough bleeding.

Cooke. Dr Baird, with the RU486 model, do you not already know that having wiped out the progesterone receptors and maintained your estradiol, you actually get a second menstruation? In other words, there is maintenance of the endometrium; in spite of an insult, it goes on and has menstruation ultimately at the predicted times. So you already have some evidence that persisting with estradiol/estrogen administration actually is an effective treatment of that intermenstrual or breakthrough bleeding.

Baird. Yes, except that the endometrium in women who have been given RU486 has received an appropriate period of unopposed estrogen for the follicular phase of that cycle, whereas the situation in women who are on progestogen-only contraception is slightly different in that, for months on end, that endometrium is exposed to low-dose progestogen. I think Dr King showed very conclusively that you require really very modest amounts of progestogen to inhibit the synthesis of progesterone receptor in postmenopausal women.

Diczfalusy. In subjects who are taking different modifications of this so-called model estrogen/progestogen pill, the endometrium is never exposed to unopposed estrogen, and the bleeding patterns in some of the studies are very good.

Baird. Well, of course, it is all a balance between the amount of estrogen and the amount of progestogen. It is not exactly true to say that they are not exposed to unopposed estrogen: when they stop the pill, they are exposed to unopposed endogenous estrogen for 7 days. But would everybody agree that long-acting progestogens induce decidualization?

Fraser. I think it is clear that they induce a degree of decidualization initially, but whether this continues for very long is uncertain. I think your comments earlier suggesting that this tissue is in fact very deficient in progesterone action is probably a very reasonable one because of a reduction in progesterone receptors. I also think there is some indirect evidence for that, even though it has not been looked for specifically in endometrium in these particular women. If we look at what has been published so far on the endometrium exposed to different types of long-acting progestogens, any evidence of decidualization disappears steadily; you get an endometrium which goes through irregular secretory changes, irregular decidualization resulting in suppressed proliferation, and even what the pathologists have called atrophy. We understand from Dr

Johannisson that, morphologically, she cannot distinguish this progestogen-exposed atrophy from the atrophy that is seen in postmenopausal uterus, so that it seems to me as if this may well be a progestogen-deprived tissue, but certainly not a decidualized one.

References

Bartelmez, G.W. (1937). Menstruation. *Physiological Review*, **17**:28–72.

Good, R.G. & Moyer, D.L. (1966). Technique of serial endometrial biopsy in the monkey through uterocutaneous fistula. *Journal of Reproduction and Fertility*, **22**:573–574.

Homma, H., Tokumura, A. & Hanahan, D.J. (1987). Binding and internalization of platelet-activating factor 1-**O**-alkyl-2-acetyl-**sn**-glycero-3-phosphocholine in washed rabbit platelets. *Journal of Biological Chemistry*, **262**:10582–10587.

Keraly, C.L. & Benveniste, J. (1982). Specific desensitization of rabbit platelets by platelet-activating factor (PAF-acether) and derivatives. *British Journal of Haematology*, **51**:313–322.

Markee, J.E. (1940). Menstruation in intraocular endometrial transplants in the rhesus monkey. *Contributions to Embryology*. Carnegie Institution of Washington Publication No. 518, **28**(No. 177):219–308.

Rees, M.C.P. (1990). Factors controlling menstrual blood volume. (In) *Contraception and Mechanisms of Endometrial Bleeding* (d'Arcangues, C., Fraser, I.S., Newton, J.R. & Odlind, V., eds.), pp.117–130. Cambridge, England, Cambridge University Press.

Sitruk-Ware, R., Yaneva, H. & Spitz, I.M. (1990). Anti-progestogens and endometrial morphology. (In) *Contraception and Mechanisms of Endometrial Bleeding* (d'Arcangues, C., Fraser, I.S., Newton, J.R. & Odlind, V., eds.), pp.325–334. Cambridge, England, Cambridge University Press.

Sixma, J.J., Christiaens, G.C.M.L. & Haspels, A.A. (1980). The sequence of haemostatic events in the endometrium during normal menstruation. (In) *Endometrial Bleeding and Steroidal Contraception* (Diczfalusy, E., Fraser, I.S. & Webb, F.T.G., eds.), pp.86–96. Bath, England, Pitman Press.

Smith, S.K. (1990). The physiology of menstruation. (In) *Contraception and Mechanisms of Endometrial Bleeding* (d'Arcangues, C., Fraser, I.S., Newton, J.R. & Odlind, V., eds.), pp.33–44. Cambridge, England, Cambridge University Press.

Tokumura, A., Homma, H. & Hanahan, D.J. (1985). Structural analogs of alkyl-acetyl-glycerophosphocholine. Inhibitory behavior on platelet activation. *Journal of Biological Chemistry*, **260**:12710–12714.

Recommendations for future work: subgroup reports

The participants reviewed the papers and discussions presented to the symposium. Recommendations for further work were grouped into four main research areas: clinical studies and treatment; steroid receptors and proteins; prostaglandins and second messengers; migratory cells, remodelling and regeneration. The recommendations from these subgroups follow.

Clinical studies and treatment

Group 1 B. Affandi, I.A. Brosens, I.D. Cooke, M.-C. Cravioto, S. Diaz, H.M. Hourihan, E. Johannisson, V. Odlind, Qiu Shu-hua, M.C.P. Rees and B.L. Sheppard.

Cooke. We identified three areas for further investigation. The first one was to look in further detail at data already available from the World Health Organization clinical studies: firstly, to look at the menstrual diaries, with the statistical package for menstrual bleeding analysis that has not been fully exploited yet. In addition, there is quite a lot of pharmacokinetic data available from the vaginal rings and from the Norplant[R] implant studies; a review of these data would give a clearer idea of the steroid profiles in relation to bleeding patterns. From studies involving endometrial biopsies or hysterectomy that have previously been carried out, there remain tissue blocks from the normal cycle and vaginal ring studies. These are well timed, and well documented, and in the light of experience gained from the discussion during this meeting, morphologists should look for new evidence.

The second item is the collection of new tissue, and there are two possible types of contraceptive users. Firstly, among patients currently being treated with Norplant[R] (we probably cannot investigate all the progestogen methods and should concentrate on one), we could look for those who might be candidates for total hysterectomy. Or we could do it the reverse way: one could take patients who were candidates for total hysterectomy who could be pretreated with Norplant[R]. One would be looking for individuals who have the two primary complications, prolonged or frequent bleeding. There is no guarantee that there will be the same morphological elements in these two categories. Having obtained these specimens, we would need a set of control data. There are really three different timed controls that would need to be selected, one in the late luteal phase, one immediately preceding menstruation, and one in early menstruation. The first two should be selected according to LH dating, day

LH + 10 and either day LH + 12 or LH + 13 would be suitable. That would then give five groups of specimens with five or ten specimens in each group. Certainly, the data should be evaluated after five have been collected in each group, and if there was major divergence or large errors on the morphometric data, then it would be preferable to continue to collect data from ten subjects. Studies should include morphometry, scanning and transmission electron microscopy.

It is important to measure the diameter of the vessels, the endothelial cells, the gap-junctions, and plasmalemmal vesicles. For light microscopy, both by cryostat and fixed preparations, leukocytic infiltration would be an important element, also gland atrophy, morphometry of the glands, spiral arteries, edema and predecidua formation. It was thought that the patients who have been treated with Norplant[R] – if that is the selected progestogen – and who are going to have hysterectomy could have a hysteroscopy immediately preceding the hysterectomy to map the focal areas of bleeding so that it would be possible to identify particular areas for closer attention and equally to provide a control area (non-bleeding) within the same uterus.

The third area for investigation was treatment. It was felt that the most promising treatment was estrogen because there were some positive data, but it was felt that it was important to extend that data base. The end-point in any statistical analysis would, of course, be an effective reduction in the amount of prolonged bleeding, or an effective reduction in the frequency of bleeding. There would need to be different ways of administering the estrogen. Oral ethinyl estradiol could be given in the form of oral contraception and the preparation one would use would depend very much on the progestogen and delivery system to be supplemented. If it was Norplant[R], it would be levonorgestrel, and of course if it was a ring, an appropriate matching progestogen would be used. If using Depo-Provera[R], then one could administer the estrogen either as estradiol cypionate or estradiol valerate. But we were reminded that there is a current WHO study looking at this, and it may in fact be possible to look at efficacy of that treatment without any further expenditure. The final treatment modality was to increase the progestogen locally by inserting a levonorgestrel-releasing IUD while having the Norplant[R] still *in situ*. That would not increase the general body load but would increase the local concentration.

Steroid receptors and proteins

Group 2 D. Archer, S.C. Bell, P. Bischof, D.L. Healy, T. Luukkainen, R. Vihko, P. Virutamasen, J. Weintraub and J.O. White.

White. Firstly, we identified areas of deficiency in our knowledge, and we felt that anything that we did on end-points of endocrine action also had to include some morphometric analysis of the tissues that we obtained, because there is still room for improvement of the methodology, and comparative analysis between normal and progestogen-treated endometrium is needed. We feel that there is a lack of basic knowledge on endocrine markers at defined times, both in normal menstruation cycles and in progestogen-treated women, and that data on the endometrial response to therapeutic interventions in women on progestogen therapy were also required.

We feel there is a lack of knowledge on autocrine and paracrine factors, the extracellular matrix and bleeding in normal and progestogen-treated women, also in the knowledge of the role of immune and inflammatory cells in endometrial bleeding. We identified gaps in knowledge with respect to sex hormone-binding globulin (SHBG) and other binding proteins in serum and tissue and their precise localization. We feel that perhaps it is dangerous totally to disregard extrauterine signals. There is also limited information on androgen and corticoid receptors and their possible role in mediating the actions of progestogens.

Our recommendations for further research are an analysis on biopsies obtained from volunteers before and after progestogen treatment. We produced a list of all the parameters that could possibly be looked at. These include: estrogen and progesterone receptors, isocitrate dehydrogenase, estradiol dehydrogenase, prolactin, macrophage markers, lymphocyte markers, glycosaminoglycans, glycoproteins, SHBG, growth factors, structural proteins, collagen IV, osteonectin, laminin, fibronectin, a_1 and a_2 pregnancy-associated endometrial globulins (PEG), and tumour necrosis factor (TNF). The analysis would obviously include morphology and electron microscopic studies as well. The initial priorities would be to measure estrogen and progesterone receptors, then to measure the products of a steroid hormone receptor interaction, e.g. estradiol dehydrogenase; prolactin, $a2$ and $a1$ PEG and a pilot study on SHBG; then to investigate the structural proteins, collagen IV and actin.

One of the difficulties that would be encountered, using immunocytochemistry, is that of fixation artefacts. There would be a need to hold a discussion on the choice of fixatives and tissue handling to avoid artefacts. There is also a great need to standardize all reagents that are to be used. The amount of tissue obtained may pose some problem due to small amounts available, and possible ethical problems regarding direct sampling at different sites. With immunocytochemistry, the problem of quantitating the data and the investigation of image analysis techniques will need to be explored and expert opinion obtained.

With respect to models that could be used for investigation, we felt that, for the present time, we should continue with studies on human endometrium, but that animal models should not be disregarded. With regard to a choice of centres, specimen collection could be achieved in selected WHO/CCRC centres, while it was felt to be advantageous to identify a single centre with known expertise to undertake the immunocytochemical analysis. For data analysis it would be useful to have multi-observer analysis.

With regard to duration of the project to compare changes in end-organ sensitivity in normal endometrium and on progestogen therapy, we considered that a 3-year project would be suitable. In terms of costs, we estimated that to fund a 3-year project would cost approximately US$265 000. We felt that in terms of the discussions we have had on animal models and how they might relate to basic science, WHO might encourage national agencies to support basic research in the area of endometrial bleeding, including the use of animal models, by granting seed money.

Prostaglandins and second messengers

Group 3 M.L. Casey, E. Diczfalusy, M.G. Elder, J. Findlay, E. Gurpide, E. Granström, M.J.K. Harper, F. Hirata, F. Naftolin, S.K. Smith, M. Toppozada.

Harper. At the outset we tried to identify those substances that we thought were likely to be the most important. It was felt in the group that there were some important substances worthy of investigation, which include the eicosanoids, all the prostaglandins and lipoxygenase products, whichever seem most important, but obviously the PGF, PGE_2 and prostacyclin and leukotrienes. Then cytokines, but specifically interleukin-1β (IL-1β) and tumor necrosis factor-α (TNFα) and also platelet-activating factor (PAF). Endothelin and free radicals were other products that we felt were important.

Rice-Evans. With regard to the measurement of free radicals, iron determination only requires a small piece of tissue, perhaps 1.5 mm by 1.5 mm. To look for reactive radicals is a different matter, because they are going to react before the tissue is taken out of the patient. But there might be a case to be made perhaps of trying to trap radicals as soon as tissue is obtained. There are specific ways of dealing with that tissue so that it can then be stored.

Harper. Certain secretory products, particularly prolactin and PP12 and/or PP14, we felt were important even though they may be secondary to the initiation; they could be used as a valuable marker of progesterone activity and, maybe, indirectly, of progesterone receptor number. At the end of the day it might be possible to use measurements of these as an indication that progesterone activity is declining in some way.

These various substances are to be assessed by a variety of different methods. Wherever appropriate or available technology exists we would recommend looking at: messenger RNA of the product, immunohistochemistry and specific activity of enzymes, substrate availability and product production; for endothelin, to include measurement of messenger RNA and peptide production and control. The secretory products could be measured by radioimmunoassays. We feel that there are certainly protocols which could be developed and be very useful for studying these various messengers or inducers of bleeding, especially in steroid-treated women who had been given progesterone and estrogen. One would need to get samples before bleeding and after an acute phase of treatment (2–4 days and later). Also important is the study of the chronic situation where people have been on long-term progestogen therapy, and here to investigate the bleeders versus the non-bleeders versus controls.

Another approach which we feel is relatively important is to investigate people who are bleeding; take samples, then treat them with the estrogen and then take samples again to see if there is some reversion of the factors thought to be important in the bleeding process. Another experimental situation is with women sampled in the luteal phase and then treated with RU486 to induce a bleeding and sampled again. You then have the two reverse situations and it is to be hoped that we might see some correlation between these two.

As to the type of tissue required for these studies, we felt, for a variety of different reasons, that the human tissue is clearly the best material. Hysterectomy specimens were preferred, basically because there is more tissue and for some of these studies you need large amounts of tissue. Another option was directed biopsies using the flexible hysteroscope with which you could take samples of areas that were bleeding and areas that were not bleeding. As a third alternative, if the other approaches are not possible, non-directed biopsies or curettage material could be used, but this was felt to be less useful. Then, only if all of these human studies fail, would we consider animal models because of the costs and the unknown factors.

Another project which we felt was worthwhile would be to investigate endothelial cells from human endometrium. Here we would like to establish cultures of endothelial cells, study the vascular strips as well and look at the action of various agents on turnover of phosphatidyl inositol products: the direct action of steroids on these cells, whether receptors are present or are necessary, and the elaboration of various cell products in response to steroid treatment. This would be in the various groups of treated patients mentioned earlier and maybe *in vitro*. We would also look at the production of PAF and PGI_2 from these endothelial cell preparations, and lastly, the production of endothelin from these cultures and strips. The actual time necessary to complete the experiments might not be too long, the constraints are probably acquiring the tissue at the right stages from the right sort of patients under the right hormonal regimens. This endothelial cell project would have a lower priority than the approaches described previously.

Migratory cells, remodelling and regeneration

Group 4 D.T. Baird, P. Böhlen, D.A. Clark, F.J. Cornillie, P. Courtoy, Y. Eeckhout, I.S. Fraser, H. Ludwig and C. Rice-Evans.

Baird. In our group, we based our plan on three underlying principles: one was that they were projects that were relevant to progestogen-induced irregular bleeding: secondly, that they were practical to carry out with present methods; and thirdly, that they should be within a budget which was practical for the sort of projects that WHO Task Forces would undertake.

Clark. We considered that our mandate was to propose practical strategies for investigating the role of migratory cells, remodelling and regeneration in progestogen-induced endometrial bleeding, i.e. breakthrough bleeding. It is clear from the presentations and papers that there are areas of lack of knowledge and controversy. Considering how to approach this, we thought that one should be careful to propose something that could be done in a fairly straightforward way and at a budget that would not be excessive. We did not feel that animal models were particularly useful in dealing with the problem. Our basic strategy would be to use tissues for the analysis of the role of cells in the problem of breakthrough bleeding that should be available as part of other on-going projects to study breakthrough bleeding.

The first project, which is the one to which we have given highest priority, is the study of those cells in the endometrium which may be involved in the initiation of bleeding – that is, by producing holes in endothelium and glandular epithelium at times when the woman would prefer that bleeding did not occur. The hypothesis that we have put forward is that the number, location and functional state of macrophages will be altered in women who are at risk of breakthrough bleeding.

Macrophages show the greatest potential to be mediators of this problem in comparison to other cell types, and this is why we selected them as the focus. Endometrial tissue from non-bleeding patients who are taking progestogens would be compared with luteal phase samples from normal women. We thought that these samples should be studied in three ways. The first and perhaps simplest way would be merely to take fixed or frozen tissue and conduct a complete morphometric assessment, including the evaluation of the number and location of macrophages using immunocytochemistry. Morphology of these cells, special stains to examine lysosomes and functional status by the use of the new techniques of in-situ messenger RNA hybridization, would allow one to assess production of factors such as TNF-α, IL-1β, transforming growth factor β (TGF-β) etc. These can be measured now on a per cell basis. Whole tissue antioxidant levels should also be checked. We thought that just accomplishing the above would begin to give us some idea as to whether altered macrophage activity was involved in breakthrough bleeding, and we considered that there might be other cells such as the endometrial granulated lymphocyte participating in the process. This is justified by the observation that these granulated cells increase in number premenstrually and could therefore be involved in the initiation of bleeding in the intermenstrual state.

However, the lack of knowledge we have concerning the endometrial granulated lymphocyte makes it difficult to propose a large number of specific experiments, and a stronger case can be made for the involvement of macrophages, at least at this time. Nevertheless, the techniques that would be used to study macrophages would give, in a parallel manner, information about endometrial granulated lymphocytes in the tissue.

The second part of this project is a logical extension to study live rather than dead tissues using explant culture techniques. This provides the opportunity to carry out an in-vitro analysis of function without many of the potential artefacts that can be induced by tissue and cell disaggregation. Using the in-vitro culture techniques with explants, we proposed that one should measure the release of cytotoxic factors such as TNF-α, as well as the release of other mediators such as IL-1β, prostaglandins, plasminogen activator and probably also PAF. This would tell us about the functional activity of macrophages in the endometrium of progestogen-treated women, and we would know whether that activity was excessive or not.

We also thought it appropriate to carry out some dynamic testing of macrophage function, for example by adding hormones to the culture, prostaglandins or recombinant cytokines to look for evidence that the cells in the endometrium of the patients might respond in a supersensitive manner and release factors that could initiate bleeding.

The third part of the project is simply to take the tissues apart and to look at the function of isolated cells, and if it were found that the dissociated and purified macrophage populations were to act differently from the way expected based on everything that had gone before, one would want to add back various other cell types to look for evidence of cell–cell interactions that could be potentially important in determining what happens at the tissue level. The results from the first project, we predict, will provide useful data concerning whether or not macrophages are abnormal in a percentage of women on gestogens such as Norplant[R].

The second project that we propose, at a slightly lower priority, would be based on the fact that many of these women suffer from prolonged bleeding and it is a hypothesis that these women have a defect in re-epithelialization, a process that appears to be involved in a stoppage of such bleeding. To test the idea that there is an abnormality in re-epithelialization, we propose to compare the endometrium from normal cycling women taken 2–4 days after the onset of menses to similarly timed samples from women who are experiencing breakthrough bleeding. We thought that it would be important to know in this set of patients and controls that the endocrine environment was the same, and therefore this would have to be measured.

In studying this tissue, we proposed that two types of experiments be done. Firstly, simply to carry out the same types of histological study as mentioned before, particularly with reference to macrophages, their number, location and their content of messenger RNA, for growth factors that are likely to be involved in epithelial growth and healing. This can be done by established techniques. Secondly, we thought that the explant culture methods should also be used and could be used profitably to examine the rate of epithelial regrowth simply by doing serial histological studies. It would also be possible to examine the direct effect of adding recombinant growth factors such as TGF-α or epidermal growth factor (EGF) to this system and, together with the data from the histology, it would then be possible to say whether there was in fact a defect in re-epithelialization that might explain prolonged bleeding. We would be able to predict, or at least infer, whether there was an intrinsic defect in the epithelial cell as a result of its exposure to progestogens, or rather a defect conditioned by the activity of altered macrophage function in the tissue slices. This we would be able to infer by having information on what this macrophage activity actually was. Of course, one could also take supernatants and determine whether or not there was a deficiency in growth factors being elaborated or an excess of cytotoxic and cytostatic cytokines.

In the second project, our primary concern was to determine if the endometrial cells of subjects taking progestogens are in some way deficient in their healing abilities, and whilst studies on the behaviour of pure epithelial cell cultures and cell lines could be done, we felt that at this time it would represent an enormous undertaking of high risk in terms of its ultimate success.

The third project was based on the view that remodelling is clearly relevant to processes involved in healing and repair, and therefore may be relevant to either the initiation or the continuation of bleeding. The studies of endothelial cells and of matrix components are more difficult than the previous two projects and hence have a slightly lower priority. Studies of endothelial cells are rather difficult, so we felt that examining the matrix would be the most productive.

Our hypothesis was that progestogen-induced abnormalities in matrix render subjects susceptible both to the initiation of breakthrough bleeding and to its continuation. Evaluation of matrix synthesis and degradation can be accomplished using established methods, and dynamic studies of estrogenic stimulation of these processes can be easily done. Therefore, we propose to compare non-bleeding progestogen-treated patient samples with comparable luteal phase samples from controls and to look at patients with bleeding at the bleeding site as well as the interbleeding sites in comparison to samples from day 2–4 of menstruating control patients.

At present, our organ culture type studies are too complex to be applied profitably to the evaluation of matrix. Identification of a defect in the matrix would lead logically to further analysis of the function of cells involved in the generation and maintenance of this matrix, and that could involve study of macrophages, granulated lymphocytes, and other cells present in the stroma. The three projects which we have outlined would require, we feel, a multicentre collaboration and interaction with those centres that would be studying the patients that are actually having the breakthrough bleeding. In this respect, we would probably need to interact with the centres in some of the third world countries where there are many women undergoing treatment.

The specific centres to be involved and the details of the collaborative studies can only be decided once a specific project (or projects) to be undertaken has been determined and a detailed research plan is written. The time-frame for the projects we would estimate to be approximately 2 years, with an estimated budget of approximately US$200000–250000 at the current rate of exchange, to be divided among the participating laboratories.

As a final postscript to our deliberations, we wish to point out that the establishment of a successful project identifying abnormalities in the cells' remodelling and healing of endometrium in progestogen-treated patients could have further benefits in attempting to deal with this problem on a worldwide basis.

For example, establishment of an effective treatment would allow us to determine if the defect we have detected in either the cells or the matrix is the one that is actually being corrected by the treatment. Further, upon identification of cell or matrix defects, we might be able to predict new types of treatments that could be tested in an attempt to stop breakthrough bleeding, either its initiation or its continuation.

Casey. I would just like to propose one other consideration for WHO. For purposes of facilitating rapid progress, the most efficient use of funds, as well as the involvement of developing countries, it seems appropriate to encourage the cooperation of physicians and investigators in developing countries with those in developed countries. Specifically, I would propose the development of cooperative, collaborative relationships between those who care for the women on progestogen contraceptive therapy with others in centres where the facilities and technology and even the reagents are more readily available. It would seem possible to encourage a team in a developing country which is able to collect adequate number of patients with records, and the other data and tissues and blood for the studies that have been proposed. Such a plan, it seems, would facilitate the training of team members from developing countries in laboratory methodology and technology transfer and may lead to enthusiastic pursuit of additional funding by the newly trained investigators from the developing country.

Newton. What you are suggesting is similar to a scheme that has been tried in another WHO Task Force. I do not know whether Dr Cooke wishes to comment on the Infertility Task Force.

Cooke. I think that what Dr Casey is suggesting is much more specific. Certainly, members of the Infertility Steering Committee were asked to go and visit other parts of the world, but there was not any tight linking of projects in the way that has just been suggested. I think this is a new departure, and maybe Dr Wilson would wish to comment as it is related to institution strengthening.

Wilson. I think it would be extremely helpful to establish collaborative links between developed country centres and developing country centres. To give an example of this, we have made some effort to establish links between the group in Melbourne and institutions in Indonesia which is near geographically. With regard to the precise details that Dr Casey outlined, you have two possibilities. You can take the tissue to the technology or you can bring the technology to the tissue, and I think you should try to do both. If you do establish such interinstitutional and international collaboration, where possible, the techniques to be used should be available in both places, and it should be achieved by exchange of personnel.

Cravioto. Actually, studies have been done in this way during the last few years because a lot of technology has been transferred to developing countries with WHO objectives. I think in many cities in developing countries, there is some technology available and they can begin with this strategy. It could be the opportunity to continue the institution strengthening in linked collaboration with developed countries.

Diczfalusy. I would like to put this in perspective. For the time being, it is estimated that the global population is about 5.2 billion. Out of this, there are 800 million couples of reproductive age. Of the 800 million couples, approximately half, that is 400 million, are using some sort of modern contraceptive. Of those 400 million, 50 million are using oral contraceptives, and something between 6 and 8 million are using long-acting steroidal contraceptive agents. Of the oral contraceptive users, there is a sharply decreasing number in the People's Republic of China, which is now probably between 25 and 30 million. The rest of the users are, with the exception of a few Latin American countries like Brazil, the so-called Western World. What is increasing in the developing countries is the use of long-acting agents, and governments of those countries are approaching WHO repeatedly for assistance. I would also like to reiterate that the mandate of the WHO programme is exclusively to assist developing countries in their problems.

On behalf of Dr Barzaletto, I would like to thank you all for the work you have done prior to the meeting and during the meeting. We are living in a very complicated world where problems tend to become global, and tend to develop very rapidly a social dimension. We hope that those of you who are working in the ivory tower of the laboratory have now a perception of what some of the problems, which were considered previously as trivialities, really are in developing countries. I think Dr Naftolin said rightly that you may also wish to devote your own laboratory to the study of some of the problems we were discussing. Mr Chairman, I would like to thank once more the organizing committee and all the contributors for their participation in this symposium.

Conclusions
J.R. Newton

We believe that the investigation of progestogen-induced bleeding, especially with long-acting methods of fertility regulation, can be completed with the present methodology and within a practical budget.

Since the last WHO meeting on endometrial bleeding held in 1979, significant progress has been made in the understanding of the underlying mechanisms involved in normal menstruation.

Methodology now exists for the identification of: estrogen and progesterone receptors in the endometrium, immunocytochemical investigations, cell signalling, second messenger identification, cytokines and other regulatory molecules, and the cytoskeleton. All these may be involved in the mechanism leading to abnormal bleeding with progestogen contraceptive methods.

Also in recent years, methods of in-vivo analysis, cell culture and the ability to investigate paracrine and autocrine control of cells have been refined.

Modern, flexible, small-diameter (3 mm) hysteroscopy now allows the repeated investigation of the human endometrium in volunteers and subjects under medication with long-acting progestogens. This procedure does not require anesthesia and is without significant morbidity. Studies using this methodology largely remove the need for animal models.

We propose a linked series of clinical and laboratory investigations to understand further the mechanisms of bleeding occurring during the administration of long-acting progestogens, and to investigate possible treatment regimens to overcome this problem.

Transfer of technology, institutional strengthening in cell biology, immunocytochemistry, morphometry and macrophage function, will need to occur to develop the proposed research area. This will allow research to occur in centres that already have large numbers of patients using progestogen for contraception.

Pairing of a developed and developing country centre with a given expertise will help in the transfer of technology and consolidation and development of research.

We feel the following laboratory and clinical priority areas are worth further investigation.

Laboratory studies

1. To study macrophages and other migratory cells that may be involved in abnormal bleeding associated with progestogen contraceptive use.
2. To study concentration of estradiol and progesterone receptors in progestogen users, the hypothesis being that these women have a chronic progesterone receptor deficiency in the absence of estrogen that causes abnormal bleeding.
3. To test substances in in-vitro systems that may be candidates for the trigger mechanism, or initiation, of bleeding. These substances to include prostaglandins, cytokines, free radicals, PAF and cell secretory products.

Outline proposals are included (preceding pages) for the study of these priority areas in the group reports which we feel require study alongside the clinical studies proposed.

Clinical studies

4. Further review of clinical data available.
   (a) Comparison of pharmacokinetic and pharmacodynamic data with menstrual diary card analysis (WHO).
   (b) Re-analysis of the tissue blocks from biopsies for new morphometry, morphology and vascular defects identified during the meeting, and the presence and type of migratory cells.
5. New studies on morphology on tissue obtained by hysteroscopy in the following groups of patients.
   (a) Current long-acting levonorgestrel progestogen users.

(b) Patients due to have a hysterectomy for gynecological reasons preprimed with long-acting methods. This will also allow comparison of endometrial biopsy specimen with the morphological examination of the whole uterus.

(c) Control patients: late luteal (day LH + 10), premenstrual (day LH + 12 or + 13) and early menstrual (day 1).

All these groups (a–c) would allow samples to be mapped for bleeding areas versus non-bleeding control areas in the same specimen. Also to use morphology to examine vascular defects and the presence and types of migratory cells identified by the meeting.

6. The investigation of treatment regimens; various modalities were recommended for investigation.

(a) Estrogen treatment for those with prolonged bleeding or irregular frequent bleeding. To the long-acting method the following could be added.

(i) Ethinyl estradiol, present in a combined low-dose oral contraceptive, but the progestogen would need to be matched to that in the long-acting method.

(ii) Estradiol cypionate or valerate.

Alternative delivery systems, e.g. transdermal, could be used.

(b) Increase local progestogen levels in the endometrium via a levonorgestrel-releasing intrauterine device.

Index

acidic fibroblast growth factor (aFGF) 469–70, 486
actin 243–4, 252
amenorrhea
  discontinuing contraceptive due to 10–11, 22
  DMPA use 15
  importance of counselling 5, 22, 24
  IUDs 22
  monthly injectables 17
  NET-EN use 16
  progestogen-only pill 14
  research 801
  subdermal implants 19
  variability between centres 9
ϵ-aminocaproic acid 124, 363
angiogenesis
  direction of growth 488
  endometrial 253, 256–7, 469
  modulators 476
  paracrine regulation of 253, 256–7
  regulation 468
  steroids and 257, 262
  triggering factors 468
angiogenic factors
  angiogenin 474
  direct/indirect 476–7
  fibroblast growth factors 469–72
  other cytokines 475–6
  recruitment 476–7
  steroid hormonal effects on 487–8
  TGF-α 474
  TGF-β 472–3
  TNF-α 473–4
angiogenin 475
anovulatory women
  bleeding disturbance in 12
  endometrial circulation 83
  sex steroid receptors and endometrial maturation 164, 167, 168–9
  treatment 516
antiestrogen receptor 155–6
antifibrinolytic agents 23, 124, 363, 497
antifibrinolytics 511

antihistamines 99, 497
antiprogestogens
  progesterone and PG synthesis 337, 339–40, 343–5
  see also RU486
antiprostaglandins 497, 511
arachidonic acid
  cyclic changes in endometrial uptake 280
  decidual activation and 308–309
  decidual PRL inhibition 216
  metabolic products
    epoxygenase products and breakthrough bleeding 284–5
    and low-dose progestogen 280–85
  oxygen radicals and altered metabolism 419–21
  release of, phospholipase activation 350, 351–3
autocrine regulators 253, 254

basic fibroblast growth factor (bFGF) 469–70, 471, 472
BN52021 295
bone resorption
  lysosomal enzymes 385
  proteinases in 435–7
breakthrough bleeding
  animal models 501, 513–14
  arachidonic acid metabolism in endometrium 280–85
  biopsy timing 514
  combined oral contraceptives 13, 34
  compliance with contraceptive 35
  endometrial surface in 512–13
  ethinyl estradiol for 516–18
  events preceding 512
  free radical generation 429–30
  functional progesterone deficiency 518–19, 520
  hysterectomy samples 512, 515–16
  IUDs and 34
  mechanism 345
  myometrium/endometrium 516
  PAF levels 297